Rheumatology in Chinese Medicine

RHEUMATOLOGY

in Chinese Medicine

Gérard Guillaume, M.D.
Mach Chieu, M.D.

EASTLAND PRESS • SEATTLE

Originally published as *Rhumatologie et Médecine Traditionnelle Chinoise,*
Edition de La Tisserande (France), 1990.

English language edition © 1996 by Gérard Guillaume and Mach Chieu

Published by Eastland Press, Incorporated
P.O. Box 12689, Seattle, WA 98111 USA
All rights reserved.

Library of Congress Card Number: 95-083689
International Standard Book Number: 0-939616-26-2
Printed in the United States of America

2 4 6 8 10 9 7 5 3 1

English language edition translated by David Vachon,
edited by David Vachon and Dan Bensky

Book design by Gary Niemeier

Abbreviated Contents

Chapter Contents

CHAPTER 35

ACUPUNCTURE FOR LOWER BACK PAIN 371

Translator's Foreword

Perspectives on the French Acupuncture Tradition

A large proportion of the Chinese medical literature available in English today is not derived from original Chinese sources, but from French texts. This is due to the fact that Chinese medicine achieved a certain status in France long before it was popularized in England and the United States. The former position of France as a colonial power in Asia induced the influx of cultural, philosophical and medical traditions from the Orient, particularly from Vietnam. The grandfather of French acupuncture, the eminent Dr. Nguyen Van Nghi, is credited with having single-handedly imported, refined and disseminated the art of acupuncture in France over the course of sixty years of teaching, writing and translating such fundamental texts as *Inner Classic (Nei jing)* and *Great Compendium of Acupuncture and Moxibustion (Zhen jiu da cheng)*. Today, French acupuncture research is highly respected worldwide for balancing a deep understanding of the Chinese classic texts with an exacting scientific attitude.

Rheumatology has traditionally been a French medical specialty. Because no Chinese book (classic or modern) has ever been devoted to this subject alone, we are indeed very fortunate to be able to present to the English-speaking public the result of the collaboration between two distinguished doctors and scholars. Dr. Gérard Guillaume, a specialist in rheumatology, immunology and sports medicine, is currently Vice-President of the French Acupuncture Association. Dr. Mach Chieu is a poet, writer and scholar of classical and modern Chinese language, calligraphy and philosophy, as well as a pediatrician. Together, they have painstakingly deciphered and translated fundamental texts, both ancient and modern, on the traditional treatment of rheumatological pathologies.

Part one of this book discusses the concept of rheumatism in terms of traditional Chinese medicine. Part two is a translation of a portion of a comprehensive and well-respected contemporary textbook that provides the context of rheumatological research and treatment in modern China, with its strong emphasis on herbal treatment. Part three presents the clinical results of the authors' practice, both as rheumatologists and acupuncturists. In the fourth and final part, the authors review the ancient Chinese medical literature, gathering a collection of references that allude to what were indeed rheumatological conditions. They also highlight the strong emphasis on acupuncture techniques in these traditional texts.

Translation Conventions

"In the right key, one can say anything.
In the wrong key, nothing; the only delicate part
is the establishment of the key."
—GEORGE BERNARD SHAW

The translation of this book represents a delicate balance among ancient Chinese thought, modern Chinese medical texts, the French acupuncture tradition and the American language and culture. A sizeable portion of the original book was a translation by Drs. Gérard Guillaume and Mach Chieu of Chinese texts into French, with the exception of *Basic Questions (Su wen),* for which the authors elected to rely on Dr. Albert Husson's translation, the 1955 version considered authoritative by most French acupuncturists. Along the way, a number of cultural and editorial concerns had to be addressed to make this translation as clear as possible to the American public, without sacrificing the idiosyncrasies of the French version.

First, the original book was designed for medical doctors, since acupuncture is primarily taught as a specialization in French medical schools. I have attempted to clarify as much as possible the terminology used, to avoid unnecessary use of medical jargon. Still, the scope of this book presupposes a fairly good understanding of conventional medical concepts by the reader.

In the same vein, the American publisher and I have chosen to eliminate several sections dealing with very basic concepts of traditional Chinese medicine such as the fundamental substances, Organs, channel pathways and acupuncture point functions, all of which can be found in numerous English-language textbooks. We have, however, retained the authors' discussion of etiological factors because they are particularly relevant to understanding the mechanisms of rheumatic pathologies, and they are not presented in this form in other textbooks.

At the insistence of the authors, and in keeping with the original French and many American works in the acupuncture literature, we have capitalized all words which have a meaning in the context of traditional Chinese medicine distinct from the everyday use of the same word (e.g., Wind as a pathogenic influence, in contrast to the climatic wind). In addition, we strived to find an English equivalent to all Chinese medical terms (e.g., panarthralgia for *lì jié bìng*), with the exception of three words which have become part of the English language today, and which we therefore left in their transliterated forms: yin, yang and Qi.

As a rule, we have inserted the *pinyin* transliteration of each Chinese medical concept, since much uncertainty and incorrect translations are associated with these elusive concepts. The *pinyin* provides an opportunity for clarification through the etymology of the word, and a point of reference for possible scholarly debate.

The individual herbs are presented by pharmaceutical name first, followed by *pinyin,* in accordance with the nomenclature established in *Chinese Herbal Medicine: Materia Medica* by Dan Bensky, Andrew Gamble et al. The classification of the formulas is derived from *Chinese Herbal Medicine: Formulas and Strategies* by Dan Bensky and Randall Barolet. Acupuncture point names are based on the nomenclature adopted by the World Health Organization in 1991, with TB- (Triple Burner) substituted for TE- (Triple Energizer). Miscellaneous (extra) channel points are identified in accordance with the system developed by the American Society of Chinese Medicine in the 1970s, and used in the English translation of the Shanghai College of Traditional Chinese Medicine's *Acupuncture: A Comprehensive Text,* translated by John O'Connor and Dan Bensky.

Certain key Chinese medical concepts have been translated into French in slightly different ways than what the English-language reader is accustomed to seeing. Although we usually followed the standard American translation for better readability, it is worth noting some of the differences in interpretation:

- *Qì,* traditionally understood as energy, is translated as "breath" *(souffle)* by the French, which better describes its genesis and dynamic nature. For a more detailed etymological explanation, please see footnote no. 1 in the first chapter of this book.
- The Chinese character for *bì* literally means painful obstruction causing numbness or paralysis; paralysis; numbness; lack of sensation; stiffness. Since there is no concept in the English language that could accurately incorporate all of its different levels of meaning, we decided to use the common American translation, "painful obstruction," although we feel that this is a restrictive interpretation. For a more detailed discussion of the original meaning and modern application of the concept of *bì*, please refer to chapter 4.
- *Jīng jīn* is typically rendered as "muscle channel" in English; the French translate the term as "tendino-muscular vessel" *(vaisseaux tendino-musculaires).* The reason is that the term "muscle channel" is an anatomical description, whereas *jing jin* actually refers to an energy

pathway. The muscle spindles only correspond to an underlying energetic structure. In this book we have chosen the term "channel sinews" in keeping with the syntax of the original Chinese, and to emphasize that these are channel-like sinews and not sinew-like channels.

Finally, the original book refers to certain techniques and models commonly used in the French acupuncture tradition, but with which most English-speaking practitioners will be unfamiliar. We therefore asked Dr. Guillaume to write certain explanatory notes in the introduction to part three of this book.

In accordance with the Council of Oriental Medical Publishers designation system, part one (CHAPTERS 1~4) and part three (CHAPTERS 8~23) of this book are original works containing connotive and functional translations. Part two (CHAPTERS 5~7) and part four (CHAPTERS 24~35) are connotive translations.

Acknowledgments

One of the biggest challenges in preparing this translation was to ensure that the nuances of each Chinese quotation and text were not lost through the double translation process, that is, in the course of translating first from Chinese into French, and then from French into English. For that, I am deeply indebted to Dan Bensky, medical editor at Eastland Press, for his tireless efforts and un-compromising standards in checking all the original Chinese texts against the English translation. The gra-ciousness, patience, ingenuity and help with which I was constantly surrounded through every step of this project is simply beyond words to describe. Dan and I are the editors referred to in the chapter notes.

I am equally grateful for Dr. Guillaume's willingness to accommodate our many requests for rewrites and explanations. It was an immensely enriching experience to share his insights into little-known aspects of the traditional Chinese medical model.

I would also like to thank Odette Vaiss of Edition de La Tisserande, publisher of the original book in France, for creating a very relaxed and resourceful environment for this whole project.

Another well-deserved credit is due Monique Fay who kindly undertook the translation of a portion of the chapter on postmenopausal osteoporosis. Part of this chapter originally appeared in the *American Journal of Acupuncture*, and we are grateful to Deborah Salisbury and her editorial board for their permission to use it. Also thanks to Peter Holmes, a respected Swiss herbalist, for his assistance in translating certain botanical and biochemical terms.

Finally, and most importantly, I wish to express my deepest gratitude and respect to my Gurudev Para-mahamsa Hariharananda, who, although not directly involved in this project, has been an inexhaustible source of inspiration and strength throughout the years, and who has helped me discover the meaning of work as sacrament.

—DAVID VACHON, L.AC.

Preface to French Edition

PREFACING A BOOK exposes the privileges and limitations of the preface writer: he opens fire, assumes the right to introduce a body of work to which he did not contribute, and provides—to the degree that he is read and believed—the tone of the reading. The authors on the other hand, encased in a modest and formal "we," await with relatively bated breath the reception that the public will eventually give them and their mentor for a day.

To preface a book of the nature and importance of Gérard Guillaume and Mach Chieu's *Rheumatology in Chinese Medicine* is to become familiar with a new enjoyable production from these authors and to discover, through their work, a new field of knowledge and practice. It is also for the preface writer, more modestly, the opportunity to describe in a few sentences what strikes him most about the fruit of this new collaboration, which already includes a number of remarkable works.

The subtle audacity of the title itself is already revealing: rheumatology is a medical specialty, particularly in France, which monitors carefully the purism of its academic discourse, as its representatives are well aware of the extent of the uncertainties which surround this subject and the control of its evolution. These questions concern the validity of etiologies which are conjured up and later abandoned; the longevity of a current symptomatology whose two clinical bases—radiological and biological—

are so difficult to reconcile and, in some cases, evolving so rapidly; the emergence of immunology and the psychosomatic dimension. The therapeutic response has been dominated by the prescription of analgesic and anti-inflammatory drugs; antibiotics play a certain part, while new perspectives are opening up with chemo- and immunotherapy. Surgical interventionism, which may create problems by its irreversible nature, has been progressively invading a pathological dimension marked by the intensity of the inflammatory signs during acute phases, and the extent of systemic involvement during processes slowly evolving toward chronicity.

Defenders of the field have therefore made it a professional duty to keep the academic discourse out of the reach of common people, and carefully isolated it from any popular traditions with which it may become dangerously associated as old wives' recipes and remedies.

Gérard Guillaume is an authentic rheumatologist—in title, deed, qualifications and practice. His knowledge of immunology prevents triggering any involuntary allergic reaction among his colleagues in this specialty. A passionate yet cautious physician, he has been applying for years his intellectual curiosity to the discovery, understanding and dissemination of Chinese medical practices while remaining up to date on the professional and medical aspects of his specialty.

Mach Chieu is just as authentic a pediatrician who has known the banks of both the Mekong and Seine rivers, and who has studied diseases, their causes and treatment according to both the traditional Chinese model in its native tongue, and the Western model. Due to their complimentary talents, collaboration between these two authors has always been fruitful, and this new offering bears ample testimony to this elegant synergy.

Beyond the title of this book—apparently so innocuous—lies a formidable challenge: bringing together rheumatology and traditional Chinese medicine, which, as the content of this book makes clear, requires both boldness and caution. It is indeed remarkable how the authors have made their way through a field strewn with stumbling blocks: "energy" concepts difficult to reconcile with current molecular-centric medical views; a symptomatology with no other common ground than a clinical picture constrained to painful signs and impairments of mobility; original therapeutic processes and resources, more justified by the internal logic of the therapeutic action than by actual validation. . . Assessing foreign practices, born out of a radically different understanding of man in his relationship with himself and his environment, is still very difficult.

Gérard Guillaume reviews fundamental concepts of traditional Chinese medicine, lists all his sources, quotes classical texts, and eventually leads the reader to the *a posteriori* inescapable conclusion that a rheumatic pathology *per se* does exist in traditional Chinese medicine. The presentation is clearly and logically laid out; in addition, the clinical cases enable the authors to describe in Western terms certain traditional Chinese medical conditions. Yet the most fascinating aspect of this traditional medicine is without any doubt the depth of its analysis of the disorder (both clinically and pathophysiologically), the methodology it uses to reposition the condition into a more general perspective, and the *continuum* leading to the treatment plan.

Setting aside the (ironic) reservations founded on established customs and practices according to which traditional Chinese medicine, and many other traditions, has strictly nothing to contribute to Western medicine, we must acknowledge that traditional Chinese medicine provides a particularly efficient therapeutic approach to rheumatic disorders. The way in which Gérard Guillaume navigates through various therapeutic modalities pertaining to Chinese medicine (not just acupuncture) attests to his extended clinical practice and knowledge.

Two parts are particularly relevant to demonstrate the value of this book and the experience of the authors: "Traditional Approaches to Rheumatology in Modern China" and "Clinical Practice of an Acupuncturist in Rheumatology." These two parts constitute, in my opinion, the major portion of this work, occupying over half of the book. Here the reader will find the elements of a renewed therapeutic approach; he will also discover what constitutes the strength and originality of this work: it speaks from experience. This is a lesson humbly given to those who are looking for an opportunity to quibble: in order to evaluate in all validity the advantages and disadvantages of both approaches, one must be able to speak both medical "languages." Gérard Guillaume and Mach Chieu know how to combine their knowledge; Gérard Guillaume knows how to speak both "languages;" this is also and above all what makes this book so easy and illuminating to read. May he be thanked for it! And so should Mach Chieu be thanked, for sharing his knowledge of the language and science of traditional Chinese medicine.

—Pierre Cornillot

PART ONE

The Concept of
Rheumatism in Traditional
Chinese Medicine

CHAPTER ONE

Energetic Body and Locomotor System

To understand the traditional Chinese medicine approach to rheumatic diseases, it is necessary to understand how the Chinese view the human organism and its organic structures. The body is never considered or described in anatomical terms, but rather as a place of circulation for the Qi (breaths[1] or energies) which give it form and function.

Human Body

The Chinese concept of the human body is far from being monolithic. The body as a whole is defined by four characteristics—four distinct ways of describing different aspects of the same reality.

Physical Structure (*tǐ* 體)

The physical structure corresponds to different layers or parts that are identifiable in a well-organized structure. The Han-dynasty work *Clarification of Terminologies (Shi ming)* provides the following definition: "Physical structure (*tǐ*) means a well-organized sequence. Bones and flesh, hair and Blood, exterior and interior, big and small follow each other in an organized fashion." The use of the number four in this quadruple division acts as a symbolic reminder of the terrestrial structure, as four is the number associated with earth.

The first pair—"bones and flesh" (*gǔ ròu*)—represents that which is hard or soft under the touch. The bones are the hard, firm, strong, rigid element of the body whereas the flesh is its soft, pliable, supple, flexible and delicate component. In this respect, the bones-flesh pair represents the body as a material—thus ephemeral—structure, which supports the movements of the various types of Qi in the body.

The second pair—"hair and Blood" (*máo xuè*)—divides the physical structure into internal and external zones (*nèi wài*), which also support the course of the Qi.

The third pair—"exterior and interior" (*biǎo lǐ*)—defines the relationship between the superficial and the deep. Exterior and interior are the two sides of the same reality, but the exterior is related more to appearance, whereas the interior is related more to organization. This pair particularly emphasizes the importance of the vitalizing exchanges that take place at all levels.

The fourth pair—"big and small" (*dà xiǎo*)—expresses the value and relative importance of human beings. Big represents that which is important, immutable, dependable, a model or a foundation. Small represents that which is changeable, ephemeral, variable. This pair particularly emphasizes distinctions, separations, hierarchies among the different layers and parts of the physical structure.

The concept of physical structure (*tǐ*) defines the unity of the body, comprising a multiplicity of components in a very well-organized sequence. It represents the material support, the backbone of the entire organization and animation system of the physical body. Man is described in his physical and mental layout.

PHYSICAL BODY (qū 軀)

According to *Clarification of Terminologies*, "The physical body (qū) means the arrangement of the body. The entire nomenclature is gathered into one bigger whole, like the detailed map of a territory." The body is here considered as an arrangement, as a territory to be governed, in which each element has its own place and function according to its proper denomination.

PHYSICAL FORM (xíng 形)

Here the physical form of the body is considered, that is, what differentiates all beings with a shape and a form. It is the appearance that one can see, feel, smell, hear; what one immediately perceives. The physical form expresses the invisible deep structure; it is where the person's normal Qi circulates, driving and producing both structure and form. It is also the place where the pathogenic Qi penetrates and where therapeutic intervention restores normalcy.

The physical form is the ground on which the various actions of life take place. It changes with time and space, which explains the influence of environment on the physical form. It is the reliable expression of an underlying reality, expressing the material physical structure (tǐ).

These two words are often combined—*xíng tǐ*—to describe the perceived human being as a whole: a deep structure covered by form. The physical form and structure are the abode of the spirit (shén).

SPIRIT (shén 神)

Spirit represents the personality of a human being interacting with heaven and earth. It expresses the organized unity of both the energies which animate the human being and the physical elements which provide the ground for these energies to circulate and operate. Spirit also includes the entire spiritual, emotional and mental dimensions of the human being.[2]

MAN (rén 人)

The term *rén* summarizes and enhances the four previous terms. Man's existence is ruled by heaven and earth, and he participates in their harmonious relationship.

We fully agree with the way Elisabeth Rochat de la Vallée concludes her remarkable work, *Symphonie corporelle*:

> An internal structure, invisible yet a determining factor (tǐ), is the primary support, the backbone and the organizing principle. This structure includes various elements and gradually takes on additional layers. Everything finds its place and its function according to its proper designation. Besides its structural guidelines, the whole is made of parts interlocking in an exact hierarchical order (qū).
>
> The appearance or tangible form is the result of this internal ordering and organization. It is that which is seen and perceived, that which alludes to the unseen forces operating inside, just as the varied relief of the landscape—mountains, plains and valleys—allude to the history of its formation and to the underground forces that have shaped it. This is the physical form (xíng).
>
> Finally, the Spirit (shén) is that which infuses the whole with life, an integral and harmonious part of the interaction between heaven and earth. Man (rén) is the final stage. The four words tǐ, qū, xíng, shén describe the progressive construction and constitutional stages of man.

Anatomical Structures

Each of the human body's anatomical structures—skin, flesh and muscles, vessels, sinews, bones—corresponds to one of the Five Phases (wǔ xíng), thereby establishing a relationship between the activities of man and the universe. The skin corresponds to Metal (Lung), the flesh and muscles to Earth (Spleen), the vessels to Fire (Heart), the sinews to Wood (Liver) and the bones to Water (Kidneys). Only the bones, muscles and sinews are relevant to our topic.

BONES (gǔ 骨)

The bones have a preferred relationship with the Water phase, with winter, with the Kidneys, and thereby with the concept of the Qi's inner withdrawal, cohesion, strength and power. Passages in chapters 5 and 44 of *Basic Questions (Su wen)* state that "The Kidneys produce the marrow and the bones" and "The bones are the property of the Kidneys." However, a passage in chapter 10 of *Divine Pivot (Ling shu)* also says that the lesser yang rules the bones. The lesser yang represents the hinge of the yang, its turning point. It represents the free-flowing quality of the yang, the yang that moves the yin. This energy level also has a preferred relationship with the outside world, particularly from a climatic point of view. For example, the yang Linking vessel has traditionally been associated with sensitivity to changes in the weather: some people who have a disturbance in this vessel can feel when it is going to rain because their bones ache.

We note that whenever there is an osseous lesion there is some sort of demineralization. Demineralization leads to a loss of structure. From this, it is clear that the diminishment of one of the deep structures involves a relatively intense loss of yin. As such, osseous lesions are always connected with Heat and/or Fire.

Bone is one of the "Eight Curious Organs." The Curious Organs have to do with durability; they store the Essence *(jīng)*. The bone itself represents the frame of the human being, its innermost and most intimate structure, which houses its most precious substance—the marrow—which in traditional terms includes the spinal cord.

FLESH AND MUSCLES (*ròu* 肉)

It is first necessary to address an ambiguity frequently found in many Western writings about traditional Chinese medicine. The word *ròu* in Chinese refers to the flesh as a palpable muscle mass, providing the form and appearance of the human body; it corresponds to the Earth Phase. On the other hand, the word *jīn* refers to the sinews and muscles from the point of view of muscular strength; it corresponds to the Wood Phase.

Moreover, the essential nature of the word *ròu* includes the notion of organization and of elasticity. Just as the bone represents the solid frame of the body and its internal structure, the flesh and muscles are by opposition its external appearance: plasticity versus rigidity. The flesh as muscle mass corresponds to the Earth Phase, the intermediary or fifth season, the Spleen, and therefore to the concept of transformation.

The Qing dynasty writer Zhang Zhi-Cong wrote in his commentaries on *Basic Questions*: "The Spleen Organ functions like a silo. It governs the transportation and transformation of the Essence of food to produce and to nourish the muscles. This is the reason why it corresponds to the flesh."

The classics also say that the Spleen nourishes the four limbs and that if it is affected, the limbs will lack nourishment, their energy will progressively diminish, and the sinews, bones and flesh will become useless due to their lack of vitality. Good muscle mass is therefore achieved by stimulating the acupuncture points that regulate the nutritive functions of the Spleen-Stomach and the Penetrating vessel.

SINEWS AND MUSCLES (jīn 筋)

Jīn is the word for muscular strength. It alludes to that which circulates with strength and power in the flesh, and infuses the form with life. Together, the strength of the bone associated with the power of the muscles and sinews give an idea of strength and sturdiness. Painful obstruction can generally be seen as a painful condition affecting the strength of the body.

The sinews and muscular strength correspond to the Wood Phase whose nature is to twist and to straighten up, and is generally characterized by its flexibility. They correspond to the spring season, and to the Liver. According to *Basic Questions*, the Liver governs, generates and brings life to the sinews. In addition, the Liver is linked to all the tissues in the body that come from the embryonic mesenchyme.

The power of the sinews is related to the strength of the Liver Blood, as noted in *Divine Pivot*: "When there is an abundance of Blood, the sinews are solid and strong; when there is a deficiency of Blood, the sinews are weak." This relationship between the sinews and Liver explains the therapeutic importance in musculoskeletal conditions of points having a particular action on the Liver Blood. One such example is LR-3 *(tai chong)*, which is indicated in cases of spasms.

JOINTS (*guān jié* 關節)

The word *guān* means barrier or gate, and *jié* means a node, knot or joint. The latter refers to such things as bamboo shoot nodes where energy concentrates, appearing in a rhythmic pattern both in space and in time. Together, these two characters evoke the idea of something that both separates and brings together, articulating in time and space, like a bamboo node.

Joints are natural obstacles to the circulation of Qi and can become pathological under certain circumstances. Physical exercises such as *taijiquan* or *qigong* promote the free circulation of Qi, and can play an important part in the prevention and treatment of joint pain.

Chapter Notes

1. We believe that from an etymological standpoint, the character for Qi should be translated as "breaths," as this gives a better sense of its genesis and dynamics.

The ancient character (气) evokes the mist rising from the earth to form clouds in the sky. The standard character (氣) represents a grain of rice bursting under the pressure of the cooking or sprouting process, releasing steam above it. Interestingly, the simplified character now used in mainland China is the same as the ancient character. Nevertheless, for easier readability, we have decided in this text to use Qi. In this we follow the usage of most books in English on traditional Chinese medicine.

2. Note that in French, *shén* is translated as personality or being (*personne*), a term that prevents confusion with the religious or spiritual concept of spirit in the English language.

CHAPTER TWO

The Channels

THE PRIMARY FUNCTION of channel theory is to explain the relationships and mutual influences among different parts of the body, and to show how physiological activities, pathology, diagnosis and therapy are all based on these relationships. This is because all the structures and functions of the body are regulated and coordinated by the channel system.

The network of channels controls and regulates all of the body's internal functions, its relationship with the external world and the macrocosm, particularly through the relationships of the Five Phases.

The channels can be thought of as immaterial vectors of Qi which organize and encompass all the body's activities, and are represented by the words channels (jīng 經), collaterals (luò 絡)—also translated as connecting vessels—and vessels (mài 脈). They are classified in accordance with particular functions of the body.

Primary and Secondary Channels

The primary channels or channel vessels (jīng mài) are the most important channels for general physiology and treatment (FIGS. 2-1~2-12). Most of the acupuncture points are distributed along these twelve main pathways. They are well-described in many texts.

The most important secondary channels are the following:

- channel sinews (jīng jīn)
- channel divergences (jīng bié)
- collaterals (luò):
    minute collaterals (sūn luò)
    superficial collaterals (bié luò)
- Curious vessels (qí jīng bā mài).

Our purpose is not to present the detail of these channels, as their descriptions are readily available in many excellent textbooks. However, a special group of channels is of particular interest in rheumatology: the channel sinews (FIGS. 2-13~2-24). It is important to remember that while these are often called muscle channels or tendinomuscular channels, that appellation is quite incorrect. They are energetic pathways rather than anatomical structures, that is, "channel-like sinews." They represent what circulates with strength in the muscle spindles connected to the pathways of the twelve primary channels.

The function of the channel sinews is to form a shield that protects the primary channels. They maintain the integrity of the whole body by connecting the "hundred bones," and they govern the movements of the joints. They all originate in the extremities at the distal well points, and end in the trunk or the head. Their wide muscle bands narrow and form points of convergence at the level of the joints, and they approximately follow the pathways of their associated primary channels.

The channel sinews end in distinct points of connection: the lower limb yang channels at the cheek, the upper limb yang on the forehead, the upper limb yin in the armpit, and the lower limb yin above the pubic area. Their primary physiological function is to govern the muscles distributed along their pathways, and they have a direct influence on motor functions, as described below.

Our clinical experience has led us to believe that the involvement of the Curious vessels (FIGS. 2-25~2-30) is also important in many rheumatic conditions. In part this is due to the relationships of the Curious vessels to the deep levels or structures of the body. Both the relatively superficial regulatory aspects of these vessels, as well as their more fundamental typology, are useful in the treatment of musculoskeletal problems.

UPPER LIMB

Shoulder

Flexion: arm greater yin, arm yang brightness
Extension: arm greater yang, arm lesser yang
Abduction: arm yang brightness, arm lesser yang
Adduction: arm terminal yin, arm lesser yin
Raising: arm lesser yang, arm yang brightness
Dropping: arm greater yang, arm yang brightness
External rotation: arm greater yang, arm lesser yang

Arm and shoulder

Adduction: arm greater yin, arm lesser yin, arm terminal yin
Internal rotation: arm greater yin, arm lesser yin, arm terminal yin
Pronation: arm lesser yin
Abduction: arm lesser yang, arm yang brightness
External rotation: arm greater yang

Elbow and forearm

Extension: arm greater yang, arm lesser yang, arm yang brightness
Flexion: arm terminal yin, arm greater yin, arm lesser yin
Supination: arm yang brightness
Pronation: arm greater yin

Wrist and hand

Flexion: arm lesser yin, arm terminal yin
Extension: arm lesser yang, arm greater yang, arm yang brightness
Abduction: arm yang brightness
Adduction: arm greater yang, arm lesser yang

Fingers

Metacarpophalangeal flexion:
    I-II: arm greater yin
    III-IV: arm terminal yin
    V: arm lesser yin
Interphalangeal flexion:
    I: arm greater yin
    II-III: arm greater yin, arm terminal yin
    IV-V: arm terminal yin, arm lesser yin
Extension:
    I: arm yang brightness
    II: arm yang brightness, arm lesser yang
    III-IV: arm lesser yang
    V: arm greater yang
Opposition (of first and fifth finger): arm greater yin, arm lesser yin

LOWER LIMB

Hip and thigh

Flexion: leg greater yin
Extension: leg greater yang
Adduction: leg lesser yin, leg terminal yin
Abduction: leg lesser yang
Internal rotation: leg lesser yang
External rotation: leg lesser yang

Leg and knee

Flexion: leg greater yang
Extension: leg yang brightness, leg lesser yang

Foot

Flexion: leg yang brightness, leg lesser yang
Extension: leg lesser yin

Toes

Metatarsophalangeal flexion: leg lesser yin
Extension: leg yang brightness, leg lesser yang

NECK

Flexion: leg greater yang, leg yang brightness, leg lesser yin
Extension: leg greater yang, arm greater yang
Sidebending and rotation: leg lesser yang, arm lesser yang, arm yang brightness

TRUNK

Flexion: yang brightness, leg lesser yin

Sidebending and rotation: leg lesser yang, leg yang
  brightness

Extension: leg greater yang

The pathology of the channel sinews is associated primarily with motor disorders, pain in the muscles, sinews and ligaments, as well as spasms, often of a traumatic origin. The well and river points on the primary channels are commonly used to treat these disorders. It is also recommended to needle the insertion zones of the ligaments distributed along the same pathway, above and below the affected area.

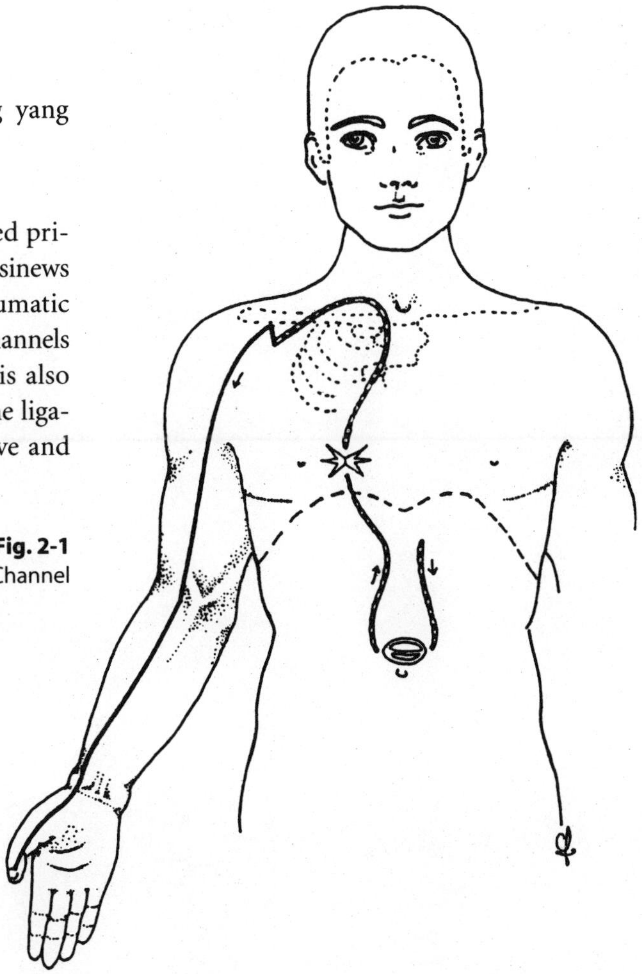

Fig. 2-1
Arm Greater Yin (Lung) Channel

 Connnection to Coupled Organ

 Pertaining Organ

 Deep Pathway

Superficial Pathway

 Connection with Channel or Point

Channel Sinew

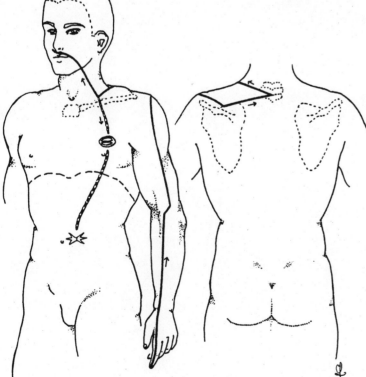

Fig. 2-2
Hand Yang Brightness (Large Intestine) Channel

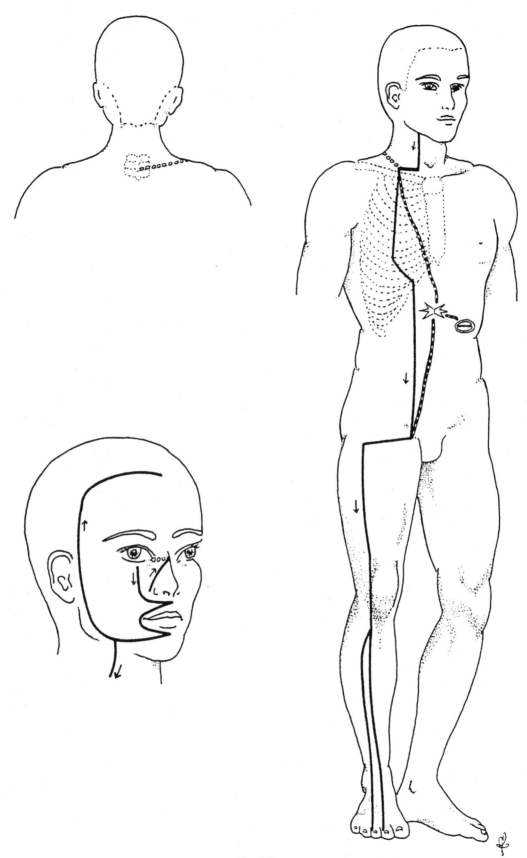

Fig. 2-3
Leg Yang Brightness (Stomach) Channel

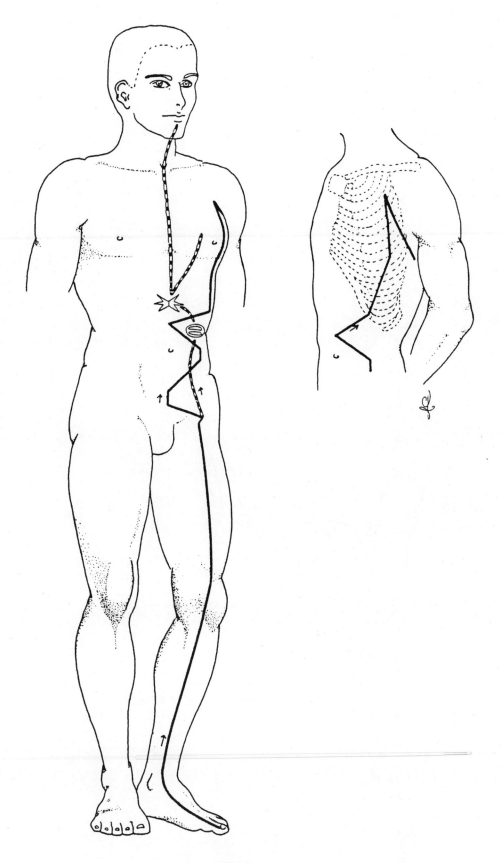

Fig. 2-4
Leg Greater Yin (Spleen) Channel

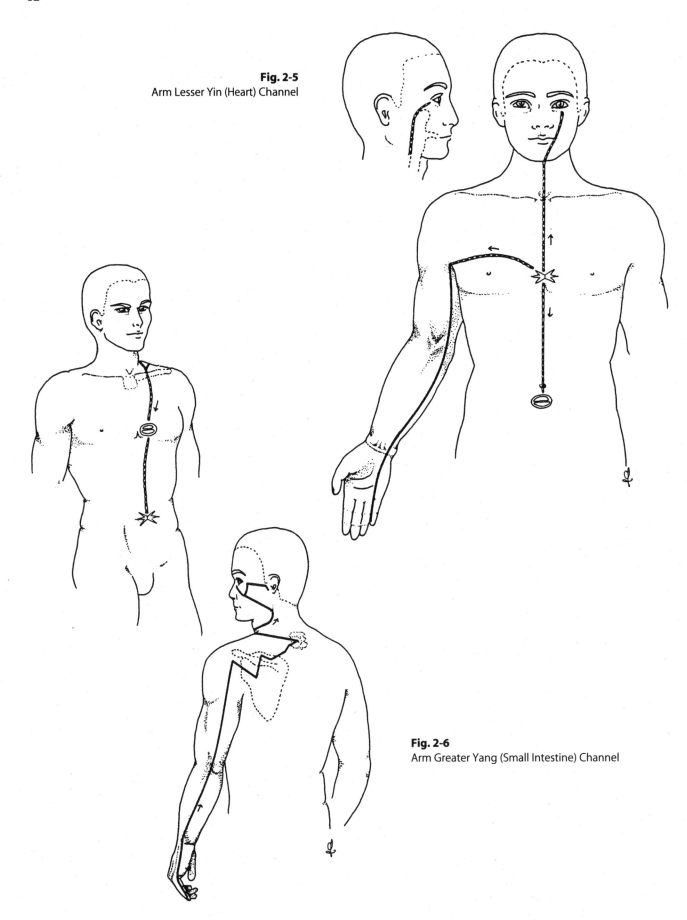

Fig. 2-5
Arm Lesser Yin (Heart) Channel

Fig. 2-6
Arm Greater Yang (Small Intestine) Channel

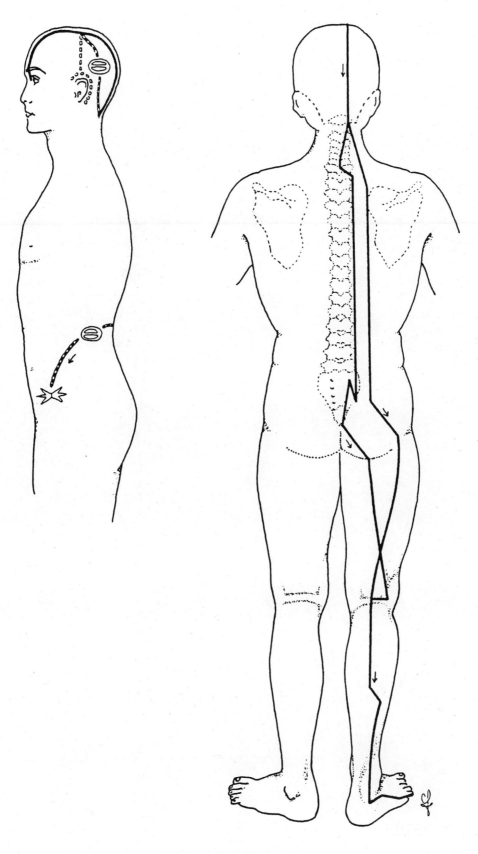

Fig. 2-7
Leg Greater Yang (Bladder) Channel

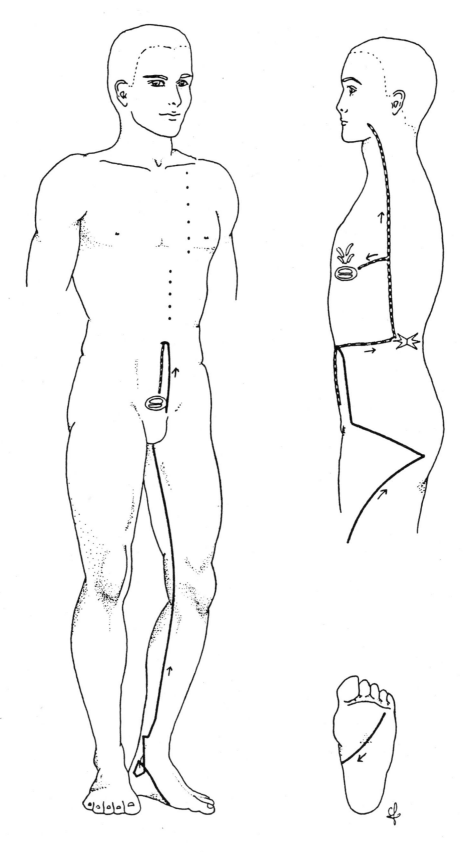

Fig. 2-8
Leg Lesser Yin (Kidney) Channel

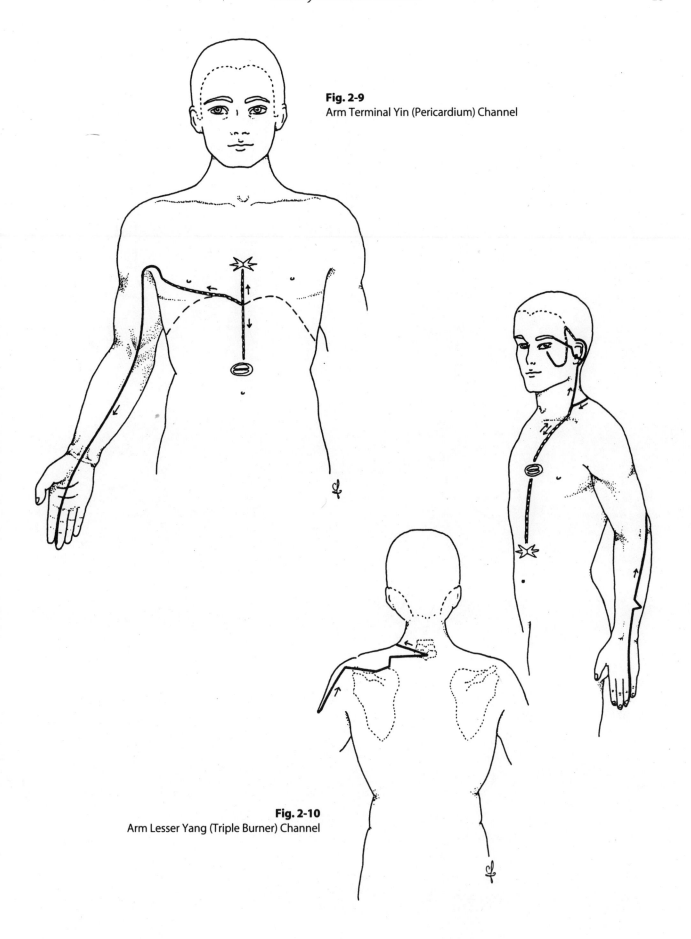

Fig. 2-9
Arm Terminal Yin (Pericardium) Channel

Fig. 2-10
Arm Lesser Yang (Triple Burner) Channel

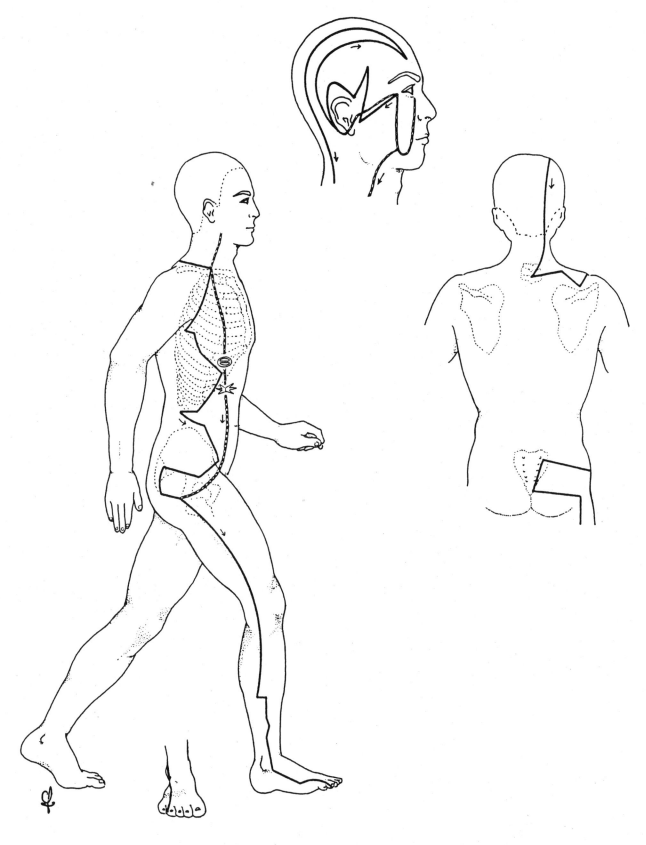

Fig. 2-11
Leg Lesser Yang (Gallbladder) Channel

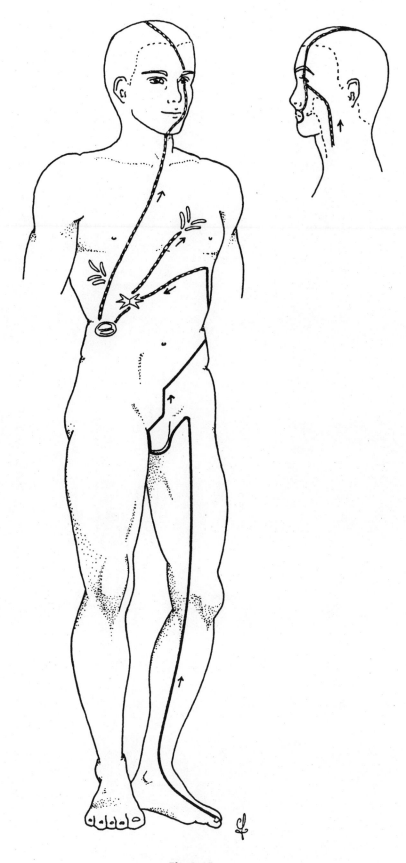

Fig. 2-12
Leg Terminal Yin (Liver) Channel

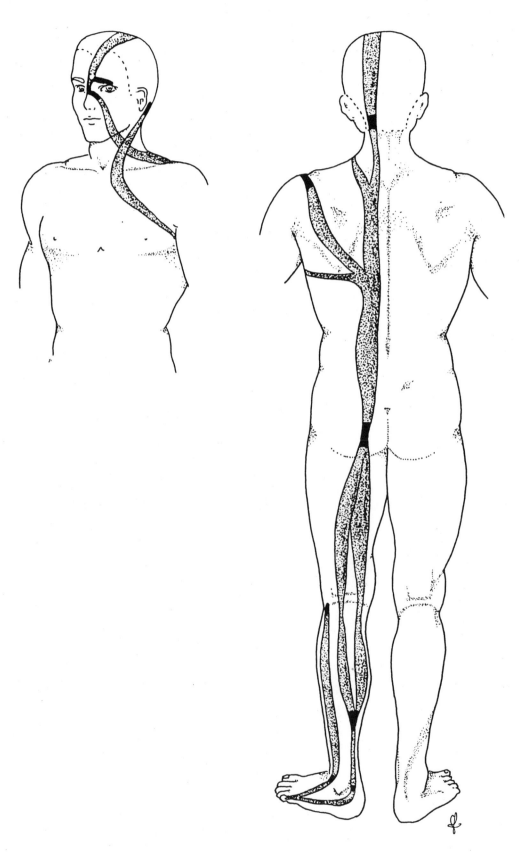

Fig. 2-13
Leg Greater Yang Channel Sinew

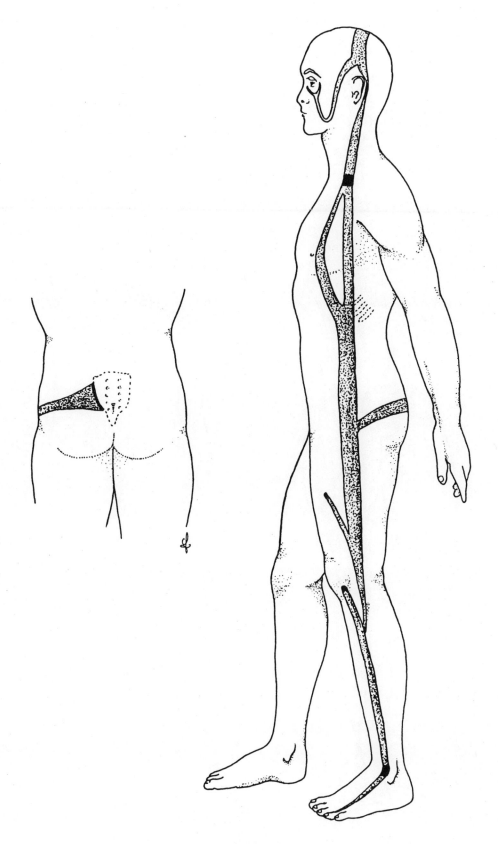

Fig. 2-14
Leg Lesser Yang Channel Sinew

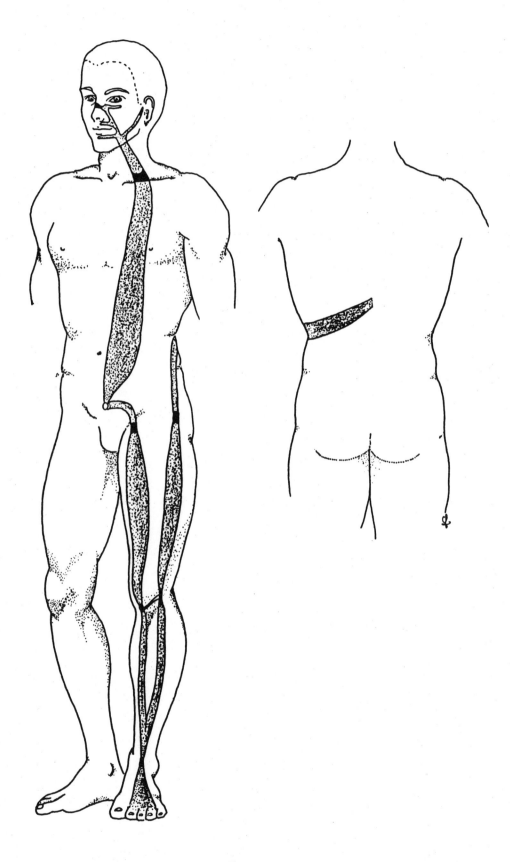

Fig. 2-15
Leg Yang Brightness Channel Sinew

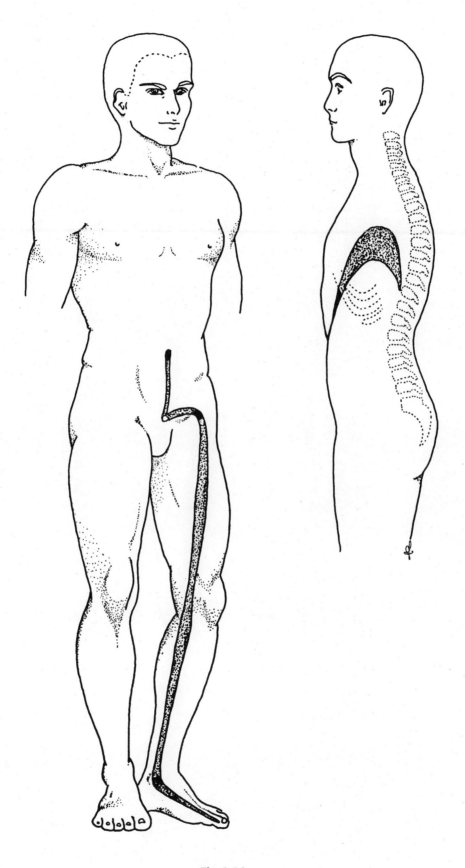

Fig. 2-16
Leg Greater Yin Channel Sinew

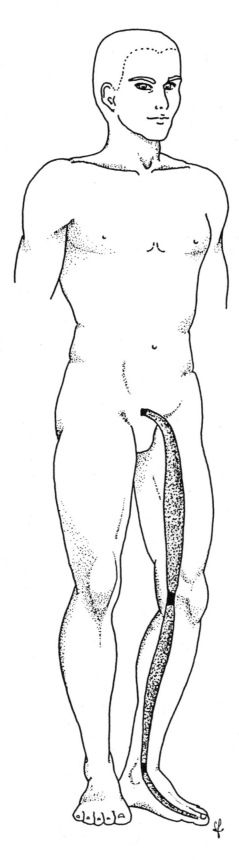

Fig. 2-17
Leg Terminal Yin Channel Sinew

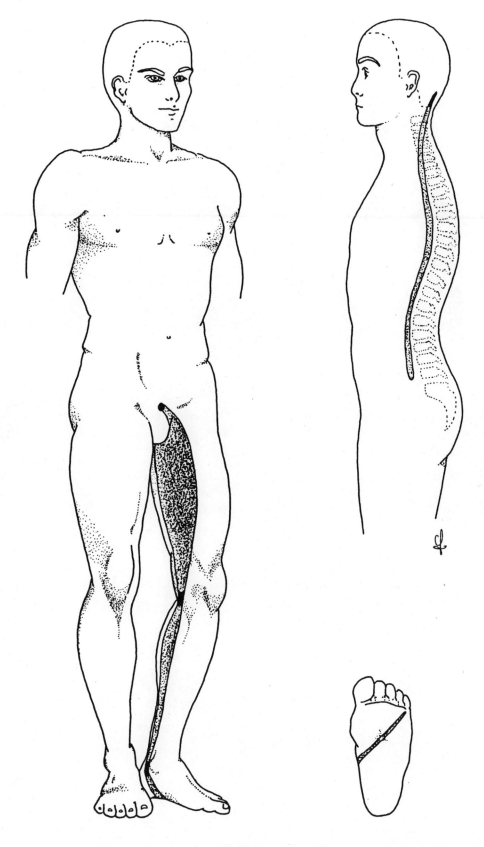

Fig. 2-18
Leg Lesser Yin Channel Sinew

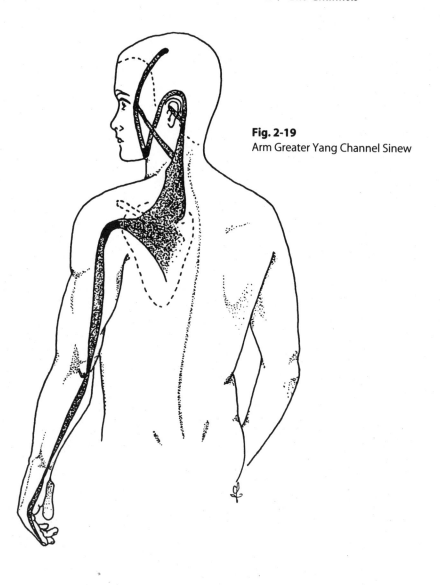

Fig. 2-19
Arm Greater Yang Channel Sinew

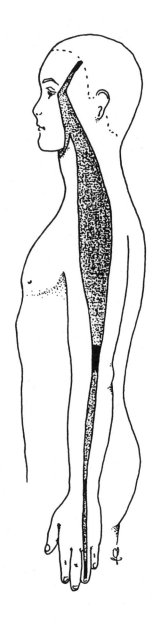

Fig. 2-20
Arm Lesser Yang Channel Sinew

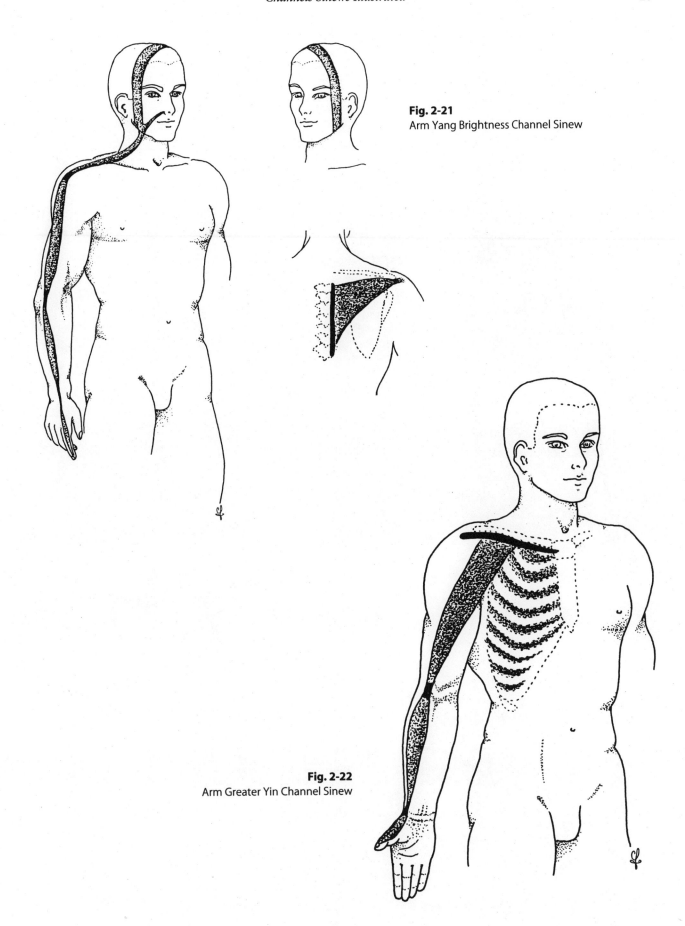

Fig. 2-21
Arm Yang Brightness Channel Sinew

Fig. 2-22
Arm Greater Yin Channel Sinew

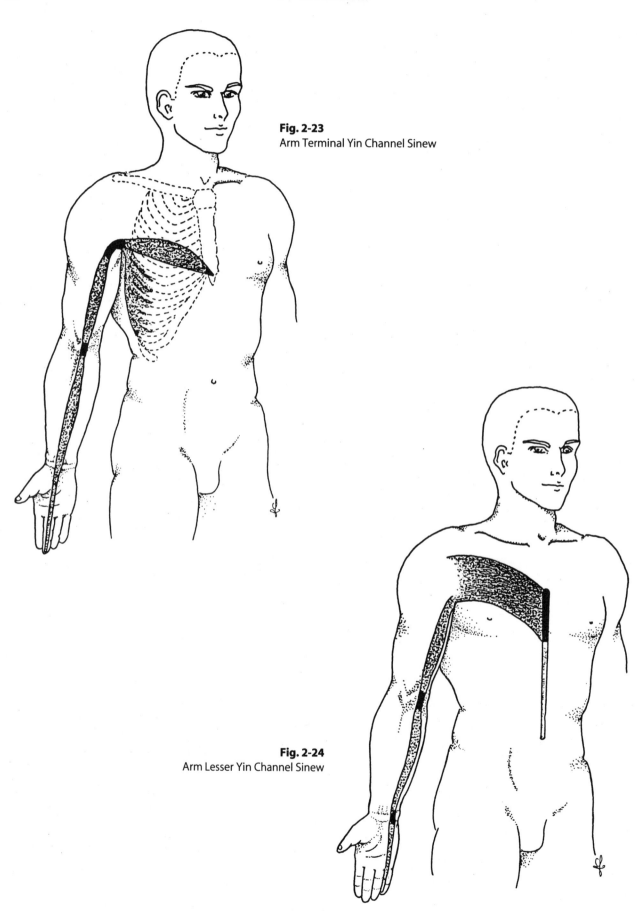

Fig. 2-23
Arm Terminal Yin Channel Sinew

Fig. 2-24
Arm Lesser Yin Channel Sinew

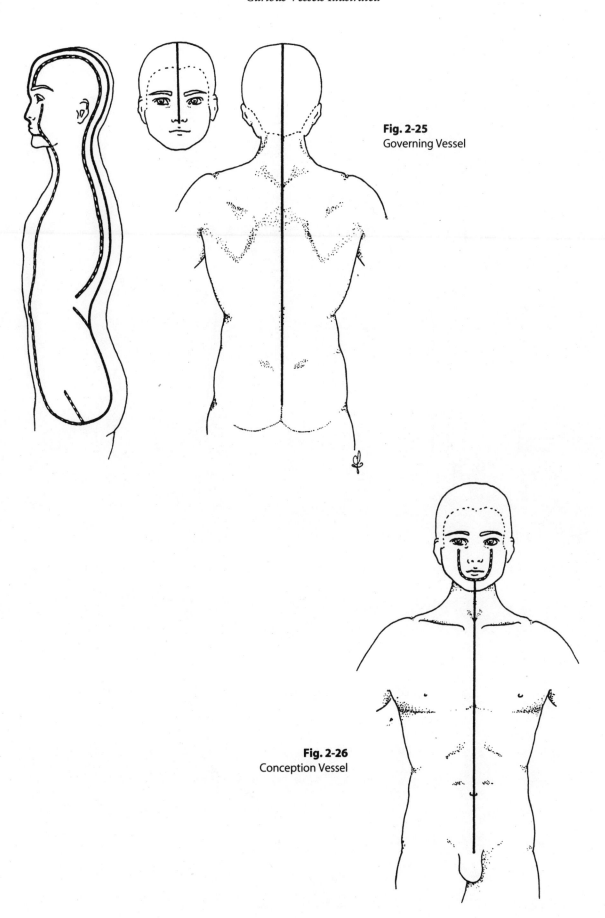

Fig. 2-25
Governing Vessel

Fig. 2-26
Conception Vessel

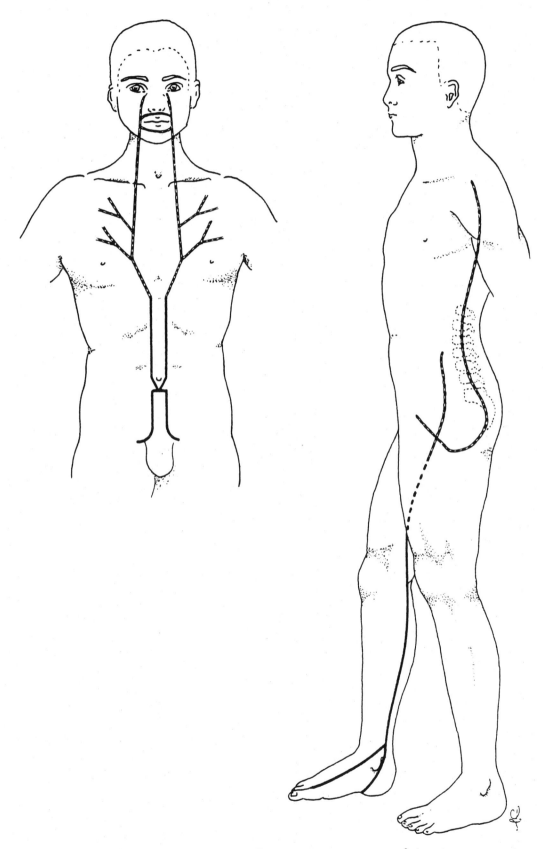

Fig. 2-27
Penetrating Vessel

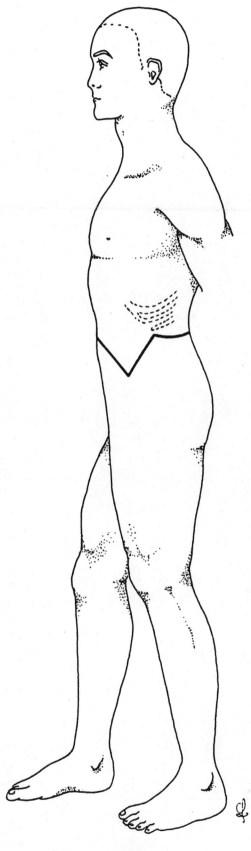

Fig. 2-28
Girdle Vessel

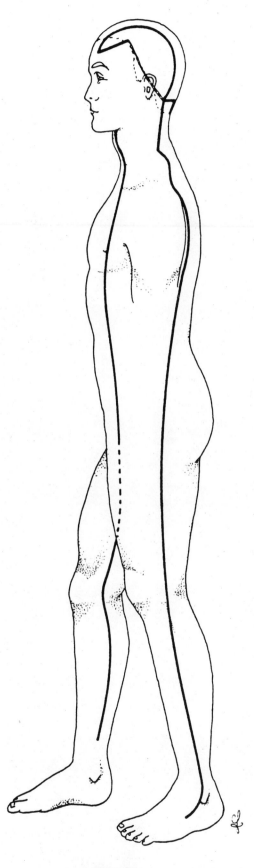

Fig. 2-29
Yin and Yang Linking Vessels

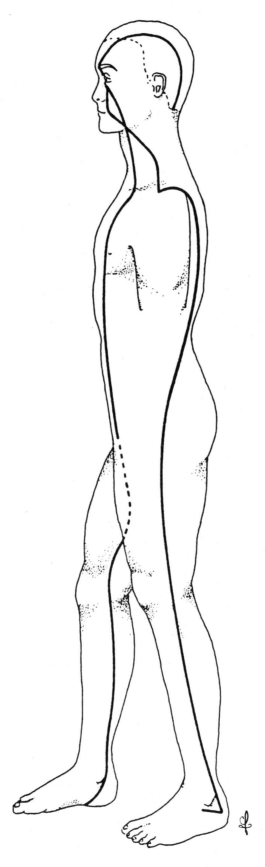

Fig. 2-30
Yin and Yang Heel Vessels

3

Etiological Factors in
Traditional Chinese Medicine

Traditional Chinese medicine defines health as the free circulation of Qi resulting from a perfect balance between the yin and the yang. This circulation can be impaired by factors that are external, internal, or neither internal nor external. The resulting yin-yang imbalance will cause excess, deficiency or stagnation of Qi.

All of these patterns are based on the struggle between the pathogenic Qi *(xié qì)* and the normal Qi *(zhēng qì)*. The intensity of this struggle determines the gravity of the symptoms for any disease. The quality of normal Qi depends on several factors:

• physical constitution
• mental state and psychological balance
• personal hygiene, habits and lifestyle
• diet
• medical history.

Since the quality of a person's normal Qi determines their state of health, the Chinese strongly emphasize certain prevention techniques—*taijiquan*, *qigong*, dietary and sexual practices—in order to strengthen it and to protect the individual from pathogenic influences. The art of traditional Chinese medicine consists of finding ways to eliminate pathogenic influences while preserving or strengthening the normal Qi.

External Factors *(wài yīn 外因)*

The importance which the Chinese attach to the concept of exogenous pathogenic factors in creating and supporting rheumatic diseases calls for a detailed analysis of these patterns of disharmony.

Six Pernicious Influences *(liù yín 六淫)*

Wind, Cold, Dampness, Dryness, Heat and Fire are the six regular energies associated with the seasonal climates. Wind is the regular Qi of spring, Heat-Fire is appropriate to summer, Dampness to the end of summer, Dryness is associated with fall, and Cold with winter.

Under normal circumstances, a healthy body is able to adapt to changes in the climate. But when climatic changes occur very suddenly, or with great intensity, or are out of synchronization with the seasons, their associated energies or Qi turn into pathogenic influences *(xié qì)*—the six pernicious energies or influences *(liù yín)*.[1] They become pathogenic agents if the normal Qi is too weak to resist: "The pathogenic flourishes where the Qi is depleted." *(Basic Questions (Su wen)*, chapter 33)

The six pernicious influences may act alone or in concert. Wind usually serves as a carrier for the other pernicious influences, and contributes to their rapid propagation. Different combinations are therefore described as Wind-Cold, Wind-Dampness, Wind-Heat, but also as Damp-Cold, Damp-Heat, etc.

A passage in chapter 66 of *Divine Pivot (Ling shu)* stipulates that the pernicious influences cannot injure the body by themselves; there must be a pre-existing insufficiency of normal Qi for the body to be affected. An example in chapter 46 illustrates this point by comparing pernicious Wind to a strong wind that uproots frail trees and strikes down people with weak constitutions: "Frequently ill people say that their joints, skin, pores and interstices lack strength. The pathogenic penetrates and stays inside. This is why they have frequent illnesses."

We must therefore distinguish three different patterns:

• When the dominant Qi corresponds to the current season (e.g., Wind in spring, Heat in summer) it is not pernicious in nature. Only those who are deficient might be affected, and the resulting illnesses are often benign.

• When the dominant Qi corresponding to the current season is excessive, its pathogenicity depends entirely on the strength of the individual's normal Qi.

• When the dominant Qi is out of synchronization with the current season, its perniciousness is all the more virulent if the dominant Heavenly Qi is of a contrary nature (e.g., Cold in summer when the Qi of the dominant Celestial Stem of the season is Heat-lesser yang), but its perniciousness is less serious if the Qi of the Celestial Stem is of an identical nature (e.g., Cold-greater yang). For more details about this process, see chapter 71 of *Basic Questions*.

A passage in chapter 46 of *Divine Pivot* explains that an attack by the same pernicious influence will affect people differently. It will induce different diseases according to the individual's constitution, that is, the quality of their nutritive Qi and defensive Qi.

These pernicious influences can transform into one another during the course of a disease. For example, an accumulation of Cold can transform into Heat, and lingering Heat can generate Dryness by burning the Fluids.

The pernicious influences' preferred routes of invasion are the upper body, the mouth or the nose, and the surface of the body, which accounts for the typical upper respiratory tract infection which occurs during the initial phase of such diseases.

In chapter 4 of *Divine Pivot*, Qi Bo explains that the pernicious influences attack people from the top, with the exception of Dampness, which usually invades from the bottom:

> The pores and interstices open up to the attack of the pathogenic influences. An attack on the face will penetrate downward through the yang brightness; an attack on the neck will penetrate downward through the greater yang; an attack on the cheek will penetrate downward through the lesser yang. Consequently, the invasion of the chest, back and both sides of the body follows an attack on the channels.

Other aspects of this process are elaborated in chapter 56 of *Basic Questions*:

> The myriad diseases always originate at the level of the skin. When pathogenic influences attack the skin, the interstices and pores open. When they open [the pathogenic influences] enter and reside in the collaterals. If they linger there and are not expelled, they will be transmitted to the primary channels. If they linger there and are not expelled, they will be transmitted to the yang Organs and gather in the Stomach and the Intestines. When a pathogenic influence starts to enter the skin, chilly piloerection occurs and there is an opening of the interstices and pores. When the pathogenic influence is in the collaterals, they are replete and the color changes. When it enters and resides in the primary channels the person will feel deficient, and furthermore there will be a collapse [of the pulse]. If it lingers between the sinews and bones and Cold is predominant, then the sinews spasm and the bones hurt. If Heat is predominant then the sinews become lax and the bones melt, the flesh liquefies, the fleshy swellings disappear, and the hair straightens and falls out.

The channel system therefore protects our most precious parts, but a deficiency in the defensive Qi allows the pernicious influences to reach the yang Organs by affecting the yang,[2] and the yin Organs by affecting the yin[3] (*Basic Questions*, chapter 29), which causes serious pathologies.

Besides spreading through the channel network, the pernicious influences can also directly invade the yin and yang Organs, for example, via the classic direct Wind-stroke *(zhòng fēng)*.

Traditional Chinese medicine basically has three different systems for tracking the spread of pernicious influences through the body. The oldest is the six stage *(liù jīng,* also known as six channel or six warp) system described in *Discussion of Cold-induced Disorders (Shang han lun)*: greater yang, yang brightness, lesser yang, greater yin, lesser yin and terminal yin. More recent systems are those progressions that deal primarily with disorders caused by Heat: the three burner system *(sān jiāo)*, or the four level *(sì fēn,* also known as four aspect or four sector) system comprised of the defensive, Qi, nutritive and Blood levels.

The presence of an external pernicious influence is detected through the pulse and the complexion, as described in the following passage from chapter 27 of *Basic Questions*:

> Whenever a pathogenic influence enters into a vessel, if it is Cold then the Blood becomes congealed and turbulent; if it is Hot then the Qi becomes all slushy and marshy. When, because of this, a deficient pathogenic influence enters and stays, it is like a gust of wind blowing on a river. The movement in the channel vessel arrives and also temporarily rises and spreads throughout its length. When it reaches the radial artery it is sometimes large [strong], sometimes small [weak]. When large, the pathogenic influence has arrived. When small, then all is in equilibrium. The course of the pathogenic influence has no place where it regularly resides. Whether it is in the yin or yang we cannot speculate. As soon as its presence can be detected in the three positions and nine places of the pulse, its route must be quickly blocked.

The relationships between these external pernicious influences and the Organs have been established in accordance with the Five Phase theory:

• Wind readily injures the Liver.
• Heat and Fire readily penetrate the Pericardium.
• Dampness readily harms the Spleen.
• Dryness readily invades the Lungs.
• Cold readily attacks the Kidneys.

Internally generated dysfunctions of the Organs can manifest the same symptoms as disorders caused by the six pernicious influences. To differentiate them, the former are described as internal Wind, internal Cold, and so forth, while the latter are called external Wind, external Cold, etc.

Wind *(fēng* 風)

Wind is the characteristic Qi of spring, but can occur in any season. Depending on its quality, it can transform into a pernicious influence and become one of the six pernicious influences. It can originate either internally or externally.

Externally generated Wind is always caused by an attack from an environmental factor on the body. Internally generated Wind always proceeds from a disturbance in a human function that creates symptoms associated with the nature of wind.

Nature of Wind

Wind is very mobile, changes suddenly, has a swift and erratic character, and appears and disappears abruptly. Its primary features are movement and transformation.

Properties of Pathogenic Wind

• Wind is the source of numerous diseases. *(Basic Questions,* chapter 19)

Wind provides a vehicle for the other pernicious influences, enabling and facilitating the penetration of Cold, Dryness, Dampness and Heat into the body, and generating symptoms of Wind-Cold, Wind-Dryness, Wind-Dampness and Wind-Heat.

• Wind is unstable, cannot be confined to a location, and tends to move upward and outward.

Wind is a yang agent and by its very nature tends to injure the upper and superficial parts of the body: "When Wind attacks the body, it starts from the top." *(Basic Questions,* chapter 29)

• Wind opens and draws out.

Wind opens the pores and interstices, enabling the sweat to come out. Wind diseases are accompanied by sweating and an aversion to wind.

• Wind moves and transforms.

A Wind-type disease is characterized by fleeting symptoms that move and change constantly. This is the case for certain types of painful obstruction where the pain in the joints does not have a fixed location, but moves from one instant to the next and fluctuates in an irregular pattern, hence its name, moving (literally "walking") painful obstruction *(xíng bì)* or Wind painful obstruction *(fēng bì)*.

• Wind appears and disappears rapidly.

The emergence of a Wind-type disease is abrupt, and its evolution is rapid.

• Movement and agitation embody the nature of Wind.

Tremors and convulsions indicate the stirring of Wind.

External Wind Diseases

Wind by itself creates a pathology which encompasses most or all of the following symptoms: fever, aversion to wind, sweating, sore throat, cough, stuffy nose, achy joints or muscles, headaches. The pulse is floating, and the tongue is pink with a thin white coating.

This clinical picture is modified when Wind combines with Cold, Heat, Dampness or Dryness. The resulting pathologies describe aspects of Wind-Cold, Wind-Heat, Wind-Dampness or Wind-Dryness. A typical example is erratic rheumatic pain in the joints, as encountered in post-streptococcal rheumatism.

Pathogenic Wind can affect the yin aspect of the body directly, that is, the yin and yang Organs. This disease—direct Wind attack or Wind-stroke *(zhòng fēng)*—is very serious from the start and presents with the clinical signs of a stroke: mental confusion, deviation of the mouth and eyes, hemiplegia, coma.

Internal Wind Diseases

The usual symptoms include such problems as dizziness, vertigo, spasms and stiffness of the limbs, tremors, faintness, agitation, sudden loss of consciousness, deviation of the mouth and eyes, and hemiplegia. This is another way in which Wind-stroke occurs.

Liver yang rebelling upward: Deficiency of Liver yin or Liver Blood creates an internal stirring of Liver Wind. Typical signs include violent headaches, vertigo, red eyes, spots in front of the eyes, tremors and paresthesia of the limbs, deviation of the mouth and eyes, speech disorders, or even coma. The pulse is wiry, and the tongue is red.

Extreme Heat generates Wind: An extreme abundance of Heat burns the Fluids, injures the Liver, produces Phlegm and stirs up Wind. Common symptoms include high fever, spasms of the limbs, stiff neck, agitation, opisthotonos, convulsions, loss of consciousness. The pulse is wiry and rapid, the tongue is red with a yellow coating.

Yin and Blood deficiency: Blood deficiency generates Wind, the Wind and the yang disrupt the upper body, and the sinews and vessels lack nourishment. The most common symptoms include contraction of the limbs, speech impairment, deviation of the mouth and eyes, hemiplegia, coma. The pulse is thin and rapid, and the tongue is red.

Dry Blood: The skin and the vessels are malnourished, and Wind stirs up. The skin is dry, rough and itchy, and the hair falls out. The pulse is choppy, and the tongue is red or purple.

Cold *(hán* 寒*)*

Chinese texts use three different words to describe Cold:

- *Hán* refers to Cold as the normal Qi of winter, which can nevertheless occur in any other season in a milder form.
- *Liáng* means cool, as opposed to warm *(wēn)*.
- *Lěng* represents the nature of Cold, as opposed to the nature of Heat *(rè)*.

In Cold diseases, the term *hán* refers either to one of the six pernicious influences, or to the result of an internal deficiency. This is the difference between external Cold and internal Cold.

External Cold is due to the invasion of the Cold pathogenic factor from the surrounding environment. It can be further differentiated as Cold-damage or Cold-attack depending on its mode of penetration.

Cold-damage *(shāng hán)* attacks the exterior of the body and is the subject of the book *Discussion of Cold-induced Disorders*. Its main symptoms are fever, chills, headache, stiffness and aversion to cold. The pulse is floating and tight, and the tongue coating is white.

Cold-attack *(zhòng hán)* attacks the interior directly—the yin and yang Organs. Its primary symptoms are vomiting clear fluids, abdominal pain, borborygmus, diarrhea and cold limbs. The pulse is sunken.

Internal Cold is always related to a yang Qi deficiency in the body. This can occur when deficiency of the yang leads to a relative excess of Cold, or when an excess of Cold in the interior exhausts the yang.

Although it is important to distinguish them, internal Cold and external Cold influence each other. People who are yang deficient—and thus have excessive internal Cold—are much more sensitive to external Cold. If the external Cold penetrates and accumulates in the body, it injures the yang and contributes to the emergence of an internal Cold pattern.

Nature of Cold

Cold slows things down, contracts, hardens and congeals. "If Cold invades a vessel, it slows down and then congeals the circulation of the Qi." (*Basic Questions*, chapter 39)

Properties of Pathogenic Cold

- Cold is a yin factor; it has the ability to injure the yang.

    An overabundance of yin generates Cold. An excess of yin or Cold injures the yang Qi. When the yang Qi can no longer perform its warming function, there is an aversion to cold and Cold diseases will appear. When the yang of the yang Organs is injured, their ability to transform is impaired, and there is a decrease in functional activity. This leads to the emergence of such symptoms as aversion to cold, general cold sensation, and diarrhea with undigested food.

• Cold generates Cold-type blockages.

Cold slows down the circulation of Blood and/or Qi, giving rise to patterns of blockage or stagnation.

"Cold can settle outside the vessels, chilling them. When the vessels are Cold they shrivel up." *(Basic Questions,* chapter 39)

"Cold can settle inside the Small Intestine membranes and vessels, congealing its Blood and preventing it from flowing toward the big channel. Its lingering presence will create swellings." *(Basic Questions,* chapter 39)

"Among the different types of Qi, Cold is the one that hardens." *(Basic Questions,* chapter 67)

• Cold attacks the Blood.

"Cold injures the Blood." *(Basic Questions,* chapter 67)

"When greater yang rules in Heaven . . . Blood deteriorates inside and produces abscesses and ulcers." *(Basic Questions,* chapter 74)

Obstruction of the Blood circulation always produces stabbing-type pains.

• Cold produces Cold-type contractions and pain.

Cold slows down the circulation of Qi: "Cold closes the skin orifices, impairs the circulation of Qi, and causes it to contract." *(Basic Questions,* chapter 39)

• The invasion of Cold in the body contracts the Qi and causes gnawing-type pains.

"When there is Cold, the Qi contracts." *(Basic Questions,* chapter 39)

Cold can settle outside the channel, chilling it and shriveling it up. The channel contracts its smaller vessels and induces a violent pain—which can be immediately alleviated by applying warmth. But repeated attacks of Cold can make the pain linger. Cold can settle inside the channel and confront its Heat; the channel in a state of excess harbors a pain that cannot tolerate any pressure. If the Cold lingers, Heat rises, the vessel swells, and the Blood and Qi become disrupted, which is why pressure is intolerably painful. *(Basic Questions,* chapter 39)

• If the Cold is in the surface, the hair follicles contract, the defensive Qi is blocked, and the following symptoms appear: aversion to cold, fever, absence of sweating, head and body aches, tight pulse.

"When the pathogenic influence penetrates the skin, the Cold induces piloerection and the pores of the skin are open." *(Basic Questions,* chapter 56)

• If the Cold reaches deeper, it causes stiffness.

"When the pathogenic influence in the muscles and the bones is very Cold, it creates stiffness of the muscles and pain in the bones." *(Basic Questions,* chapter 56)

External Cold Diseases

Either excessive external Cold or deficient defensive Qi promotes the invasion of Cold inside the body, according to the six stage system. This condition presents with three primary symptoms: (1) chills, due to the invasion of Cold, with a desire for warm drinks and warm clothes; (2) feverishness, due to the struggle between the normal and pathogenic Qi; and (3) pain, due to the slowing down and obstruction in the circulation of Blood and Qi, which is alleviated by warmth.

When Wind combines with Cold in a Wind-Cold pattern, the following signs and symptoms are present: severe chills, slight fever, headaches, stuffy and runny nose, painful joints, thin and white tongue coating, floating and tight pulse.

Painful obstruction due to penetration of Cold is characterized by violent pains and is therefore known as severe (literally "painful") painful obstruction *(tòng bì).* It is alleviated by warmth and aggravated by cold, and is in a fixed location.

When Cold injures the Stomach and Spleen there is epigastric pain, vomiting of clear fluids, lack of appetite, borborygmus and diarrhea.

Internal Cold Diseases

Internal Cold is always due to yang deficiency at the level of the yin and yang Organs. As the [French] *Dictionnaire de médecine traditionnelle* puts it: "Deficiency and depletion of the yin Organs and yang Organs disrupts the circulation and transformation of the Water and Fluids, and the turbid yin stays with the empty yang; the vigorous yin therefore generates internal Cold."

This syndrome is also known as deficiency Cold, or Cold from deficiency. Its main signs and symptoms are aversion to cold, cold limbs, feeling cold inside, vomiting clear fluids, diarrhea with undigested food, frequent urination, fatigue, dull complexion, sleeping in a curled-up position, sunken and slow pulse, and a white and wet tongue coating.

In the particular case of Kidney yang deficiency (deficiency of the Fire of the gate of vitality), the body's source of yang is depleted, which manifests as a loss of the Qi's warming and transformative functions. This causes cold extremities, sexual impotence, and an overflow of pathogenic Water with such problems as frequent urination, edema, lower back pain and sterility.

Summerheat (*shǔ* 暑)

The concept of Heat can be expressed with four different words in Chinese:

- *Rè* refers to the Hot nature of something, as opposed to a Cold nature. This concept is independent of the cycle of the seasons.
- *Shǔ* is the dominant Qi of summer, manifesting between the summer solstice and the autumn equinox.
- *Wēn* is that which is warm as opposed to cool; it describes certain types of Hot diseases, that is, the warm-febrile diseases *(wēn bìng)* which classically occur before the summer solstice.
- *Huǒ* is Fire, the most extreme expression of Heat.

Summerheat causes exogenous diseases only during summer. There is no such thing as Summerheat diseases outside the summer season.

Nature of Heat

Heat warms up, dilates, circulates, spreads, and tends to rise. Its nature is yang.

Properties of Summerheat

- Summerheat belongs to yang, and its nature is excessive Heat.

    "In Summerheat-induced diseases there is sweating, choking and thirst. When there is no agitation, there is delirious speech. The body is like a blazing fire that can be dispersed by sweating." *(Basic Questions,* chapter 3)

- The chief characteristic of Summerheat is that it rises and spreads.

    When Summerheat penetrates the body it rises and spreads; it opens the pores and interstices of the skin and induces intense sweating; it dries up the Fluids and causes excessive thirst, oliguria and a stifling sensation in the chest. Qi and Fluids are lost through sweating, and the resulting deficiency causes asthenia and dyspnea, and can even lead to loss of consciousness.

    "Summerheat opens the cutaneous orifices, activates the circulation of the nutritive Qi and defensive Qi, and draws sweat out, which leads to a leakage of Qi." *(Basic Questions,* chapter 39)

- Extreme Heat generates Wind and agitates the Blood.

    The telltale signs are hyperthemia, delirious speech, spasms of the limbs, loss of consciousness, turned-up eyes, stiff neck, opisthotonos.

- Heat speeds up the circulation of Blood.

    Heat causes reckless movement of the Blood, such that it travels outside the vessels. This can lead to various types of hemorrhage including epistaxis, hematemesis, hematuria, rectal bleeding and metrorrhagia.

- Summerheat readily combines with Dampness.

    This is not surprising since the summer season is often accompanied by a high degree of humidity due to the evaporation of water. The usual clinical signs are fever, thirst, diarrhea, nausea, heavy limbs and a stifling sensation in the chest.

Summerheat-stroke

The common clinical signs are headaches, hyperthermia, thirst, oliguria, sweating, anxiety, and a big and rapid pulse. In severe cases there is restlessness, delirium and loss of consciousness.

There are two clinical aspects to Summerheat-stroke *(zhòng shǔ)*, which is also known as Heat-stroke *(zhòng rè)*. The differentiation depends on whether it is due to an overexposure to the sun (yang) or to an overabundance of coolness (yin).

Yang Heat-stroke: This condition is directly related to a prolonged exposure to the sun. The classical signs are accompanied by redness of the skin, excessive sweating, vertigo, and even loss of consciousness. When especially severe, the symptoms may indicate that the Heat is attacking the Heart and Pericardium, with such signs as an elevation of body and skin temperature, absence of sweating, stifling sensation in the chest with signs of anxiety, a red tongue with a yellow coating, and a flooding pulse.

Yin Heat-stroke: This is actually an invasion of pathogenic Cold, as a result of seeking some way to cool down, such as sleeping outside, exposing oneself to wind or air conditioning, or ingesting an excessive amount of cold drinks, raw foods or ice cream. Symptoms include fever, aversion to cold, headaches, absence of sweating, abdominal pain and diarrhea.

Summerheat often combines with Dampness, either because the Heat of heaven embraces the Dampness of the earth, which stagnates and then evaporates, or because of latent Dampness due to an overconsumption of fruit and raw foods. Both of these conditions occur often during the summer.

Clinically, Summerheat diseases are often observed to be accompanied by Damp signs of constriction, such as fatigue with a sensation of heaviness in the whole body, stifling sensation in the chest, turban-type headaches, nausea, vomiting and diarrhea. That is why the ancient Chinese used to recommend treating Summerheat and Dampness diseases simultaneously.

When Heat combines with Wind it injures the surface, then progresses toward the upper burner and causes such symptoms as aversion to wind and cold, fever, headaches, spontaneous sweating, and a flooding, big and yet frail pulse.

Finally, the combination of Heat and Dampness is often the cause of dysentery with tenesmus, or of sudden turmoil,[4] characterized by vomiting, nausea, diarrhea and abdominal pain.

Dampness (shī 濕)

Dampness is the dominant Qi of Indian summer, which in China corresponds to the season of Dampness. According to *Dictionnaire de médecine traditionnelle*:

> Dampness is one of the six pernicious influences, belonging to the category of yin pernicious influences. It is heavy and turbid by nature, and can obstruct the dynamics of the Qi. It is controlled by the transformative and transportive functions of the Spleen.

Dampness may also refer to the consequence of a disruption in the Spleen's transformative and transportive functions, causing stagnation of the body's Water and Fluids. These two aspects establish a clear distinction between externally and internally caused Dampness.

External Dampness is caused by climatic dampness, a prolonged exposure to rain, or a damp environment. Internal Dampness is caused by dietary imbalances due to an overconsumption of fatty foods, sweet and processed foods, raw foods or alcohol, which disrupts the Spleen's functions in water metabolism.

These two pathologies often influence one another: the initial external Dampness disease impairs the proper functioning of the Spleen, which then cannot perform its transformative and transportive functions, and Dampness accumulates in the body. If the Spleen's yang is depleted, the Water-Dampness cannot be transformed, which facilitates the invasion of external Dampness.

Nature of Dampness

Dampness is heavy and turbid by nature; it tends to accumulate, stagnate and lodge itself in a fixed location. It is difficult to eliminate.

Properties of Pathogenic Dampness

• Dampness has a heavy and turbid character.

When external Dampness penetrates the surface, the nutritive Qi and defensive Qi are no longer in harmony. This causes heaviness of the head, fatigue and general weakness, and stiff limbs. If the pathogenic Dampness stays in the channels and the joints, the yang Qi cannot circulate, the skin and the muscles feel numb, and the joints are stiff and painful.

The turbid, impure nature of Dampness creates symptoms such as prurigo, impetigo, eczema, sticky stools, mucus in the eyes, turbid urine, and leukorrhea.

• Dampness sticks and stagnates.

These features explain why Dampness inside the body tends to linger, and why Damp diseases often have a chronic character, are aggravated by a change in weather, and are difficult to treat. This is the reason why Damp-type painful obstruction is also called fixed or lingering painful obstruction (*zhuó bì*) and why eczema is difficult to completely cure.

• Dampness (a yin agent) readily obstructs the circulation of Qi and injures the yang Qi.

Dampness is viscous and sticky; it stagnates in the Organs and the channels where it impairs the circulation and functioning of the Qi, and disrupts its ascending and descending activities. Symptoms appear such as a stifling sensation in the chest, oliguria and dysuria, and difficult bowel movements. Dampness can also be marked by a sensation of a ball or mass in the abdomen, stomach or throat, as in the "plum-pit Qi" syndrome.

Because of its yin nature, Dampness depletes the yang Qi, particularly the Spleen yang, which can no longer ascend. As a result there is diarrhea, distention of the abdomen and a loss of appetite.

• Dampness oozes and saturates.

The affected parts swell and retain water, and there is edema, dull pain, swelling and paresthesia. This is also why eczema is usually considered to be due to Dampness.

External Dampness Diseases

The general symptomatology includes fever with sweating, heavy and achy head, difficulty in moving around, fixed, deep and dull pain, a sensation of heaviness in the whole body, stifling sensation in the chest, tired upper and lower limbs, sticky white tongue coating, floating and moderate pulse.

Dampness is often associated with other pernicious influences: Wind, Cold or Heat.

Wind-Dampness: evening fevers, clamminess, fetid sweating which does not lower the temperature, aversion to wind, heavy head and body, stiffness and numb sensation in the limbs, and a floating and moderate pulse.

Damp-Cold: fever with aversion to cold, absence of sweating, heavy sensation in the body, painful joints, and a floating and slow pulse.

Damp-Heat: asthenia, stifling and heavy sensation in the chest, despondent mood, warm body, aversion to cold at first, followed by constant fever, thirst, and a greasy and yellow tongue coating.

"In diseases due to Dampness the head feels hemmed in. If Damp-Heat cannot be eliminated, the big muscles contract and there are spasms. The small muscles become flaccid and there is atrophy." (*Basic Questions,* chapter 3)

Damp warm-febrile diseases *(shī wēn)* represent a special case. They are infectious diseases that occur in summer and at the beginning of autumn. They injure the functions of the Spleen and Stomach.

If Dampness predominates the Spleen is injured, and there is constant fever that is not relieved by sweating, thirst with no desire to drink or preference for warm drinks, sensation of fullness in the chest, nausea, tired upper and lower limbs, heaviness of the head and body, turbid urine, soft stool, thick and white tongue coating, and a moderate pulse.

If Heat predominates the Stomach is injured, and there is high fever, a bitter taste in the mouth, thirst with little desire to drink, nausea, dark urine, constipation or soft and scanty stool, anxiety, dry, thick and yellow tongue coating, red tip and edges, and a rapid pulse.

Internal Dampness Diseases

If Dampness settles in the upper body there is heaviness in the head, nasal obstruction, yellowish conjunctiva, stifling sensation in the chest, dyspnea, fullness in the chest and profuse phlegm.

If Dampness settles in the mid-portion of the body there is dyspepsia, heavily coated tongue, nausea, vomiting, no appetite, and fullness in the epigastrium or sensation of an abdominal mass.

If Dampness settles in the lower body there is abdominal bloating, oliguria, soft or liquid diarrhea, turbid urine, leukorrhea, swollen skin, and edema at the top of the foot.

Dryness *(zào 燥)*

Dryness is the dominant Qi of autumn. External Dryness refers to an attack of the pernicious climatic Dryness. It invades mostly through the nose and mouth, and the resulting diseases often originate in the Lungs and affect the defensive Qi. External Dryness is often linked to the residual heat of summer or to the premature cold of winter.

Internal Dryness results from a severe loss of Fluids, an insufficient supply of Fluids, inappropriate use of the sweating, emetic or purging techniques, or an attack of Heat or Fire—in which case Dryness corresponds to the residual Fire Qi.

Nature of Dryness

Dryness withers, dehydrates, retracts and is astringent.

Properties of Pathogenic Dryness

• Dryness is dry and astringent.

Dryness is yang by nature. It has the ability to injure the Fluids and cause a pattern of exhaustion of the yin Fluids characterized by dryness of the nose, mouth and throat, thirst, withered and dry skin, dull hair, dry stool or constipation, oliguria, dry tongue and a thin pulse.

• Dryness readily injures the Lungs.

Dry Lungs are no longer moistened by the Fluids, and their functions of transportation, downward distribution, purification and cooling of the Qi are disrupted. The following symptoms are indicative of this condition: a dry cough or one which produces scanty amounts of either viscous sputum which is hard to expectorate, or blood-streaked sputum, dyspnea, and chest pain.

External Dryness Diseases

Warm-Dryness (wēn zào): fever, sweating, thirst, dry nose and throat, dry cough with little sputum or blood-streaked sputum, chest pain, anxiety.

Cool-Dryness (liáng zào): fever, aversion to cold, absence of sweating, headaches, dry mouth, dry nose with a sensation of obstruction, and a dry and scantily productive cough.

Internal Dryness Diseases

Internal Dryness diseases indicate an exhaustion of the yin due to an excessive loss of Fluids through profuse sweating, vomiting, diarrhea, polyuria or hemorrhage. They can also be caused by improper therapeutic prescriptions or a chronic illness.

The main symptoms are intense thirst, dry mouth and throat, dry and wrinkled skin, dull complexion and hair, chapped lips, oliguria, constipation or dry and hard stools, weight loss and a thin and choppy pulse.

Heat (rè 熱) and Fire (huǒ 火)

Heat and Fire correspond to an abundance of yang. External Heat usually belongs to the yang-type excess category, as in Wind-Heat, Summerheat, Damp-Heat or Dry-Heat, and is induced by the pathogenic Heat of warm-febrile diseases. Internal Heat is due to a dysfunction of the yin and yang Organs, of the yin and yang, or of the Qi and Blood.

Fire is caused by an exacerbation of a Hot disease. It arises inside the body and induces such patterns as Heart Fire flaming upward, Liver Fire blazing upward, and Gallbladder Fire rebelling. Internal Fire is most often the result of yin deficiency (Fluids or Blood), stagnation (of Qi, Blood, food or Phlegm), attack by one of the pernicious influences (Wind, Cold, Dampness, Summerheat, Dryness) or disruption in one of the five emotions. This is summarized in the adages "The five Qi transform into Fire" and "The five emotions transform into Fire."

As a normal Qi, Fire is contained in the Organs and performs a warming and transforming function. It is the yang Qi that the *Inner Classic* refers to as the lesser Fire *(shǎo huǒ)* or young Fire *(shào huǒ)*. If the yang is too abundant, it turns into blazing Fire, which depletes and disperses the normal Qi and becomes pathogenic. The *Inner Classic* refers to this as strong Fire *(zhuàng huǒ)*.

Nature of Heat and Fire

Heat warms, dilates, relaxes, softens the hard, leads and circulates the Qi. Fire burns, rises and tends to spread rapidly.

Properties of Pathogenic Heat and Fire

• Heat-Fire is yang; its nature is to flare up and rise.

At the peak of its activity, the rising Heat-Fire burns and consumes everything. The resulting symptoms are fever, aversion to heat, thirst, restlessness, sweating, red and dry tongue, and a flooding and rapid pulse. When the spirit is affected, there is restlessness with anxiety, insomnia, dementia, mental confusion and delirium.

The resulting diseases manifest primarily in the upper body. Heart Fire blazing upward causes mouth and tongue ulcerations. Abundant and consuming Stomach Fire leads to painful swelling of the gums. Liver Fire rebelling upward manifests as headaches and red, swollen and painful eyes.

• Heat-Fire depletes the Fluids.

Heat-Fire injures and dries the yin and burns the Fluids, leading to a desire for cold drinks, dry mucous membranes, oliguria and dry and hard stools.

• Fire generates Wind and agitates the Blood.

Heat stirs up the Liver Wind, extreme Heat generates Wind with fever, loss of consciousness, delirium, spasms and contracture of the limbs, upturned eyes, stiff neck, and opisthotonos.

Fire-Heat agitates the Blood, causing blood extravasation and hemorrhage of various sorts including hematomas, purpura, hemoptysis and hematuria. The accumulation of Fire-Heat in the Blood level leads to the formation of abscesses and pus.

External Fire-Heat Diseases

Clinically, Fire is the result of the transformation of the five pathogenic influences (Wind, Cold, Heat, Dampness and Dryness). Common signs are fever, headaches, throat swelling, dry mucous membranes, thirst, red eyes, red tongue with a dark yellow coating, oliguria. At a more advanced stage there is restlessness, anxiety, insomnia, possible skin or mucous membrane ulcerations, and a floating or flooding and rapid pulse. In contagious febrile diseases, this symptomatology can occur when Heat spreads through the four levels and reaches the Blood level.

Internal Fire-Heat Diseases

Excess Fire is a yang excess and manifests in the pathological patterns of Heart, Liver, Lung or Stomach Fire. The telltale symptoms are tongue and mouth ulcerations, red eyes, bitter taste in the mouth, restlessness, anxiety, dry and sore throat, desire for cold drinks, dry stools, oliguria and dark urine.

Deficiency Fire is the result of yin deficiency, mostly of the Kidneys, Liver or Heart. Besides the usual Heat symptoms, there are signs of deficiency such as five-center Heat (Heat in the soles of the feet, the palms of the hands and in the chest).

LATENT PATHOGENIC INFLUENCES (*fú xié* 伏邪)

The invading pathogenic influences can hide (*fú*) in a latent state inside the body, waiting to spring into action at the appropriate time. This concept dates back at least to the *Inner Classic*:

> A very sudden onset of Wind generates Cold and Heat. This is why when someone is injured by Wind in spring, the pathogenic Qi is retained and there is urgent morning diarrhea in summer. When someone is injured by Summerheat in summer, they will have malarial conditions in autumn. When someone is injured by Dampness in autumn, they will have rebellion and cough in winter and later develop paralysis of the lower limbs. When someone is injured by Cold in winter, they will definitely have a warm disease in spring. The Qi of the four seasons, when they contend, injure the five yin organs. (*Basic Questions*, chapter 3)

Similarly, the statement in chapter 5 of *Basic Questions* that an overabundance of yin manifests within the yang, and vice versa, underscores the latency of clinical manifestations in contrast to the invasion of pathogenic influences.

The period of incubation differentiates the latent pathogenic influence conditions from the seasonal pernicious influence conditions. This is illustrated in chapter 58 of *Divine Pivot*, when the Yellow Emperor wonders why certain illnesses erupt suddenly even though the patients have not been exposed to any external pathogenic factor or internal pathogenic emotion. Qi Bo replies that "the retention of the pathogenic influence is the cause," and that certain recurrent factors will activate it, such as an unbalanced diet, trauma, the change of seasons, emotions. Another significant indication is the absence of any sign of an external attack at the beginning of the illness, except when a new invasion activates the hidden pathogenic influence.

The disease progresses according to an internal Heat pattern and can rapidly injure the Fluids. Thus, according to A. Husson in his remarks accompanying the translation of *Basic Questions*, chapter 31, a winter cold which emerges immediately is a Cold-damage disorder (*shāng hán*); later in spring, it is a Warm disease (*wēn bìng*); and much later in summer, it is a Summerheat disease (*shǔ bìng*).

We have very little information about the concept of latent pathogenic influences, and yet we feel that they play a fundamental role in the genesis and recurrence of rheumatic conditions. This approach bears a close relationship with the immunological concept of rheumatism.

EPIDEMIC PATHOGENIC INFLUENCES (*yì lì* 疫癘)

These abnormal, toxic, harmful influences are spread throughout a population. Their effects are not influenced by differences in people's constitutions, general health or age. Their clinical manifestations are always similar, contrary to those of the six pernicious influences, which vary according to the seasons. They are carried by air, and they invade through the nose or the mouth. Their diseases are triggered only by abnormal climatic conditions (excessive Dampness, flooding, prolonged drought), poor hygiene or improper nutrition. These toxic influences affect the upper respiratory tract, penetrate the Stomach and the Intestines, trigger abrupt clinical manifestations and spread very rapidly. They correspond to modern biomedicine's description of contagious diseases (bacterial or viral), such as the plague, smallpox, cholera, diphtheria and typhoid.

Internal Factors (*nèi yīn* 內因)

THE SEVEN EMOTIONS (*qī qíng* 七情)

The concept of the emotions in traditional Chinese medicine covers all psycho-emotional stresses which, if in a state of excess, can disrupt the circulation of the Blood and Qi and the harmony of the yin and yang Organs.

There are seven emotions: elation (also known as joy[5]—*xǐ*), anger (*nù*), worry (*yōu*), pensiveness (*sī*), sadness (*bēi*), fear (*kǒng*) and fright (*jīng*). They are all involved in the exchanges between people and their environment, and are the psychological manifestations of a Qi movement perceived as an emotion or expressed as a feeling. There are seven Qi mechanisms that are as much the agents of emotion as their manifestations. Fear, for instance, lowers the Qi, but it also indicates a descent of Qi.

Physiologically speaking, the Seven Emotions are part of the psychic activity of the Organ Qi, and are not inherently pathogenic factors. Due to violent, prolonged or repeated stresses, they can disrupt the circulation of the Blood and Organ Qi and induce disease. They can also result from the impairment of one of the Organ's functions. Therefore its cause and pattern of disharmony will need to be determined.

The Seven Emotions have a direct action on the Organs, which is why they are considered to be the main pathogenic factors for internal injury *(nèi shāng):* "All external pathogenic influences having been ruled out … the physician cannot ignore the emotional state of the patient." *(Basic Questions,* chapter 77)

CORRESPONDENCES BETWEEN EMOTIONS AND ORGANS

According to the theory of the Five Phases, each of five emotions is related to an Organ, and they are collectively called the Five Emotions or Wills *(wǔ zhì).* The emotion related to the Heart is elation, the Spleen pensiveness, the Lungs sadness, the Kidneys fear, and the Liver anger. When one of the emotions is in a state of excess, it injures its corresponding Organ.

EMOTIONS AS PATHOLOGICAL AGENTS

Excessive emotion disrupts the circulation of Qi; it affects the functional activity of the Organs, disrupts the ascending or descending, inward or outward movements of the Qi, and destroys the balance between Qi and Blood.

- Excessive elation scatters the Qi, and harms the Heart and the spirit.
- Excessive anger causes the Qi and Blood to ascend, and harms the Liver and the Kidneys.
- Excessive worry results in stagnation of the Qi, and harms the Lungs.
- Excessive pensiveness and obsessiveness congeals the middle Qi, and harms the Spleen yang.
- Excessive sadness weakens the Qi, and harms the five yin Organs.
- Excessive fear lowers the Qi, and harms the Kidneys and the Liver.
- Excessive fright disrupts and flusters the Qi, and confuses the spirit.

All excessive emotion affects the Heart, the Liver and the spirit. In a state of excess, the presence of these emotions can indicate a disruption in the circulation of Qi.

Elation: Heart disorders, disruption of the spirit-clarity
Anger: Liver Qi rebellion, excess Blood
Worry: Blood and Qi deficiency, Lung yin deficiency
Pensiveness: Spleen yang disorders, insufficient Blood production
Sadness: upper and middle burner disorders
Fear: upper burner blockage, Blood deficiency, downward movement of Qi
Fright: spirit confusion, Heart Qi disorders

Any excessive emotion can transform into Fire. Fire in itself is a pathological factor: it burns the Fluids, dries the Blood (which is then unable to nourish the Heart) and causes such disturbances of the spirit as irritability, restlessness, worry, anxiety, insomnia.

Neither Internal nor External Factors
(bú nèi wài yīn 不内外因)

DIETARY IRREGULARITIES

Food—a source of flavors and energy—is the chief provider of Qi to nourish and maintain the Essence of each Organ. Any dietary imbalance, whether from a quantitative or a qualitative point of view, will affect the dynamics of the body's Qi. In the same respect, food that is improper for consumption, due to poor hygiene or the presence of toxins, can generate parasitic, infectious or toxic disorders.

The quantitative aspect is that malnutrition or underfeeding causes a deficiency in Blood and Qi production. Furthermore, a diminution in the Stomach's and Spleen's functions leads to signs of malabsorption, due to an insufficient production of Blood and Qi.

The qualitative aspect is that overconsumption of fatty, rich foods and alcohol creates Damp-Heat patterns, with production of Phlegm and Blood and Qi stagnation. Ingesting raw foods or an excessive amount of cold food or drink injures the Spleen's yang Qi and contributes to the formation of Damp-Cold. Eating excessive amounts of hot or spicy foods can lead to an accumulation of Heat in the Stomach and Intestines, and injure the Fluids. Spoiled or stale foods produce signs of Damp-Heat, which may turn into Fire.

An imbalance in the harmony of the flavors affects the dynamics of the Qi, the Organs and their correspondences, as follows:

- Acrid (spicy), sweet, and bland flavors—yang in nature—assist the ascending and descending movement of the Qi.

  The acrid flavor disperses, tonifies, moistens and circulates. In excess, it dissipates the muscles and vessels and disperses the Essence and the spirit.

  The sweet flavor tonifies, scatters, slows down, harmonizes, and regulates the middle burner. In excess, it smothers the Heart and disrupts the function of the Kidneys, darkening the complexion.

  The bland flavor is diuretic.

• Sour, bitter, salty, and astringent flavors—yin in nature—assist the descending and inward movement of the Qi.

The sour flavor is astringent; it gathers, collects and immobilizes. In excess, it causes the Liver to overflow and the Spleen to become too dry.

The bitter flavor dries, hardens and strengthens, and drains. In excess, it dehydrates the Spleen and thickens the Stomach Fluids.

The salty flavor softens and relaxes, moisturizes and lowers, and is a laxative. In excess, it contracts the flesh, taxes the long bones and checks the Heart.

The acrid flavor is astringent.

FATIGUE AND OVEREXERTION

These two elements exhaust the Blood and Qi. On the other hand, lack of exercise can lead to Blood and Qi stagnation.

EXCESSIVE SEXUAL ACTIVITY

According to traditional Chinese medicine, excessive sexual activity and repeated pregnancies exhaust the Essence of the Kidneys and weaken the lower back and knees.

MISCELLANEOUS FACTORS

Injuries, traumatic lesions, burns, insect stings, animal bites, worms and parasites are all pathogenic factors. One aspect of the concept of hereditary diseases is discussed in chapter 47 of *Basic Questions* under the title "Diseases of the Top" (*diān jí*).

Pathogenesis

The pathogenesis of diseases in traditional Chinese medicine rests on two fundamental concepts: (1) the quality of the normal Qi, which reflects the physical and mental constitution of the patient; and (2) the presence and strength of pathogenic influences.

A diseased state shows a struggle between these two elements and will determine a state of deficiency, excess or stagnation, of a yin or a yang type, of a Cold or Hot nature, on the surface or deep inside. The resulting disruption of the circulation of energies can be local, distant or general and cause pathogenic productions.

The pathogenic productions can also be thought of as internal pathogenic factors. These are Phlegm and Congested Fluids, and Blood stasis. They play a critical part in chronic rheumatic pathologies.

PHLEGM AND CONGESTED FLUIDS (*tán yǐn* 痰飲)

In traditional Chinese medicine, Phlegm and Congested Fluids define a dysfunction of fluid metabolism. Phlegm (*tán*) is thick and indicates a more aggravated stage than Congested Fluids (*yǐn*), which are thinner. With Spleen deficiency, the transportive and transformative functions are weak. This causes Dampness which, when it stagnates, gives rise to Phlegm and Congested Fluids. Another mechanism in their formation is related to Heat. Under the influence of Heat, the Fluids turn into Congested Fluids, and, if the process continues, coagulate into Phlegm, which can concentrate in any part of the body, but especially in the joints.

This terminology does not merely imply sputum and bronchial mucus; it also refers to all the obstructing mechanisms that impair the circulation of the Fluids or disrupt the proper functioning of the Organs responsible for Water and Fluid metabolism.

Phlegm and Congested Fluids can be caused by three factors:

1. Excessive consumption of alcohol and fatty or sweet foods, which coalesce and generate Damp-Heat.
2. Emotion-induced internal injury causing Qi stagnation, which can turn into Fire, dry the Fluids, and transform them into Phlegm and Congested Fluids. A typical example is Liver Qi stagnation, which prevents the Liver Qi from smoothing and distributing the Qi. The Qi cannot circulate, but stagnates, turns into Fire and coagulates the Fluids.
3. Functional disorder of the Organs involved in the metabolism of the Fluids:

   • If the Spleen cannot perform its yang function of transporting and transforming the Fluids, they accumulate and concentrate.
   • If the Lungs cannot lower and purify the Fluids, they condense.
   • If the Kidneys—"master of the Fluids"—cannot control the Water and the Fluids, Congested Fluids appear.
   • If the Triple Burner—"Organ of the Water pathways"—cannot control the circulation of Fluids, they stagnate and condense.

BLOOD STASIS (*yū xuè* 瘀血)

The slowing down of Blood circulation, or blood extravasation, generates a group of patterns that the Chinese identify as Blood stasis or Blood masses.

Exogenous pathogenic Cold slows down the Blood circulation and makes it stagnate, whereas Heat promotes the formation of masses. A trauma-induced hemorrhage or hematoma can lead to similar consequences.

Endogenous deficient or stagnant Qi is unable to move the Blood. The cause must be investigated to determine whether it is dysfunction of the Liver (stores the Blood), the Heart (governs the Blood) or the Spleen (keeps the Blood in the vessels).

These patterns must be explored in rheumatology when there is stabbing pain or localized red, hot swellings that worsen at night.

Chapter Notes

1. While we have been careful to distinguish these terms, the words pathogenic *(xié)* and pernicious *(yín)* are often used interchangeably.
2. We think this may refer to the yang brightness.
3. We think this may refer to the greater yin.
4. Sudden turmoil *(huò luàn)* is a traditional Chinese term that was adopted for the biomedically-defined disease cholera. Some books on traditional Chinese medicine also use this term.
5. While this term is usually translated as "joy," it more properly refers to the feelings of elation, exhilaration, excitement, exultation (what is felt after winning a contest) rather than to sublime feelings of joy or bliss.

CHAPTER FOUR

Pain

The concept of rheumatism in modern bio-medicine includes all the bone and joint medical conditions that share a number of common signs, pain undoubtedly being the most important one. In China, rheumatism belongs to the painful obstruction or *bì* category, as described in chapter 43 of *Basic Questions (Su wen)*. The word *bì* means painful obstruction which causes such symptoms as pain, numbness, paralysis, lack of sensation and stiffness.

In classical literature, the painful obstruction category covers a number of conditions caused by the invasion of the pathogenic influences Wind, Cold, Dampness and sometimes Heat into the body. When the bones, joints, ligaments, sinews and muscles are affected by these pathogenic influences, the resulting pathologies are similar to the biomedical concept of rheumatism, but in a broader sense, since the concept of painful obstruction includes organic locations such as painful obstruction of the Liver and Spleen, even though these could be viewed as possible complications of rheumatism. On the other hand, it is not easy to rule out neurological conditions, as these distinctions have not been clearly established in Chinese texts.

The distinction between degenerative rheumatism (degenerative joint disease) and inflammatory rheumatism (inflammatory joint disease) is not made clear in traditional Chinese medicine texts, which only describe the progression of different stages of the same pathology according to different patterns of induction and different terrains or constitutions. The Chinese approach linking rheumatism to external agents deserves to be taken into account, if we consider possible viral causes and resulting autoimmune dysfunction.

To attempt to go beyond this and match two vastly different nosologies would only prove confusing. Close comparison of these two distinct yet complementary approaches, however, yields some interesting observations.

Eight Diagnostic Parameters
(*bā gāng* 八綱)

In traditional Chinese medicine, pain—a master symptom in rheumatology—is considered to be the result of a dysfunction in the circulation of Qi and/or Blood. This is a yin-yang conflict which is consciously perceived by the individual.

In order to be interpreted accurately, this warning symptom must be analyzed according to the eight parameters (also known as the eight principles)—interior-exterior, Cold-Heat, deficiency-excess, yin-yang—which will define its essential features, in order to determine its etiology and prognosis. Without going into these in great detail, a few points relating to pain must be made here, as appropriate treatment depends on their proper understanding.

Interior–Exterior (biǎo lǐ 表裡)

This parameter specifies the location of pain—relatively superficial or deep. It can reside in one of the anatomical layers—skin, vessels, muscles, bones—or in an Organ, at the level of the primary or secondary channels, and so on. This parameter also deals with the progression of pain. If the pain is said to be rebellious or insurgent (nì), it becomes deeper and worsens. Pain is said to be favorable or smooth (shùn) if it becomes progressively more superficial and improves.

Cold–Heat (hán rè 寒熱)

This parameter establishes the nature of pain. Cold pain indicates either deficiency of yang Qi with vigorous yin, or an attack of pathogenic Cold slowing down the circulation of Qi and/or Blood and promoting the emergence of painful symptoms. One important marker of Cold pain is that it is alleviated by warmth.

Hot pain suggests either yin deficiency with vigorous yang, or an attack of pathogenic Heat. Pain due to Heat is alleviated by cold.

Deficiency–Excess (xū shí 虛實)

This parameter reflects the state of the normal Qi and of the pathogenic Qi. Pain from deficiency, which improves upon pressure or local support, means that the normal Qi is locally deficient. Pain from excess, which is aggravated by pressure, indicates that the pernicious factors are in a state of local excess. One particular aspect of excess is *stagnation*. Stagnation manifests like excess, except that in all cases it is ameliorated by warmth, movement or massage, regardless of whether it is stagnation of yin or yang.

The distinction between deficiency and excess is the fundamental basis for applying the therapeutic principles of tonifying deficiency and draining[1] excess, while always supporting the normal Qi (TABLE 4-1).

Yin–Yang

This general parameter qualifies the type of pain:

- A yin-type pain is dull, throbbing, constant, of moderate intensity, chronic, occurring or aggravated at night, deep.
- A yang-type pain is sharp, violent, paroxysmal, stabbing, burning, intense, acute, diurnal, superficial.

These two parameters incorporate and synthesize the six previous parameters and allow the physician to pinpoint the origin of the symptom.

TABLE 4-1 EIGHT PARAMETERS & STAGNATION		
Parameter	**Characteristic**	**Stagnation**
Yin-Yang	Yin: dull, continuous, deep pain Yang: sharp, intense, superficial pain	Same
Cold-Hot	Cold: improves with warmth, worsens with cold Heat: improves with cold, worsens with warmth	Same
Interior-Exterior	Interior: external or internal pathogenic influence; deep location Exterior: external pathogenic influence; superficial location	Same
Deficiency-Excess	Deficiency: improves with pressure Excess: worsens with pressure	Improves with movement or massage

An analytical approach to pain must not exclude or isolate any of these parameters. For example, the synthesis of the diagnosis must specify whether it is a yin, deep, excess, Cold-type pain, or a yang, superficial, excess, Hot-type pain. This synthesis is only the first step, because the progression of different types of painful obstruction is usually multidimensional. There are many complex aspects, which bring to mind the following observations:

- The eight parameters cannot be divided into four independent, unrelated pairs. They must be studied in relation to one another in order to distinguish deficiency and excess in relation to Cold and Heat, to interior-exterior, to yin-yang.
- During the progression of a disease, symptoms can change into their opposite: Cold-type pain can transform into Hot-type pain; it can move from a superficial location to a deep one; and it can change from deficiency to excess.
- At different stages of a disease, symptoms of an opposite nature can occur simultaneously. For example, there can be *both* Cold-type and Hot-type pain, and *both* superficial and deep pain.

All the determining symptoms and developments of a

pathology must fit within the framework of the eight diagnostic parameters. Knowledge of these parameters requires thorough analysis of the warning symptom (pain), careful monitoring of its development, and integration of all the associated signs. It is a vital diagnostic and therapeutic methodology.

Energetic Mechanisms of Pain

EXCESS-TYPE PAIN (*shí tòng* 實痛)

Main Features

This is an acute and continuous pain, sometimes with a sensation of local distention, and is aggravated by pressure and local support. It can be accompanied by hyperesthesia.

Triggering Factors

Deficiency of defensive Qi will permit the pernicious influences of Wind, Cold, Dampness or (rarely) Heat to penetrate the body and impair the circulation of the Qi and/or Blood.

Pain from invasion of pathogenic Cold: The pain does not move much. It is acute, deep, aggravated by cold and alleviated by topical application of warmth. The tongue coating is thin and white, and the pulse is sunken and wiry.

Pain from invasion of pathogenic Wind: The pain is moving, fleeting, random and rather superficial. The tongue coating is thin or absent, and the pulse is floating.

Pain from invasion of pathogenic Dampness: The pain is fixed, and sensitive to climatic conditions (especially dampness). It can be accompanied by swelling in the joints, a sensation of numbness, and paresthesia. At a later stage, the joints become deformed. The pulse is floating and soggy.

Hot-type pain: In general, Heat is the result of the transformation of the previously described invasive pathogenic influences stagnating in the body. This pain is characterized by the presence of inflammatory signs such as redness, swelling and a local sensation of heat. It is alleviated by cold and aggravated by warmth. The tongue coating is yellow, and the pulse is floating and rapid.

Pathogenesis

Excess yin pain: The pain is dull, accompanied by spasms or contractions. It is aggravated by pressure and cold, and alleviated by warmth. It is either due to invasion of external pathogenic Cold, or to yang deficiency.

Excess yang pain: The pain is sharp, intense, stabbing, tearing. It is aggravated by pressure and warmth, and alleviated by cold. It indicates either the presence of local pathogenic influences in excess, or an underlying yin deficiency.

Excess Blood pain: The pain is dull, throbbing, pulsating, like being pricked. It is aggravated by pressure.

DEFICIENCY–TYPE PAIN (*xū tòng* 虛痛)

Main Features

This is a rather chronic and intermittent pain, aggravated by exertion, alleviated by rest, pressure or local support.

Pathogenesis

This pain occurs after a protracted illness, when the normal Qi is weakened.

Yang deficiency pain: The pain is dull, heavy, with a sensation of fatigue. It is aggravated by movement or exertion, and by cold. It is alleviated by pressure and warmth.

Yin deficiency pain: The pain has a burning sensation. It is alleviated by cold and pressure, and is aggravated by warmth. Its presence often indicates that the Fluids have been injured by Heat.

Blood deficiency pain: The pain is intense, alleviated by pressure, and sensitive to wind and cold. It often leads to a sensation of crawling of the skin or other skin sensitivity. The tongue body is pale, without coating, and the pulse is rapid and thin.

STAGNATION–TYPE PAIN (*yū tòng* 瘀痛)

Main Features

Stagnation is a special form of excess which is particularly alleviated by movement or massage and local warmth. This type of pain worsens when the person rests, is cold, or just at the beginning of movement. For example, shoulder pain of this type worsens when the person begins to move their shoulder, but diminishes as the movement continues.

Pathogenesis

Yang stagnation pain: This sharp pain occurs primarily during the second half of the night, or upon awakening.

It forces the patient to get up, but rapidly disappears after getting started. According to our observations, most of the time it indicates the invasion of a pernicious influence into the lesser yang stage. This is the intermediary yang stage or system which is responsible for setting the various types of Qi in motion. This type of pain includes stagnation of Qi.

Yin stagnation pain: This dull pain improves toward the end of the day if it is due to yang deficiency or stagnation, which impairs movement. It occurs mostly in the morning upon awakening, and is accompanied by a sensation of distention, numbness and topical cold, and requires a long period of gradual warming up. The remaining three types of pain are actually subsets of yin stagnation.

Blood stasis pain: This pain is characterized by a sensation of being pricked or paroxysmal stabbing, and indicates a separation of the Qi and Blood due to trauma or strain. Lower back pain due to excessive exertion is a typical example. When the Qi, which governs the Blood, is in a state of deficiency, Blood becomes static. The resulting pain takes on a chronic character that can be accompanied by peripheral circulation disorders.

Phlegm stagnation pain: The production of Phlegm, resulting from a disruption of Fluid metabolism, can occur in any part of the body. When it does, the circulation of Qi is impaired and there is a dull pain with a sensation of heaviness, "stuckness" and numbness.

Fluid stagnation pain: When fluid stagnation occurs, it is more often a matter of swelling or local edema than frank pain.

Traditional Terminology for Pain

Heavy pain (zhòng tòng 重痛)
  This type of pain is accompanied by a heavy, distended sensation, and is most often associated with an invasion of Dampness.

Cold pain (lěng tòng 冷痛)
  This type of pain gives a local sensation of cold, and is relieved by warmth. If externally contracted, it is caused by pathogenic Cold impairing the circulation in the channels. If internally generated, it indicates a yang deficiency.

Latent pain (yǐn tòng 隱痛)
  Literally "hidden pain," this type of pain is constant yet bearable. It is due to interior deficiency, usually Cold from deficiency, or Qi or Blood deficiency.

Stabbing pain (cì tòng 刺痛)
  This sharp, needle-like pain corresponds to Blood stasis.

Pain with fatigue (suān tòng 痠痛)
  Literally "soreness pain," this aching pain, like heavy pain, indicates an accumulation of Dampness impairing the circulation of Qi, especially at the muscle level.

Violent pain (jiǎo tòng 絞痛)
  This type of pain is caused by the intense or "true" pathogenic influences, which block the circulation of Qi, and by the freezing and coagulating action of pathogenic Cold.

Pain with swelling (zhàng tòng 脹痛)
  Literally "distention pain," this type of pain is characteristic of the obstruction of Qi circulation. It occurs primarily at the level of the abdomen.

Spastic pain (chě tòng 扯痛)
  Literally "pulling pain," spastic pain is associated either with Liver deficiency, in which the Liver is unable to nourish the muscles and sinews, or with the invasion of pathogenic Cold in the exterior.

Random pain (zǒu cuàn tòng 走竄痛)
  Literally "running and escaping pain," this is a Wind-type rheumatic pain or a Qi stagnation pain.

Empty pain (kōng tòng 空痛)
  This pain is accompanied by a sensation of emptiness, caused by a loss of Qi, Blood, Essence or Marrow.

Chapter Notes

1. *Editors' note:* This concept is often translated in English as disperse or sedate. The word *xiè* in Chinese simply means to drain, as in drain off or drain out. It is the counterpart of *bǔ,* to tonify or supplement. Note that another function of acupuncture, the Chinese word *sǎn,* is properly translated as disperse or scatter.

PART TWO

Traditional Approaches to Rheumatology in Modern China

PART TWO

Introduction

IN THIS PART we present the ways in which rheumatic diseases are treated in contemporary China. We have chosen the approach published in *Practical Traditional Chinese Internal Medicine*,[1] which covers the subject exhaustively. We have translated the appropriate parts of this text in their entirety, with minimal editing.[2]

A few preliminary remarks are necessary:

• In the first part, the Chinese authors introduce selections from traditional texts on which they base their observations. Some selections relevant to rheumatology are presented with more context in part four of our book. Reading them will help you better understand the approach used here.

• Following a trend that started as early as the last century, the Chinese authors have simplified their approach by dividing rheumatic diseases into painful obstruction *(bì)* and panarthralgia *(lì jié bìng)* disorders. Lower back pain is always dealt with separately.

• This presentation by pattern *(zhèng)* is modeled after modern biomedical nosology, but we need to make an additional distinction. A *zhèng* is a theoretical clinical framework which explains the evolution of a pathological process. It is defined by the compilation of significant clinical signs (obtained from, among other things, the pulse and tongue) that determine a state of excess or deficiency, Cold or Heat, interior or exterior, yin or yang. For the sake of convenience, some books improperly translate the term *zhèng* as "syndrome."

The purpose of this classification system is to break down a clinical picture into theoretical patterns to demonstrate the relationship between the pathogenic agent and the host, and show how these patterns can occur successively or simultaneously. It thus becomes obvious that any pathology identified from a biomedical nosology must be "translated" into patterns if we want to understand the underlying energetic mechanisms and select the most appropriate therapeutic response. Using the pattern option could, however, lead to rigidity and oversimplification, and overlook some of the pathogenic modalities of the pathological process. This is what we have attempted to demonstrate in part three of this book through our personal approach to rheumatic diseases.

• However interesting and seductive it may seem, the comparisons with biomedical syndromes lack specific diagnostic elements to provide an accurate picture. The overly positive results reported by the Chinese authors (e.g., over 90 percent success rate) make us wonder about their choice of methodology, or the accuracy of the biomedical diagnosis.

• The suggested therapeutic interventions rely almost

entirely on the use of herbs, as is the case in most contemporary Chinese texts. The use of acupuncture is extremely limited and typically symptomatic. This provides a striking contrast with the wealth of acupuncture treatments described in the ancient texts that are also included in this book. The number of political and social upheavals that have adversely affected acupuncture in the course of the last two or three centuries may have something to do with this unfortunate situation.

• The age-old knowledge of the Chinese about herbal prescriptions is to be viewed with deep respect; we believe that it will provide modern biomedicine with an important research field in its quest for new medicines. However, the frequent use of toxic plants (e.g., aconite, nux vomica) must prompt the practitioner to exercise utmost caution in prescribing these traditional formulas.

Notes

1. Huang Wen-Dong, et al., *Practical Traditional Chinese Internal Medicine (Shi yong zhong yi nei ke xue)* (Shanghai: Shanghai Science and Technology Press, 1985). Chapter 5 of the present text is drawn from pages 554-66, chapter 6 from 566-69 and chapter 7 from 301-7.
2. *Editors' note:* The only significant editing that we have done is to omit treatments based on materia medica that are unavailable outside of local areas of China. We have also supplemented some of the bibliographic materials.

CHAPTER FIVE

Painful Obstruction

PAINFUL OBSTRUCTION[1] *(bì 痹)* disorders develop after an attack by pathogenic Wind, Cold, Dampness or Heat. The main symptoms include pain, soreness, numbness and paresthesia *(má mù)*, heaviness and impaired movement of the limbs and joints.

Clinically, painful obstruction is characterized by progressive degeneration or by frequent relapses. The main pattern of disharmony is one of obstruction and lack of flow of the Blood and Qi, which prevents nourishment from reaching the sinews, vessels and joints.

History

The term painful obstruction first appeared in *Yellow Emperor's Inner Classic (Huang di nei jing)*. One entire chapter (43) of *Basic Questions (Su wen)* is devoted to this problem, a passage from which observes that

> The three influences Wind, Cold and Dampness arrive in various ways, intermingle and constitute painful obstruction. When the Wind influence predominates it is a moving painful obstruction *(xíng bì)*; when the Cold influence predominates it is a severe painful obstruction *(tòng bì)*; when the Dampness influence predominates it is a fixed painful obstruction *(zhuó bì)*. . . . As for those things that are considered painful obstruction, each occurs when a person contracts severe Wind, Cold or Dampness at its particular season.

Elsewhere in the same chapter the relationship between the emergence of painful obstruction disorders and diet and lifestyle is noted: "Diet and the place of residence are the root cause of these diseases." These are the most ancient and systematic passages that can be found regarding the etiology and pathogenesis of painful obstruction disorders.

Chapter 43 describes the progression of painful obstruction disorders as follows. When pathogenic Wind-Damp-Cold stagnates in the sinews and bones, the pain is difficult to arrest; when the disease lingers and worsens, the circulation of nutritive Qi and protective Qi is impaired, the skin is not nourished, and there is numbness and paresthesia; when the pathogenic Qi penetrates deeper into the body, it invades the five yin Organs and the six yang Organs, and causes painful obstruction of the Organs.

"The vessels fail to afford passage *(mài bù tōng)*, there is irritability *(fán)* with epigastric throbbing, sudden, violent rising of Qi causing panting, dryness of the throat with a tendency to sigh, and when inversion Qi *(jué qì)* ascends there is fear"—this constitutes Heart painful obstruction.

"When there is a tendency toward bloating, such that the buttocks are in the place of the feet and the back in the place of the head"—this constitutes Kidney painful obstruction. Similar descriptions are found for the other yin Organs.

This chapter further identifies painful obstruction of the skin, flesh, vessels, sinews and bones in accordance with the seasons and the particular sites in the body that are invaded by Wind, Cold and Damp pathogenic influences. The description incisively summarizes a great deal of clinical experience, and demonstrates that the author(s) had a relatively advanced level of understanding of the painful obstruction disorder.

HAN DYNASTY (221 B.C.–220 A.D.)

In the chapter on greater yang diseases in *Discussion of Cold-induced Disorders (Shang han lun)*, Zhang Zhong-Jing discusses the treatment of Wind and Dampness in the greater yang stage (§174-75):

> At the eighth or ninth day of Cold-damage, when Wind and Dampness contend with each other, there is pain and irritability throughout the body, it is difficult to turn oneself over, no vomiting, lack of thirst, and the pulse is floating, deficient and choppy, use Cinnamon Twig and Prepared Aconite Decoction *(gui zhi fu zi tang)*. If the stools are hard and urination is without difficulty, use Remove Cinnamon Twig plus Atractylodes Decoction *(qu gui jia zhu tang)*.
>
> When Wind and Dampness contend with each other, the bones and joints are painful to the point that flexion-extension is impossible, pain is aggravated by pressure, there is sweating, shortness of breath, difficult urination, and aversion to wind with reluctance to get undressed. The body may become slightly swollen. Use Licorice and Prepared Aconite Decoction *(gan cao fu zi tang)*.

Cinnamon Twig and Prepared Aconite Decoction *(gui zhi fu zi tang)* is prescribed when the exterior yang is deficient, pathogenic Wind predominates, and Wind and Dampness sustain each other in the exterior. The decoction in which Rhizoma Atractylodis Macrocephalae *(bai zhu)* is used instead of Ramulus Cinnamomi Cassiae *(gui zhi)* is prescribed when the exterior yang is deficient and Dampness is abundant interiorly. Licorice and Prepared Aconite Decoction *(gan cao fu zi tang)* is used when both the exterior and interior yang are deficient and the pathogenic Wind, Cold and Damp influences obstruct the joints, sinews and vessels. Although quite simple, this shows how people use the methods of differentiating patterns and discussing treatments.

In chapter 2 (§14) of *Essentials from the Golden Cabinet (Jin gui yao lue fang lun)*, Zhang Zhong-Jing also talks about the symptomatology and treatment of Damp painful obstruction:

> When with a greater yang disease the joints are painful, there is irritability, and the pulse is submerged and thin,[2]

this is called Damp painful obstruction. With the symptoms of Damp painful obstruction there is difficulty with urination, but the stool comes unexpectedly quickly. Still, in such a situation one must promote the patient's urination.

The term panarthralgia *(lì jié bìng)* appears in chapter 5 of the same text. This condition presents with "generalized joint pain with inability to flex or extend the joints"(§11); "flashing pain" (§10); "various joints of the limbs are sore and painful, the body is crooked and gaunt, the legs are swollen as if they are about to fall off" (§8). (For a detailed discussion of this disorder, see chapter 6 below.)

Many of Zhang Zhong-Jing's prescriptions for panarthralgia, Wind-Dampness in the greater yang stage, or Damp painful obstruction—such as Licorice and Prepared Aconite Decoction *(gan cao fu zi tang)*, Aconite Decoction *(wu tou tang)*, and Cinnamon Twig, Peony, and Anemarrhena Decoction *(gui zhi shao yao zhi mu tang)*—were considered effective, and have been commonly used, down to the present day.

SUI DYNASTY (581–618)

In *Discussion of the Origins of Symptoms of Disease (Zhu bing yuan hou lun)*, Chao Yuan-Fang takes the fundamental concept of painful obstruction developed in *Basic Questions* even further, and distinguishes among such conditions as Wind-Damp painful obstruction *(fēng shī bì)*, Wind painful obstruction *(fēng bì)*, Wind numbness *(fēng bù rén)*, Wind coolness *(fēng lěng)* and "Wind-induced contractions of the four limbs with inability to flex or extend them."

In article 22 of the first division, Wind-Damp-Cold painful obstruction is described as follows:

> [Its] symptomatology may either be a thickening of the skin or muscle aches and pain. Wind, Cold and Dampness come together to form painful obstruction. If Wind and Dampness predominate over Cold, it is Wind-Damp painful obstruction. It is because the Blood and Qi are deficient that the person is susceptible to Wind-Dampness and this disease develops. If it persists for a long time and is not healed, it enters into the channels and collaterals, fights in the yang channels, and may lead to a functional disability of the body, hands and feet.

This passage reflects a definite understanding of the pathological mechanisms, clinical manifestations and progression of Wind-Damp painful obstruction.

In article 6 of the same division, "bandit" Wind *(zéi fēng)* is described as follows:

When it [bandit Wind] attacks the patient, while there is pain it cannot be pressed [heavily], motion and rotation are impossible, and there is no heat at the painful location. When there is injury from Wind and Cold, there is deep pain in the bones and joints, which are sore to the touch; there is a sensation of alarming cold inside the body, with a desire to put something warm on the painful area to gain some relief. Occasionally there is sweating.

Bandit Wind is just the cause of this disease; in reality, however, this is a vivid description of the symptoms and features of painful obstruction disorder.

In article 1 of the second division, panarthralgia *(li jié bìng)* is equally well-characterized:

[Its] symptomatology is shortness of breath, spontaneous sweating, excruciating pain in all the joints, and inability to flex or extend them. When Wind invades the joints, it contends with the Blood and Qi and they attack each other; this is why there is pain. When the Blood and Qi are deficient, sweating appears. When Wind and Cold contend at the level of the sinews, flexion and extension are impossible.

These writings had a considerable influence on the great masters of the Tang and Song dynasties.

Tang (618–907) and Song (960–1279) Dynasties

In books from the Tang era, such as *Supplement to the Thousand Ducat Prescriptions (Qian jin yi fang)* and *Arcane Essentials from the Imperial Library (Wai tai bi yao)*, as well as such works from the Song era as *Sagelike Prescriptions from the Taiping Era (Tai ping sheng hui fang)* and *Imperial Encyclopedia of Medicine (Sheng ji zong lu)*, the authors followed Chao Yuan-Fang's approach; that is, they distinguished painful obstruction from panarthralgia, but included both of them in the Wind disease category. They based their understanding of etiology and pathogenesis on Chao Yuan-Fang's concepts.

For instance, in the eighth division of *Supplement to the Thousand Ducat Prescriptions*, entitled "The Various Winds," Sun Si-Miao writes:

When panarthralgic Wind settles in a person who is not treated for a prolonged period, it can create a dysfunction of the bones and joints. . . . From ancient times to the present, no matter whether noble or base, there are always those who suffer from it. This is because the Wind Toxin harms them.

When Sun Si-Miao says that after a while there is a dysfunction of the bones and joints, he is referring to the joint deformation that occurs during the chronic stage of the disease, when the pathogenic influence penetrates the bones and joints.

From a therapeutic standpoint, *Supplement to the Thousand Ducat Prescriptions* and *Arcane Essentials from the Imperial Library* were compilations of numerous ancient and new prescriptions that broadened the field of therapeutic modalities with the addition of, among other things, moxibustion, medicated wines and the use of ointments in massage.

Moreover, the thirteenth division of *Arcane Essentials from the Imperial Library* added a new condition to painful obstruction and panarthralgia: "white tiger disease" *(bái hǔ bìng)*:

White tiger disease occurs mostly when the Toxins of Wind, Cold, Summerheat and Dampness take advantage of deficiency to arrive. When the inner pattern of the body's functions is disturbed and the Wind pathogen attacks, the channels and vessels are clumped and stagnant. The Blood and Qi do not move [but] pile up in the areas between the bones and between the joints or in the four limbs. The color of the flesh does not change and the condition is dormant during the daytime, but becomes active at night. When active, it affects the marrow and the pain is comparable to being bitten by a tiger, hence its name: white tiger disease.

Two books from the Song era, *Sagelike Prescriptions from the Taiping Era* and *Imperial Encyclopedia of Medicine*, describe painful obstruction disorders, panarthralgia and white tiger disease. While the relevant portions of these works deal mostly with ancient theories, in addition to the notion of Wind-Damp-Cold painful obstruction they introduce the new concept of Hot painful obstruction *(rè bì)*. Herbs commonly prescribed for this condition include Radix Rehmanniae Glutinosae *(sheng di huang)*, Rhizoma Cimicifugae *(sheng ma)*, Cornu Rhinoceri *(xi jiao)*, Cornu Antelopis *(ling yang jiao)*, Tuber Ophiopogonis Japonici *(mai men dong)*, Gypsum *(shi gao)*, and Radix et Rhizoma Rhei *(da huang)*. These are sweet and cold or bitter and cold herbs that are based on the therapeutic methods developed for the use of Rhinoceros Horn Decoction *(xi jiao tang)* from *Thousand Ducat Prescriptions*.

Song era prescriptions rely more than their predecessors on the use of animal products. This is especially true of insect and snake products such as Scolopendra Subspinipes *(wu gong)*, Buthus Martensi *(quan xie)*, Zaocys Dhumnades *(wu shao she)*, Agkistrodon seu Bungarus *(bai hua she)* and Lumbricus *(di long)*. Among

the representative formulas of this style is Silkworm Cocoon Powder *(yuan can e san)* listed in the tenth division
of *Sagelike Prescriptions from the Taiping Era*, which
consists of silkworm cocoon *(yuan can e)*, Bombyx
Batryticatus *(jiang can)*, Periostracum Cicadae *(chan tui)*
and Lumbricus *(di long)*. Another is Scorpion Pill *(yi lang
wan)* from the nineteenth division of the same work,
which is simply Buthus Martensi *(quan xie)*. Finally, there
is Musk Pill *(she xiang wan)* from Xu Shu-Wei's *Formulas
of Universal Benefit from My Practice (Pu ji ben shi fang)*.
These are all rather special formulas that were based on
the experience of the physician authors.

JIN DYNASTY (1115–1234)

In *Discussion Illuminating the Yellow Emperor's Basic
Questions (Huang di su wen xuan ming lun fang)*, Liu He-
Qian (also known as Liu Yuan-Su), based on the painful
obstruction chapter in *Yellow Emperor's Inner Classic*,
identifies different types of formulas according to the
predominance of Wind, Cold or Dampness. For these
three patterns he prescribes Ledebouriella Decoction
(fang feng tang), Poria Decoction *(fu ling tang)* and Poria
and Ligusticus Decoction *(fu ling chuan xiong tang)*
respectively. For Hot painful obstruction, he recommends
Cimicifuga Decoction *(sheng ma tang)*.

In chapter 2 of *Confucians' Duties to Their Parents (Ru
men shi qin)*, Zhang Zi-He (also known as Zhang Cong-
Zheng) criticizes the confusion caused by grouping Wind
painful obstruction, atrophy, inversion and leg Qi disorders altogether under the rubric of Wind, a practice which
was established during the Sui and Tang eras. He claims
that these disorders

> are fundamentally different, yet many contemporary
> [doctors] cannot make any distinction among them and
> treat all of them as patterns of Wind-Cold and tonify what
> is deficient below. This is why there are those that are not
> cured for interminable days and endless years.

He goes on to say that "the main source of painful
obstruction is Damp-Heat; Wind and Cold are of
secondary importance. When the three pathogenic influences combine, they create painful obstruction."

At the onset of disease Zhang recommends the three
strong therapeutic methods (sweating, purging and
vomiting) for attacking painful obstruction. He does not
use the Tang and Song era term "white tiger disease," nor
Zhang Zhong-Jing's term panarthralgia *(lì jié bìng)*.
Instead, Zhang Zi-He revered the term painful obstruction from *Yellow Emperor's Inner Classic*.

On the other hand, Li Dong-Yuan and Zhu Dan-Xi
discarded all the terms painful obstruction, panarthralgia
and white tiger disease, and in their stead established the
name "painful Wind" *(tòng fēng)*. For example, in a chapter entitled "On Painful Wind" in *Supplementary
Discussions for the Perfection of Understanding through
Investigation of Phenomena (Ge zhi yu lun)*, Zhu Dan-Xi
wrote:

> Painful Wind is usually related to the Blood receiving Heat
> that bubbles and boils by itself. If later the patient walks
> through cold water, stands in a damp place, uses a fan to
> cool himself, or exposes himself to wind in his sleep, then
> Cold and coolness contend externally. The Hot Blood
> congeals and flows roughly when it meets turbid sweat, and
> pain appears. This pain is more intense at night because it
> proceeds through the yin.

In *Secrets from the Orchid Chamber (Lan shi mi cang)*, Li
Dong-Yuan suggests that painful Wind is primarily due to
Blood deficiency. On the other hand, Zhu Dan-Xi distinguished among Blood deficiency, Blood Heat, Wind,
Dampness, Phlegm and stasis. Consider, for example, the
following passage from *Teachings of [Zhu] Dan-Xi (Dan xi
xin fa)*:

> When an overweight person suffers from painful joints, it is
> often due to Wind-Dampness and Congested Fluids
> streaming through and remaining in the channels. When a
> lean person suffers from painful joints, it is due to Blood
> deficiency.

These comments indicate that the patient's constitution
was already considered to be a significant factor. Zhu
Dan-Xi recommended Generally Useful Formula for
Painful Wind *(tong feng tong yong tang)* to treat this disorder, and differentiated between upper and lower limb
problems in the selection of herbs. This had a great influence on subsequent practice.

MING (1368–1644) AND
QING (1644–1911) DYNASTIES

Faced with increasing complexity in disease terminology,
the majority of physicians agreed to group the identified
disorders under the names painful obstruction, panarthralgia, white tiger disease and painful Wind. For
example, in the first chapter of *Remnants of the Purposes of
Medicine (Yi zhi xu yu)*, Sun Yi-Kui criticizes Li Dong-
Yuan's and Zhu Dan-Xi's painful Wind theories: "The
reality is lost because of the names. This has already been
harmful for a long time." Similarly, in *Comprehensive
Medicine According to Master Zhang (Zhang shi yi tong)*,

Zhang Lu-Yu notes that "Painful Wind disorder is called bandit Wind in *Divine Pivot*, painful obstruction in *Basic Questions*, panarthralgia in *Essentials from the Golden Cabinet*, and later white tiger panarthralgia." Yet the causes and etiological mechanisms are fundamentally identical in that "they often result from Wind, Cold and Damp Qi taking advantage of an underlying state of deficiency to attack the channels and collaterals. It is caused by Qi and Blood congealing and becoming stagnant."

From the standpoint of etiology and pathogenesis, the physicians of this era developed the Heat and deficiency aspects of painful obstruction. Yu Chang is one the authors who classified painful obstruction in the deficiency category. In *Precepts for Physicians (Yi men fa lü)* he wrote:

> In treating painful obstruction, those who are not clear on its principles and lump all the various types together, indiscriminately treating them as if they were all Wind problems, are medical criminals. . . . The old prescriptions often use Herba Ephedrae *(ma huang)* and Radix Angelicae Dahuricae *(bai zhi)* because Herba Ephedrae *(ma huang)* can unblock the yang Qi and Radix Angelicae Dahuricae *(bai zhi)* can promote the movement of the nutritive and protective [Qi]. When they are added to such medicines as Four-Substances Decoction *(si wu tang)* and Four-Gentlemen Decoction *(si jun zi tang)*, it is not solely because they can release the exterior.

For chronic painful obstruction with deformation and stiffness of the joints, Yu emphasized the need to nourish the Blood and Qi first, before treating the painful obstruction. He further claimed that crane's knee-Wind disorder in children "is not necessarily due to Wind-Damp-Cold painful obstruction, but is often related to prenatal Kidney Qi deficiency with Cold yin stagnation at the level of the lower back and knees that cannot be released."

Feng Zhao-Zhang, in *Feng's Brocade Bag (Feng shi jin nang)*, wrote that crane's knee-Wind is essentially a case of Kidney deficiency: the Kidneys govern the bones, and when the Kidney Qi is depleted and weak, pathogenic influences take advantage and generate disease. *Medical Revelations (Yi xue xin wu)*, by Cheng Guo-Peng, suggests that this condition is due to "exhaustion of the root of the three yin with invasion of the channels and collaterals by vile pathogenic influences."

Zhang Jing-Yue (also known as Zhang Jie-Bing) is one of the authors who associated painful obstruction with Heat. In the painful obstruction chapter of *Collected Treatises of [Zhang] Jing-Yue (Jing yue quan shu)*, he noted that although painful obstruction is based on the general principle that the obstruction is caused by the combination of Wind, Cold and Dampness, it is necessary to differentiate between yin patterns and yang patterns. The yang pattern is Hot painful obstruction. "Those with Cold should be approached by warming up and heating. Those with Fire should be approached by clearing and cooling." But Zhang acknowledged that in cases of painful obstruction, "Cold patterns are common and Hot patterns rare."

The great specialists on Warm-febrile diseases have different opinions about this disorder. In the second division of *Systematic Differentiation of Warm Diseases (Wen bing tiao bian)*, Wu Ju-Tong emphatically states that "Painful obstruction certainly often starts with Cold, but its association with Heat is not infrequent either." He says that the improper use of hot and spicy herbs produces immediate undesirable effects.

In the seventh division of *Case Histories from the Compass of Clinical Patterns (Lin zheng zhi nang yi an)*, Ye Tian-Shi appropriately elaborates on the pathological mechanisms and treatment of Hot painful obstruction disorders:

> Painful obstruction has always been primarily treated as the mixture of the three influences Wind, Cold and Dampness. However, the diseases are different. There is Damp-Heat from the superimposition of external Summerheat, or that from the internal collecting of water and grains. Pathogenic influences coming from the outside settle in the channels and collaterals, whereas internal pathogenic influences invade the collaterals of the yang Organs. This is why with acrid, releasing herbs [although] there is sweating, the Hot painful obstruction is not diminished. What is needed is a rapid clearing of the yang brightness.

This passage clearly demonstrates that the etiologies of Damp-Hot painful obstruction and Wind-Damp-Cold painful obstruction are different, and call for different treatments.

In *Mirror of Medicine (Yi jing)*, Gu Song-Yuan further develops these concepts. He suggests that Hot painful obstruction may result not only from pathogenic Heat or Dampness, but also from Wind-Damp-Cold painful obstruction in which the "pathogenic influences stagnate and the disease is long-lasting. Wind transforms into Fire, Cold transforms into Heat, and Dampness transforms into Phlegm" thus generating Hot painful obstruction. Gu's therapeutic prescription is to unblock the channels, invigorate the Blood, disperse the stagnant pathogenic influences, direct Fire downward, clear the Heat, and dislodge the Phlegm.

In addition, Wang Qing-Ren in *Correction of Errors among Physicians (Yi lin gai cuo)* suggests that painful obstruction can be due to Blood stasis. The prescription Drive Out Blood Stasis from a Painful Body Decoction *(shen tong zhu yu tang)* is typical of this therapeutic approach. Other books, such as Tang Rong-Chuan's *Discussion of Blood Patterns (Xue zheng lun)* and Zhang Xi-Chun's *Records of Heart-felt Experiences in Medicine with Reference to the West (Yi xue zhong zhong can xi lu)*, follow the same orientation and further develop the concept that painful obstruction can be due to Blood stasis.

Physicians of the Ming and Qing eras also developed their own understandings and treatments of Wind-Damp-Cold painful obstruction. For example, in *Essential Readings for those in the Medical Lineage (Yi zong bi du)*, Li Shi-Cai writes that when the three pathogenic influences of Wind, Cold and Dampness give rise to disease, although they each have their own features, they often combine to form painful obstruction. One cannot sharply differentiate them. To treat moving painful obstruction, dispersing Wind is the primary therapeutic principle, with the help of expelling Cold and regulating Dampness. In addition, in order to release Wind, it is first necessary to treat the Blood; when the Blood moves, Wind will automatically be extinguished. So, in turn, it is necessary to use preparations that tonify the Blood. To treat severe painful obstruction, dispersing Cold is primary, with the help of dispersing Wind and drying Dampness. In turn, it is necessary to use preparations that tonify Fire, utilizing strongly acrid and strongly warming herbs to counteract the harmful effects of congealing Cold. To treat fixed painful obstruction, resolving Dampness is primary, with the help of expelling Wind and dispersing Cold. In turn, it is necessary to regulate the Spleen and tonify the Qi; when Earth is strong it can overcome Dampness.

Zhang Jing-Yue thought that Cold painful obstruction and Hot painful obstruction not only deserved different treatments, but that in the case of Blood deficiency and Blood Heat, "one must nourish the Blood and Qi." Ye Tian-Shi applied his idea that "long-term diseases enter the collaterals" in discussing long-term refractory painful obstruction. He recommended invigorating the Blood, transforming stasis, and using reptile and insect substances to search for and dig out stagnation in order to unblock and open the collaterals and vessels. He also proposed the idea that "Recent pathogenic influences must be quickly dispersed, but those that have taken up residence must be gradually attacked." For deficient patients with chronic painful obstruction, Ye recommended the general method of nourishing the Liver and Kidneys along with the Qi and Blood. These concepts greatly influenced later generations of practitioners.

In order to simplify the clinical classification of painful obstruction, many physicians suggested grouping them into large categories. For example, *Golden Mirror of the Medical Tradition (Yi zong jin jian)* classified painful obstruction according to deficiency and excess: "Painful obstruction deficiency refers to painful obstruction in patients with Qi and Blood deficiency. . . . Painful obstruction excess refers to painful obstruction in patients with Qi and Blood excess." Wu Ju-Tong also wrote, "In general, we cannot get beyond the two poles of Cold and Heat and the different treatments for deficiency and excess."

In summary, the traditional Chinese medical literature relating to painful obstruction is abundant. *Basic Questions* was the first work to establish its broad features; in later centuries, these were expanded and enhanced through the clinical experience of numerous physicians, which made our understanding more complete. Since Liberation [1949], the satisfactory results obtained by treating the biomedically-defined diseases of degenerative arthritis and rheumatoid arthritis within the traditional Chinese medical framework of painful obstruction have been sufficient to demonstrate the value of the theories and experiences of our predecessors. They are worth pursuing further to raise our awareness and competence at all levels of practice.

Scope

By observation and study of the etiologies, pathogenic patterns and clinical manifestations of painful obstruction, modern Chinese physicians have established that this condition encompasses such biomedical disorders as rheumatoid arthritis, degenerative joint disease, sciatica and osteoproliferative diseases (hyperplastic spine diseases, cervical spine diseases, bone spurs of the heel, and osteoarthritis deformans). In addition, when such diseases as brucellosis, thrombophlebitis, scleroderma, erythema nodosum, polyarteritis nodosa, systemic lupus erythematosus and polymyositis present with clinical symptoms of painful obstruction, the present chapter can be used as a reference both for identification and treatment.

Etiology and Pathology

The word *bì* means obstructed and blocked. The pathogenic influences Wind, Cold, Dampness and Heat take advantage of deficiency to invade the body. When this occurs, the movement of Blood and Qi is not smooth and the channels and collaterals become obstructed and stagnant. Another pattern is the accumulation of turbid Phlegm or Blood stasis in the channels that penetrates deep into the joints, sinews or channels, thus giving rise to disease.

Much of the literature and clinical research has demonstrated that the emergence of painful obstruction is closely related to the strength or weakness of a person's constitution, as well as environmental factors and climatic changes. Each of these factors will be examined in the following sections.

DEFICIENT ORGANISM CONTRACTING PATHOGENIC INFLUENCES

When one's constitution is weak with insufficient Qi and Blood and a laxity in the pores and interstices, external pathogenic influences can easily invade the body. Once the disease has appeared, because the patient is not strong enough to expel them, pathogenic Wind, Cold, Dampness or Heat can gradually penetrate deeper, settling in the sinews, bones and Blood vessels where they give rise to painful obstruction. This is why the weakness of the organism is an internal determining factor in the development of this type of disease.

If a patient's yang is deficient, his external defenses are weak and he is readily injured by pathogenic Wind, Cold and Dampness; the most common pattern to emerge is Wind-Damp-Cold painful obstruction. If a patient's yin is deficient, the yang Qi is in a state of relative predominance. The Organs and channels will first experience a buildup of Heat. In such cases the emerging pattern is Wind-Damp-Hot painful obstruction.

INVASION OF EXTERNAL PATHOGENIC INFLUENCES

Pathogenic Wind, Cold, Dampness and Heat are the typical external pathogenic factors that lead to this disorder. Those with weak constitutions are readily subject to invasion by external pathogenic influences. There are also those with relatively strong constitutions who, for a number of reasons, develop this disorder. Such reasons include living for long periods in very cold areas, lacking adequate protection against the cold; prolonged exposure to cold at work; sleeping in areas affected by snow or fog; living in damp areas; sleeping while exposed to the wind; getting caught in the wind and rain; working in water; exposure to cold or dampness after physical exertion; going into the water when sweating. Disease can also be caused by the repeated attack of pathogenic Wind-Damp-Cold when the protective Qi is deficient, or by the transformation of these pathogenic influences into Heat after stagnating in the body over a long period of time.

TARRYING OF PHLEGM AND LODGING OF BLOOD STASIS

In the chronic phase of the disease, Blood and Qi circulation is impaired, which can lead to "Blood tarrying, which constitutes stasis, and Dampness congealing, which constitutes Phlegm." Phlegm and Blood stasis can clump together or combine with external pathogenic influences to obstruct the channels and penetrate the bones to such an extent that the deep roots of the disease become very difficult to pull out. The swelling and deformation of the joints that occurs during the later stages of painful obstruction is due either to Phlegm obstruction or to Blood stasis at the level of the joints.

The important thing to note is that when painful obstruction develops, the internal factor is most often insufficiency of yang Qi and yin Essence, while the external factor is the influence of pathogenic Wind, Cold, Dampness and Heat. In the beginning, the focus is on the excess of the pathogenic influence; the disease is located in the limbs, skin, flesh and channels. Long-term illness is more often a case of deficiency of normal Qi with retention of the pathogenic influences, or enmeshment of deficiency and excess. The location of the disease is then deeper in the sinews, bones or Organs.

Clinical Manifestations and Differential Diagnosis

CLINICAL MANIFESTATIONS

The chief clinical manifestations of painful obstruction are pain, aching, numbness and paresthesia, heaviness and reduced range of motion in the limbs and joints. Pain, in different degrees of intensity, is typical of all forms of painful obstruction disorders, along with some reduced range of motion.

Painful obstruction disorders usually have a slow and progressive onset. Some patients may complain initially of fever, thirst, sweating, sore throat and general discomfort, which progresses and develops into the appearance of joint symptoms. However, in the vast majority of cases, the onset is insidious. The pain can move about or remain in a fixed location for a long period of time. There can be sharp pain, numbness and paresthesia, or swelling.

Painful obstruction disorders are characterized by a progressive evolution, or by relapses on an irregular basis. These recurrences can cause nodules or spotted eruptions in some patients. The nodules are usually located around the knuckles, are as big as a sesame seed, and are hard, tenacious and not tender. *Thousand Ducat Prescriptions* classifies them as a sign of panarthralgia. *Record of Classifications, Patterns, and Treatments (Lei zheng zhi zai)* describes the symptoms as follows:

> Wind-induced pain of panarthralgia has no fixed point. It moves through all the bones and joints, its intensity is that of a tiger bite. . . . When there is severe painful Wind, the fingers have contractions and there are many nodules on the body.

The spotted eruptions are located on the volar aspects of the limbs and on the trunk. Their color is pale red, their shape is vaguely circular but irregular, and they appear intermittently. The appearance of these nodules and spotted eruptions not only has a certain diagnostic value, their number and duration are also an indication of the severity of the disease and are related to its progression or regression.

DIFFERENTIAL DIAGNOSIS

It is important to differentiate painful obstruction from atrophy. Although both of these disorders affect the limbs, they have different clinical manifestations, etiologies and pathologies.

Atrophy disorder *(wěi)* is characterized by a decrease in muscular strength of the limbs with atrophy. In severe cases, the hands can no longer grasp objects and the feet can no longer support the patient. There is usually no pain in the joints and limbs, and the usual location is in the lower limbs.

Painful obstruction disorder is mainly characterized by pain in the limbs, trunk, joints and muscles. It is not limited to the limbs, but can affect the shoulders, back, spine and other structures of the trunk.

The pathological mechanism of painful obstruction is a blockage of the channels by pathogenic influences, which impair the flow of Blood and Qi. The key phrase is "with painful obstruction there is no passage *(bù tōng)*." By contrast, the pathological mechanism of atrophy disorder is exhaustion of and harm to the Essence and Blood of the five yin Organs, such that there is nothing to moisten the peripheral flow, resulting in a loss of nourishment in the channels and vessels. The key phrase is "with atrophy there is weakness and no use *(bù yōng)*." Clinically speaking, these two patterns are actually quite easy to differentiate.

Pattern Differentiation and Discussion of Treatment

PATTERN DIFFERENTIATION

New versus Old and Deficient versus Excessive

The onset of painful obstruction disorder is usually related to pathogenic Wind, Cold, Dampness and Heat taking advantage of deficiency to penetrate into the body, where they obstruct the flow of Qi and Blood in the channels and collaterals. The chief feature is pathogenic excess.

After many recurrent attacks or progressive evolution, obstruction of the channels by long-term pathogenic Qi disrupts the flow of nutritive and protective Qi; Dampness accumulates and transforms into Phlegm; the collaterals are obstructed by stasis; and the Phlegm and Blood stasis become lumped together. In most cases the chief features are a combination of deficiency of normal Qi and pathogenic excess.

When the disease is prolonged it penetrates deeply inside the body. By this time the Blood and Qi are exhausted and depleted, the Liver and Kidneys are deficient, and the sinews and bones lack nourishment. This condition is characterized by deficiency of normal Qi with retention of the pathogenic influences. The chief feature is deficiency of normal Qi.

Acute diseases usually belong to the excess category, whereas chronic conditions are usually deficient. However, these are only generalizations. Clinically, there can be pre-existing Liver and Kidney Blood and Qi deficiency which is followed by an attack of an external pathogenic influence. In such cases, deficiency is the chief feature from the onset. Frequently one also sees cases in which the "root" is one of deficiency and the "branch" is one of excess. If, on the other hand, the condition has been progressing for several months or years, Damp-Cold may have become a chronic fixture, Damp-Heat may have accumulated, or Blood stasis and Phlegm may have melded together. When this occurs, excess and deficiency have formed a complex, and thus one finds chronic cases where the chief feature is pathogenic excess.

DIFFERENTIATION OF CONSTITUTIONS

The strength or weakness of the patient's constitution has a definite influence on the clinical manifestations of the disease.

Patients with a yang deficient constitution have a tendency to be fat and weak. They have a shiny or sallow complexion, sweat profusely, have an aversion to wind, are easily fatigued, have loose or frequent bowel movements, a thick, wide and pale tongue, and a deficient pulse. The emergence of painful obstruction disorder in patients with this type of constitution would most likely be of a Wind-Damp-Cold type.

When there is yin or Blood insufficiency, the patient is typically thin, with a greyish complexion or a yellow complexion with malar flush. They experience tidal fevers and night sweats, insomnia with dream-disturbed sleep, constipation, and have a thin red tongue and a faint, rapid pulse. When patients with this type of constitution develop painful obstruction disorder, it is usually of the Wind-Damp-Hot type.

PATHOGENIC INFLUENCES: SPECIAL CHARACTERISTICS

Painful obstruction disorders are differentiated according to the predominance of pathogenic Wind, Cold, Heat or Dampness. Each has its own clinical characteristics.

Wind is light in nature, and readily moves. The associated pain is erratic and moves around: sometimes it is in the shoulder, sometimes in the elbow; sometimes it is in the upper extremities, sometimes in the lower. It does not have a specific, set location. The tongue coating is thin and white, and the pulse is floating. Clinically, Wind-induced diseases are generally found in the upper limbs and back. A passage in chapter 4 of *Divine Pivot* notes that "When the upper part of the body is affected, it indicates an attack of [Wind] pathogen."

Cold is congealing and stagnant by nature. Pain associated with Cold is fixed, tight and severe. It is often compared to being cut or stabbed. It is aggravated by cold and relieved by warmth. The tongue coating is white, and the pulse is tight.

Dampness is sticky and cloying by nature. When the aches and pains are intense, Dampness resides in the joints and makes them swell. The tongue coating is white and greasy, and the pulse is soggy. Clinical manifestations often appear in the lower extremities, low back and knees: "When the lower part of the body is affected, it indicates an attack of Dampness." (*Divine Pivot*, chapter 4)

Heat is urgent and pressing by nature. It readily burns away the Fluids and thereby promotes stagnation, which can transform into a pathogenic influence. The normal Fluids do not circulate, depriving the sinews and vessels of nourishment, and they become tense. Redness, swelling, heat and pain in the joints then ensue. The pain is intense and there is an intolerance to touch. Patients often have high fever and thirst, with a yellow, dry tongue coating and a slippery, rapid pulse.

The various pathogenic influences often "come sooner or later in no particular order" and "intermingle and form painful obstruction." A good grasp of their special characteristics enables us to clearly differentiate what is primary from what is secondary, and thereby focus on what is most important in therapy.

PHLEGM AND BLOOD STASIS: SPECIAL CHARACTERISTICS

Blood stasis and turbid Phlegm are commonly generated during the course of painful obstruction, as a result of the long-term impairment to the flow of Blood and Qi in the channels due to pathogenic factors.

Phlegm lodges in the joints, and Blood stasis obstructs the collaterals. This further aggravates the painful obstruction and interferes with the delivery of nourishment from the Blood and Qi. Pain, numbness, impaired movement and swelling, or even joint deformation will ensue. Owing to the depth of penetration of the pathogenic influence, commonly used formulas that expel Wind, disperse Cold and eliminate Dampness often prove inadequate. This is why a thorough analysis is necessary to assess the role played by Phlegm and Blood stasis in generating the disease:

- The chronic phase of a disease is often accompanied by Blood stasis and Phlegm accumulation, in accordance with the mechanisms discussed above. Because of this, any case of painful obstruction where the pain does not respond to commonly used therapeutic methods must be evaluated in terms of possible Blood stasis or the presence of Phlegm.
- Joint swelling and pain is often the result of simultaneous obstruction caused by both Phlegm and Blood stasis. Swelling of the joints is often linked to a physical

manifestation of the pathogenic influences (also known as "formed" pathogenic influences) lingering inside the joint. When Dampness has not yet turned into Phlegm, the edema will be diffuse and soft to the touch, and the pain will not really be excruciating. On the other hand, when Phlegm and Blood stasis combine, the swelling will feel harder to the touch, the limbs will be numb, and the pain excruciating.

- Blood stasis patterns are characterized by a thin and choppy pulse, and by purple spots on the tongue. Turbid Phlegm patterns present with a soggy and moderate pulse, and a white and greasy tongue coating.

Presentation

Painful obstruction disorders present many different aspects. They can be identified as old or recent, excessive or deficient, or with a predominance of Wind, Cold, Heat or Dampness. In order to clarify the clinical therapeutics, in this chapter we have divided painful obstruction disorders into two general categories: excessive painful obstruction and deficient painful obstruction.

Excessive painful obstruction disorders include those in which Wind, Cold or Dampness predominates. (These are also known as moving painful obstruction, severe painful obstruction, and fixed painful obstruction respectively.) Hot painful obstruction and stubborn painful obstruction are other types of excess.

Deficient painful obstruction disorders include Qi and Blood deficient painful obstruction, yin deficient painful obstruction, and yang deficient painful obstruction.

EXCESSIVE PAINFUL OBSTRUCTION (shí bì 實痺)

Moving Painful Obstruction (xíng bì 行痺) or Wind-predominant Painful Obstruction (fēng bì 風痺)

Presentation

The pain and aching is in the muscles and joints of the limbs; the pain is migratory and is not restricted to a particular location. The joints have a limited range of motion. Parts most affected are the upper limbs, shoulders and back. At the onset of the disease, there are often exterior signs such as fever with an aversion to wind. The tongue coating is thin and white, and the pulse is floating and lax (huǎn).

Analysis

Moving painful obstruction is the result of pathogenic Wind taking advantage of a condition in which the protective Qi and yang are unsecured, and the pores and interstices are flaccid, to penetrate the skin, muscles and channels. The nature of Wind is migratory, hence the name and primary characteristic of the pain, which moves about.

Wind is a yang pathogenic influence: "When the disease is in the upper part [of the body], it is the yang that is affected." The upper limb is where the six arm channels meet; when pathogenic Wind invades here, it moves through the Blood vessels and the channels, blocks the collaterals and obstructs the flow of Blood and Qi. This is why there are aches and pains and impaired movement.

At the onset of the disease, the aversion to wind, and the fever and body soreness, reflect the struggle between the normal and pathogenic Qi. The floating and lax pulse, and the thin and white tongue coating, indicate that the pathogenic influence is located in the exterior.

Severe Painful Obstruction (tòng bì 痛痺) or Cold-predominant Painful Obstruction (hán bì 寒痺)

Presentation

The pain in the limbs, joints and muscles is excruciating and feels as if one is being cut by a knife or stabbed by needles. It is aggravated by cold, relieved by warmth, and has a relatively stable location. The pain increases at night and diminishes during the day. The joints cannot be flexed or extended. The painful area is neither red nor hot, and often feels cold to the patient. The tongue coating is white, and the pulse is wiry and tight.

Analysis

The main feature of severe painful obstruction disorder is excruciating pain in a fixed location. This is because Cold is a yin pathogenic influence that tends to linger and cause stagnation. When the Blood and Qi are disrupted by pathogenic Cold, the channels are affected; there is pain and spasms like when one is exposed to very cold water. In addition, the pain is so intense that flexion or extension becomes difficult.

Topical application of warmth momentarily disperses the pathogenic Cold and moves the Blood and Qi, thereby temporarily alleviating the pain. Cold slows downs the circulation of Blood and Qi, which congeal. Their flow becomes choppy, which aggravates the pain.

Pathogenic Cold readily injures the yang Qi, causing the Blood and Qi to stagnate. Stasis of Blood and Phlegm-Dampness ensue, which further aggravates the symptoms. Clinically, severe painful obstruction is often accompanied by Blood stasis with stabbing pain in the limbs and joints, numbness and loss of limb motility. Cold and Dampness frequently combine, causing pain with a sensation of cold, heaviness or superficial swelling in the joints. The pathogenic combination of Cold and Dampness mostly affects the lower back and lower limbs. The pain associated with Cold and Phlegm entering the four limbs is not confined to any specific place, and the painful area feels heavy.

Fixed Painful Obstruction (*zhuó bì* 著痹) or Damp-predominant Painful Obstruction (*shī bì* 濕痹)

Presentation

The pain in the joints and muscles of the extremities has a relatively fixed location. In addition, there is an obvious sensation of heaviness. The skin and muscles may be numb, or there may be edema in the affected area. Range of motion is limited, and the pain is alleviated by pressure and warmth. The tongue is pale with a white and greasy coating, and the pulse is slow, lax and soggy.

Analysis

Dampness is a yin pathogenic factor. It is heavy, turbid, sticky and stagnant by nature, hence the name fixed painful obstruction. The pain is mostly in a fixed location; the stagnation of pathogenic Dampness and impairment in the circulation of the Blood and Qi create a sensation of heaviness and numbness. Although the pain is not excruciating, it lingers and is hard to get rid of; it is characterized by heaviness and numbness. As the limbs and joints feel heavy and numb, movement becomes limited, allowing less activity.

Pathogenic Dampness is generated either by an invasion of external Dampness through the flaccid pores and interstices, or by a pooling of body Fluids under pathological conditions. Whether exogenous or endogenous, it has a direct relationship with dysfunction of the Spleen's transportive and transformative functions. This is why fixed painful obstruction is often accompanied by a stifling sensation in the chest, reduced appetite, indigestion, abdominal distention, semi-liquid stools, a pale tongue with a greasy coating, and a lax and soggy pulse. All of these are signs of Spleen deficiency with encumbering Dampness. The peripheral joints often show signs of edema, which indicates a local accumulation of pathogenic Dampness.

When Dampness is vigorous, the yang diminishes, hence the desire to seek warmth and avoid cold. Topical application of warmth and massage momentarily circulates and spreads the yang Qi and reduces the pain and numbness; however, pathogenic Dampness quickly returns and the same symptoms reappear.

Hot Painful Obstruction (*rè bì* 熱痹)

Presentation

The pain is in the joints of the limbs, with local redness and heat; there is a very intense sensation of tightness, pain and swelling. The sinews and vessels are tight and painful to the touch, and there is severe loss of motility such that it is difficult to get out of bed and move around. The pain decreases during the day and increases at night, and is often accompanied by thirst, fever, irritability and a desire to seek cold and avoid warmth. The tongue body is red with a yellow and dry coating, and the pulse is slippery and wiry.

Analysis

Heat is a yang pathogenic influence, and is insistent and pressing by nature. When it penetrates the channels and joints, it struggles with the body's Qi and Blood. There is intense pain due to the tightness of the sinews and vessels, and of the stagnation in the channels. Local heat and redness, fever, thirst, irritability, the rapid pulse and red tongue with a yellow coating are all typical signs of Fire and Heat, which characteristically injure the Fluids.

Stubborn Painful Obstruction (*wán bì* 頑痹)

Presentation

This type of painful obstruction has already undergone a long evolution and a number of recurrences. The joints are stiff and deformed, the areas surrounding the joints are slightly dull and purplish, the pain is excruciating, the location does not change, range of motion is severely impaired, and in some cases there is a painful numbness. The affected joint can be red, swollen and painful with accompanying signs of fever, thirst, and dark and scanty urine. On the other hand, the joint could feel icy cold with the symptoms varying with changes in the weather, such that the pain is aggravated during cold spells. With warmth the pain diminishes. There are often purple spots on the tongue, and the pulse is thin and choppy.

Analysis

When painful obstruction is chronic, the channels' Blood and Qi are slowed down and obstructed by the presence of external pathogenic influences. This causes stasis of Blood and turbid Phlegm, which settle deeply in the joints. At this point they are very difficult to eradicate.

Phlegm and Blood stasis meld together, further aggravating the blockage caused by painful obstruction, and the pain becomes stabbing and excruciating. When the Blood and Qi can no longer circulate, numbness appears. Since the turbid Phlegm and Blood stasis tend to settle in a fixed location, the pain is localized. The area surrounding the joint is dull and purplish, the tongue exhibits purple spots (petechiae), and the pulse is thin and choppy. These are all manifestations of Blood stasis. If there are additional signs of redness of the joints, fever, excessive thirst, dark urine, a greasy tongue coating and a rapid pulse, this indicates that Damp-Heat has settled at the ends of the channels and combined with Blood stasis. If cold aggravates the pain and warmth soothes it, and if the tongue coating is white and the pulse is slow, then the pathogenic Wind, Cold and Dampness have penetrated deeply to the sinews and bones, and have combined with Phlegm and Blood stasis.

DEFICIENT PAINFUL OBSTRUCTION (*xū bì* 虛痺)

Deficient Blood and Qi Painful Obstruction (*qì xuè xū bì* 氣血虛痺)

Presentation

As the painful obstruction progresses over time, the bones and joints become sore and painful. The intensity of the pain varies: it is most acute when movement is involved. There may also be spasms or contractures of the muscles and sinews. The facial complexion is dull and yellowish. There are palpitations, asthenia, shortness of breath, spontaneous sweating, weight loss, poor appetite, diarrhea, and a pale tongue with either no coating or a white coating. The pulse is soggy and frail, or thin and faint.

Analysis

When painful obstruction becomes chronic, the Blood and Qi are depleted and insufficient, the normal Qi is weak, and the pathogenic influence is retained. Under these conditions, the sinews and bones become malnourished, the pain lingers, and there are spasms and twitches

of the sinews and flesh. At this time, although the pain in the joints and muscles is not severe, it drags on and is difficult to eliminate. At the same time, because of the Blood and Qi deficiency, external pathogenic influences readily penetrate the body; or patients may unwisely expose themselves to wind or rain. Under these circumstances they may again contract pathogenic Wind-Damp-Cold. This, in turn, would reactivate the painful obstruction symptoms, giving rise to a pattern of deficient normal Qi and excessive pathogenic influence.

Deficient Blood and Qi painful obstruction is often the consequence of a constitutional Blood and Qi insufficiency, severe hemorrhage, Kidney and Spleen yang deficiency, or the after effects of a chronic disease. It can also be due to a pattern of excessive painful obstruction transforming into deficient Blood and Qi painful obstruction after a long period of time.

Deficient Yang Painful Obstruction (*yáng xū bì* 陽虛痺)

Presentation

The painful obstruction is chronic, the joints are painful, numb and deformed, there is a distinct local sensation of cold, and the muscles and sinews are atrophied. The face is pale and lusterless, the body and limbs are cold, the spine is bent forward so that the patient hunches over, the lower back and knees are sore and weak, and there is profuse urination, watery stools or daybreak diarrhea. The tongue is pale and white, and the pulse is submerged and frail.

Analysis

When the patient has been ill for a long time, the yang Qi becomes insufficient, the exterior and the protective Qi are not secured, pathogenic influences readily penetrate the body, and the bones and joints are painful with varying degrees of intensity. When the pathogenic influences remain inside for a long time, the Blood and Qi fail to provide nourishment, the joints become stiff and deformed, and the sinews and muscles atrophy.

The lower back is the dwelling of the Kidneys, and the knees are the dwelling of the sinews. When the knees and lower back become sore, soft and weak, or when a person takes on a hunched posture, it indicates that the disease has affected the Liver and Kidneys. These are signs of exhaustion and deficiency of those Organs. A poor appetite, watery stools, lack of strength and shortness of breath show that the Spleen yang is also deficient, and that the source of generation and transformation is insufficient. Coldness in the body and limbs, cold sensation in the joints, spontaneous sweating and aversion to wind all indicate yang deficiency and external Cold.

Deficient Yin Painful Obstruction
(*yīn xū bì* 陰虛痹)

Presentation

The painful obstruction is prolonged without improvement, the bones and joints are painful, the sinews and vessels are tense and tight, and the pain and contraction are always aggravated by movement. There is general soreness and weakness, irritability and restlessness, night sweats, vertigo, tinnitus, facial flushing, hot flashes or unremitting low-grade fever. The temperature may be normal during the day and rise at night, the lower back may be sore and the knees weak. The joints are often red, swollen, hot and sometimes deformed, with a significant decrease in the range of motion. The symptoms worsen at night and improve during the day. There is also dryness of the mouth, irritability, lack of appetite, dry and hard stools, a red tongue with little coating, and a thin pulse.

Analysis

When the illness is chronic, the yin will become weak and there will be insufficiency of the Liver and Kidneys. Continual or excessive consumption of hot and drying herbs injures the Liver and Kidney yin, interfering with the nourishment of the sinews and bones. When Blood becomes deficient it can generate internal Wind, which may lead to tension and tightness of the sinews and vessels. The lack of nourishment leads to pain in the bones and joints, which is aggravated by movement. The yin is exhausted and the yang is overactive, hence the vertigo, tinnitus, night sweats, redness of the face, chronic low-grade fever, dryness of the mouth and irritability. Lower back soreness and weakness of the knees indicate that the Essence and Blood of the Kidneys and Liver are insufficient.

Treatment

Principles and Prescriptions

In treating painful obstruction, one generally does not depart from the principles of warming what is Cold, clearing what is Hot, eliminating what is lodged (pathogenic influences with form such as Dampness, Phlegm or Blood stasis) and tonifying what is deficient. A distinction should be drawn, however, between recent and old conditions, and between deficiency and excess.

During the early stages or when the disorder is recent and the general state of health is relatively good, if warming herbs are to be used, those that warm and disperse or warm and unblock should be prescribed. When the illness is chronic, the normal Qi is weak and the pathogenic influence is retained, and the resulting pattern generally belongs to the category of Cold from deficiency. In these cases the primary treatment principle should be to warm and tonify.

Excessive Heat conditions call for sweet and cold or bitter and cold formulas to clear the Heat. For Damp-Heat, one should clear the Heat and simultaneously promote the draining of Dampness. When there is Heat from deficiency, it is important to enrich the yin and clear the Heat. When expelling excesses, the state of the normal Qi (vigorous or weak) must be considered so as to prevent further weakening. When tonifying deficiency, care must be taken to avoid trapping the pathogenic influence inside, thereby aggravating the excess.

Pain is the chief manifestation of painful obstruction disorders: its presence reflects a blockage to the circulation of the Blood and Qi in the channels. There is an adage, "With no passage there is pain *(bù tōng zé tòng)*." This is why disbanding and unblocking *(xuān tōng)* is the preferred therapeutic method for all types of painful obstruction disorders. When the Blood and Qi flow freely, the nutritive and protective Qi will be in harmony, and the pain associated with painful obstruction will gradually disappear.

For Wind-Damp-Cold painful obstruction, acrid herbs should be used to warm the body in order to stimulate the yang Qi so that the pathogenic Qi can be expelled. For Wind-Damp-Hot painful obstruction, one should disperse the Wind, clear the Heat and transform the Dampness. In cases of stubborn painful obstruction, the Phlegm and Blood stasis meld together. In these cases one must break up the Blood stasis and transform the Phlegm, perhaps at the same time adding reptile and insect substances that search for and dig out the stagnation. All of these principles include disbanding and unblocking. For chronic painful obstruction in cases of deficiency, if the yang is deficient, use warming-dispersing, warming-unblocking and tonifying herbs. For patients with yin deficiency, the soft, yin formulas must embody the principle of movement within quiescence (*jìng zhōng yǒu dòng*).[3] If the yin is deficient, light herbs should be used to promote peaceful movement.

Many painful obstruction disorders are characterized by irregular attacks. The general course of action during these attacks is to expel the pathogenic influence; in between attacks, the main treatment principle is to strengthen the nutritive and protective Qi, nourish the Blood and Qi, and tonify the Liver and Kidneys.

EXCESSIVE PAINFUL OBSTRUCTION

Moving Painful Obstruction, Severe Painful Obstruction, Fixed Painful Obstruction

Treatment Principle

The treatment principle is to expel Wind, disperse Cold, drain Dampness and warm and unblock the channels.

Prescriptions

The principal formula used to disperse Wind-Damp-Cold painful obstruction is Remove Painful Obstruction Decoction from *Medical Revelations (juān bì tāng)*. Among the ingredients of this formula, Radix et Rhizoma Notopterygii *(qiang huo)*, Radix Angelicae Pubescentis *(du huo)*, Ramulus Cinnamomi Cassiae *(gui zhi)* and Radix Gentianae Qinjiao *(qin jiao)* expel Wind, disperse Cold and overcome Dampness; Radix Angelicae Sinensis *(dang gui)*, Radix Ligustici Chuanxiong *(chuan xiong)*, Radix Aucklandiae Lappae *(mu xiang)* and Gummi Olibanum *(ru xiang)* harmonize the Qi as well as nourish and invigorate the Blood.

Overall this formula is warming without being drying, and unblocks without injuring.

When Wind is predominant, add Radix Ledebouriallae Divaricatae *(fang feng)*. When Cold is predominant, add Herba Ephedrae *(ma huang)*, Radix Aconiti Carmichaeli Praeparata *(zhi chuan wu)*, Radix Aconiti Kusnezoffii Praeparata *(zhi cao wu)*, Herba cum Radice Asari *(xi xin)* and Minor Invigorate the Collaterals Special Pill *(xiao huo luo dan)*. When Dampness is predominant, add Radix Stephaniae Tetrandrae *(fang ji)*, Rhizoma Atractylodis *(cang zhu)*, Semen Coicis Lachryma-jobi *(yi yi ren)* and Excrementum Bombycis Mori *(can sha)*. For fever, add Rhizoma Anemarrhenae Asphodeloidis *(zhi mu)*, Radix Scutellariae Baicalensis *(huang qin)*, Flos Lonicerae Japonicae *(jin yin hua)* and Fructus Forsythiae

Suspensae *(lian qiao)*. For pain in the upper limbs, add Radix Clematidis *(wei ling xian)*, Rhizoma Curcumae Longae *(jiang huang)* and Fructus Tribuli Terrestris *(bai ji li)*.For pain in the lower limbs, add Radix Achyranthis Bidentatae *(niu xi)*, Fructus Chaenomelis Lagenariae *(mu gua)* and Radix Dipsaci Asperi *(xu duan)*.

Whenever Cold and Dampness combine, but Cold predominates—as when the sensation of cold is intense and the pain severe—one can use Aconite Decoction *(wu tou tang)* to warm the channels, disperse Cold, expel the painful obstruction and alleviate the pain. In this prescription, the combination of Radix Aconiti *(wu tou)* and Herba Ephedrae *(ma huang)* can search for and dig out the Wind-Cold that has entered the bones. Add to this combination Radix Astragali Membranacei *(huang qi)* to augment the Qi and secure the protective Qi, Radix Paeoniae *(shao yao)* to nourish the Blood, and Radix Glycyrrhizae Uralensis *(gan cao)* and honey to soothe the pain and relieve Toxicity.

Radix Aconiti *(wu tou)* comes in two different varieties: Radix Aconiti Carmichaeli *(chuan wu)*, which is from Sichuan, and Radix Aconiti Kusnezoffii *(cao wu)* . The effect of the latter is much more intense than the former. This is due to the fact that soil conditions vary between the north and south, as does climatic humidity. The choice is guided by the physician's experience, the patient's tolerance and feedback, and the accuracy of the diagnosis. When prepared forms of these types of aconite do not yield the expected results, the dried forms can be used. They must first be simmered with honey over a low flame for two hours. This eliminates the toxicity that might otherwise produce side effects. The dosage can be slowly increased; the practitioner must know how much to use with the particular patient. The length of treatment should be kept short. If the patient develops signs of toxicity after ingesting these herbs—numbness of the tongue, dizziness, palpitations, bradycardia, or skipped beats—its ingestion must immediately be discontinued, and the patient should quickly be given frequent administrations of Mung Bean and Licorice Decoction *(lu dou gan cao tang)*. If there is any question as to the patient's safety, they should be taken to an emergency room.

At the onset of painful obstruction disorder, when pathogenic Wind-Damp-Cold is still in the exterior, and there is no sweating (exterior excess condition), one can use Ephedra Decoction plus Atractylodes *(ma huang jia zhu tang)* to induce light sweating. Five-Accumulation Powder *(wu ji san)* can also be prescribed in the form of sesame-seed sized pills to be taken one or two times daily,

20 to 30 grams each time. For exterior deficiency conditions with sweating, use Cinnamon Twig and Prepared Aconite Decoction (*gui zhi fu zi tang*).

Hot Painful Obstruction

Treatment Principle

The treatment principle is to clear Heat, relieve Toxicity, invigorate the Blood and unblock the collaterals. When Heat combines with Wind and Dampness, the additional principle is to disperse Wind and overcome Dampness. If Heat combines with Dampness alone, the main focus is to clear Heat and promote the elimination of Dampness.

Prescriptions

When at the onset of the disease the joint symptoms are accompanied by fever, aversion to wind, dysphagia and cough, add to Ephedra, Apricot Kernel, Gypsum, and Licorice Decoction (*ma xing shi gan tang*) herbs that disperse Wind, invigorate the collaterals and clear Heat: Herba seu Flos Schizonepetae Tenuifoliae (*jing jie*), Fructus Arctii Lappae (*niu bang zi*), Semen Sojae Praeparatum (*dan dou chi*), Herba Menthae Haplocalycis (*bo he*), Rhizoma Belamcandae Chinensis (*she gan*), Radix Platycodi Grandiflori (*jie geng*), Flos Lonicerae Japonicae (*jin yin hua*), Fructus Forsythiae Suspensae (*lian qiao*), Radix Scutellariae Baicalensis (*huang qin*), Ramus Lonicerae Japonicae (*ren dong teng*), Bombyx Batryticatus (*jiang can*), Ramulus Mori Albae (*sang zhi*), Radix Gentianae Qinjiao (*qin jiao*) and Radix Paeoniae Rubrae (*chi shao*). Six-Miracle Pill (*liu shen wan*) may also be prescribed.

When the disease moves from the exterior to the interior with accompanying signs of high fever, thirst, sweating, irritability, a stifling sensation in the chest and racing pulse, use White Tiger Decoction (*bai hu tang*) as the main formula to strongly clear Heat from the Qi level, in combination with such Heat-clearing and Toxicity-relieving herbs as Cortex Phellodendri (*huang bai*), Rhizoma Coptidis (*huang lian*), Fructus Gardeniae Jasminoidis (*zhi zi*) and Radix et Rhizoma Polygoni Cuspidati (*hu zhang*).

When the fever is unremittingly high and is accompanied by constipation, add Mirabilitum (*mang xiao*) and Radix et Rhizoma Rhei (*da huang*), with the addition of Purple Snow Special Pill (*zi xue dan*), to clear Heat and Toxins and unblock the bowels.

If the Hot painful obstruction causes pain in the joints, muscles and sinews with contractions, the follow-

ing herbs invigorate the Blood, unblock the collaterals, disband painful obstruction and alleviate pain: Ramulus Mori Albae (*sang zhi*), Ramulus Cinnamomi Cassiae (*gui zhi*), Radix Gentianae Qinjiao (*qin jiao*), Herba Siegesbeckiae (*xi xian cao*), Rhizoma Curcumae Longae (*jiang huang*), Radix Clematidis (*wei ling xian*), Ramulus et Folium Tamaricis (*cheng liu*), Ramus Lonicerae Japonicae (*ren dong teng*) and Gummi Olibanum (*ru xiang*).

If the joints are red, swollen and excruciatingly painful, accompanied by contraction of the sinews occurring mostly at night, high fever, intense thirst, a red and dry tongue, and a wiry and rapid pulse, Toxic Heat has transformed into Fire and penetrated to the depth of the sinews and bones. Combine Rhinoceros Horn Decoction (*xi jiao tang*) with White Tiger Decoction (*bai hu tang*) to clear Heat and Toxins. Cornu Rhinoceri (*xi jiao*) and Cornu Antelopis (*ling yang jiao*) can be replaced by Carapax Amydae Sinensis (*bie jia*) and Cornu Bubali (*shui niu jiao*) respectively. The following may also be added: Ramus Lonicerae Japonicae (*ren dong teng*), Lumbricus (*di long*), Radix Achyranthis Bidentatae (*niu xi*), Ramulus Sangjisheng (*sang ji sheng*), Gummi Olibanum (*ru xiang*), Radix Gentianae Qinjiao (*qin jiao*), Rhizoma Imperatae Cylindricae (*bai mao gen*), Radix Rehmanniae Glutinosae (*sheng di huang*) and Radix et Rhizoma Polygoni Cuspidati (*hu zhang*).

For pronounced Heat from deficiency, add Increase the Fluids Decoction (*zeng ye tang*) with Herba Dendrobii (*shi hu*), Rhizoma Anemarrhenae Asphodeloidis (*zhi mu*), Cortex Moutan Radicis (*mu dan pi*) and Cortex Lycii Radicis (*di gu pi*).

For macular-type eruptions of the skin, add herbs that cool the Blood and relieve Toxicity: Radix Rehmanniae Glutinosae (*sheng di huang*), Radix Paeoniae Rubrae (*chi shao*) and Radix Salviae Miltiorrhizae (*dan shen*).

Hot painful obstruction can also be caused by Wind-Damp-Cold painful obstruction that collects inside over a long period of time and transforms into Heat. When this occurs the treatment principle is the same as that discussed immediately above. When pathogenic Wind-Damp-Cold begins to transform into Heat, such signs and symptoms appear as aversion to wind, thirst, irritability and a stifling sensation in the chest, local sensation of heat in the joints with pain and swelling. In these cases, when the pathogenic Wind-Damp-Cold is still present, use Ephedra, Forsythia, and Aduki Bean Decoction (*ma huang lian qiao chi xiao dou tang*) with additions as indicated below.

In this formula, Herba Ephedrae *(ma huang)* causes sweating and opens up the exterior, Fructus Forsythiae Suspensae *(lian qiao)* clears Heat, Semen Phaseoli Calcarati *(chi xiao dou)* and Cortex Catalpae Ovatae Radicis *(zi bai pi)* (usually Cortex Mori Albae Radicis *[sang bai pi]* is substituted for this herb) drain Dampness, Semen Pruni Armeniacae *(xing ren)* promotes the movement of Qi, honey-toasted Radix Glycyrrhizae Uralensis *(zhi gan cao)* and Fructus Zizyphi Jujubae *(da zao)* harmonize the middle burner.

For thirst, add Gypsum *(shi gao)* and Talcum *(hua shi)*; for fever add Rhizoma Anemarrhenae Asphodeloidis *(zhi mu)* and Cortex Phellodendri *(huang bai)*; for red, swollen, painful joints, add Rhizoma Dioscoreae Hypoglaucae *(bei xie)*, Radix Aristolochiae Fangchi *(fang ji)*, Semen Coicis Lachryma-jobi *(yi yi ren)*, Ramus Lonicerae Japonicae *(ren dong teng)* and Radix et Rhizoma Polygoni Cuspidati *(hu zhang)*; for aversion to wind, add Radix Ledebouriellae Divaricatae *(fang feng)* and Radix et Rhizoma Notopterygii *(qiang huo)*.

When Cold and Heat are melded together, the joint pain is severe, there is swelling and local heat, the patient has an aversion to wind and cold, and there is unremitting fever. The treatment principle is to combine warming and cooling herbs, as in the commonly used Cinnamon Twig, Peony, and Anemarrhena Decoction *(gui zhi shao yao zhi mu tang)*.

In this formula, Herba Ephedrae *(ma huang)* and Ramulus Cinnamomi Cassiae *(gui zhi)* expel Wind-Cold and unblock the channels and collaterals; Radix Lateralis Aconiti Carmichaeli Praeparata *(fu zi)* warms the yang, opens up areas of painful obstruction, and alleviates pain; Rhizoma Atractylodis Macrocephalae *(bai zhu)* and Radix Ledebouriellae Divaricatae *(fang feng)* eliminate Dampness and expel Wind; Radix Paeoniae *(shao yao)* and Rhizoma Anemarrhenae Asphodeloidis *(zhi mu)* clear heat and nourish the yin; Radix Glycyrrhizae Uralensis *(gan cao)* and Rhizoma Zingiberis Officinalis Recens *(sheng jiang)* harmonize the Stomach and regulate the middle burner.

For mental and physical fatigue, add Radix Astragali Membranacei *(huang qi)*; for yin deficiency and intense internal Heat, add Radix Rehmanniae Glutinosae *(sheng di huang)*; for poor appetite, add Pericarpium Citri Reticulatae *(chen pi)* and Massa Fermentata *(shen qu)*; for fever, add Gypsum *(shi gao)* and Cortex Phellodendri *(huang bai)*; for Blood deficiency with edema in the joints of the limbs, add Radix et Caulis Jixueteng *(ji xue teng)* and Herba Pyrolae Rotundifoliae *(lu xian cao)*; for

pronounced Dampness with swelling of the joints, add Rhizoma Dioscoreae Hypoglaucae *(bei xie)*, Rhizoma Alismatis Orientalis *(ze xie)*, Radix Aristolochiae Fangchi *(fang ji)* and Semen Coicis Lachryma-jobi *(yi yi ren)*.

When pathogenic Heat combines with Damp-Heat, generating Damp-Hot painful obstruction with red and painful joints, use Disband Painful Obstruction Decoction *(xuan bi tang)* to clear and resolve Damp-Heat, while unblocking the channels and collaterals.

In this formula, Radix Aristolochiae Fangchi *(fang ji)* clears Heat, resolves Dampness, unblocks the collaterals, and alleviates pain; Talcum *(hua shi)* and Semen Coicis Lachryma-jobi *(yi yi ren)* are bland herbs that drain and resolve Dampness; Semen Pruni Armeniacae *(xing ren)* disseminates and promotes the proper movement of the Lung Qi; Excrementum Bombycis Mori *(can sha)*, Rhizoma Pinelliae Ternatae *(ban xia)* and Semen Phaseoli Calcarati *(chi xiao dou)* eliminate Dampness and transform turbidity; Fructus Forsythiae Suspensae *(lian qiao)* and Fructus Gardeniae Jasminoidis *(zhi zi)* drain Heat from constraint.

When the Dampness is drained, the Heat is eliminated and the channels and collaterals are unblocked, the pain associated with painful obstruction will simply disappear.

For excessive or severe pain, add such substances as Cortex Erythrinae *(hai tong pi)*, Rhizoma Curcumae Longae *(jiang huang)*, Fructus Xanthii Sibirici *(cang er zi)*, Rhizoma Dioscoreae Hypoglaucae *(bei xie)* and Lumbricus *(di long)* to unblock the collaterals, expel Wind and drain Dampness. Three-Marvel Powder *(san miao san)* can also be added to strengthen the Heat-purging and Dampness-draining effects.

Stubborn Painful Obstruction

Treatment Principle

The primary treatment principle is to invigorate the Blood, transform stasis, transform Phlegm and unblock the collaterals. Secondarily, it is important to support the normal Qi by tonifying the Kidneys and nourishing the Liver.

Prescriptions

The basic formulas used for this pattern are Drive Out Blood Stasis from a Painful Body Decoction *(shen tong zhu yu tang)*, Minor Invigorate the Collaterals Special Pill *(xiao huo luo dan)*, Major Invigorate the Collaterals Special Pill *(da huo luo dan)* and Augment the Kidneys and Remove Painful Obstruction Pill *(yi shen juan bi wan)*.

The first of these formulas, Drive Out Blood Stasis from a Painful Body Decoction *(shen tong zhu yu tang)*, includes Semen Persicae *(tao ren)*, Flos Carthami Tinctorii *(hong hua)* and Radix Angelicae Sinensis *(dang gui)* to invigorate the Blood and transform stasis; Excrementum Trogopterori seu Pteromi *(wu ling zhi)* and Lumbricus *(di long)* to expel Phlegm and open the collaterals; Radix Ligustici Chuanxiong *(chuan xiong)*, Myrrha *(mo yao)* and Rhizoma Cyperi Rotundi *(xiang fu)* to regulate the Qi, invigorate the Blood and alleviate pain; Radix et Rhizoma Notopterygii *(qiang huo)* and Radix Gentianae Qinjiao *(qin jiao)* to expel Wind and Dampness; Radix Cyathulae Officinalis *(chuan niu xi)* to strengthen the sinews and bones; and Radix Glycyrrhizae Uralensis *(gan cao)* to harmonize the actions of the different substances.

This formula can be used for severe painful obstruction of long duration without improvement due to the melding together of Phlegm and Blood stasis.

Minor Invigorate the Collaterals Special Pill *(xiao huo luo dan)* warms and disperses Wind and Cold, while also transforming Phlegm and Blood stasis. Major Invigorate the Collaterals Special Pill *(da huo luo dan)* contains many ingredients. Together in this formula are substances that expel Wind, invigorate the Blood, disperse Cold, clear Heat and support the normal Qi. It is used for patients with chronic pain due to painful obstruction in the collaterals.

Augment the Kidneys and Remove Painful Obstruction Pill *(yi shen juan bi wan)* is a formula that treats both the branch and root of the disease. In this formula, Radix Rehmanniae Glutinosae *(sheng di huang)*, Radix Rehmanniae Glutinosae Conquitae *(shu di huang)*, Radix Angelicae Sinensis *(dang gui)*, Herba Epimedii *(yin yang huo)* and Radix et Caulis Jixueteng *(ji xue teng)* nourish and invigorate the Blood; Herba Pyrolae Rotundifoliae *(lu xian cao)*, Rhizoma seu Herba Aristolochiae Mollissimae *(xun gu feng)* and Radix et Rhizoma Polygoni Cuspidati *(hu zhang)* expel and disperse Damp-Wind. The formula also includes seven ingredients derived from the animal kingdom: Buthus Martensi *(quan xie)*, Scolopendra Subspinipes *(wu gong)*, Zaocys Dhumnades *(wu shao she)* or Agkistrodon seu Bungarus *(bai hua she)*, Nidus Vespae *(lu feng fang)*, Eupolyphaga seu Opisthoplatia *(tu bie chong)*, Cartharsius *(qiang lang)* and Bombyx Batryticatus *(jiang can)*. These are all strong and effective substances that invigorate the Blood, transform Blood stasis, expel pathogenic influences and unblock the collaterals.

This formula is especially useful for stubborn painful obstruction with deficient normal Qi and excessive pathogenic Qi of long duration. This type of painful obstruction does not respond to the usual formulas that expel Wind, disperse Cold, dry Dampness and unblock the collaterals. Here the Blood stasis has invaded the collaterals, and there is Blood deficiency and Kidney exhaustion.

DEFICIENT PAINFUL OBSTRUCTION

Qi and Blood Deficient Painful Obstruction

Therapeutic Principle

The primary treatment principle is to harmonize and tonify the Blood and Qi.

Prescriptions

A commonly used prescription is Astragalus and Cinnamon Twig Five-Substance Decoction *(huang qi gui zhi wu wu tang)* plus Radix Angelicae Sinensis *(dang gui)*. This formula harmonizes stagnation of the nutritive Qi and promotes the movement of the protective Qi. The early nineteenth-century writer Chen Xiu-Yuan, in *Subtle Uses of Latter-Day Formulas (Shi fang miao yong)*, viewed this script as the general formula for all deficient painful obstruction disorders. The addition of Radix Angelicae Sinensis *(dang gui)* strengthens the formula's action in nourishing and invigorating the Blood, in accordance with the adages, "When tonifying there should be some stirring; when promoting movement there should be some tonification," and "To treat Wind, treat the Blood first; when the Blood moves, Wind will be extinguished naturally." The combination of Radix Astragali Membranacei *(huang qi)* and Radix Angelicae Sinensis *(dang gui)* both augments the Qi and generates Blood.

When Qi deficiency predominates, use Tonify the Middle and Augment the Qi Decoction *(bu zhong yi qi tang)* with the addition of Radix Lateralis Aconiti Carmichaeli Praeparata *(fu zi)* and two or three of the following herbs to disperse, unblock and open up the painful obstruction: Ramulus Mori Albae *(sang zhi)*, Rhizoma Curcumae Longae *(jiang huang)*, Radix Ledebouriellae Divaricatae *(fang feng)*, Radix Clematidis *(wei ling xian)*, Radix Gentianae Qinjiao *(qin jiao)* and Herba Siegesbeckiae *(xi xian cao)*.

When Blood deficiency predominates, use Four-Substance Decoction *(si wu tang)* as a base formula and add other herbs as needed.

For Blood and Qi deficiency with Liver and Kidney deficiency, use Angelica Pubescens and Sangjisheng Decoction (*du huo ji sheng tang*). In this formula, Radix Rehmanniae Glutinosae Conquitae (*shu di huang*),[4] Radix Paeoniae Lactiflorae (*bai shao*), Radix Angelicae Sinensis (*dang gui*) and Radix Ligustici Chuanxiong (*chuan xiong*) nourish and invigorate the Blood; Radix Ginseng (*ren shen*), or more commonly Radix Codonopsitis Pilosulae (*dang shen*), as well as Sclerotium Poriae Cocos (*fu ling*) and Radix Glycyrrhizae Uralensis (*gan cao*), tonify the Qi and strengthen the Spleen; Ramulus Sangjisheng (*sang ji sheng*), Cortex Eucommiae Ulmoidis (*du zhong*) and Radix Achyranthis Bidentatae (*niu xi*) tonify the Liver and Kidneys, strengthen the sinews and bones, and fortify the lower back and knees. Together with these herbs, Radix Angelicae Pubescentis (*du huo*), Herba cum Radice Asari (*xi xin*), Radix Ledebouriellae Divaricatae (*fang feng*) and Radix Gentianae Qinjiao (*qin jiao*) expel Wind-Dampness to alleviate the pain associated with painful obstruction.

In this way, both the root and branch of the disease are attended to, the normal Qi is supported, and the pathogenic influence is dispersed. This formula is prescribed when the course of the disease is so long that it is classified as chronic, there are frequent relapses, the Liver and Kidney Blood and Qi are insufficient, the joints are painful, and the lower back and thighs are sore.

When Cold predominates, add Radix Lateralis Aconiti Carmichaeli Praeparata (*fu zi*); when Heat predominates, add Radix Gentianae Qinjiao (*qin jiao*) and substitute Radix Rehmanniae Glutinosae (*sheng di huang*) for Radix Rehmanniae Glutinosae Conquitae (*shu di huang*), and Ramulus Mori Albae (*sang zhi*) for Ramulus Cinnamomi Cassiae (*gui zhi*);[5] for pronounced Dampness with loose stools, remove Radix Rehmanniae Glutinosae Conquitae (*shu di huang*) and add Rhizoma Atractylodis (*cang zhu*) and Rhizoma Atractylodis Macrocephalae (*bai zhu*); for Blood stasis, add Semen Persicae (*tao ren*) and Flos Carthami Tinctorii (*hong hua*).

When Radix Dipsaci Asperi (*xu duan*) is substituted for Ramulus Sangjisheng (*sang ji sheng*) and Radix Astragali Membranacei (*huang qi*) is added, the resulting formula is Three Painful Obstruction Decoction (*san bi tang*) from *Fine Formulas for Women (Fu ren liang fang)*, which basically has the same indications.

There is a Revised Three Painful Obstruction Decoction (*gai ding san bi tang*) listed in *Comprehensive Medicine According to Master Zhang (Zhang shi yi tong)*. This formula removes Radix Dipsaci Asperi (*xu duan*), Cortex Eucommiae Ulmoidis (*du zhong*), Radix Gentianae Qinjiao (*qin jiao*), Radix Rehmanniae Glutinosae Conquitae (*shu di huang*), Radix Angelicae Pubescentis (*du huo*) and Radix Achyranthis Bidentatae (*niu xi*), and adds Rhizoma Atractylodis Macrocephalae (*bai zhu*), Radix Aristolochiae Fangchi (*fang ji*) and Radix Aconiti (*wu tou*). This formula is used to treat a combination of the Wind-Damp-Cold pathogenic influences that cause congealing and stagnation of Qi and Blood with contractions and spasms of the hands and feet. Besides its fundamental actions of tonifying the Qi and nourishing the Blood, the formula also expels Wind, disperses Cold and drives out Dampness. It is prescribed for patterns of deficiency of the normal qi and pathogenic excess.

For Blood and Qi deficient painful obstruction disorders, we also recommend Mutton Stew with Tangkuei and Fresh Ginger (*dang gui sheng jiang yang rou tang*) with the addition of Ramulus Cinnamomi Cassiae (*gui zhi*) and Radix Paeoniae Lactiflorae (*bai shao*). This has the therapeutic action of regulating and nourishing.

Yang Deficient Painful Obstruction

Treatment Principle

The primary treatment principle is to warm the yang and augment the Qi.

Prescriptions

True Warrior Decoction (*zhen wu tang*) is commonly used, often with additions. In this formula, Radix Lateralis Aconiti Carmichaeli Praeparata (*fu zi*) and Rhizoma Zingiberis Officinalis Recens (*sheng jiang*) warm the channels and disperse Cold; Sclerotium Poriae Cocos (*fu ling*) and Rhizoma Atractylodis Macrocephalae (*bai zhu*) tonify the Spleen and eliminate Dampness; and Radix Paeoniae Lactiflorae (*bai shao*) nourishes the Blood, alleviates pain and softens the harsh characteristics of Radix Lateralis Aconiti Carmichaeli Praeparata (*fu zi*).

For Qi deficiency, substitute Radix Ginseng (*ren shen*) for Rhizoma Zingiberis Officinalis Recens (*sheng jiang*). The resulting formula is Prepared Aconite Decoction (*fu zi tang*), in which the combination of Radix Lateralis Aconiti Carmichaeli Praeparata (*fu zi*) and Radix Ginseng (*ren shen*) warms and tonifies the basal yang.

Adding Ramulus Cinnamomi Cassiae (*gui zhi*), Rhizoma Zingiberis Officinalis (*gan jiang*) and Radix Glycyrrhizae Uralensis (*gan cao*) gives you Eight-Substance Decoction with Prepared Aconite (*fu zi ba wu tang*), a formula indicated for yang Qi deficiency with a preponderance of Cold yin, manifested by unbearable stabbing pain in the limbs.

After the pain has been alleviated with one of the above formulas, add as needed such herbs as Radix Astragali Membranacei *(huang qi)*, Radix Angelicae Sinensis *(dang gui)*, Herba Epimedii *(yin yang huo)*, Ramulus Sangjisheng *(sang ji sheng)*, Radix Dipsaci Asperi *(xu duan)*, Radix Morindae Officinalis *(ba ji tian)*, Rhizoma Cibotii Barometz *(gou ji)*, Cortex Eucommiae Ulmoidis *(du zhong)*, Radix Achyranthis Bidentatae *(niu xi)* and Lignum Pini Nodi *(song jie)* to tonify and augment the Blood and Qi, warm and nourish the Liver and Kidneys, and fortify and strengthen the sinews and bones.

When the pain associated with the obstruction is severe, use Augment the Kidneys and Remove Painful Obstruction Pill *(yi shen juan bi wan)* or Minor Gold Special Pill *(xiao jin dan)*. The latter is a prepared medicine recommended in *Standards of Patterns and Treatments in External Medicine (Wai ke zheng zhi zhun sheng)* for yin-type sores, abscesses and oozing cutaneous ulcerations.

In this formula, Radix Angelicae Sinensis *(dang gui)*, Flos Carthami Tinctorii *(hong hua)*, Myrrha *(mo yao)*, Excrementum Trogopterori seu Pteromi *(wu ling zhi)* and Resina Liquidambaris *(bai jiao xiang)* invigorate the Blood and dispel stasis; Lumbricus *(di long)* and Semen Momordicae Cochinchinensis *(mu bie zi)* transform Phlegm and unblock the collaterals; and Radix Aconiti Carmichaeli Praeparata *(zhi chuan wu)* and Radix Aconiti Kusnezoffii Praeparata *(zhi cao wu)* expel Wind-Cold and alleviate pain.

Secretio Moschus *(she xiang)* is acrid, warm and so intensely penetrating that it releases that which is hidden. It is therefore particularly effective in unblocking the collaterals and alleviating pain.

Yin Deficient Painful Obstruction

Treatment Principle

The primary treatment principle is to enrich the Kidneys and nourish the Liver.

Prescriptions

Use Six-Ingredient Pill with Rehmannia *(liu wei di huang wan)* with the addition of Radix Angelicae Sinensis *(dang gui)* and Radix Paeoniae Lactiflorae *(bai shao)*. The main formula enriches the Kidney yin, and the two addi-

tions nourish the Liver Blood. Other herbs can be added to tonify and augment the Liver and Kidneys and strengthen and fortify the sinews and bones, among them: Herba Dendrobii *(shi hu)*, Fructus Chaenomelis Lagenariae *(mu gua)*, Gelatinum Corii Asini *(e jiao)*, Fructus Lycii *(gou qi zi)*, Ramulus Sangjisheng *(sang ji sheng)*, Cortex Eucommiae Ulmoidis *(du zhong)*, Radix Dipsaci Asperi *(xu duan)*, Semen Astragali *(sha yuan ji li)*, Semen Coicis Lachryma-jobi *(yi yi ren)*, Ramulus Mori Albae *(sang zhi)*, Caulis Trachelospermi Jasminoidis *(luo shi teng)*, Radix Achyranthis Bidentatae *(niu xi)*, Radix Polygoni Multiflori *(he shou wu)* and Rhizoma Polygonati Odorati *(yu zhu)*.

For yin deficiency with ascendant yang and internal movement of Liver Wind, add ingredients like Concha Haliotidis *(shi jue ming)*, Concha Ostreae *(mu li)*, Folium Mori Albae *(sang ye)*, Ramulus cum Uncis Uncariae *(gou teng)*, Flos Chrysanthemi Morifolii *(ju hua)* and Two-Ultimate Pill *(er zhi wan)* to pacify the Liver and anchor the yang.

For shaking sensations and tremors in the sinews and muscles, add ingredients like Fructus Tribuli Terrestris *(bai ji li)* and Rhizoma Gastrodiae Elatae *(tian ma)* to disperse Wind.

For pain in the joints, add two or three of the following ingredients to invigorate the Blood and unblock the collaterals: Radix Salviae Miltiorrhizae *(dan shen)*, Radix et Caulis Jixueteng *(ji xue teng)*, Caulis Trachelospermi Jasminoidis *(luo shi teng)*, Fructus Chaenomelis Lagenariae *(mu gua)*, Herba Siegesbeckiae *(xi xian cao)*, Rhizoma Dioscoreae Nipponicae *(chuan shan long)*, Ramulus Mori Albae *(sang zhi)*, Herba cum Radice Lycopodii Clavati *(shen jin cao)*, Caulis Piperis Futokadsurae *(hai feng teng)*.

CAUTIONS AND CONTRAINDICATIONS

In the treatment of painful obstruction, traditional Chinese medicine prohibits the use of purgatives, astringents or substances that are sour and cold or bitter and cold, while encouraging the use of acrid and dispersing substances, those that promote the movement of Qi, those that dry Dampness, and sweet and bland herbs that leach out Dampness. This advice is found in the Ming work *Annotated Classic of Materia Medica (Ben cao jing shu)*.

However, these guidelines only apply in cases where the Wind-Damp-Cold painful obstruction has not yet transformed into Heat. They should not be rigidly followed in cases that have already transformed into Heat.

Ran Xue-Feng[6] has pointed out in *A Peek at the Eight Methods and Efficacious Formulas (Ba fa xiao fang ju yu)* that

> The detailed description of the pathology of Hot painful obstruction is in *Basic Questions*, but its treatment was first described in *Classic of Materia Medica*. Wind, Cold and Dampness can be said to be the causes of the disease; over a period of time Cold transforms into Heat, Dampness into Dryness, the presentation changes and so do the treatment methods. Not only can sweet and cold [substances] be used, but it is also essential to add bitter and cold formulas to have practical results.

Moreover, as noted in *Precepts for Physicians (Yi men fa lü)*, "In treating painful obstruction, those who are not clear on its principles and lump all the various types together, indiscriminately treating them as if they were all Wind problems, are medical criminals." *Confucians' Duties to Their Parents (Ru men shi qin)* also criticizes physicians who treat painful obstruction disorders without identifying which channels are affected, or differentiating yin from yang Organs, or exterior from interior, and who facilely throw at patients such drying and warming substances as Radix Aconiti (wu tou), Radix Lateralis Aconiti Carmichaeli Praeparata (fu zi), Gummi Olibanum (ru xiang) and Myrrha (mo yao). On top of this they add different kinds of external therapeutic methods to forcefully attack the painful obstruction, which weakens the normal Qi in the process. "Painful obstruction itself is not terminal; death is due to the mistakes of physicians."

Other Therapeutic Methods

Acupuncture, moxibustion and other external therapeutic methods can be used in combination with herbal prescriptions to increase the efficacy of painful obstruction treatment. Folk remedies can likewise be adapted according to circumstances.

FOLK REMEDIES

Prescriptions For Internal Use

Wind-Damp-Cold Painful Obstruction

1. Decoction of 30g Herba Erodii seu Geranii (lao guan cao) and 30g Herba Herba Siegesbeckiae (xi xian cao).
2. Cook 60g of Rhizoma Drynariae (gu sui bu) in a double boiler with dog meat.

3. Decoction of 18-24g Radix et Caulis Jixueteng (ji xue teng), 18-30g Radix Rehmanniae Glutinosae (sheng di huang), 9g Radix Ledebouriellae Divaricatae (fang feng), 9g Radix Gentianae Qinjiao (qin jiao), 9g Myrrha (mo yao), 12-18g Herba Leonuri Heterophylli (yi mu cao), 12g Radix Clematidis (wei ling xian), 9g Cortex Eucommiae Ulmoidis (du zhong), 12g Radix Aristolochiae Fangchi (fang ji) and 9g Gummi Olibanum (ru xiang).
4. Decoction of 30g Herba Pyrolae Rotundifoliae (lu xian cao).
5. Decoction of 24-30g Herba cum Radix Cynanchi Paniculati (xu chang qing), 200g lean pork, and 70g of aged spirits, to be taken twice daily.
6. Decoct a five-inch piece of Radix Notoginseng Recens (xian san qi), with the leaves, and 100g brown sugar. Add two chicken eggs before drinking. To be taken over two consecutive days.
7. Decoction of 15g each of Ramus Tinosporae Sinensis (kuan jin teng), Caulis Trachelospermi Jasminoidis (luo shi teng), Radix et Caulis Jixueteng (ji xue teng), Ramus Lonicerae Japonicae (ren dong teng) and Caulis Piperis Futokadsurae (hai feng teng).
8. Siegesbeckia and Clerodendron Pill (xi tong wan), which is made of equal parts of Herba Siegesbeckiae (xi xian cao) and Folium Clerodendri Trichotomi (chou wu tong). The dosage is 3-6g taken three times a day with water.
9. Decoction of 10g Radix Angelicae Pubescentis (du huo), 30g Ramulus Sangjisheng (sang ji sheng), 12g Radix Gentianae Qinjiao (qin jiao), 10g Radix Achyranthis Bidentatae (niu xi), 10g Cortex Eucommiae Ulmoidis (du zhong), 12g Radix Angelicae Sinensis (dang gui) and 6g Radix Glycyrrhizae Uralensis (gan cao).

Hot or Damp-Hot Painful Obstruction

1. Decoction of 30g Ramulus Mori Albae Extremitas (sang zhi jian), 10g Radix Achyranthis Bidentatae (niu xi), 10g Radix Stephaniae Tetrandrae (han fang ji), 30g Fasciculus Vascularis Luffae (si gua luo).
2. Decoction of 15g Caulis et Rhizoma Sinomenii Acuti (qing feng teng) and 10g Radix Stephaniae Tetrandrae (han fang ji).
3. Decoction of 250g Ramulus Mori Albae (sang zhi) and 250g Ramulus et Folium Tamaricis (cheng liu). Strain and add 250g of honey, and cook on a low flame until it thickens into a syrup. Take 12g diluted in water, twice a day.

4. Decoction of 10g Cortex Acanthopanacis Gracilistylus Radicis *(wu jia pi)* and 30g Ramus Lonicerae Japonicae *(ren dong teng)*.

5. Decoction of 12g Cortex Erythrinae *(hai tong pi)*, 3g Herba Menthae Haplocalycis *(bo he)*, 3g Radix Cyathulae Officinalis *(chuan niu xi)*, 3g Radix et Rhizoma Notopterygii *(qiang huo)*, 15g Radix Rehmanniae Glutinosae *(sheng di huang)*, 15g Semen Coicis Lachryma-jobi *(yi yi ren)*, 9g Cortex Acanthopanacis Gracilistylus Radicis *(wu jia pi)* and 9g Cortex Lycii Radicis *(di gu pi)*.

6. Decoction of 30g Radix et Rhizoma Polygoni Cuspidati *(hu zhang)* and one tablespoon of alcohol, once daily.

7. Decoction of 60g Radix Puerariae *(ge gen)*, 45g Ramus Lonicerae Japonicae *(ren dong teng)*, 15g Fasciculus Vascularis Luffae *(si gua luo)*, 12g Fructus Liquidambaris Taiwanianae *(lu lu tong)*. Divide into three doses, and take three doses daily.

Prescriptions For External Use

1. Decoction of 200g Folium Artemisiae Argyi *(ai ye)* as a bath; avoid subsequent exposure to drafts.

2. Decoction of 30g each of Cortex Erythrinae *(hai tong pi)*, Ramulus Cinnamomi Cassiae *(gui zhi)*, Caulis Piperis Futokadsurae *(hai feng teng)*, Fructus Liquidambaris Taiwanianae *(lu lu tong)*, Ramus Tinosporae Sinensis *(kuan jin teng)* and Radix seu Ramulus et Folium Zanthoxyli Nitidi *(ru di jin niu)*. The painful joints are positioned over the steam rising from the decoction, and then washed in the decoction for 10-20 minutes once or twice daily, for one month.

3. Powder 30g of each of the following: Radix Aconiti Carmichaeli Praeparata *(zhi chuan wu)*, Radix Aconiti Kusnezoffii Praeparata *(zhi cao wu)*, Lignum Pini Nodi *(song jie)*, untreated Rhizoma Arisaematis *(sheng nan xing)* and untreated Rhizoma Pinelliae Ternatae *(sheng ban xia)*. Soak in alcohol and apply topically. Do *not* use internally.

4. Dry-fry 500g of table salt and 140g of Fructus Foeniculi Vulgaris *(xiao hui xiang)*. Wrap in cloth, and apply topically while hot.

5. Dry-fry 500g of either Semen Gossypii *(mian hua zi)* (cotton seed) or Excrementum Bombycis Mori *(can sha)* until hot. Add an appropriate amount of alcohol and use as a poultice.

6. Dry-fry together 120g Rhizoma Acori Graminei *(shi chang pu)*, 60g Fructus Foeniculi Vulgaris *(xiao hui xiang)* and 500g table salt until hot. Wrap in cloth, and apply topically while hot.

7. Take 60g of fresh taro, add an appropriate amount of ginger, chives and vinegar, and grind up. Apply topically as a poultice. If taro is not available, potato can be substituted.

8. Put in small packages (25cm x 15cm) 3g Rhizoma Zingiberis Officinalis *(gan jiang)*, 2g Ramulus Cinnamomi Cassiae *(gui zhi)*, 2g Radix Paeoniae Rubrae *(chi shao)*, 2g Radix Angelicae Sinensis *(dang gui)*, 1g Radix et Rhizoma Notopterygii *(qiang huo)*, 1g Radix Puerariae *(ge gen)*, 1g Radix Ligustici Chuanxiong *(chuan xiong)*, 1g Cortex Erythrinae *(hai tong pi)*, 1g Rhizoma Curcumae Longae *(jiang huang)* and 1g Gummi Olibanum *(ru xiang)*. Steam the packages until the steam permeates them. Wait until their temperature drops to 40°C, then apply them topically, sometimes also applying direct electrical current to the packages.

9. Soak for two weeks 30g of Radix Clematidis *(wei ling xian)* in 500ml of aged vinegar, then strain and apply topically with the addition of direct current .

MEDICINAL TINCTURES AND WINES

1. Shi Guo-Gong Medicinal Wine *(shi guo gong yao jiu)*. Ingredients include 120g Os Tigris *(hu gu)* (Os Leopardis *[bao gu]* or Os Canis *[gou gu]* can be substituted), 60g Radix Angelicae Sinensis *(dang gui)*, 60g ginger juice-fried Cortex Eucommiae Ulmoidis *(jiang zhi chao du zhong)*, 60g Radix Achyranthis Bidentatae *(niu xi)*, 60g dry-fried Rhizoma Atractylodis Macrocephalae *(chao bai zhu)*, 60g Fructus Lycii *(gou qi zi)*, 60g deep-fried Carapax Amydae Sinensis *(jiu su bie jia)*, 60g Radix Ledebouriellae Divaricatae *(fang feng)*, 60g Radix et Rhizoma Notopterygii *(qiang huo)*, 60g Lignum Pini Nodi *(song jie)*, 60g dry-fried Excrementum Bombycis Mori *(chao can sha)*, 60g Rhizoma Dioscoreae Hypoglaucae *(bei xie)*, 120g Fructus Xanthii Sibirici *(cang er zi)*, 120g Radix Gentianae Qinjiao *(qin jiao)* and 120g dried cooked Radix Solani Melongenae *(qie gen)*. Coarsely grind all the ingredients together, soak in 30ml of white wine in a sealed container for 10 days, then strain and add 500g of white coarse-grained sugar. Drink one small glass (30-50ml) twice daily.

2. White Flower Snake Wine *(bai hua she jiu)*. Ingredients include 90g Agkistrodon seu Bungarus *(bai hua she)*, 30g Radix et Rhizoma Notopterygii *(qiang huo)*, 30g Radix Ledebouriellae Divaricatae *(fang feng)*, 30g Radix Gentianae Qinjiao *(qin jiao)*, 30g Radix Angelicae Sinensis *(dang gui)*, 30g Cortex Acanthopanacis Gracilistylus Radicis *(wu jia pi)* and 24g Rhizoma Gastrodiae Elatae *(tian ma)*. Soak in 3 to 5 liters of spirits for about one month. Drink 17 to 70ml two to three times daily.

3. Cook in a double boiler for one hour, with 500ml of alcohol, 30g each of Caulis et Rhizoma Sinomenii Acuti *(qing feng teng)*, Caulis Piperis Futokadsurae *(hai feng teng)*, Squama Manitis Pentadactylae *(chuan shan jia)* and Cortex Acanthopanacis Gracilistylus Radicis *(wu jia pi)*. Strain out the herbs and save the wine. Take 30 to 50ml in the morning and evening.

4. Soak 9g each of Flos Lonicerae Japonicae *(jin yin hua)*, Fructus Pruni Mume *(wu mei)*, Radix Aconiti Kusnezoffii Praeparata *(zhi cao wu)*, Radix Aconiti Carmichaeli Praeparata *(zhi chuan wu)*, Radix Glycyrrhizae Uralensis *(gan cao)* and Flos Carthami Tinctorii *(hong hua)* for 12 days in one liter of alcohol. Take 5 to 10ml three times daily.

5. Add to one liter of alcohol equal parts of Flos Carthami Tinctorii *(hong hua)*, Rhizoma Homalomenae Occultae *(qian nian jian)*, Radix Ligustici Chuanxiong *(chuan xiong)*, Ramulus Sangjisheng *(sang ji sheng)*, Radix Cyathulae Officinalis *(chuan niu xi)*, Radix et Rhizoma Notopterygii *(qiang huo)*, Radix Angelicae Pubescentis *(du huo)*, Pericarpium Citri Reticulatae *(chen pi)*, Cortex Acanthopanacis Gracilistylus Radicis *(wu jia pi)*, Radix Angelicae Sinensis *(dang gui)*, Fructus Chaenomelis Lagenariae *(mu gua)*, Rhizoma Polygonati Odorati *(yu zhu)* and Fructus Gardeniae Jasminoidis *(zhi zi)*. Take 30 to 50ml two to three times daily.

6. Add to some alcohol equal parts of Herba Erodii seu Geranii *(lao guan cao)*, Radix et Caulis Erycibes Obstusifoliae *(ding gong teng)*, Ramulus Mori Albae *(sang zhi)* and Herba Siegesbeckiae *(xi xian cao)*. Take 15 to 30ml three times daily.

ACUPUNCTURE

Treatment of painful obstruction with acupuncture is quite effective when performed according to the following guidelines:

1. The practitioner must have a good grasp of tonification and draining needling techniques.

2. If there is stiffness, pain, weakness and paresthesia, use more moxibustion than needling. If there is only local distention, pain, swelling and redness, use acupuncture without moxibustion.

3. For severe conditions, the main points are needled on the healthy side first, and then on the affected side. When the condition has improved, the points on the affected side can be needled first.

4. Needle retention time is generally 10-15 minutes.

Commonly Used Points for Joint Pain

Shoulder: LI-15 *(jian yu)*, TB-14 *(jian liao)*, SI-10 *(nao shu)*, M-UE-48 *(jian qian)*,[7] "Shoulder Back"*(jian hou)*,[8] tender points in the deltoid muscle

Elbow: LI-11 *(qu chi)*, LI-10 *(shou san li)*, LI-4 *(he gu)*, PC-5 *(chi ze)*

Wrist: TB-4 *(yang chi)*, TB-5 *(wai guan)*, LI-4 *(he gu)*

Hip: BL-54 *(zhi bian)*, ST-32 *(fu tu)*, GB-30 *(huan tiao)*

Knee: ST-32 *(fu tu)*, GB-34 *(yang ling quan)*, ST-35 *(du bi)*

Ankle: LR-4 *(zhong feng)*, GB-40 *(qiu xu)*, BL-60 *(kun lun)*, KI-3 *(tai xi)*, ST-41 *(jie xi)*

Other Point Selections

Main points for shoulder, elbow and scapula: LI-15 *(jian yu)*, LI-11 *(qu chi)*, LI-4 *(he gu)*, BL-15 *(fei shu)*. Secondary points: TB-6 *(zhi gou)*, SI-3 *(hou xi)*, PC-5 *(chi ze)*, PC-3 *(qu ze)*, TB-10 *(tian jing)*, TB-15 *(tian liao)*

Main points for wrist, hand and fingers: TB-5 *(wai guan)*, LI-11 *(qu chi)*, LI-4 *(he gu)*. Secondary points: LI-5 *(yang xi)*, TB-4 *(yang chi)*, SI-5 *(yang gu)*, TB-3 *(zhong zhu)*, M-UE-8 *(ba feng)*, M-UE-1 *(shi xuan)*, LU-8 *(jing qu)*, LU-9 *(tai yuan)*, SI-4 *(wan gu)*

Main points for spine: GV-16 *(feng fu)*, GV-14 *(da zhui)*, GV-2 *(yao shu)*, BL-13 *(fei shu)*, BL-14 *(jue yin shu)*. Secondary points: GB-30 *(huan tiao)*, BL-40 *(wei zhong)*, BL-60 *(kun lun)*

Main points for lower limbs: BL-23 *(shen shu)*, BL-25 *(da chang shu)*, BL-31~34 *(ba liao)*, GV-2 *(yao shu)*, GB-30 *(huan tiao)*, GB-34 *(yang ling quan)*, ST-36 *(zu san li)*. Secondary points: GB-31 *(feng shi)*, ST-32 *(fu tu)*, ST-33 *(yin shi)*, LR-2 *(xing jian)*, ST-41 *(jie xi)*, BL-40 *(wei zhong)*, BL-57 *(cheng shan)*, GB-44 *(zu qiao yin)*, GB-39 *(xuan zhong)*, BL-60 *(kun lun)*, KI-6 *(zhao hai)*, KI-2 *(ran gu)*, ST-44 *(nei ting)*, PC-9 *(zhong chong)*, "Jade Yin" *(yu yin)*,[9] LR-4 *(zhong feng)*

Prognosis

At the onset of a painful obstruction disorder, because the normal Qi is not yet in a state of great deficiency and the pathogenic influence is relatively mild and superficial, it is not difficult to obtain a cure if treatment is given in a timely manner. If, however, the opportunity for early treatment is lost, improper treatment is administered, or treatment is neglected during the maintenance stage, the pathogenic influence can shift from the channels, muscles and skin level and penetrate deeply into the vessels and Blood, sinews and bones, before reaching the internal Organs and generating different pathological patterns.

IMPROPER OR POORLY-TIMED TREATMENT

Failure to treat painful obstruction disorder at the onset, thereby allowing it to reach the interior, is to neglect taking advantage of the body's ability to expel the pathogenic influences while they are still in the exterior and the muscles.

It is said that Wind, Cold and Damp pathogenic influences usually "arrive in various ways" and "intermingle to constitute painful obstruction." "Arrive in various ways" means that a pathogenic influence may come sooner or later to attack the body. If, for example, an individual lives in a damp place, works in water, gets caught in the rain, or if he sweats and then exposes himself to wind or goes in the water, he is said to be attacked first by Dampness, and then by Wind-Cold. Or, if a person lives in a very cold area, the muscles and skin are first affected by pathogenic Cold, and then possibly exposed thereafter to Wind or Dampness.

Pathogenic Dampness is stagnant, sticky and tenacious; it cannot be compared to Wind or Cold, which can be eliminated through diaphoresis. These differences are often neglected by patient and physician alike, thereby promoting the settling of pathogenic Dampness inside the body, which may then interact with other external factors.

People who have previously been attacked by Wind-Damp-Cold often re-contract them. This commonly occurs if the person gets wet or is exposed to Dampness when the pathogenic influence has not yet been fully expelled, or during the convalescent stage when the protective Qi is not yet stable.

When Wind-Damp-Cold reside in the body for a long time, they become constrained and can transform into Heat. This can lead to pathogenic Wind-Damp-Cold-Heat in which all the pathogenic influences bind together.

In this form, each pathogenic influence is hard to distinguish and very difficult to eliminate.

Inducing excessive diaphoresis during the early stages of the disease injures the normal Qi. This can harm the yang Qi of both the interior and exterior. When physicians do not differentiate excess from deficiency or acute from chronic diseases, they may (mistakenly) use high doses of herbs to expel Wind, dry Dampness and disperse Cold over a long period of time. This can cause serious injury to the Qi, Blood and Fluids.

When patients fail to rest, are unable to improve their lifestyles or work habits, do not protect themselves from Wind, Cold and Dampness, do not control their sexual activities or their fondness for heavy, rich foods, this can also disrupt the proper functioning of the body. These things will prevent the normal Qi from becoming strong enough to expel the pathogenic influences.

PATHOLOGICAL CHANGES IN LATER STAGES

Changes noted in later stages of painful obstruction are a decline in the general state of health, with the painful obstruction either failing to improve or frequently recurring.

Bone and joint deformation is another late-stage pathological change. This can progress to the point of rotoscoliosis of the thoracic and lumbar spine, or gradual impairment of walking and in using the hands, such that the patient cannot perform daily living activities.

At the same time as the joints become painful, swollen and deformed, there is gradual depletion of and injury to the internal Organs. Symptoms include palpitations, fatigue, shortness of breath, sweating, lower back pain, spermatorrhea, reduced appetite and loose stools. In such cases the prognosis is often poor.

Precautions and Preventive Measures

The first thing in treating painful obstruction disorders is to be sure that the body is protected from Cold and Dampness. This is particularly important when the patient lives in damp and cold areas. The patient must know that if he sweats when exercising, he should avoid exposure to wind; or when her clothes get damp, she must change them. Patients should not bathe or shower immediately after exercising or working while they are still hot and sweaty. It is also important that their bedding be clean and dry. Whenever a person is attacked by external pathogenic influences, they should seek immediate and thorough treatment to prevent progression of the disease to the interior. If the general state of health shows signs of deterioration, sufficient rest must be provided.

Since most painful obstruction disorders are cases of "surplus in the midst of insufficiency," patients must follow rules of proper lifestyle. These include control of sexual activity, moderation of diet, sufficient rest and so on. They should also engage in appropriate physical exercise to increase immunity.

Current Research

CHINESE HERBAL MEDICINE FOR RHEUMATOID ARTHRITIS

Classification of Rheumatoid Arthritis in Traditional Chinese Medicine

Cases of rheumatoid arthritis generally belong to the category of painful obstruction. Since rheumatoid arthritis affects the bones and joints and can cause joint deformation, some authors believe it should be classified as panarthralgia, as described in *Essentials from the Golden Cabinet*. But because panarthralgia also falls within the purview of painful obstruction, this is not really a topic of contention. (Panarthralgia is discussed in the next chapter.)

Classification of Painful Obstruction

Most people base their differentiation of the types of painful obstruction on chapter 43 of *Basic Questions* ("On Painful Obstruction"). There the different clinical manifestations are classified as moving (*xíng*) or Wind-predominant, severely painful (*tòng*) or Cold-predominant, and fixed (*zhuó*) or Damp-predominant painful obstruction. Hot (*rè*) painful obstruction is often added to make a total of four types.

Zhu Dan-Xi also identified three types. He collapsed Wind, Cold and Damp painful obstruction into a single category, to which he added Hot painful obstruction (which includes Wind-Damp-Hot painful obstruction) and stubborn (*wán*) painful obstruction (Kidney deficiency is the root, and Blood stasis is the branch).

There are other ways of differentiating painful obstruction. It can be differentiated into Hot or Cold types. The Hot type can further be divided into yang brightness Heat, yin deficiency with internal Heat, and internally

vigorous Damp-Heat. The Cold type includes Wind, Cold and Damp painful obstructions. Some authors classify painful obstruction according to its stage of progression: Cold, Heat and Cold-Heat complex types can be seen during acute phases, while Liver and Kidney deficiency or harboring of Phlegm and Blood stasis can be identified during phases of stability. Other authors distinguish among mild, moderate and severe conditions. In the mild type, the protective yang is weak and pathogenic Cold attacks the channels. In the moderate type, the Blood and Qi are exhausted and deficient and Damp-Cold obstructs the collaterals. In the severe type, the Liver, Kidneys and Spleen are deficient and turbidity congeals in the joints.

We [the Chinese authors of this text] tend to classify painful obstruction according to deficiency and excess, which seems to better fit clinical reports. This is why we clearly label some cases of painful obstruction as deficient. This includes Blood and Qi deficient painful obstruction, yin deficient painful obstruction, and yang deficient painful obstruction. However, rheumatoid arthritis often presents a complex condition of deficient root with an excessive branch, or enmeshment of deficiency and excess together. Therefore the distinctions between the two types should be regarded as relative, and not taken dogmatically.

Pattern Analysis and Therapeutic Conclusions

Treatment of rheumatoid arthritis is usually based on the differentiation of patterns, with the addition of special substances and formulas. For example, Dr. Fang's[10] approach, based on the theory that "the Liver governs the sinews and the Kidneys govern the bones," considers this disease to be located in the Liver and Kidneys. In character he considers the root to be yin deficiency or yang deficiency; its branches additionally harbor such influences as Wind, Cold, Dampness, Heat, Blood stasis or Phlegm.

When the symptoms of Wind, Cold, Dampness and Heat are rather acute and severe, the prescription is commonly based on Major Gentiana Qinjiao Decoction (*da qin jiao tang*).

When both the normal Qi is deficient and the pathogenic influence is excessive, the focus of treatment is to strengthen the normal Qi and simultaneously to eliminate the pathogenic influence. The basic formula is a modification of Tangkuei, Peony, and Rehmannia Decoction (*dang shao di huang tang*) containing Radix Angelicae Sinensis (*dang gui*), Radix Paeoniae Lactiflorae (*bai shao*), Radix Rehmanniae Glutinosae (*sheng di huang*), Rhizoma

Atractylodis *(cang zhu)*, Fructus Chaenomelis Lagenariae *(mu gua)*, Cortex Moutan Radicis *(mu dan pi)*, Sclerotium Poriae Cocos *(fu ling)*, Rhizoma Alismatis Orientalis *(ze xie)*, Radix Achyranthis Bidentatae *(niu xi)*, Semen Plantaginis *(che qian zi)*, Ramulus Cinnamomi Cassiae *(gui zhi)*, Radix Clematidis *(wei ling xian)* and Rhizoma Dioscoreae Nipponicae *(chuan shan long)* .

For Cold, add Radix Lateralis Aconiti Carmichaeli Praeparata *(fu zi)*; for Heat, add Gypsum *(shi gao)*. For severe yin deficiency, increase the dosage of Radix Rehmanniae Glutinosae *(sheng di huang)* (up to 60g). For Qi deficiency, add Radix Ginseng *(ren shen)* and Radix Astragali Membranacei *(huang qi)*.

Based on the theories that "its root is located in the Kidneys" and "long-term pain enters the collaterals," Dr. Zhu[11] advocates tonifying the Kidneys and fortifying the Governing vessel to address the root, while using insect and reptile substances that invigorate the Blood and unblock the collaterals to treat the branch. Using a formula he developed called Augment the Kidneys and Remove Painful Obstruction Pill *(yi shen juan pi wan)*, Dr. Zhu treated 155 patients and obtained a 71 percent rate of success or marked improvement with an overall effectiveness rate of 96 percent.

Dr. Dai[12] used large amounts of the three Aconites—Radix Aconiti Carmichaeli Praeparata *(zhi chuan wu)*, Radix Aconiti Kusnezoffii Praeparata *(zhi cao wu)* and Radix Lateralis Aconiti Carmichaeli Praeparata *(fu zi)*—as the chief herbs. He added Rhizoma Zingiberis Officinalis *(gan jiang)*, Herba cum Radice Asari *(xi xin)*, Herba Ephedrae *(ma huang)* and Ramulus Cinnamomi Cassiae *(gui zhi)* to make a special formula to warm the channels and alleviate pain. For Damp-Heat painful obstruction, herbs to clear Heat and resolve Dampness were used as adjuncts to Radix Aconiti Carmichaeli Praeparata *(zhi chuan wu)* and Radix Aconiti Kusnezoffii Praeparata *(zhi cao wu)*.

There are also reports of using Cinnamon Twig, Peony, and Anemarrhena Decoction *(gui zhi shao yao zhi mu tang)* as the main formula.[13] To this formula, Gypsum *(shi gao)* is added for fever, Radix et Caulis Jixueteng *(ji xue teng)* for Blood deficiency, Radix Stephaniae Tetrandrae *(fang ji)* and Rhizoma Dioscoreae Hypoglaucae *(bei xie)* for severe Dampness with swelling of the limbs, and Radix Astragali Membranacei *(huang qi)* for Qi deficiency.

Other authors use a basic formula comprised of Rhizoma et Radix Notopterygii *(qiang huo)*, Radix Angelicae Pubescentis *(du huo)*, Ramulus Cinnamomi Cassiae *(gui zhi)*, Radix Ledebouriallae Divaricatae *(fang feng)*, Rhizoma Atractylodis *(cang zhu)*, Radix Angelicae Sinensis *(dang gui)* and Flos Carthami Tinctorii *(hong hua)*. For Cold, add Radix Aconiti Carmichaeli Praeparata *(zhi chuan wu)* and Radix Aconiti Kusnezoffii Praeparata *(zhi cao wu)*. For Heat, replace Radix et Rhizoma Notopterygii *(qiang huo)* and Radix Angelicae Pubescentis *(du huo)* with Rhizoma Anemarrhenae Asphodeloidis *(zhi mu)* and Radix Scutellariae Baicalensis *(huang qin)*. For Qi deficiency, add Radix Astragali Membranacei *(huang qi)*. For insufficient Blood, add Radix Paeoniae Lactiflorae *(bai shao)*. The addition of herbs to dispel Wind and unblock the collaterals may also be considered, such as Radix Gentianae Qinjiao *(qin jiao)*, Ramulus Mori Albae *(sang zhi)*, Fasciculus Vascularis Luffae *(si gua luo)*, Rhizoma Curcumae Longae *(jiang huang)*, Cortex Erythrinae *(hai tong pi)*, Caulis Trachelospermi Jasminoidis *(luo shi teng)* and Rhizoma Homalomenae Occultae *(qian nian jian)*.

Other reports mention Angelica Pubescens and Sangjisheng Decoction *(du huo ji sheng tang)* as the basic prescription. For Cold, add Radix Lateralis Aconiti Carmichaeli Praeparata *(fu zi)*; if the Cold is severe, increase the dosage of Radix Ledebouriallae Divaricatae *(fang feng)* and Ramulus Cinnamomi Cassiae *(gui zhi)*. For intense Heat, increase the dosage of Radix Gentianae Qinjiao *(qin jiao)* and Radix Rehmanniae Glutinosae *(sheng di huang)*; replace Radix Paeoniae Lactiflorae *(bai shao)* with Radix Paeoniae Rubrae *(chi shao)* and Ramulus Cinnamomi Cassiae *(gui zhi)* with Ramulus Mori Albae *(sang zhi)*; and add Radix Scutellariae Baicalensis *(huang qin)*, Radix Aristolochiae Fangchi *(fang ji)* and Ramus Lonicerae Japonicae *(ren dong teng)*. For pronounced Dampness, remove Radix Rehmanniae Glutinosae *(sheng di huang)* and add Rhizoma Atractylodis *(cang zhu)*, Semen Coicis Lachryma-jobi *(yi yi ren)* and Rhizoma Atractylodis Macrocephalae *(bai zhu)*. For Blood stasis, add Semen Persicae *(tao ren)*, Flos Carthami Tinctorii *(hong hua)* and Radix Paeoniae Rubrae *(chi shao)*. For problems in the upper limbs, add Rhizoma Curcumae Longae *(jiang huang)* and Radix Clematidis *(wei ling xian)*. For pain in the lower limbs, add Radix Achyranthis Bidentatae *(niu xi)* and Fructus Chaenomelis Lagenariae *(mu gua)*.

A review of the experimental literature suggests that modern practitioners have made some progress in understanding and treating Hot painful obstruction (Wind-Damp-Heat and Damp-Heat painful obstructions). In terms of pathology, more than a few authors believe that the etiology of painful obstruction cannot be limited to the "three influences Wind, Cold and Dampness [which] arrive in various ways, intermingle and constitute painful obstruction."[14] They further believe that the concept of Hot painful obstruction resulting from a transformation of constrained Wind, Cold and Dampness, or from an internal accumulation of Heat with accompanying attack by an external pathogenic influence, simply does not correspond to reality. They emphasize the fact that pathogenic Heat can penetrate through the mouth and nose and attack the patient directly, thereby giving rise to painful obstruction.

Dr. Zhang believes that in the clinic, many more cases of rheumatoid arthritis belong to the Hot than to the Cold category. Traditional Chinese medicine is also more effective in treating Hot-type rheumatoid arthritis than Cold type. For pronounced Heat and relatively mild Dampness, the basic prescription is White Tiger plus Cinnamon Twig Decoction *(bai hu jia gui zhi tang)*, with the addition of such substances as Ramus Lonicerae Japonicae *(ren dong teng)*, Ramulus et Folium Tamaricis *(cheng liu)*, Radix Paeoniae Rubrae *(chi shao)*, Radix Rehmanniae Glutinosae *(sheng di huang)*, Radix Stephaniae Tetrandrae *(han fang ji)* and Calcitum *(han shui shi)*. For Damp-Heat, use Four-Marvel Powder *(si miao san)* as the main formula.

In another clinical series, Wind-Damp-Heat was treated with Wind-Dampness Formula No. 1 *(feng shi fang I)*, which contains Flos Lonicerae Japonicae *(jin yin hua)*, Radix Rehmanniae Glutinosae *(sheng di huang)*, Rhizoma Smilacis Glabrae *(tu fu ling)*, Radix Cynanchi Baiwei *(bai wei)*, Cortex Moutan Radicis *(mu dan pi)*, Herba Dendrobii *(shi hu)*, Radix Clematidis *(wei ling xian)*, Herba Artemisiae Annuae *(qing hao)*, Radix Gentianae Qinjiao *(qin jiao)*, Radix Achyranthis Bidentatae *(niu xi)* and Ramulus Mori Albae *(sang zhi)*.

When both Dampness and Heat are vigorous, Wind-Dampness Formula No. 2 *(feng shi fang II)* was used. This formula consists of Rhizoma Smilacis Glabrae *(tu fu ling)*, Rhizoma Atractylodis *(cang zhu)*, Cortex Phellodendri *(huang bai)*, Cortex Erythrinae *(hai tong pi)*, Semen Coicis Lachryma-jobi *(yi yi ren)*, Sclerotium Poriae Cocos *(fu ling)*, Radix Stephaniae Tetrandrae *(han fang ji)*, Radix Clematidis *(wei ling xian)*, Rhizoma Dioscoreae Hypoglaucae *(bei xie)*, Radix Angelicae Pubescentis *(du huo)*, Radix Paeoniae Rubrae *(chi shao)* and Lignum Pini Nodi *(song jie)*.

Using the above methods, a success rate of 90 percent was reported in a sample of 116 cases.[15]

Dr. Dai's team, on the other hand, believes that most cases of rheumatoid arthritis belong to the Cold category. Based on 149 clinical cases, 142 of which were caused by Wind-Damp-Cold with Cold predominating, they advocate administering large doses of Radix Lateralis Aconiti Carmichaeli Praeparata *(fu zi)* and Radix Aconiti *(wu tou)* to warm the channels and attack the painful obstruction.

The divergence between these two points of view [Dr. Zhang's and Dr. Dai's] could be explained by the different geographic origins of the authors.

Besides these considerations, many physicians pay special attention to deficient painful obstruction disorders. They believe that such disorders should not be treated as patterns of excess; that they should be removed from the Wind-Damp-Cold framework; and that therapeutic methods such as dispersing Wind, eliminating Cold and draining Dampness should not be used in their treatment, as they risk further injury to the Qi and Blood.

For yang deficiency, some authors recommend Yang-Heartening Decoction *(yang he tang)* with the addition of Radix Lateralis Aconiti Carmichaeli Praeparata *(fu zi)* and Radix Angelicae Sinensis *(dang gui)* as the primary formula. Herbs to tonify the Kidneys and fortify the Governing vessel can also be added, such as Rhizoma Cibotii Barometz *(gou ji)*, Ramulus Sangjisheng *(sang ji sheng)*, Radix Morindae Officinalis *(ba ji tian)*, Fructus Psoraleae Corylifoliae *(bu gu zhi)* and Radix Dipsaci Asperi *(xu duan)*.

For yin deficiency, the treatment principle is to nourish the Blood and make the sinews supple. Frequently, large doses of such herbs as Radix Rehmanniae Glutinosae *(sheng di huang)*, Herba Dendrobii *(shi hu)*, Radix Paeoniae Lactiflorae *(bai shao)*, Radix Adenophorae seu Glehniae *(sha shen)*, Tuber Ophiopogonis Japonici *(mai men dong)*, Fructus Chaenomelis Lagenariae *(mu gua)*, Radix Salviae Miltiorrhizae *(dan shen)*, Rhizoma Polygonati Odorati *(yu zhu)*, Radix Achyranthis Bidentatae *(niu xi)*, Cortex Moutan Radicis *(mu dan pi)*, Ramulus cum Uncis Uncariae *(gou teng)*, Fructus Tribuli Terrestris *(bai ji li)* and Ramus Lonicerae Japonicae *(ren dong teng)* are used. Most of these are sweet, cold substances that soften and moisten. They are commonly combined with such herbs as Radix et Caulis Jixueteng *(ji xue teng)*, Herba Erodii seu Geranii *(lao guan cao)*, Herba Siegesbeckiae *(xi xian cao)* and Ramulus Sangjisheng *(sang ji sheng)* to remove the painful obstruction and unblock the collaterals.

For internal stirring of Liver Wind, substances that

anchor and sedate should be added. All this knowledge and experience deserves serious consideration.

The Use of Radix Aconiti *(wu tou)* and Radix Lateralis Aconiti Carmichaeli Praeparata *(fu zi)*

The use of Radix Aconiti *(wu tou)* and Radix Lateralis Aconiti Carmichaeli Praeparata *(fu zi)* raises several issues, including patterns for which they are suitable, dosage, combination with other substances, and preparation.

Dr. Zhu[16] states that "Radix Aconiti *(wu tou)* has demonstrated a proven efficacy for treating joint pain; it is, however, unsuitable when there is local heat, redness and swelling, or when there is fever and thirst." This means that Radix Aconiti *(wu tou)*—and also Radix Lateralis Aconiti Carmichaeli Praeparata *(fu zi)*—is suitable for Wind-Damp-Cold painful obstruction disorders.

Clinically, most early and middle stage cases of rheumatoid arthritis are of the Wind-Damp-Cold type. The yang deficient type is characteristic of later stages. There are thus many opportunities for prescribing Radix Aconiti *(wu tou)* and Radix Lateralis Aconiti Carmichaeli Praeparata *(fu zi)*.

Radix Aconiti Carmichaeli Praeparata *(zhi chuan wu)* and Radix Aconiti Kusnezoffii Praeparata *(zhi cao wu)* are prescribed to warm the channels and alleviate pain. Radix Lateralis Aconiti Carmichaeli Praeparata *(fu zi)* is used to tonify the yang Qi. However, these substances are frequently combined for their synergistic effect. Dr. Dai,[17] for example, often prescribes his personal formula Aconite, Lateral Aconite, Ephedra, Asarum, Cinnamon Twigs, Ginger, and Licorice Decoction *(wu fu ma xin gui jiang cao tang)*, which is comprised of 15-60g Radix Aconiti Carmichaeli Praeparata *(zhi chuan wu)*, 15-60g Radix Aconiti Kusnezoffii Praeparata *(zhi cao wu)*, 30-120g Radix Lateralis Aconiti Carmichaeli Praeparata *(fu zi)*, 12-20g Herba Ephedrae *(ma huang)*, 6-12g Herba cum Radice Asari *(xi xin)*, 30-60g Ramulus Cinnamomi Cassiae *(gui zhi)*, 30-90g Rhizoma Zingiberis Officinalis *(gan jiang)* or Rhizoma Zingiberis Officinalis Recens *(sheng jiang)* , and 30-60g of either honey-toasted Radix Glycyrrhizae Uralensis *(zhi gan cao)* or Radix Glycyrrhizae Uralensis *(gan cao)*.

Dr. Li[18] commonly uses a formula comprised of 30g Radix Aconiti Carmichaeli Praeparata *(zhi chuan wu)*, 60g Radix Lateralis Aconiti Carmichaeli Praeparata *(fu zi)*, 9g Herba cum Radice Asari *(xi xin)*, 15g Ramulus Cinnamomi Cassiae *(gui zhi)*, 12g Radix Ledebouriallae Divaricatae *(fang feng)*, 24g Rhizoma Atractylodis *(cang zhu)*, 15g Caulis Trachelospermi Jasminoidis *(luo shi teng)*, 15g Lignum Pini Nodi *(song jie)*, 12g Radix Ligustici Chuanxiong *(chuan xiong)*, 15g Radix Paeoniae Lactiflorae *(bai shao)*, 15g Cortex Acanthopanacis Gracilistylus Radicis *(wu jia pi)*, 24g Radix Angelicae Sinensis *(dang gui)*, 30g Cornu Cervi Degelatinatium *(lu jiao shuang)*, 15g Cortex Eucommiae Ulmoidis *(du zhong)*, 15g Ramulus Sangjisheng *(sang ji sheng)*, 12g Radix Angelicae Pubescentis *(du huo)*, 12g Radix Achyranthis Bidentatae *(niu xi)*, 30g Semen Coicis Lachryma-jobi *(yi yi ren)*, 30g Radix Codonopsitis Pilosulae *(dang shen)*, 12g Rhizoma Alpiniac Officinari *(gao liang jiang)*, 10g honey-toasted Radix Glycyrrhizae Uralensis *(zhi gan cao)*, 9g Fructus Amomi *(sha ren)* and 25g Fructus Zizyphi Jujubae *(da zao)*.

All of these authors advocate that, for long-term severe disease, it is necessary to use high dosages of Radix Aconiti Carmichaeli Praeparata *(zhi chuan wu)*, Radix Aconiti Kusnezoffii Praeparata *(zhi cao wu)* and Radix Lateralis Aconiti Carmichaeli Praeparata *(fu zi)*. Low dosages are ineffective.

In Dr. Dai's experience, Radix Aconiti *(wu tou)* is a mandatory herb regardless of whether the painful obstruction is a Cold or Hot variety. For Damp-Cold painful obstruction, use the formulas described above. For Damp-Hot painful obstruction, continue to rely on the strengths of Radix Aconiti Carmichaeli Praeparata *(zhi chuan wu)* in alleviating pain and eliminating painful obstruction, and combine it with such herbs as Cortex Phellodendri *(huang bai)*, Talcum *(hua shi)*, Semen Coicis Lachryma-jobi *(yi yi ren)*, Herba Lophatheri Gracilis *(dan zhu ye)*, Fructus Forsythiae Suspensae *(lian qiao)*, Fructus Amomi Kravanh *(bai dou kou)* and Cortex Poriae Cocos *(fu ling pi)*.

Dr. Zhu often uses capsules of Secretio Moschus *(she xiang)* along with decoctions of such herbs as Radix Aconiti Carmichaeli Praeparata *(zhi chuan wu)*, Ramulus Cinnamomi Cassiae *(gui zhi)*, Herba Epimedii *(yin yang huo)*, Radix Angelicae Sinensis *(dang gui)*, Herba cum Radice Asari *(xi xin)* and Radix Angelicae Pubescentis *(du huo)*. When the Cold pathogenic influence is relatively mild and the patient's constitution is weak, he uses Radix Aconiti Carmichaeli Praeparata *(zhi chuan wu)*; when the Cold pathogenic influence is severe, he uses untreated Radix Aconiti Carmichaeli *(sheng chuan wu)*. In addition, Dr. Zhu notes that the effect of Radix Aconiti Kusnezoffii *(cao wu)* on painful obstruction and pain is greater than that of Radix Aconiti Carmichaeli *(chuan wu)*, and that they can be used together in treating severe conditions.

For adults, start with a dosage of 3 to 5g, and increase gradually to 10 to 15g a day. This is a safe and effective way to use these herbs.

Dr. Zhang[19] has used Aconite Decoction (*wu tou tang*) to treat Wind-Cold painful obstruction, but the formula he generally uses is comprised of 4-9g Radix Aconiti Carmichaeli Praeparata (*zhi chuan wu*), 3-6g Herba Ephedrae (*ma huang*), 6-9g Radix Angelicae Pubescentis (*du huo*), 15-30g Radix Aristolochiae Fangchi (*fang ji*), 6g Caulis Mutong (*mu tong*), 12-18g Radix Astragali Membranacei (*huang qi*), 15g Radix Angelicae Sinensis (*dang gui*) and 45g Radix Glycyrrhizae Uralensis (*gan cao*). Other herbs are added according to whether Wind, Cold or Dampness predominates, and whether there is Heat, Phlegm or Blood stasis.

Some authors, however, believe that Radix Aconiti Carmichaeli Praeparata (*zhi chuan wu*) and Radix Lateralis Aconiti Carmichaeli Praeparata (*fu zi*) should not be prescribed in high dosages, as their effects might extend beyond the location of the disease, and prolonged use could exhaust the Qi and injure the Blood.

Different points of view have always existed on this question. They might be due to differences in geographic location influencing patient tolerance for these herbs, or to differences in the prescription habits of the physicians. This leads to marked differences in the dosages of Radix Aconiti (*wu tou*) and Radix Lateralis Aconiti Carmichaeli Praeparata (*fu zi*), and is the reason why we [the Chinese authors] share Dr. Zhu's recommendation of gradually increasing the dosage to meet the threshold of efficacy, and to lower it step by step once the desired result is achieved.

To prepare these herbs in decoctions, they must be boiled for a long time to eliminate their toxicity without destroying their therapeutic properties. The unprepared herb must be boiled for three hours; the prepared form for two hours. This process should not be considered complete until there is no numbing sensation when the liquid is placed on the tongue.

According to modern research, the toxicity of all these aconite products is related to their alkaloids (such as aconitine), especially their effect on intra-cardiac conduction. Because these constituents are water-soluble and dispersed by heat, all it takes to eliminate this problem is boiling the herb for a sufficient period of time. Experiments conducted outside of China have shown that heat and high pressure eliminate the toxicity of Radix Aconiti (*wu tou*) and Radix Lateralis Aconiti Carmichaeli Praeparata (*fu zi*) while maintaining their cardiotonic and diuretic properties.

The type of combinations used with Radix Aconiti (*wu tou*) and Radix Lateralis Aconiti Carmichaeli Praeparata (*fu zi*) are also very important. Generally speaking, the addition of high dosages of Radix Glycyrrhizae Uralensis (*gan cao*), honey and Rhizoma Zingiberis Officinalis (*gan jiang*) strengthen the analgesic effect, and also further control toxicity. If, after ingesting Radix Aconiti (*wu tou*) or Radix Lateralis Aconiti Carmichaeli Praeparata (*fu zi*), the patient experiences such signs of toxicity as paresthesia of the tongue or vertigo, the treatment must be immediately discontinued and large quantities of honey (90 to 120g) and rice water, or high doses of Radix Ledebouriallae Divaricatae (*fang feng*), Radix Glycyrrhizae Uralensis (*gan cao*) or mung bean soup, must be prescribed as antidotes. If signs of tachycardia, coma or a slow or irregular pulse appear, emergency intervention is required.

Single Herbs: Current Research and Use

Recently, some Chinese herbs that are relatively effective in treating this condition have been discovered. One example is Radix Folium et Flos Tripterygii Wilfordi (*lei gong teng*), found in Hubei and other regions of China. It has been tested as a monotherapy, either in decoctions or tinctures, to treat rheumatoid arthritis. In the beginning, research was done on 116 cases and the overall rate of effectiveness was 91.8 percent. Later this work was extended throughout that province and over 500 cases were reported. The rate of effectiveness was 91 to 95 percent. The daily dosage was usually 10 to 20g, and even the highest daily dosage did not exceed 30g. Tripterygium tablets have been made from the original herb. Thay have been used for rheumatoid arthritis, Wind-Damp-Hot painful obstruction, chronic nephritis and systemic lupus erythematosus, with a certain degree of success.

Later, other regions such as Fujian, Guilin and Nanjing conducted therapeutic experiments on rheumatoid arthritis using this herb, with good preliminary results. However, the chemical composition of this herb has not yet been completely identified.[20] It would appear to be able to regulate the immunological functions of the body. Whether fresh or in prepared form, this herb has definite toxic side effects, and its safety margin is rather narrow; signs of poisoning or even death can occur beyond a certain dosage. In some reports of poisoning the mortality rate has reached 41.8 percent. This herb must therefore be used with extreme caution. Extensive additional research is needed.

In Kunming, Herba Radix seu Fructus Begoniae Yunnanensis *(shan hai tang)* has been used to treat rheumatoid arthritis with very significant results. This herb can alleviate pain, swelling and range of motion difficulties. It has relatively few side effects. In one study of 15 cases (with the longest duration of disease being 15 years), the results were excellent in five cases, and good in seven cases, with a prescribed dosage of two 25mg pills three times daily, usually for one month (the longest treatment lasted one year).

In addition, the pharmacology of other herbs are being studied as they relate to rheumatoid arthritis. These include Radix Rehmanniae Glutinosae *(sheng di huang)*, Radix Gentianae Qinjiao *(qin jiao)*, Radix Ginseng *(ren shen)*, Herba cum Radice Asari *(xi xin)*, Radix Angelicae Pubescentis *(du huo)*, Radix Ligustici Chuanxiong *(chuan xiong)*, Radix Angelicae Sinensis *(dang gui)*, Radix Ledebouriellae Divaricatae *(fang feng)* and Radix Glycyrrhizae Uralensis *(gan cao)*.

It has been reported that all the measures of blood viscosity in patients with rheumatoid arthritis are higher than normal. After appropriate herbal therapy these measurements, which include sedimentation rate, significantly return to normal. This supports the theory that the effect of Chinese herbs on this disease is likely to be, at least in part, mediated by their effect on blood viscosity and sedimentation rates. Other researchers believe that Chinese herbs which tonify the Qi, Blood or Kidneys, or that are made of insects and reptiles, act on this disease by strengthening the organism's immunity while dampening the immune response.

CHINESE HERBAL MEDICINE FOR RHEUMATIC FEVER

Generally speaking, acute rheumatic fever[21] is classified in the Hot painful obstruction category. The formula commonly used for this disorder is White Tiger plus Cinnamon Twig Decoction *(bai hu jia gui zhi tang)*, to which are added, as needed, Ramulus Mori Albae *(sang zhi)*, Radix Gentianae Qinjiao *(qin jiao)* and Ramus Lonicerae Japonicae *(ren dong teng)*,

For Heat excess, add Calcitum *(han shui shi)*, Rhizoma Anemarrhenae Asphodeloidis *(zhi mu)*, Gypsum *(shi gao)*, Radix Gentianae Longdancao *(long dan cao)*, Flos Lonicerae Japonicae *(jin yin hua)* and Fructus Forsythiae Suspensae *(lian qiao)*. For Damp excess, add Rhizoma Atractylodis *(cang zhu)*, Talcum *(hua shi)* and Excrementum Bombycis Mori *(can sha)*. For severe pain,

add Gummi Olibanum *(ru xiang)*, Myrrha *(mo yao)*, Rhizoma Corydalis Yanhusuo *(yan hu suo)* and Fructus Rhododendri Mollis *(liu zhou zi)*. When Dampness and Heat are both vigorous, Three-Nut Decoction *(san ren tang)* and Four-Marvel Powder *(si miao san)* can be used. Signs such as heart palpitations, red tongue and rapid pulse often indicate that the yin has been injured by a combination of the pathogenic influences Wind, Dampness and Heat. When this occurs, it is also necessary to nourish the Heart yin.

The Traditional Chinese Medicine Research Group of the Sichuan Medical School has reported that in cases of rheumatic fever and rheumatic carditis, the pattern must be analyzed from the perspective of the four levels (protective, Qi, nutritive and Blood). The fundamental pathogenic pattern is linked to the invasion of the pathogenic influences from the exterior to the interior, from the protective level to the Qi level, and then on to the nutritive and Blood levels. Clinically, the vast majority of patients have problems at either the Qi level or the nutritive/Blood levels. The treatment principle is therefore to clear Heat, cool the Blood, and relieve Toxicity.

When Heat spreads through the Qi level, White Tiger Decoction *(bai hu tang)* is the main formula, with the addition of Flos Lonicerae Japonicae *(jin yin hua)*, Fructus Forsythiae Suspensae *(lian qiao)*, Ramulus Mori Albae *(sang zhi)*, Radix Achyranthis Bidentatae *(niu xi)*, Fructus Chaenomelis Lagenariae *(mu gua)*, Radix Aristolochiae Fangchi *(fang ji)*, Radix Gentianae Qinjiao *(qin jiao)*, Ramulus Cinnamomi Cassiae *(gui zhi)*, Rhizoma Atractylodis *(cang zhu)*, Herba Siegesbeckiae *(xi xian cao)*, Rhizoma Curcumae Longae *(jiang huang)* and Ramulus et Folium Tamaricis *(cheng liu)*.

When exterior symptoms are also present, add Herba seu Flos Schizonepetae Tenuifoliae *(jing jie)*, Herba Menthae Haplocalycis *(bo he)*, Fructus Arctii Lappae *(niu bang zi)* and Semen Sojae Praeparatum *(dan dou chi)*. For severe sore throat, add Radix Scutellariae Baicalensis *(huang qin)*, Radix Sophorae Tonkinensis *(shan dou gen)*, Fructificatio Lasiosphere seu Calvatiae *(ma bo)*, Rhizoma Belamcandae Chinensis *(she gan)* and Radix Platycodi Grandiflori *(jie geng)*. For high fever, add Rhizoma Coptidis *(huang lian)*, Cortex Phellodendri *(huang bai)*, Fructus Gardeniae Jasminoidis *(zhi zi)* and Purple Snow Special Pill *(zi xue dan)*.

For Heat blazing in both the Qi and nutritive levels, use such formulas as Clear the Nutritive Level Decoction *(qing ying tang)*, Rhinoceros Horn and Rehmannia Decoction *(xi jiao di huang tang)* or Clear Epidemics and

Overcome Toxin Decoction (qing wen bai du yin). For fever with profuse sweating, or during the post-febrile stage when the Qi and yin are insufficient, use such formulas as Generate the Pulse Powder (sheng mai san), Benefit the Stomach Decoction (yi wei tang) or Lophatherus and Gypsum Decoction (zhu ye shi gao tang). For uneasiness in the precordium with palpitations, use honey-toasted Radix Glycyrrhizae Uralensis (zhi gan cao) to Generate the Pulse Powder (sheng mai san). This formula tonifies the Heart and calms the Spirit. For localized infections, use Six-Miracle Pill (liu shen wan) and, topically, apply Borneal and Borax Powder (bing peng san).

There are reports that a formula comprised of Flos Lonicerae Japonicae (jin yin hua), Radix Isatidis seu Baphicacanthi (ban lan gen), Radix Gentianae Qinjiao (qin jiao), Radix Clematidis (wei ling xian), Ramulus Cinnamomi Cassiae (gui zhi), Radix et Rhizoma Notopterygii (qiang huo) and Radix Angelicae Pubescentis (du huo) has been used successfully in treating active rheumatic fever. Each packet is decocted and then divided into two doses. When the heart rate is increased, add Semen Biotae Orientalis (bai zi ren) and Semen Zizyphi Spinosae (suan zao ren). For fever, add Radix Bupleuri (chai hu) and Radix Scutellariae Baicalensis (huang qin). For high fever, add Gypsum (shi gao).

There are also reports of using the formula Augmented Stephania and Rehmannia Decoction (jia wei fang ji di huang tang), which includes Radix Stephaniae Tetrandrae (han fang ji), Radix Rehmanniae Glutinosae (sheng di huang), Radix Ledebouriellae Divaricatae (fang feng), Ramulus Cinnamomi Cassiae (gui zhi), Radix Glycyrrhizae Uralensis (gan cao), Herba Taraxaci Mongolici cum Radice (pu gong ying), Flos Chrysanthemi Indici (ye ju hua), Ramus Lonicerae Japonicae (ren dong teng), Ramulus et Folium Tamaricis (cheng liu) and Radix et Rhizoma Notopterygii (qiang huo). This formula has bitter, cold herbs that relieve Toxicity and acrid, warm herbs to unblock painful obstruction and relieve the joint symptoms. If the tongue is red, the throat sore and the joints red, swollen and hot, and there are skin macules, remove Ramulus Cinnamomi Cassiae (gui zhi) and Radix et Rhizoma Notopterygii (qiang huo), and increase the dosage of Radix Rehmanniae Glutinosae (sheng di huang) to 60-90g. Also add Cortex Moutan Radicis (mu dan pi), Radix Paeoniae Rubrae (chi shao), Cornu Bubali (shui niu jiao) and Radix Arnebiae seu Lithospermi (zi cao). If the fever is very high, add Gypsum (shi gao). Take one packet a day.

However, as noted in various reports, sometimes patients with a modern biomedical diagnosis of rheumatic fever will have a traditional diagnosis of Wind-Damp-Cold painful obstruction. Our diagnosis must therefore not be bound by biomedical nosology, but should be based on the differentiation of patterns. Patients who suffer from rheumatic fever usually have febrile symptoms. However, fever does not necessarily correspond to the presence of a Hot pathogenic influence, but is commonly due to the combination of Dampness and Heat. Constrained Damp-Cold transforming into Heat, or a yin deficiency-induced internal Heat, are not uncommon either. If a high fever occurs in the context of Damp-Cold painful obstruction, Aconite Decoction (wu tou tang), with some additional ingredients, is still the treatment recommended for the root condition. This illustrates how a biomedical diagnosis must be re-evaluated in accordance with traditional Chinese medicine theory through the analysis of symptoms.

A team led by Dr. Bei[22] presented the results of a survey of 60 cases of rheumatic arthritis, distributed between Wind-Damp-Hot and Wind-Damp-Cold painful obstruction categories. In the first group, the prescribed therapeutic method was to clear Heat and unblock the collaterals, while adjunctively dispersing Wind and dispelling Dampness. For this group, a modified form of Aristolochia Decoction (mu fang ji tang) was used. In the second group, the treatment principle was to unblock the painful obstruction by invigorating the collaterals, with the addition of herbs that dispel Wind, disperse Cold and drive out Dampness. For this group, the formula prescribed was Remove Painful Obstruction Decoction from Medical Revelations (juan bi tang). The results were as follow: 3 were basically cured, 25 had significant improvement, 14 had some improvement, and 8 experienced no change.[23] In both groups the sedimentation rate, antistreptolysin O titers and other laboratory markers significantly decreased toward normal levels. According to Dr. Zhu,[24] when warming and heating herbs are used for treating Cold painful obstruction, and those that clear Heat in cases of Hot painful obstruction, the relevant biochemical markers are lowered and become more normal.

In treating rheumatic fever, some authors further recommend that differentiation of patterns and diagnosis of disease must be combined. This is because while arthritis can be detected during clinical exams, the diagnosis of cardiac problems often requires the use of imaging techniques and electrocardiography. Although the redness and swelling of the joints can diminish after treatment, along with the associated pain, improvement in myocarditis takes a certain amount of time. For this reason one cannot discontinue treatment just because the joint symptoms have improved. The authors believe that treatment during the recovery period should focus on regulating and tonifying the Qi and Blood. Most patients need to be followed for at least three months.

CHINESE MEDICAL TREATMENT OF SCIATICA

The clinical symptoms of sciatica are continuous dull pain, stabbing pain, or gripping pain in the lower back and lower limbs. It is often triggered by changes in the weather, exposure to cold, and overwork. Pain is particularly severe during these attacks. Because there is no local heat, or only a subjective sensation of heat that cannot be felt by others, this condition can be interpreted and treated as Wind-Damp-Cold painful obstruction or as stubborn painful obstruction.

According to the experience of Dr. Gong,[25] Cinnamon Twig, Peony, and Anemarrhena Decoction (*gui zhi shao yao zhi mu tang*) is useful in treating this condition. However, the dosage must be large, for if you treat a serious condition with a mild formula it is hard to get results. Dr. Gong's usual dosages for this formula are as follows: Ramulus Cinnamomi Cassiae (*gui zhi*) 24g, Radix Ledbouriallae Divaricatae (*fang feng*) 24g, Radix Paeoniae Lactiflorae (*bai shao*) 18g, Herba Ephedrae (*ma huang*) 12g, Rhizoma Zingiberis Officinalis Recens (*sheng jiang*) 30g, Rhizoma Atractylodis Macrocephalae (*bai zhu*) 30g, Rhizoma Anemarrhenae Asphodeloidis (*zhi mu*) 24g, and Radix Lateralis Aconiti Carmichaeli Praeparata (*fu zi*) 60g (boiled for two hours before adding the other ingredients). One packet is prescribed daily, with a normal course of treatment being three to twenty days. In addition, coarsely grind 30g each of untreated Radix Aconiti Carmichaeli (*sheng chuan wu*) and untreated Radix Aconiti Kusnezoffii (*sheng cao wu*), and 9g of Fructus Evodiae Rutaecarpae (*wu zhu yu*). Fry with table salt until black, and, while still hot, place it in a cheesecloth bag and apply locally.

There are also reports of using a compound variation of Aconite Decoction (*wu tou tang*). Soak the following in two liters of white wine for ten days: Radix Aconiti Carmichaeli Praeparata (*zhi chuan wu*) 30g, Radix Aconiti Kusnezoffii Praeparata (*zhi cao wu*) 30g, Flos Lonicerae Japonicae (*jin yin hua*) 30g, Radix Arnebiae seu Lithospermi (*zi cao*) 30g, Fructus Pruni Mume (*wu mei*) 30g, and white sugar 500g. Filter and take 15ml twice daily. Administered in 50 cases of sciatica, this formula gave satisfying results. In the best cases, an improvement was felt within two weeks, and the condition was resolved in four weeks. The longest cases took twelve weeks to resolve.

In addition, prepared formulas based on Aconite Decoction (*wu tou tang*), and others based on Radix Aconiti (*wu tou*) or Radix Lateralis Aconiti Carmichaeli Praeparata (*fu zi*), have been used to treat this disease with good effect. These include such formulas as Musk Capsules (*she xiang yuan*), Minor Gold Special Pill (*xiao jin dan*), Major Invigorate the Collaterals Special Pill (*da huo luo dan*), Minor Invigorate the Collaterals Special Pill (*xiao huo luo dan*), Aconite and Cinnamon Twig Decoction (*wu tou gui zhi tang*), Atractylodes Macrocephala and Prepared Aconite Decoction (*bai zhu fu zi tang*) and Licorice and Prepared Aconite Decoction (*gan cao fu zi tang*).

There are also reports regarding the use of Semen Strychni (*ma qian zi*) as the main herb in the treatment of sciatica and various types of arthralgia. For instance, the *Compendium of Chinese Medical Therapies (Zhong yi zhi liao hui bian)*, published by the Zhengzhou City Health Department, mentions Astragalus and Polygonum Decoction (*huang qi shou wu tang*), which is composed of Radix Astragali Membranacei (*huang qi*) 30g, Radix Polygoni Multiflori (*he shou wu*) 30g, Semen Strychni Praeparata (*zhi ma qian zi*) 1-3g, Buthus Martensi (*quan xie*) 2-5g, Radix et Caulis Jixueteng (*ji xue teng*) 30g, and Radix Glycyrrhizae Uralensis (*gan cao*) 30g. Shanghai's Yangpu Hospital of Traditional Chinese Medicine uses Wind Pain Powder (*feng tong san*) prepared in the following manner: equal parts of Semen Strychni (*ma qian zi*) and Herba Ephedrae (*ma huang*) are decocted together, after which the latter herb is discarded. Semen Strychni (*ma qian zi*) is then toasted by itself and fried together with sand or oil, and then ground into powder. The powder is taken every night with yellow wine or lukewarm water, starting with 0.06g and gradually increasing to 0.15g daily. This powder should be taken with caution, as it contains a toxic compound (strychnine); if signs of vertigo and spasms appear within twelve hours after ingestion, the patient should be given plenty of water to drink or some phenobarbitol.

Many authors insist on the need to differentiate the patterns of those diagnosed by modern biomedicine as having sciatica. According to some, these conditions usually reflect Qi or Blood deficiency, or Liver and Kidney deficiency, as the root of the disease. For Liver and Kidney deficiency, use Angelica Pubescens and Sangjisheng Decoction (du huo ji sheng tang). For severe pain, use Three Painful Obstruction Decoction (san bi tang) as modified by Dr. Zhang.[26] In the case of underlying Blood deficiency, formulas to warm the channels and disperse Cold are prescribed, with the addition of substances to nourish the Blood and unblock the vessels; or use Tangkuei Decoction for Frigid Extremities (dang gui si ni tang) as the base formula, and add Fructus Chaenomelis Lagenariae (mu gua), Radix Achyranthis Bidentatae (niu xi), Herba cum Radice Lycopodii Clavati (shen jin cao), Radix Salviae Miltiorrhizae (dan shen) and Radix et Caulis Jixueteng (ji xue teng). When Cold predominates, add Radix Aconiti Carmichaeli Praeparata (zhi chuan wu), Radix Aconiti Kusnezoffii Praeparata (zhi cao wu) and Radix Lateralis Aconiti Carmichaeli Praeparata (fu zi). When Dampness predominates, add Rhizoma Atractylodis (cang zhu) and Radix Aristolochiae Fangchi (fang ji). If Wind predominates, add Radix Ledebouriellae Divaricatae (fang feng) and Radix Clematidis (wei ling xian). For long-term diseases with intense pain due to a combination of Phlegm and Blood stasis, add Semen Persicae (tao ren), Flos Carthami Tinctorii (hong hua), Excrementum Trogopterori seu Pteromi (wu ling zhi), Radix Salviae Miltiorrhizae (dan shen), Carapax Amydae Sinensis (bie jia), Gummi Olibanum (ru xiang) and Myrrha (mo yao). For accompanying lower back pain with clear paraspinal tenderness, add Rhizoma Cibotii Barometz (gou ji), Radix Dipsaci Asperi (xu duan), Cortex Eucommiae Ulmoidis (du zhong), Fructus Lycii (gou qi zi), Ramulus Sangjisheng (sang ji sheng), Radix Morindae Officinalis (ba ji tian), Herba Epimedii (yin yang huo) and Eupolyphaga seu Opisthoplatia (tu bie chong). For those with Qi deficiency, add Radix Astragali Membranacei (huang qi) and Radix Codonopsitis Pilosulae (dang shen).

Some people use Tonify the Middle and Augment the Qi Decoction (bu zhong yi qi tang), with the addition of Radix Paeoniae Lactiflorae (bai shao), Fructus Chaenomelis Lagenariae (mu gua), Cortex Eucommiae Ulmoidis (du zhong), Radix Cyathulae Officinalis (chuan niu xi) and Ramulus Cinnamomi Cassiae (gui zhi), to tonify the Spleen, augment the Qi, invigorate the Blood, transform stasis, warm the channels and unblock the collaterals. For stabbing pain, add Radix Salviae Miltiorrhizae (dan shen), Radix et Caulis Jixueteng (ji xue teng) and Radix Notoginseng (san qi). If the pain is worse at night, add Radix Polygoni Multiflori (he shou wu) and Gelatinum Corii Asini (e jiao). If Dampness predominates, add Fructus Chaenomelis Lagenariae (mu gua) and Semen Coicis Lachryma-jobi (yi yi ren). If the patient has a poor appetite, add Fructus Amomi (sha ren) and a dark-toasted combination of Massa Fermentata (shen qu), Fructus Crataegi (shan zha) and Fructus Hordei Vulgaris Germinantus (mai ya).

Others prescribe an augmented form of Tonify the Yang to Restore Five-tenths Decoction (bu yang huan wu tang), which is made up of Radix Astragali Membranacei (huang qi) 60g, Radix Angelicae Sinensis (dang gui) 30g, Radix Codonopsitis Pilosulae (dang shen) 30g, Radix Paeoniae Rubrae (chi shao) 18g, Lumbricus (di long) 15g, Ramulus Cinnamomi Cassiae (gui zhi) 15g, Radix Ligustici Chuanxiong (chuan xiong) 20g, Radix et Caulis Jixueteng (ji xue teng) 20g, Semen Persicae (tao ren) 9g, Flos Carthami Tinctorii (hong hua) 9g, and Radix Glycyrrhizae Uralensis (gan cao) 9g. This is adjusted as circumstances dictate.

After using this decoction (one packet daily divided into four doses) on a sample of 100 patients, 89 were clinically cured (disappearance of signs and symptoms with no recurrence within one year), 7 showed definite improvement (significant decrease in pain or its elimination with stability after herbs were discontinued), and 2 people showed moderate improvement. Overall, this is a 98 percent success rate.

According to other authors, sciatica disorders do not always fall in the category of Cold and deficiency, as some will present a Hot or Damp-Heat etiology. This is often seen after prolonged or excessive use of drying, Wind-expelling herbs, or when the individual's constitution tends toward Heat excess. This pattern is one of internal Heat scorching the sinews. The main symptoms are a local sensation of heat and severe pain. The treatment is a high dosage of White Tiger Decoction (bai hu tang) with the addition of Rhizoma Imperatae Cylindricae (bai mao gen), Rhizoma Dioscoreae Hypoglaucae (bei xie), Caulis Bambusae in Taeniis (zhu ru), Semen Coicis Lachryma-jobi (yi yi ren) and Ramulus Mori Albae (sang zhi). For Damp-Heat, add Fructus Chaenomelis Lagenariae (mu gua), Rhizoma Atractylodis (cang zhu) and Excrementum Bombycis Mori (can sha). For Fluid deficiency, add Radix Rehmanniae Glutinosae (sheng di huang) and Tuber Ophiopogonis Japonici (mai men dong). For spasms of the sinews and vessels, add Lumbricus (di long) and Radix Achyranthis Bidentatae (niu xi).

When Wind-Damp-Cold is constrained for a long period and transforms into Heat, or for Damp-Heat invading the collaterals, use Four-Marvel Powder (*si miao san*) with the addition of Fructus Chaenomelis Lagenariae (*mu gua*), Excrementum Bombycis Mori (*can sha*), Herba Artemisiae Yinchenhao (*yin chen hao*), Radix Aristolochiae Fangchi (*fang ji*), Radix Sophorae Flavescentis (*ku shen*), Rhizoma Dioscoreae Hypoglaucae (*bei xie*), Cortex Erythrinae (*hai tong pi*), Caulis Piperis Futokadsurae (*hai feng teng*), Caulis Trachelospermi Jasminoidis (*luo shi teng*), Radix Clematidis (*wei ling xian*) and Ramulus Mori Albae (*sang zhi*).

When the pathology is related to trauma, use Four-Substance Decoction (*si wu tang*) with the addition of Radix Achyranthis Bidentatae (*niu xi*), Gummi Olibanum (*ru xiang*), Myrrha (*mo yao*), Fasciculus Vascularis Luffae (*si gua luo*), Semen Persicae (*tao ren*), Flos Carthami Tinctorii (*hong hua*), Herba cum Radice Lycopodii Clavati (*shen jin cao*) and Radix Dipsaci Asperi (*xu duan*).

For late-stage conditions, focus on prescriptions that enrich the Kidneys, nourish the Liver, and include sweet, cold and moistening herbs. Examples are modifications of such formulas as Hidden Tiger Pill (*hu qian wan*) and Gathered Spirits Paste (*ji ling gao*). The main ingredients of these formulas include Radix Rehmanniae Glutinosae (*sheng di huang*), Radix Rehmanniae Glutinosae Conquitae (*shu di huang*), Tuber Ophiopogonis Japonici (*mai men dong*), Tuber Asparagi Cochinchinensis (*tian men dong*), Fructus Ligustri Lucidi (*nu zhen zi*), Herba Ecliptae Prostratae (*han lian cao*), Cortex Eucommiae Ulmoidis (*du zhong*), Rhizoma Polygonati Odorati (*yu zhu*), Cortex Phellodendri (*huang bai*), Gelatinum Corii Asini (*e jiao*), Gelatinum Cornu Cervi (*lu jiao jiao*), Gelatinum Plastri Testudinis (*gui ban jiao*), Fructus Lycii (*gou qi zi*), Radix Angelicae Sinensis (*dang gui*) and Radix Paeoniae Lactiflorae (*bai shao*).

CHINESE MEDICAL TREATMENT OF BONE SPURS

This condition, which generally appears after the age of forty, is characterized by pain and a loss of strength. The joints most frequently involved are the knees and spine, which are weight-bearing joints. There is no local redness, no migrating sensation of pain, and no systemic symptomatology. X-rays show calcium deposits around the joints and osteophytes. The general state of health is usually good.

Because, according to traditional theory, the Liver governs the sinews, the Kidneys govern the bones, and the lower back is the abode of the Kidneys, the principle of treatment for this condition is to tonify the Kidneys and nourish the Liver, as well as invigorate the Blood and transform Blood stasis. There have been many recent writings on this subject. In general they report that traditional Chinese medicine is effective in eliminating the symptoms and inhibiting the growth of new osteophytes, but has no significant effect on pre-existing osteophytes.

One study reports using Peony and Chaenomeles Decoction (*bai shao mu gua tang*) in the treatment of 160 cases. This formula consists of Radix Paeoniae Lactiflorae (*bai shao*) 30 to 60g, Fructus Chaenomelis Lagenariae (*mu gua*) 12g, Radix Glycyrrhizae Uralensis (*gan cao*) 12g, Radix et Caulis Jixueteng (*ji xue teng*) 13g, and Radix Clematidis (*wei ling xian*) 13g. For problems of the cervical vertebrae and those below the knees, add Cortex Eucommiae Ulmoidis (*du zhong*) and Radix Achyranthis Bidentatae (*niu xi*). For diarrhea, add dry-fried Rhizoma Atractylodis Macrocephalae (*chao bai zhu*) and Sclerotium Poriae Cocos (*fu ling*). Of the 160 cases in the study, 85 involved the cervical spine, 60 had osteophytic disease of the lumbar spine, and the remainder involved other joints. A total of 109 cases were completely cured, 42 showed definite improvement, and 9 had some improvement.

Other studies reported on the use of Yang-Heartening Decoction (*yang he tang*) with the addition of Rhizoma Drynariae (*gu sui bu*) and Pyritum (*zi ran tong*) in the treatment of ten cases of vertebral osteophytes. Of the seven cases involving the lumbar spine, four showed clear effects and three improved. One case each of thoracic spine disease, lumbar disc disease and sacralization showed some improvement.

The associated hospital of the Shanghai Number Two Medical School used Anti-Osteophyte Tablets (*kang gu zhi zeng sheng pian*) to treat 121 cases. The tablets consisted of Radix Aconiti Carmichaeli Praeparata (*zhi chuan wu*), Radix Lateralis Aconiti Carmichaeli Praeparata (*fu zi*), Gummi Olibanum (*ru xiang*), Semen Strychni Praeparata (*zhi ma qian zi*), Cortex Cinnamomi Cassiae (*rou gui*), Radix Angelicae Sinensis (*dang gui*), Radix Paeoniae Lactiflorae (*bai shao*), Radix Codonopsitis Pilosulae (*dang shen*) and Herba Epimedii (*yin yang huo*). The overall success rate was 91.7 percent. Physical manipulation was used in combination with the herbal treatment in 21 cases of cervical degenerative joint disease.

Dr. Liu[27] gathered 34,571 case histories, of which 1,181 were systematically reviewed. There were 820 cases of spinal inflammation, 120 cases of cervical spine disease, 110 bone spurs of the calcaneus and 131 cases of large joint disease. All were treated with a concentrated pill of his own design called Osteophyte Pill (*gu zhi zeng sheng wan*). This formula is composed of Radix Rehmanniae Glutinosae Conquitae (*shu di huang*), Herba Pyrolae Rotundifoliae (*lu xian cao*), Rhizoma Drynariae (*gu sui bu*), Herba Cistanches (*rou cong rong*), Radix et Caulis Jixueteng (*ji xue teng*), Herba Epimedii (*yin yang huo*) and Semen Raphani Sativi (*lai fu zi*). One month's course of treatment consisted of 5g taken two or three times a day. The longest course of treatment before any effect was seen was five months, the shortest five days. In most cases the effects were felt after one or two months of treatment, with the cases of spinal inflammation obtaining the fastest and most stable results. According to Dr. Liu, these afflictions are due to deficiency of the Kidneys, which are unable to generate marrow to fill the bones, causing bone problems. Osteophyte Pill (*gu zhi xeng sheng wan*) clearly controls the generation of osteophytes and alleviates pain. The altered bone mass is somewhat restored to normalcy, and the opening of the channels and collaterals plays an analgesic function.

The Heilongjiang Research Center of Our Motherland's Medicine reports using Bone-Gold Special Pill (*gu jin dan*) in the treatment of 213 cases. Those with Blood stasis types were treated with Bone-Gold No. 8 Formula (*gu jin ba hao*), which consists of honey-toasted Semen Strychni (*zhi ma qian zi*) 9g, Radix Paeoniae Lactiflorae (*bai shao*) 10g, Rhizoma Corydalis Yanhusuo (*yan hu suo*) 15g, Radix Notoginseng (*san qi*) 9g, Radix Aucklandiae Lappae (*mu xiang*) 15g, Myrrha (*mo yao*) 15g, Flos Carthami Tinctorii (*hong hua*) 15g, Tuber Curcumae (*yu jin*) 10g, Radix Gentianae Qinjiao (*qin jiao*) 20g, Gummi Olibanum (*ru xiang*) 15g, Sanguis Draconis (*xue jie*) 9g, Radix Achyranthis Bidentatae (*niu xi*) 15g, and Ramulus Cinnamomi Cassiae (*gui zhi*) 15g. These herbs are toasted in sand; Semen Strychni (*zhi ma qian zi*) must be toasted until brown. They are then powdered and prepared into honey-based pills of 6g each, to be taken twice daily, mornings and evenings, on an empty stomach.

Bone-Gold No. 14 Formula (*gu jin shi si hao*) was prescribed for bone spurs associated with Damp-Cold, and consists of honey-toasted Semen Strychni (*zhi ma qian zi*) 15g, honey-toasted Radix Aconiti Carmichaeli (*zhi chuan wu*) 15g, honey-toasted Radix Aconiti

Kusnezoffii (*zhi cao wu*) 15g, Radix Clematidis (*wei ling xian*) 30g, Gummi Olibanum (*ru xiang*) 30g, Myrrha (*mo yao*) 30g, Ramulus Sangjisheng (*sang ji sheng*) 30g, Radix Paeoniae Rubrae (*chi shao*) 30g, Herba Siegesbeckiae (*xi xian cao*) 20g, and Radix et Caulis Erycibes Obstusifoliae (*ding gong teng*) 20g. It is prepared and taken in the same manner as Bone-Gold No. 8 Formula, described above. Of the 213 cases in the study, a 93 percent efficacy rate was reported, broken down as follows: 198 showed some improvement (54 were significantly improved and 144 were moderately improved) and there were 15 failures. Semen Strychni (*ma qian zi*) sometimes caused minor gastric upset, vertigo, dryness of the mouth and purpura, but no significant toxic reactions were observed. The dosage of strychnine in this formula is 3mg, which places it well within the safety margin (6mg maximum). Moreover, the fact that Semen Strychni (*ma qian zi*) is toasted in sand and its preparation is simple makes it easy to control the toxicity of the herb. Analysis has shown that the proportion of strychnine is between 0.71 and 1.28 percent, which is comparable to what was achieved using older methods of preparation.

With respect to external treatment, Dr. Shi[28] of the physical therapy department at the General Hospital of the Beijing Command used aged vinegar, or Radix Clematidis (*wei ling xian*) soaked in vinegar, as a conductor for direct electrical current to treat foot pain from bone spurs, arthritis and hip pain. Of the 450 cases monitored, 93.11 percent showed some improvement.

The Friendship Hospital and Hospital No. 263 prescribed warm plasters, through which a direct electrical current was run, with satisfactory results in the treatment of osteophytic joint disease and cervical spine disease. The plaster is made with dried Rhizoma Zingiberis Officinalis (*gan jiang*), Ramulus Cinnamomi Cassiae (*gui zhi*), Radix Paeoniae Rubrae (*chi shao*), Radix Angelicae Sinensis (*dang gui*), Rhizoma et Radix Notopterygii (*qiang huo*), Radix Puerariae (*ge gen*), Radix Ligustici Chuanxiong (*chuan xiong*), Cortex Erythrinae (*hai tong pi*), Rhizoma Curcumae Longae (*jiang huang*) and Gummi Olibanum (*ru xiang*).

There are also reports of successfully alleviating local pain by applying small bags consisting of 60g of powdered Radix Ligustici Chuanxiong (*chuan xiong*) and 30g of Radix Clematidis (*wei ling xian*). The bags are placed on the painful areas and changed once a week, for 30 to 45 days.

Application of Painful Obstruction Diagnostic and Treatment Principles to Other Diseases

Since painful obstruction includes a broad range of disorders, pathologies other than those previously mentioned may fit within this framework. At a minimum, one or more stages in the development of several diseases discussed below can be understood and treated by applying principles based on the treatment of painful obstruction.

THROMBOPHLEBITIS

During the end stages (necrotic phase) of this disease there are manifestations similar to those called "sloughing ulcer" *(tuō jū)* in old texts. In the early and middle stages (local ischemic phase, dystrophic phase) the symptoms include cold in the affected limbs, paresthesia, numbness, pain and intermittent limping. These match the diagnosis of painful obstruction and can be treated in a similar fashion.

The Xuanwu Hospital in Beijing reported on 1,290 cases, which were treated as follows:

For those with yin deficiency and Toxic Heat the prescription was composed of Flos Lonicerae Japonicae *(jin yin hua)* 15-30g, Radix Scutellariae Baicalensis *(huang qin)* 10-15g, Flos Chrysanthemi Indici *(ye ju hua)* 15-30g, Herba Dendrobii *(shi hu)* 15-30g, Herba Begoniae Fimbristipulatae *(zi bei tian kui)* 15-30g, Herba Taraxaci Mongolici cum Radice *(pu gong ying)* 15-30g, Herba cum Radice Violae Yedoensitis *(zi hua di ding)* 15-30g, Radix Scrophulariae Ningpoensis *(xuan shen)* 15-30g, Radix Paeoniae Rubrae *(chi shao)* 15-30g, Radix et Caulis Jixueteng *(ji xue teng)* 15-30g and Radix Astragali Membranacei *(huang qi)* 12-30g. For thirst, Radix Trichosanthis Kirilowii *(tian hua fen)* was added, and for severe pain, Rhizoma Corydalis Yanhusuo *(yan hu suo)*. When the Toxic Heat was severe, Fructus Forsythiae Suspensae *(lian qiao)* was added. When the upper limbs were affected, Rhizoma Cimicifugae *(sheng ma)* was used, and for the lower limbs, Radix Achyranthis Bidentatae *(niu xi)*.

For cases of deficiency Cold the prescription was composed of Radix Angelicae Sinensis *(dang gui)* 15-30g, Radix Rehmanniae Glutinosae Conquitae *(shu di huang)* 12-24g, Gelatinum Cornu Cervi *(lu jiao jiao)* 12-30g,

Semen Sinapis Albae *(bai jie zi)* 15-30g, Flos Carthami Tinctorii *(hong hua)* 10-15g, Herba Ephedrae *(ma huang)* 3-10g, Ramulus Cinnamomi Cassiae *(gui zhi)* 10-15g, Semen Persicae *(tao ren)* 15-30g, Rhizoma Zingiberis Officinalis *(gan jiang)* 15-30g, Lumbricus *(di long)* 10-18g and Radix Glycyrrhizae Uralensis *(gan cao)* 10-15g. For frigid extremities, Radix Lateralis Aconiti Carmichaeli Praeparata *(fu zi)* was added, and for Qi deficiency, Radix Codonopsitis Pilosulae *(dang shen)*.

Where both the Qi and Blood were exhausted the prescription consisted of Radix Codonopsitis Pilosulae *(dang shen)* 10-15g, Sclerotium Poriae Cocos *(fu ling)* 12-30g, Radix Angelicae Sinensis *(dang gui)* 15-30g, Radix Astragali Membranacei *(huang qi)* 12-30g, Radix Salviae Miltiorrhizae *(dan shen)* 12-30g, Radix Ligustici Chuanxiong *(chuan xiong)* 12g, Rhizoma Atractylodis Macrocephalae *(bai zhu)* 12-30g, Radix Glehniae *(bei sha shen)* 12-30g, Radix Paeoniae Lactiflorae *(bai shao)* 12-30g and Radix Rehmanniae Glutinosae Conquitae *(shu di huang)* 12-30g.

For Blood stasis the prescription consisted of Ramus Lonicerae Japonicae *(ren dong teng)* 15-30g, Rhizoma Sparganii Stoloniferi *(san leng)* 10-15g, Eupolyphaga seu Opisthoplatia *(tu bie chong)* 10-15g, Lacca Sinica Exsiccatae *(gan qi)* 10-24g, Flos Carthami Tinctorii *(hong hua)* 10-15g, Rhizoma Curcumae Ezhu *(e zhu)* 10-15g, Appendix Euonymi Alati *(gui jian yu)* 10-15g, Radix Anemones Raddeanae *(zhu jie xiang fu)* 12-30g, Lumbricus *(di long)* 10-15g, Radix Angelicae Sinensis *(dang gui)* 12-30g, Radix Ligustici Chuanxiong *(chuan xiong)* 12g, and Radix Salviae Miltiorrhizae *(dan shen)* 10-30g. For inflammation of the veins, Radix Arnebiae seu Lithospermi *(zi cao)* and Radix Rubiae Cordifoliae *(qian cao)* were added.

Of the 1,290 cases in the study, 526 (48 percent) were cured, 330 (25.5 percent) showed significant improvement, 401 (31.1 percent) had some improvement, and 33 cases (2.6 percent) showed no effect.

Chongqing No. 1 Traditional Chinese Hospital reported a study of 89 cases, which were divided into two categories: clumped Heat Toxin and Damp-Cold stagnation. In the first group, the treatment principle was to nourish the yin, clear the Heat, relieve Toxicity and unblock the collaterals. The formulas used were Four-Valiant Decoction for Well Being *(si miao yong an tang)*, Anemarrhena, Phellodendron, and Rehmannia Decoction *(zhi bai di huang tang)* or a modified Four-Substance Decoction with Safflower and Peach Pit *(tao hong si wu tang)*. In the second group, the treatment principle was to warm the channels, disperse Cold, eliminate Dampness and remove the painful obstruction. Treatment was based on the formulas Tangkuei Decoction for Frigid Extremities (*dang gui si ni tang*) and True Warrior Decoction (*zhen wu tang*), with the addition of Radix Aconiti Carmichaeli Praeparata (*zhi chuan wu*) and Radix Aconiti Kusnezoffii Praeparata (*zhi cao wu*) along with external therapeutic methods. The results were satisfactory.

The Guananmen Hospital of the Academy of Traditional Chinese Medicine differentiates this condition as follows:

- Cold deficiency type (corresponding to the ischemic phase), for which modified Yang-Heartening Decoction (*yang he tang*) is prescribed.
- Blood stasis type (corresponding to the dystrophic phase), for which Invigorate the Blood and Transform Stasis Decoction (*huo xue hua yu tang*) is prescribed. This formula is composed of Radix Angelicae Sinensis (*dang gui*), Radix Achyranthis Bidentatae (*niu xi*), Semen Persicae (*tao ren*), Flos Carthami Tinctorii (*hong hua*), Lumbricus (*di long*), Eupolyphaga seu Opisthoplatia (*tu bie chong*), Hirudo seu Whitmaniae (*shui zhi*), Rhizoma Acori Graminei (*shi chang pu*) and Squama Manitis Pentadactylae (*chuan shan jia*).
- Heat Toxin type (corresponding to the ulceration phase), for which modified Four-Valiant Decoction for Well-Being (*si miao yong an tang*) and Management of Walking Decoction (*gu bu tang*) are prescribed.
- Qi and Blood deficiency type (corresponding to the convalescence phase), for which modified All-Inclusive Great Tonifying Decoction (*shi quan da bu tang*) and Ginseng Decoction to Nourish the Nutritive Qi (*ren shen yang ying tang*) are prescribed.

Recently, many hospitals and researchers report treating this condition by applying the general principles of invigorating the Blood and transforming stasis, and adding herbs according to the presence or absence of Cold or Heat. For example, the Academy of Medical Sciences treated 103 cases with Effective Formula to Unblock the Vessels (*tong mai ling*). The main ingredients of this formula invigorate the Blood and transform stasis. Most of the patients experienced either an elimination of or significant improvement in pain and lameness after treatment. There was also improvement in the peripheral pulses and circulation of the affected limb, increase in skin humidity, and either healing or near-closure of the lesions.

The Tianjin School of Medicine used a formula consisting of Radix Angelicae Sinensis (*dang gui*), Radix Salviae Miltiorrhizae (*dan shen*), Radix et Caulis Jixueteng (*ji xue teng*), Radix Ligustici Chuanxiong (*chuan xiong*) and Radix Paeoniae Rubrae (*chi shao*) as the basic substances, with the addition of other herbs according to pattern differentiation. Of 102 cases, the general success rate was 76.17 percent, with a corrected efficacy rate of 84 percent.

Some authors, however, believe that invigorating the Blood and transforming Blood stasis must be done in moderation, taking into account whether the condition is recent or chronic, deficient or excessive. In other words, this method should not be used indiscriminately.

The Huashan Hospital associated with the Shanghai No. 1 Medical School suggests that in the acute stage of thrombophlebitis, the collaterals and vessels are often affected by pathogenic Cold, Dampness and Heat, which must therefore be eliminated. After the acute phase there is a rather long period of ischemia. During this stage herbs that invigorate the Blood, dispel stasis and renew what is old can be added to basic prescriptions that support the normal Qi. This limits the progression of lesions, shortens their evolution and minimizes the number of amputations.

POLYMYOSITIS

This disease consists of inflammation of the muscles; its etiology is still unknown. Onset is often characterized by problems with the distal muscles of the limbs, which then spreads to the other muscles. The muscular strength of the four limbs is diminished, movement is impaired, the muscles are swollen and painful both to the touch and spontaneously, the joints are painful, and temperature varies. When combined with erythematic skin eruptions, the condition is called dermatomyositis.

The onset phase often corresponds to Wind-Damp-Hot painful obstruction, which calls for modified versions of such formulas as Major Gentiana Qinjiao Decoction (*da qin jiao tang*), Ledebouriella Decoction (*fang feng tang*) and Ephedra, Forsthyia, and Aduki Bean Decoction (*ma huang lian qiao chi xiao dou tang*).

The chronic phase usually falls in the category of either yin deficiency with internal Heat, or Qi and Blood deficiency. Formulas used for this phase of the disease include Six-Ingredient Pill with Rehmannia (*liu wei di huang wan*) with the addition of Radix Angelicae Sinensis (*dang gui*), Radix Paeoniae Lactiflorae (*bai shao*), Radix

Codonopsitis Pilosulae *(dang shen)* and Rhizoma Polygonati *(huang jing)*; Two-Ultimate Pill *(er zhi wan)*; Anemarrhena, Phellodendron, and Rehmannia Pill *(zhi bai di huang wan)*; Hidden Tiger Pill *(hu qian wan)*; and modified Four-Substance Decoction *(si wu tang)*.

The dermatology department at the Xiyuan Hospital of the Academy of Traditional Chinese Medicine considers Spleen deficiency to be the root of this disorder, along with stagnation of Liver Blood. Over time the Kidneys are affected and there is yin deficiency with internal Heat. The treatment principle is to enrich and nourish the Kidney yin, supported by the principles of tonifying the Qi, clearing the Heat, cooling the Blood, invigorating the Blood and unblocking the collaterals.

SYSTEMIC LUPUS ERYTHEMATOSUS

Lupus erythematosus is a collagen disease which takes either a localized discoid form or a systemic form. The latter has especially complex clinical manifestations. The multiplicity of symptoms can involve many different organ systems. Among the main symptoms is polyarticular arthralgia, which can be treated as painful obstruction and differentiated accordingly.

According to Dr. Gu,[29] the acute stage of this disorder usually corresponds to Hot painful obstruction, which is often the result of pathogenic Wind, Cold and Dampness being constrained over a long period of time and then transforming into Heat. The nutritive and protective Qi are not in harmony, the channels and collaterals are obstructed by Blood stasis, and the movement of Blood and Qi are not smooth. The main treatment principle is to clear Heat, aided by the principles of dispersing Wind, transforming Dampness, invigorating the Blood and unblocking the collaterals. The recommended formula is an augmented form of White Tiger and Cinnamon Twig Decoction *(bai hu gui zhi tang)*. Dr. Gu believes that the chronic stage often corresponds to moving painful obstruction with external pathogenic Wind-Damp-Cold obstructing the channels and impairing the circulation of Qi and Blood. The principles of treatment are to harmonize the nutritive Qi, unblock the collaterals, disperse Cold and resolve Dampness, using a modified version of Remove Painful Obstruction Decoction *(juan bi tang)*.

BRUCELLOSIS

Dr. Fang[30] interprets this disease as a form of deficient painful obstruction, and prescribes his own formula called Control Brucellosis No. 2 *(yi bu er hao fang)*. This is composed of Rhizoma Atractylodis *(cang zhu)*, Ramulus Cinnamomi Cassiae *(gui zhi)*, Fructus Schisandrae Chinensis *(wu wei zi)*, Radix Glycyrrhizae Uralensis *(gan cao)*, Radix Rehmanniae Glutinosae *(sheng di huang)*, Radix Astragali Membranacei *(huang qi)*, Fructus Zizyphi Jujubae *(da zao)* and Semen Tritici Aestivi Levis *(fu xiao mai)*. In one study of 512 cases, the efficacy rate exceeded 90 percent.

ERYTHEMA NODOSUM, ERYTHEMA INDURATUM, POLYARTERITIS NODOSA

These conditions are usually due to an obstruction of Qi and Blood, with the addition of an attack by an external pathogenic influence. The dermatology departments at the Capital Hospital, the Guanganmen Hospital and the Chinese Academy of Traditional Chinese Medicine have treated these conditions with satisfying results by invigorating the Blood, dispersing stasis, promoting the circulation of Qi and unblocking the collaterals. The most commonly prescribed formula is Four-Substance Decoction with Safflower and Peach Pit *(tao hong si wu tang)* with the addition of such substances as Radix Salviae Miltiorrhizae *(dan shen)*, Radix et Caulis Jixueteng *(ji xue teng)*, Radix Achyranthis Bidentatae *(niu xi)*, Rhizoma Cyperi Rotundi *(xiang fu)*, Pericarpium Citri Reticulatae Viride *(qing pi)*, Caulis Piperis Futokadsurae *(hai feng teng)* and Herba Lycopi Lucidi *(ze lan)*.

For flaming red nodes, yellow urine, constipation, red tongue and rapid pulse, add Cortex Moutan Radicis *(mu dan pi)*, Folium Daqingye *(da qing ye)* and Flos Lonicerae Japonicae *(jin yin hua)*; for dark, dull purple lesions, pale tongue and slow pulse, add Herba Ephedrae *(ma huang)* and Ramulus Cinnamomi Cassiae *(gui zhi)*; for red lesions that linger, add Squama Manitis Pentadactylae *(chuan shan jia)* and Pseudobulbus Shancigu *(shan ci gu)*; for protracted ulcerations that do not heal, add Radix Codonopsitis Pilosulae *(dang shen)*, Radix Astragali Membranacei *(huang qi)* and Radix Rehmanniae Glutinosae Conquitae *(shu di huang)*; for sore and painful joints, add Radix Gentianae Qinjiao *(qin jiao)*, Fructus Chaenomelis Lagenariae *(mu gua)*, Radix Clematidis *(wei ling xian)*, Radix et Rhizoma Notopterygii *(qiang huo)* and Radix Angelicae Pubescentis *(du huo)*.

SCLERODERMA

This disease is generally due to insufficiency of Kidney yang together with Qi deficiency and Blood stasis, with the addition of externally contracted pathogenic influences obstructing the skin and muscles. There is painful obstruction and blockage that leads to a loss of harmonious exchange between the nutritive and protective Qi. At the Longhua Hospital in Shanghai, the principles of treatment are to warm the channels, support the yang and regulate and harmonize the nutritive and protective Qi.

The most commonly used decoctions are Yang-Heartening Decoction *(yang he tang)* or Tangkuei Decoction to Tonify the Blood *(dang gui bu xue tang)* with the addition of Radix Aconiti Carmichaeli Praeparata *(zhi chuan wu)*, Herba cum Radice Asari *(xi xin)*, Radix et Rhizoma Notopterygii *(qiang huo)*, Radix Angelicae Pubescentis *(du huo)* and Radix Paeoniae Rubrae *(chi shao)*. For Kidney yang deficiency, add Radix Morindae Officinalis *(ba ji tian)*, Herba Epimedii *(yin yang huo)* and Herba Cistanches *(rou cong rong)*. For Blood stasis, add Flos Carthami Tinctorii *(hong hua)*, Semen Persicae *(tao ren)*, Semen Vaccariae Segetalis *(wang bu liu xing)* and Radix Paeoniae Rubrae *(chi shao)*.

When upper limb symptoms predominate, add Ramulus Mori Albae *(sang zhi)* and Radix et Caulis Jixueteng *(ji xue teng)*; when lower limb symptoms predominate, add Radix Achyranthis Bidentatae *(niu xi)* and Caulis et Rhizoma Sinomenii Acuti *(qing feng teng)*. For hot skin, add Flos Lonicerae Japonicae *(jin yin hua)*, Fructus Forsythiae Suspensae *(lian qiao)* and Cortex Moutan Radicis *(mu dan pi)*.

In the associated hospital of the Medical Department, the treatment principle is to invigorate the Blood and transform Blood stasis. In one study, 84 cases of localized scleroderma were satisfactorily treated with Effective Formula to Unblock the Vessels *(tong mai ling)*, which is based on Blood-invigorating herbs.

These preliminary results tend to show that herbs that invigorate the Blood and transform stasis can improve microcirculation and lead to recovery of proliferaive or degenerative connective tissue.

Summary

The etiological and pathological changes associated with painful obstruction disorders usually occur under conditions of an underlying insufficiency of normal Qi. This allows the Wind-Damp-Cold external pathogenic influences to invade the body and obstruct the circulation of Qi and Blood.

At the onset, painful obstruction disorder affects the channels, muscles and exterior. If it lingers in the body over a long period of time it will affect the sinews and bones, and penetrate deeply into the yin and yang Organs, leading to pathological changes throughout the body. The pathological processes of painful obstruction are thus rather prolonged. Clinically, they are either progressive in nature or occur in irregular crises.

Painful obstruction most often presents patterns where the normal Qi is deficient and the pathogenic influences are excessive. To facilitate differentiation of deficient patterns from those of excess, this chapter was divided between patterns of excessive painful obstruction (Wind-Damp-Cold painful obstruction, Wind-Damp-Hot painful obstruction, stubborn painful obstruction) and patterns of deficient painful obstruction (deficient Blood and Qi painful obstruction, deficient yang painful obstruction, deficient yin painful obstruction).

For patterns of excessive painful obstruction, the main principle of treatment is to attack the painful obstruction:

- For Wind-Damp-Cold painful obstruction, warm the yang while disseminating and unblocking.
- For Wind-Damp-Hot painful obstruction, clear the Heat, resolve the Dampness and expel the Wind.
- For stubborn painful obstruction, invigorate the Blood, transform the Blood stasis, transform the Phlegm and unblock the collaterals.

For patterns of deficient painful obstruction, the main principle is to harmonize and tonify the Liver, Kidneys, Qi, Blood, yin and yang. The therapeutic methods of dispersing and attacking should be used with caution to avoid further injury to the normal Qi.

- For deficient Qi and Blood painful obstruction, tonify the Qi and Blood simultaneously.
- For deficient yang painful obstruction, warm and tonify the yang Qi.
- For deficient yin painful obstruction, rely on sweet, cold, softening and moistening formulas.
- For deficient normal Qi and excessive pathogenic Qi, support the normal and simultaneously expel the pathogenic.

The practitioner must be able to distinguish painful obstruction disorder from atrophy disorder; the main differentiating factor is the presence or absence of pain. Pain is the primary feature of painful obstruction disorder, whereas atrophy disorder is characterized by atrophy, weakness and loss of function.

Painful obstruction can become a systemic condition. As the duration of the disorder lengthens, it penetrates deeper and can lead to pathological changes involving many Organs. For better results, it is therefore preferable to treat it in the early stages.

Formulas[31]

Aconite Decoction (*wū tóu tāng*)

烏頭湯

Herba Ephedrae (*ma huang*)
Radix Paeoniae Lactiflorae (*bai shao*)
Radix Astragali Membranacei (*huang qi*)
Radix Aconiti Praeparata (*zhi wu tou*)
Radix Glycyrrhizae Uralensis (*gan cao*)
Honey

Angelica Pubescens and Sangjisheng Decoction
(*dú huó jì shēng tāng*)

獨活寄生湯

Ramulus Sanjisheng (*sang ji sheng*)
Radix Angelicae Pubescentis (*du huo*)
Radix Gentianae Qinjiao (*qin jiao*)
Radix Ledebouriellae Divaricatae (*fang feng*)
Herba cum Radice Asari (*xi xin*)
Radix Angelicae Sinensis (*dang gui*)
Radix Paeoniae Lactiflorae (*bai shao*)
Radix Ligustici Chuanxiong (*chuan xiong*)
Radix Rehmanniae Glutinosae (*sheng di huang*)
Cortex Eucommiae Ulmoidis (*du zhong*)
Radix Achyranthis Bidentatae (*niu xi*)
Radix Ginseng (*ren shen*)
Sclerotium Poriae Cocos (*fu ling*)
Radix Glycyrrhizae Uralensis (*gan cao*)
Cortex Cinnamomi Cassiae (*rou gui*)
SOURCE: *Thousand Ducat Prescriptions*

Astragalus and Cinnamon Twig Five-Substance Decoction (*huáng qí guì zhī wǔ wù tāng*)

黃蓍桂枝五物湯

Radix Astragali Membranacei (*huang qi*)
Ramulus Cinnamomi Cassiae (*gui zhi*)
Radix Paeoniae Lactiflorae (*bai shao yao*)
Rhizoma Zingiberis Officinalis Recens (*sheng jiang*)
Fructus Zizyphi Jujubae (*da zao*)
SOURCE: *Essentials from the Golden Cabinet*

Augment the Kidneys and Remove Painful Obstruction Pill (*yì shèn juān bì wán*)

益腎蠲痺丸

Radix Rehmanniae Glutinosae Conquitae (*shu di huang*)
Radix Angelicae Sinensis (*dang gui*)
Herba Epimedii (*yin yang huo*)
Herba Pyrolae Rotundifoliae (*lu xian cao*)
Buthus Martensi (*quan xie*)
Scolopendra Subspinipes (*wu gong*)
Zaocys Dhumnades (*wu shao she*)
Radix Ledebouriallae Divaricatae (*fang feng*)
Eupolyphaga seu Opisthoplatia (*tu bie chong*)
Bombyx Batryticatus (*jiang can*)
wine-toasted Cartharsius (*jiu qiang lang*)
Radix Rehmanniae Glutinosae (*sheng di huang*)
Radix et Caulis Jixueteng (*ji xue teng*)
Herba Erodii seu Geranii (*lao guan cao*)
Rhizoma seu Herba Aristolochiae Mollissimae (*xun gu feng*)
Radix et Rhizoma Polygoni Cuspidati (*hu zhang*)
SOURCE: *Journal of Traditional Chinese Medicine* (12:1,1980)

Cinnamon Twig and Prepared Aconite Decoction
(*guì zhī fù zǐ tāng*)

桂枝附子湯

Ramulus Cinnamomi Cassiae (*gui zhi*)
Radix Glycyrrhizae Uralensis (*gan cao*)
Radix Aconiti Carmichaeli (*fu pian*)
Fructus Zizyphi Jujubae (*da zao*)
Rhizoma Zingiberis Officinalis Recens (*sheng jiang*)
SOURCE: *Discussion of Cold-induced Disorders*

Cinnamon Twig, Peony, and Anemarrhena Decoction (*guì zhī sháo yào zhī mǔ tāng*)

桂枝芍藥知母湯

Ramulus Cinnamomi Cassiae (*gui zhi*)
Radix Paeoniae Lactiflorae (*bai shao yao*)
Rhizoma Anemarrhenae Asphodeloidis (*zhi mu*)
Herba Ephedrae (*ma huang*)
Rhizoma Atractylodis Macrocephalae (*bai zhu*)
Radix Ledebouriallae Divaricatae (*fang feng*)
Radix Lateralis Aconiti Carmichaeli Praeparata (*fu zi*)
Rhizoma Zingiberis Officinalis Recens (*sheng jiang*)
Radix Glycyrrhizae Uralensis (*gan cao*)
SOURCE: *Essentials from the Golden Cabinet*

Disband Painful Obstruction Decoction
 (xuān bì tāng)

宣痺湯

Radix Stephaniae Tetrandrae (fang ji)

Semen Pruni Armeniacae (xing ren)

Talcum (hua shi)

Fructus Forsythiae Suspensae (lian qiao)

Fructus Gardeniae Jasminoidis (zhi zi)

Semen Coicis Lachryma-jobi (yi yi ren)

Rhizoma Pinelliae Ternatae (ban xia)

Excrementum Bombycis Mori (can sha)

Semen Phaseoli Calcarati (chi xiao dou)

Rhizoma Curcumae Longae (jiang huang)

Cortex Erythrinae (hai tong pi)

SOURCE: Systematic Differentiation of Warm Diseases

Drive Out Blood Stasis from a Painful Body Decoction (shēn tòng zhú yū tāng)

身痛逐瘀湯

Semen Persicae (tao ren)

Flos Carthami Tinctorii (hong hua)

Radix Angelicae Sinensis (dang gui)

Radix Glycyrrhizae Uralensis (gan cao)

Excrementum Trogopterori seu Pteromi (wu ling zhi)

Rhizoma Cyperi Rotundi (xiang fu)

Lumbricus (di long)

Radix Gentianae Qinjiao (qin jiao)

Gummi Olibanum (ru xiang)

Radix et Rhizoma Notopterygii (qiang huo)

Radix Achyranthis Bidentatae (huai niu xi)

SOURCE: Correction of Errors Among Physicians

Ephedra Decoction Plus Atractylodes
 (má huáng jiā zhú tāng)

麻黄加朮湯

Herba Ephedrae (ma huang)

Semen Pruni Armeniacae (xing ren)

Ramulus Cinnamomi Cassiae (gui zhi)

Rhizoma Atractylodis Macrocephalae (bai zhu)

Radix Glycyrrhizae Uralensis (gan cao)

SOURCE: Essentials from the Golden Cabinet

Ephedra, Apricot Kernel, Gypsum, and Licorice Decoction (má xìng shí gān tāng)

麻杏石甘湯

Herba Ephedrae (ma huang)

Semen Pruni Armeniacae (xing ren)

Gypsum (shi gao)

Radix Glycyrrhizae Uralensis (gan cao)

SOURCE: Discussion of Cold-induced Disorders

Ephedra, Forsythia, and Aduki Bean Decoction
 (má huáng lián qiáo chì xiǎo dòu tāng)

麻黄連翹赤小豆湯

Herba Ephedrae (ma huang)

Fructus Forsythiae Suspensae (lian qiao)

Semen Pruni Armeniacae (xing ren)

Fructus Zizyphi Jujubae (da zao)

Cortex Catalpae Ovatae Radicis (zi bai pi)

Semen Phaseoli Calcarati (chi xiao dou)

Rhizoma Zingiberis Officinalis Recens (sheng jiang)

Radix Glycyrrhizae Uralensis (gan cao)

SOURCE: Discussion of Cold-induced Disorders

Five-Accumulation Powder (wǔ jī sǎn)

五積散

Herba Ephedrae (ma huang)

Rhizoma Atractylodis (cang zhu)

Radix Angelicae Dahuricae (bai zhi)

Radix Angelicae Sinensis (dang gui)

Radix Paeoniae Lactiflorae (bai shao yao)

Radix Ligustici Chuanxiong (chuan xiong)

Fructus Citri Aurantii (zhi ke)

Radix Platycodi Grandiflori (jie geng)

Ramulus Cinnamomi Cassiae (gui zhi)

Rhizoma Zingiberis Officinalis (gan jiang)

Sclerotium Poriae Cocos (fu ling)

Radix Glycyrrhizae Uralensis (gan cao)

Cortex Magnoliae Officinalis (hou po)

Pericarpium Citri Reticulatae (chen pi)

Rhizoma Pinelliae Ternatae (ban xia)

Rhizoma Zingiberis Officinalis Recens (sheng jiang)

SOURCE: Imperial Grace Formulary of the Tai Ping Era

Four-Substance Decoction (sì wù tāng)

四物湯

Radix Rehmanniae Glutinosae Conquitae (shu di huang)

Radix Angelicae Sinensis (dang gui)

Radix Ligustici Wallichii (chuan xiong)

Radix Paeoniae Lactiflorae (bai shao yao)

SOURCE: Imperial Grace Formulary of the Tai Ping Era

Increase the Fluids Decoction (zēng yè tāng)

曾液湯

Radix Rehmanniae Glutinosae (sheng di huang)

Radix Scrophulariae Ningpoensis (xuan shen)

Tuber Ophiopogonis Japonici (mai men dong)

SOURCE: *Systematic Differentiation of Warm Diseases*

Mutton Stew with Tangkuei and Fresh Ginger

  (dāng guī shēng jiāng yáng ròu tāng)

當歸生薑羊肉湯

Radix Angelicae Sinensis (dang gui)

Rhizoma Zingiberis Officinalis Recens (sheng jiang)

Mutton (yang rou)

SOURCE: *Essentials from the Golden Cabinet*

Prepared Aconite Decoction (fù zǐ tāng)

附子湯

Radix Lateralis Aconiti Carmichaeli Praeparata (fu zi)

Rhizoma Atractylodis Macrocephalae (bai zhu)

Radix Ginseng (ren shen)

Sclerotium Poriae Cocos (fu ling)

Radix Paeoniae Lactiflorae (bai shao yao)

SOURCE: *Discussion of Cold-induced Disorders*

Remove Painful Obstruction Decoction (juān bì tāng)

蠲痺湯

Rhizoma et Radix Notopterygii (qiang huo)

Radix Angelicae Pubescentis (du huo)

Ramulus Cinnamomi Cassiae (gui zhi)

Radix Gentianae Qinjiao (qin jiao)

Radix Angelicae Sinensis (dang gui)

Radix Ligustici Chuanxiong (chuan xiong)

Radix Glycyrrhizae Uralensis (gan cao)

Caulis Piperis Futokadsurae (hai feng teng)

Ramulus Mori Albae (sang zhi)

Gummi Olibanum (ru xiang)

Radix Aucklandiae Lappae (mu xiang)

SOURCE: *Medical Revelations*

Rhinoceros Horn Decoction (xī jiǎo tāng)

犀角湯

Cornu Rhinoceri (xi jiao)

Cornu Antelopis (ling yang jiao)

Radix Scutellariae Baicalensis (huang qin)

Fructus Gardeniae Jasminoidis (zhi zi)

Radix Peucedani (qian hu)

Rhizoma Cimicifugae (sheng ma)

Radix et Rhizoma Rhei (da huang)

Rhizoma Belamcandae Chinensis (she gan)

Semen Sojae Praeparatum (dan dou chi)

SOURCE: *Thousand Ducat Prescriptions*

Six-Ingredient Pill with Rehmannia

  (liù wèi dì huáng wán)

六味地黄丸

Radix Rehmanniae Glutinosae Conquitae (shu di huang)

Fructus Corni Officinalis (shan zhu yu)

Radix Dioscoreae Oppositae (shan yao)

Rhizoma Alismatis Orientalis (ze xie)

Cortex Moutan Radicis (mu dan pi)

Sclerotium Poriae Cocos (fu ling)

SOURCE: *Craft of Medicinal Treatment for Childhood
  Disease Patterns*

Three-Marvel Powder (sān miào sǎn)

三妙散

Rhizoma Atractylodis (cang zhu)

Cortex Phellodendri (huang bai)

Radix Achyranthis Bidentatae (niu xi)

SOURCE: *True Lineage of Medicine*

Tonify the Middle and Augment the Qi Decoction

  (bǔ zhōng yì qì tāng)

補中益氣湯

Radix Astragali Membranacei (huang qi)

Radix Codonopsis Pilosulae (dang shen)

Rhizoma Atractylodis Macrocephalae (bai zhu)

Radix Glycyrrhizae Uralensis (gan cao)

Radix Angelicae Sinensis (dang gui)

Rhizoma Cimicifugae (sheng ma)

Radix Bupleuri (chai hu)

Pericarpium Citri Reticulatae (chen pi)

SOURCE: *Discussion of the Spleen and Stomach*

True Warrior Decoction (zhēn wǔ tāng)

眞武湯

Radix Lateralis Aconiti Carmichaeli Praeparata (fu zi)

Sclerotium Poriae Cocos (fu ling)

Rhizoma Atractylodis Macrocephalae (bai zhu)

Radix Paeoniae Lactiflorae (bai shao yao)

Rhizoma Zingiberis Officinalis Recens (sheng jiang)

SOURCE: *Discussion of Cold-induced Disorders*

White Tiger Decoction (*bái hǔ tāng*)

白虎湯

Gypsum *(shi gao)*
Rhizoma Anemarrhenae Asphodeloidis *(zhi mu)*
Nonglutinous rice *(geng mi)*
Radix Glycyrrhizae Uralensis *(gan cao)*
SOURCE: *Discussion of Cold-induced Disorders*

Chapter Notes

1. *Editors' note:* The word *bì* means an obstruction to the free circulation of Qi and Blood, and the word by itself can simply mean obstruction. The expression "painful obstruction" has become one of the standard translations in English language texts and will be used throughout this book, as it is basically a satisfactory translation. However, we wish to acknowledge that this is a slightly restrictive interpretation: while most forms of *bì* are painful, some are not.

2. One edition says loose *(huǎn)*.

3. *Editors' note:* "Quiescence" here refers to nourishment of the yin, "movement" to disbanding and unblocking the painful obstruction.

4. *Editors' note:* The original formula prescribes Radix Rehmanniae Glutinosae *(sheng di huang)*.

5. *Editors' note:* The original formula prescribes Cortex Cinnamomi Cassiae *(rou gui)*.

6. *Editors' note:* A famous traditional Chinese physician who lived from 1877-1962.

7. *Editors' note:* Literally "shoulder front." This point is more commonly known as *jiān nèi líng*, "shoulders' front mound."

8. *Editors' note:* We have been unable to determine which point is meant by *jiān hòu*.

9. *Editors' note:* We have been unable to determine which point is meant by *yù yīn*.

10. *Editors' note:* The full name of Dr. Fang is not disclosed in the original text. It is possible that this reference should be to Dr. Wang, as the following article is included in the references under the name Wang Ren-Zhang: "Discussion of pattern analysis and therapeutic conclusions for rheumatoid arthritis, with appended report of an analysis of 100 examples," *New Medicine and Materia Medica (Xin yi yao xue)* 3, 1979.

11. Zhu Liang-Chun, "Experiences in treating painful obstruction," *Journal of Traditional Chinese Medicine (Zhong yi za zhi)* 12:1, 1980. The ingredients for his formula are listed at the end of this chapter.

12. *Editors' note:* The full name of Dr. Dai is not disclosed in the original text.

13. Zhang Mo-Duan, "Clinical analysis of 32 cases of rheumatoid arthritis treated with cinnamon twig, peony, and anemarrhena decoction," *Journal of Traditional Chinese Medicine (Zhong yi za zhi)* 1:38, 1981.

14. *Basic Questions,* chapter 43.

15. Zhang Ming-He, "Summary of the effectiveness of combined Chinese-Western treatment of 116 cases of rheumatoid arthritis," *Collection of Papers on Traditional Chinese Medicine from Shandong Province (Shangdong sheng zhong yi xue shu lun wen ji)*, 1979.

16. *Editors' note:* This appears to refer to Zhu Liang-Chun, previously mentioned in n. 11.

17. *Editors' note:* Dr. Dai is not further identified.

18. Li Xiao-Pu, *Reference for Diagnosis and Treatment* (Kunming: Yunnan College of Traditional Chinese Medicine, 1978).

19. Zhang Bo-Yu, *Case Histories of Zhang Bo-Yu* (Shanghai: Shanghai Science and Technology Press, 1979).

20. *Editors' note:* To date, the primary identified components include wilfordine, wilforine, wilforgine, wilfortrine, wilforzine, celastrol.

21. *Editors' note:* The Chinese term for rheumatic fever is *fēng shī rè*. This is also the term for the traditional disorder Wind-Damp-Heat. Even when, as here, it is used in the biomedical sense, it can refer to post-streptococcal rheumatism as well as rheumatic fever proper.

22. Bei Shu-Ying, "Traditional Chinese herbal treatment of rheumatoid arthritis with appended survey of 60 cases," *Jiangsu Traditional Chinese Medicine (Jiangsu zhong yi)* 1:35, 1980.

23. *Editors' note:* It is not stated what happened to the other ten cases. There is probably a misprint in the original text.

24. *Editors' note:* This appears to refer to Zhu Liang-Chun, previously mentioned in n. 11 above.

25. *Editors' note:* The original text does not indicate who this particular Dr. Gong is, or otherwise identify his report.

26. *Editors' note:* It is unclear who Dr. Zhang is, and what specific modifications he made to the formula.

27. Liu Bai-Ling, "Using osteophyte pills in the treatment of 1,181 cases of osteophytes," *New Traditional Chinese Medicine (Xin zhong yi)* 2:11, 1973.

28. Shi Yong-Ming, "Aged vinegar with direct current therapy for 58 cases of bone spurs, arthritis, and diseases of large joints," *New Herbal Medicine (Xin yi yao xue)* 7:41, 1974.

29. Gu Bo-Hua, *Selected Experiences of External Medicine* (Shanghai: Shanghai Science and Technology Press, 1976).

30. Fang Yao-Zhong, "Summary of 512 cases of brucellosis," unpublished research, 1975.

31. *Editors' note:* Included here are only those formulas that appear in this section of the original text, which is by no means all of the formulas noted in the chapter itself. The only change that we have made is to arrange the formulas in alphabetical order by English name. For more detailed information regarding most of these formulas, see Dan Bensky and Randall Barolet, *Chinese Herbal Medicine: Formulas & Strategies* (Seattle: Eastland Press, 1990).

CHAPTER SIX

Panarthralgia Disorder

THE CLINICAL CHARACTERISTICS of panarthralgia disorder are joint pain, swelling and deformity to the point of inability to move the joints. Because its pain spreads throughout all the joints in the body, it is called panarthralgia *(lì jié bìng 歷節病)*, or literally, "disease that goes through all the joints."

History

In chapter 5 of the Han work *Essentials from the Golden Cabinet (Jin gui yao lue)*, Zhang Zhong-Jing describes this disorder in a relatively systematic manner. In the pertinent sections of that book, the primary etiology of panarthralgia is given as insufficiency in one's natural endowment, incautious regulation of one's life, or lack of moderation in one's desires. All this can lead to injury and exhaustion of the Qi, Blood, Liver and Kidneys. The Liver governs the sinews and the Kidneys govern the bones. When these two Organs are deficient, there is nothing with which to nourish the sinews and bones. A place with intense deficiency is a place that welcomes a pathogenic influence. Pathogenic Wind, Cold and Dampness take advantage of the deficiency and enter the body. When there are pathogenic influences both externally and internally, this disease results. Zhang Zhong-Jing noted the following clinical manifestations: "The various joints of the limbs are sore and painful, the body is crooked and gaunt, and the legs are swollen as if they are about to fall off. . . . The body is crooked and gaunt, only the feet are swollen and enlarged." With respect to treatment, based on differences in the condition, Zhang developed two formulas: Cinnamon Twig, Peony, and Anemarrhena Decoction *(gui zhi shao yao zhi mu tang)* and Aconite Decoction *(wu tou tang)*. In terms of the principles and methods of treatment, as well as the specific herbs and formulas, he laid a good foundation for later generations of physicians.

After the Han period this disorder was known by such names as "panarthralgic wind" *(lì jié fēng)*, "white tiger disorder" *(bái hǔ bìng)*, or "white tiger panarthralgic wind" *(bái hǔ lì jié fēng)*. Over time a deeper understanding was gained of its etiology and clinical manifestations, along with more abundant treatment modalities.

The Tang physician Sun Si-Miao wrote, in the third chapter of the eighth division of his *Thousand Ducat Prescriptions (Qian jin yao fang)*, "When panarthralgia strikes an individual and the condition is not treated, it can invade the joints and cause loss of one's footing and [one] falls." This is a very appropriate illustration of the characteristic stages of development of this disease. Sun Si-Miao also added to the etiology of panarthralgia the concept of "Heat Toxin circulating in the four limbs."

The eighth-century writer Wang Dao linked the different etiologies in the thirteenth division of *Arcane Essentials from the Imperial Library (Wai tai bi yao)*:

Generally speaking, the disease is due to penetration of Toxic Wind, Cold, Heat and Dampness acting on an underlying deficiency. The control function is disrupted, the body is attacked by the pathogenic Wind, there is clumping and stagnation in the channels and vessels, which builds up between the bones and joints or resides in the four limbs.

Wang also emphasized the characteristic symptoms of this disease, that the pain is excruciating, and that it diminishes during the day and increases at night: "This disease subsides during the day and is aggravated at night; the pain pierces the marrow and lets go suddenly, like a white tiger bite, hence its name."

Later, during the Ming dynasty, in a chapter in *Formulas of Universal Benefit (Pu ji fang)* entitled "Panarthralgia Disorder," the phrase "the fingers are crooked and bent" appeared. The Qing dynasty work *Comprehensive Medicine According to Master Zhang (Zhang shi yi tong)* noted that when this disease lasts a long time without a cure, "limb joints like mallets" can be observed.

From a diagnostic and therapeutic point of view, *Formulas to Aid the Living (Ji sheng fang)* divided this disease into three categories, Wind, Cold and Dampness:

> Those for whom the pain is like an awl have more Cold. Those who are so swollen and full that it is like the limb is going to fall off have more Dampness. Those who sweat have more Wind.

Different texts, such as *Thousand Ducat Prescriptions, Arcane Essentials from the Imperial Library, Imperial Grace Formulary of the Tai Ping Era (Tai ping hui min he ji ju fang), Comprehensive Recording of Sage-like Benefit from the Zheng He Era (Zheng he sheng ji zong lu), Formulas of Universal Benefit from My Practice (Pu ji ben shi fang)*, have described the various treatments for panarthralgia: decoctions, plasters, pills, powders, medicinal wines, acupuncture and massage.

As far as the relationship between panarthralgia and painful obstruction is concerned, it is commonly held that painful obstruction is a more general concept and that panarthralgia is just one aspect of it.

Panarthralgia is specifically related to joint pathologies; its chief features are joint deformation, pain, impaired motion and stiffness. The biomedical disorders of rheumatoid arthritis and gout share similarities with this condition, and this chapter as well as the previous one on painful obstruction can therefore be used as a reference for diagnosis and treatment.

Etiology and Pathology

The etiology and pathology of panarthralgia fall into one of two categories: exhausted and harmed Liver and Kidneys, and penetration of pathogenic influences.

EXHAUSTED AND HARMED LIVER AND KIDNEYS

As previously noted by Zhang Zhong-Jing, the Liver governs the sinews and the Kidneys govern the bones. The sinews and bones rely on the Liver, Kidneys, Essence, Blood and Fluids for nourishment. They also rely on the warmth of the Liver and Kidney yang Qi. These can be compromised by various factors including congenital constitutional insufficiency, excessive sexual activity, overconsumption of acidic or salty foods, emotional experiences such as fright and terror or frustration and anger, or a poor convalescent routine. Each of these factors can eventually exhaust and harm the Kidney and Liver essential Qi, or directly harm the yang Qi, or first harm the yin Essence which, as it progresses, harms the yang. "Where the pathogenic has attacked, the person's Qi must be deficient."[1]

A state of exhaustion in the Liver and Kidneys can induce stagnation of the Qi and Blood, the nutritive and the protective, which collects in the areas around the joints and transforms into Heat, ferments into Phlegm, causes the Blood to stagnate and form stasis, and thus leads to joint swelling, deformation, pain and impaired movement.

On the other hand, since the external protective Qi is not firm, external pathogenic influences can easily attack the body. The pathogenic influences of Wind, Cold, Dampness and Heat take advantage of this underlying deficiency to invade the body, impair the circulation of the nutritive and protective Qi, clog and stagnate the channels and collaterals, penetrate the sinews and bones, and aggravate the condition.

PENETRATION OF PATHOGENIC INFLUENCES

When the normal Qi is insufficient, pathogenic influences can easily attack. Exposing oneself to wind after drinking alcoholic beverages, going in the water while sweating, falling asleep in a cool place, or living in a damp and cool environment are all factors that can promote the invasion of Wind, Cold, Dampness and Heat.

Since pathogenic Wind moves freely, undergoes frequent transformations and circulates throughout the body, it can affect several joints simultaneously or successively. Pathogenic Cold freezes, slows down and congeals. Besides impairing movement in the joints and sinews, it can also cause stagnation of the Blood and Qi and the nutritive and protective Qi, accompanied by violent pain. Pathogenic Dampness sticks, stagnates, impairs the movement of the Qi and Blood and prevents smooth circulation, causing the affected areas to become swollen, painful and heavy; the pathology is chronic and it is difficult for the patient to get better quickly. Pathogenic Heat settles in the channels and vessels, spreads throughout the body and exhausts the Fluids and Blood. When the Blood is dry, Blood stasis and Heat combine. When the Fluids are depleted, they transform into Phlegm. The joints and channels become obstructed by the Heat, Phlegm and Blood stasis. This combination generates Toxins, the Essence and Qi are seriously injured, and the progression of the illness accelerates.

Pathogenic Wind, Cold, Dampness and Heat often combine to trigger a disease; on the other hand, a lingering Wind-Damp-Cold disorder may eventually transform into Heat. That is why the symptoms' characteristics must be closely analyzed in order to prevent misdiagnosis.

In addition to these factors, we must bear in mind that this condition can also result from strain (i.e., lifting a heavy object) or from a fall, either of which can cause Blood stasis and Qi stagnation.

Diagnosis and Treatment

Clinical manifestations will show whether the disorder can be considered latent or in the process of getting worse (exacerbation). This must be taken into account for purposes of treatment. During latency the disease is in a relatively quiescent stage, and the picture is one of deficient normal Qi with retained pathogenic influences, primarily either a weak and deficient yang Qi or an insufficiency of yin Blood. There are often no significant joint problems during this period, and when they occur they are not intense.

During exacerbations, joint pain is intensified and may be accompanied by such exterior signs as aversion to cold, and fever. The dominant picture is one of an excess of pathogenic Qi. This usually occurs when one has not been careful in protecting oneself, which allows pathogenic Wind, Cold and Dampness to invade the body.

LATENT STAGE

Weak and Deficient Yang Qi

Symptomatology

After frequent recurrences of joint pain, the joints become stiff, motion is impaired and the pain becomes mild, dull or nonexistent. At the same time the patient has a pale complexion, lightheadedness, tinnitus, fear of cold, spontaneous sweating, soreness and weakness of the lower back and legs, profuse and clear urine, frequent urination at night and posturinary drip. The pulse is submerged, thin and frail, and the tongue is pale with a thin white coating.

Pathology

A deficient yang constitution comes about either from chronic Cold and Damp stagnation or a long-term disease that first harms the yin and then the yang. With yang Qi deficiency, the skin and hair are not stable, the Protective Qi fails in its assignment to protect the exterior, and the person feels cold, has an aversion to wind, and sweats profusely. When the outside fence[2] has holes in it, external pathogenic influences penetrate easily. When the holding, stabilizing and containing functions falter, urination is frequent and clear, and there is frequent urination at night. If there is yang Qi deficiency, the ascending and rising motions in the body are without force, manifesting in lightheadedness and a pale complexion. The lower back is the abode of the Kidneys; if the Kidney Qi is insufficient, it can no longer perform its warming and nourishing functions, which can cause weakness of the lower back and knees, and coldness of the four limbs. The pale tongue and thin pulse are both manifestations of yang Qi deficiency.

Treatment

The treatment principle is to warm the yang and augment the Qi.

For signs of intense Cold, combine yang-warming and Cold-dispersing methods. For severe pain, also invigorate the Blood and open the collaterals.

Prescriptions

The basic formula is Kidney Qi Pill from *Golden Cabinet (jin gui shen qi wan)*, with the addition of Radix Codonopsitis Pilosulae *(dang shen)* and Radix Astragali Membranacei *(huang qi)*. In this formula, Radix Codonopsitis Pilosulae *(dang shen)*, Radix Astragali Membranacei *(huang qi)*, Radix Lateralis Aconiti Carmichaeli Praeparata *(fu zi)* and Ramulus Cinnamomi Cassiae *(gui zhi)* warm the yang and augment the Qi; Radix Rehmanniae Glutinosae Conquitae *(shu di huang),* Fructus Corni Officinalis *(shan zhu yu)* and Radix Dioscoreae Oppositae *(shan yao)* augment the Kidneys and supplement the Essence; Sclerotium Poriae Cocos *(fu ling),* Rhizoma Alismatis Orientalis *(ze xie)* and Cortex Moutan Radicis *(mu dan pi)* resolve Dampness and drain the pathogenic influences.

For Spleen deficiency with excess Dampness, add Rhizoma Atractylodis *(cang zhu),* Rhizoma Atractylodis Macrocephalae *(bai zhu),* Semen Coicis Lachryma-jobi *(yi yi ren),* Caulis Mutong *(mu tong)* and Herba Plantaginis *(che qian cao).* For insufficiency of Liver Blood, add Radix Angelicae Sinensis *(dang gui)* and Radix Paeoniae Lactiflorae *(bai shao).* For symptoms of intense Cold, add Herba cum Radice Asari *(xi xin)* and Radix Aconiti Carmichaeli Praeparata *(zhi chuan wu).* To invigorate the Blood and unblock the collaterals, choose from among such herbs as Radix et Caulis Jixueteng *(ji xue teng),* Radix Clematidis *(wei ling xian),* Rhizoma Dioscoreae Nipponicae *(chuan shan long),* Radix Angelicae Pubescentis *(du huo),* Ramulus Sangjisheng *(sang ji sheng)* and Cortex Acanthopanacis Gracilistylus Radicis *(wu jia pi).*

If there is a Wind-Cold invasion with an underlying yang deficiency, Minor Prolong Life Decoction *(xiao xu ming tang)* can be prescribed. In this formula, Radix Ginseng *(ren shen),* Radix Paeoniae Lactiflorae *(bai shao)* and Radix Ligustici Chuanxiong *(chuan xiong)* nourish the Blood and tonify the deficiency; Ramulus Cinnamomi Cassiae *(gui zhi),* Herba Ephedrae *(ma huang)* and Radix Lateralis Aconiti Carmichaeli Praeparata *(fu zi)* warm the channels and unblock the yang; Radix Ledebouriallae Divaricatae *(fang feng)* and Radix Stephaniae Tetrandrae *(fang ji)* eliminate Wind-Dampness to unblock the collaterals; Semen Pruni Armeniacae *(xing ren)* regulates the Qi; Radix Glycyrrhizae Uralensis *(gan cao)* harmonizes the middle burner. If there is no Heat stagnation, Radix Scutellariae Baicalensis *(huang qin)* can be deleted. For excessive sweating, Herba Ephedrae *(ma huang)* is replaced by Radix Astragali Membranacei *(huang qi).*

In cases of long-standing yang deficiency, pathogenic Dampness invades the joints and transforms into Phlegm; the joints become swollen, painful and cold. Yang-Heartening Decoction *(yang he tang)* should then be prescribed. In this formula, Gelatinum Cornu Cervi *(lu jiao jiao)* — or Cornu Cervi Degelatinatium *(lu jiao shuang)* — and Radix Rehmanniae Glutinosae Conquitae *(shu di huang)* intensely tonify the Blood and Essence. Herba Ephedrae *(ma huang),* Quick-fried Rhizoma Zingiberis Officinalis *(pao jiang)* and Cortex Cinnamomi Cassiae *(rou gui)* unblock the yang and unbind the painful obstruction. Semen Sinapis Albae *(bai jie zi)* eliminates Phlegm.

Herbs such as the following can be added to invigorate the Blood and transform Blood stasis, warm the channels and unblock the collaterals: Herba Epimedii *(yin yang huo),* Nidus Vespae *(lu feng fang),* Buthus Martensi *(quan xie),* Radix Angelicae Sinensis *(dang gui),* Gummi Olibanum *(ru xiang),* Myrrha *(mo yao),* Flos Carthami Tinctorii *(hong hua)* Semen Persicae *(tao ren).*

For Qi and Blood deficiency, add Radix Astragali Membranacei *(huang qi)* and Radix Angelicae Sinensis *(dang gui).* For yang deficiency, add Radix Lateralis Aconiti Carmichaeli Praeparata *(fu zi).*

Yin Blood Deficiency

Symptomatology

Following a prolonged history of recurrent attacks of joint pain, the joints feel contracted, motion is limited, and there is often a slight topical burning sensation with redness and swelling. Pain is usually more significant at night. In some cases there may be no clear joint problems. Accompanying signs may include lightheadedness, vertigo, ringing in the ears, dry mouth, irritability, warm palms and soles, insomnia with vivid dreams, weakness of the lower back and knees, thin and rapid pulse, and shiny red tongue.

Pathology

This condition can arise in a person with an underlying yin-deficient constitution, following a loss of Blood, chronic disease or persistent Damp-Heat, or contraction of Toxic Heat, or Wind-Damp-Cold causing long-term constraint and transforming into Heat. In all these scenarios the pathogenic Heat injures the yin and leads to an insufficiency of yin Blood. The deficient yin Blood cannot nourish the sinews and bones, causing joint dysfunction and weakness and soreness in the lower back and knees. Yin deficiency generates internal Heat, which stirs up and rises, causing vertigo, vivid dreams, irritability, dryness of the throat and ringing in the ears. Heat burns the sinews and vessels, causing local redness and heat, as well as pain that worsens at night. The pulse and tongue characteristics confirm the diagnosis of yin Blood deficiency and internal Heat.

Treatment

The principle of treatment is to enrich the yin, clear the Heat, nourish the Blood and harmonize the Blood. For pronounced internal Heat, the treatment principle is to enrich the yin and cause the Fire to descend.

Prescriptions

The basic formula is a combination of Six-Ingredient Pill with Rehmannia *(liu wei di huang wan)* and Four-Substance Decoction *(si wu tang)*.

For internal Heat, add Cortex Phellodendri *(huang bai)* and Rhizoma Anemarrhenae Asphodeloidis *(zhi mu)*. For impaired movement of the joints, add Ramulus Mori Albae *(sang zhi)*, Herba cum Radice Lycopodii Clavati *(shen jin cao)*, Radix Achyranthis Bidentatae *(niu xi)*, Herba Herba Siegesbeckiae *(xi xian cao)*, Lumbricus *(di long)* and Bombyx Batryticatus *(jiang can)*. For weakness and pain in the lower back and knees, add Semen Cuscutae Chinensis *(tu si zi)*, Radix Achyranthis Bidentatae *(niu xi)*, Cortex Eucommiae Ulmoidis *(du zhong)*, Radix Dipsaci Asperi *(xu duan)* and Cortex Lycii Radicis *(di gu pi)*. For pain that worsens at night, add Radix Paeoniae Rubrae *(chi shao)*, Semen Persicae *(tao ren)*, Flos Carthami Tinctorii *(hong hua)* and Radix Angelicae Sinensis *(dang gui)*.

For redness and swelling of the joints, combine Two-Marvel Powder *(er miao san)* with Rhizoma Dioscoreae Hypoglaucae *(bei xie)*, Semen Coicis Lachryma-jobi *(yi yi ren)*, Radix Achyranthis Bidentatae *(niu xi)* and Lumbricus *(di long)*. Another possibility is to take 3-5g of powdered Cortex Phellodendri *(huang bai)*. This is known as Slinking Powder *(qian xing san)*.

EXACERBATION STAGE

Cold Pattern

Symptomatology

The principal signs are fever, aversion to cold, absence of sweating or fever unabated by sweating, severe joint pain appearing successively or simultaneously in more than one location, and reduced range of motion. Pain is aggravated by exposure to wind and cold, and is alleviated by topical application of warmth. The tongue is pale with a thin white coating, and the pulse is tight and either floating or submerged.

Pathology

Panarthralgia is caused by an invasion of pathogenic

Wind-Damp-Cold. When these three pathogenic influences combine, Cold is predominant. At the onset the pathogenic influences settle in the exterior, as indicated by the fever and aversion to cold.

When Wind and Cold predominate, the fever is high and there is no sweating. When Wind and Dampness predominate, the fever is mild, there is sweating but the sweating does not disperse the pathogenic influences, and the fever lingers on. When pathogenic influences attack they progress toward the interior. At this time they stir up any pathogenic influences that were previously harbored inside.

The nature of Cold is to contract, Wind is characteristically migratory, and the nature of Dampness is heavy and turbid. When these pathogenic influences clog the joints they obstruct the circulation of Blood and Qi, causing severe joint pain (alleviated by the application of warmth) and limiting the range of motion. The pale tongue with a thin white coating is a sign of Cold, and the tight pulse indicates pain.

Treatment

The principle of treatment is to warm the yang, dispel the Cold and alleviate the pain.

Prescriptions

The basic formula is Aconite Decoction *(wu tou tang)*. In this formula, Herba Ephedrae *(ma huang)* promotes sweating, releases the exterior, disperses Cold and unblocks the painful obstruction; Radix Aconiti *(wu tou)* tracks down Wind, disperses Cold, warms the channels and alleviates pain; Radix Astragali Membranacei *(huang qi)* augments the protective Qi; Radix Paeoniae Lactiflorae *(bai shao)* regulates the Blood and painful obstruction; Radix Glycyrrhizae Uralensis *(gan cao)* harmonizes the various ingredients in this formula. The decoction is prepared with honey, which not only augments the Blood and nourishes the sinews, moderates the spasms and alleviates the pain, but also counteracts the Dry and Hot Toxicity of the aconite.

For joint swelling and excess Dampness, use Five-Accumulation Powder *(wu ji san)*. For Blood stasis, add Semen Persicae *(tao ren)*, Flos Carthami Tinctorii *(hong hua)*, Radix Paeoniae Rubrae *(chi shao)*, Squama Manitis Pentadactylae *(chuan shan jia)* and Spina Gleditsiae Sinensis *(zao jiao ci)*, as well as Major Invigorate the Collaterals Special Pill *(da huo luo dan)*.

Hot Pattern

Symptomatology

The patient will present with an aversion to wind, fever, and sweating that does not affect the fever. The joints are red, hot, swollen and painful, and cannot tolerate any pressure. There is irritability, thirst with desire to drink, dark urine, red tongue with a yellow coating, and a rapid, forceful pulse.

When the Toxic Heat is intense, the joint pain, swelling and heat will be excruciating, comparable to being cut or bitten by a tiger. It intensifies at night and lessens during the day. The patient loses weight and may develop scaly skin, the tongue is red with little moisture and a dry yellow coating, and the pulse is thin and rapid.

Pathology

This condition is caused by the Toxic Qi of pathogenic Heat, Damp-Heat transforming into Fire, or the constraint of Wind-Damp-Cold for a prolonged period, which then transforms into Fire. The nature of Fire is violent; it sears the sinews and vessels such that the joints become red, hot and severely painful. Fire condenses the Fluids, causing irritability, thirst and dark urine. Signs indicative of exterior disorders, such as aversion to wind and a floating pulse, often accompany the early stages of this condition. When the pathogenic Heat enters the interior, the blazing Fire injures the Fluids, the tongue becomes red with little saliva, and with a dry yellow coating, and the pulse becomes thin and rapid.

Treatment

The principle of treatment is to clear the Heat, relieve the Toxicity, invigorate the Blood and unblock the collaterals.

Prescriptions

Rhinoceros Horn Decoction *(xi jiao tang)* is recommended, with the addition of Semen Persicae *(tao ren)* and Flos Carthami Tinctorii *(hong hua)*. In this formula, Cornu Rhinoceri *(xi jiao)* and Cornu Antelopis *(ling yang jiao)* relieve Toxicity and clear Heat; Radix et Rhizoma Rhei *(da huang)*, Radix Scutellariae Baicalensis *(huang qin)* and Fructus Gardeniae Jasminoidis *(zhi zi)* drain the excessive Fire; Rhizoma Cimicifugae *(sheng ma)* and Rhizoma Belamcandae Chinensis *(she gan)* relieve Heat Toxicity; Radix Peucedani *(qian hu)* and Semen Sojae Praeparatum *(dan dou chi)* release the exterior and disperse pathogenic influences; Semen Persicae *(tao ren)* and Flos Carthami Tinctorii *(hong hua)* invigorate the Blood and unblock the collaterals.

Cornu Rhinoceri *(xi jiao)* and Cornu Antelopis *(ling yang jiao)* can be replaced by Flos Lonicerae Japonicae *(jin yin hua)*, Fructus Forsythiae Suspensae *(lian qiao)*, Herba cum Radice Violae Yedoensitis *(zi hua di ding)*, Flos Chrysanthemi Indici *(ye ju hua)*, Rhizoma Imperatae Cylindricae *(bai mao gen)* and Rhizoma Phragmitis Communis *(lu gen)*.[3]

For vigorous Heat, add Gypsum *(shi gao)*, Rhizoma Anemarrhenae Asphodeloidis *(zhi mu)* and Ramus Lonicerae Japonicae *(ren dong teng)*. For Heat injuring the yin, add Radix Rehmanniae Glutinosae *(sheng di huang)*, Radix Scrophulariae Ningpoensis *(xuan shen)* and Tuber Ophiopogonis Japonici *(mai men dong)*.

Other herbs to expel Wind and open the collaterals can also be added, such as Ramulus Sangjisheng *(sang ji sheng)*, Radix Gentianae Qinjiao *(qin jiao)*, Ramulus Mori Albae *(sang zhi)*, Radix Clematidis *(wei ling xian)*, Radix Paeoniae Rubrae *(chi shao)*, Lumbricus *(di long)* and Excrementum Bombycis Mori *(can sha)*.

OTHER PREMODERN TREATMENTS

1. For panarthralgia with swelling due to Wind-Heat attacking the fingers such that they become red, swollen, numb and have paresthesia, take Fructus Arctii Lappae *(niu bang zi)* 90g, Semen Sojae Praeparatum *(dan dou chi)* 30g, and toasted Rhizoma et Radix Notopterygii *(chao qiang huo)* 30g. Powder and take 6g each time with boiled water. From *Prescriptions of Universal Benefit from My Practice (Pu ji ben shi fang)*.

2. For panarthralgia due to Wind with pain in the bones and joints that is unremitting, both night and day, take powdered Myrrha *(mo yao)* 20g, with toasted and powdered Os Tigris *(hu gu)* 90g. Take 6g each time with warm wine. From *Illustrated Classic of the Materia Medica (Tu jing ben cao)*

3. For those with joint pain as intense as a tiger bite for whom there is a scary pain in the bones and joints, take equal parts of a sufficient quantity of Semen Sinapis Albae *(bai jie zi)*, Semen Momordicae Cochinchinensis *(mu bie zi)*, Radix Euphorbiae Kansui *(gan sui)*, Gummi Olibanum *(ru xiang)* and Radix Aconiti Carmichaeli Praeparata *(zhi chuan wu)*. Grind the ingredients into a fine powder, and use rice paste to

prepare pills the size of a small grain. Take 70 to 80 pills each time with wine. From *Fine Formulas of Extraordinary Effectiveness (Qi xiao liang fang).*

4. For white tiger panarthralgic Wind, apply moxibustion at both the internal and external malleoli. From *Outline of Medicine (Yi xue gang mu).*

5. For panarthralgic Wind of the limbs with pain so excruciating it is like being pounded by a hammer, take Aconite Eight-Substance Decoction *(fu zi ba wu tang).* The ingredients are 90g each of Radix Lateralis Aconiti Carmichaeli Praeparata *(fu zi),* Rhizoma Zingiberis Officinalis *(gan jiang),* Radix Paeoniae *(shao yao),* Sclerotium Poriae Cocos *(fu ling),* Rhizoma Pinelliae Ternatae *(ban xia),* Cortex Cinnamomi Cassiae *(rou gui)* and Radix Ginseng *(ren shen),* together with 120g of Rhizoma Atractylodis Macrocephalae *(bai zhu).* Grind into a powder and take 12g decocted with two small glasses of water until seven-tenths of a glass is left. Strain and take before meals. From *Outline of Medicine (Yi xue gang mu).*

6. For white tiger panarthralgia, use Augmented Four-Substance Decoction *(jia wei si wu tang).* This formula includes Radix Rehmanniae Glutinosae *(sheng di huang),* Radix Angelicae Sinensis *(dang gui),* Radix Ligustici Chuanxiong *(chuan xiong)* and Radix Paeoniae Lactiflorae *(bai shao)* with the addition of Semen Persicae *(tao ren),* Radix Achyranthis Bidentatae *(niu xi),* Pericarpium Citri Reticulatae *(chen pi),* Sclerotium Poriae Cocos *(fu ling),* Radix Glycyrrhizae Uralensis *(gan cao),* Radix Angelicae Dahuricae *(bai zhi)* and Radix Gentianae Longdancao *(long dan cao).*

If the pain is primarily in the upper part of the body, indicating that Wind predominates, add Radix et Rhizoma Notopterygii *(qiang huo),* Ramulus Cinnamomi Cassiae *(gui zhi)* and Radix Clematidis *(wei ling xian).* If the pain is primarily in the lower extremities, indicating that Dampness predominates, add Radix Achyranthis Bidentatae *(niu xi),* Radix Aristolochiae Fangchi *(fang ji),* Caulis Mutong *(mu tong)* and Cortex Phellodendri *(huang bai).* When there is Phlegm, add Pulvis Arisaemae cum Felle Bovis *(dan nan xing),* Rhizoma Pinelliae Ternatae *(ban xia)* and Rhizoma Zingiberis Officinalis Recens *(sheng jiang).* For Blood deficiency, double the amounts of Radix Ligustici Chuanxiong *(chuan xiong)* and Radix Angelicae Sinensis *(dang gui),* and add Flos Carthami Tinctorii *(hong hua).* Take as a decoction. From *True Lineage of Medicine (Yi xue zheng chuan).*

Prognosis

Periods of latency and exacerbation tend to alternate in panarthralgia disorder. When the nutritive and protective Qi are deficient and the body is invaded by an external pathogenic influence, this can exacerbate a pre-existing condition after a period of latency. Early and appropriate treatment will eliminate the external pathogenic influence and restore the original state of relative balance.

Because the latent phase of panarthralgia is characterized by a state of deficiency, there are few symptoms; on the other hand, the exacerbation phase represents a state of excess, with an acute symptomatology. The shift from one phase to the other illustrates the alternation between manifestation (branch) and root, deficiency and excess, moderation and urgency.

The development of this disease depends first on the internal progression of the pathogenic influences, and second on the timing of the treatment. That is why it is essential for patients to protect themselves against external pathogenic influences during the latent phase in order to prevent a relapse or an aggravation of the condition, and to treat the condition early and efficiently during the exacerbation phase in order to reverse the evolution.

There can also be transformation back and forth between different types of patterns during the exacerbation phase of this disorder. Hot types are generally the most severe, hence the need to prevent the contraction and accumulation of Wind-Damp-Cold, which can transform into Heat.

During the evolution of panarthralgia, it is often difficult to bring swollen and deformed joints fully back to normal in the short term. The changing nature of this disorder and the frequent relapses can cause permanent damage, or even lead to death.

Prevention

Internal injury is often the source of panarthralgia. It is therefore important to maintain harmonious emotions and desires, a balanced diet, and to avoid working to the point of exhaustion. Another fundamental aspect of prevention is to protect and strengthen the normal Qi, regularly practice some therapeutic physical exercise, and keep the sinews and joints of the limbs mobile.

From a preventive point of view, it is also recommended that patients with this condition dress warmly in order to guard themselves against external pathogenic influences, and so avoid catching colds. In case of joint stiffness and obvious limitation in the range of motion, it is necessary to curtail activities appropriately.

Modern Research

The clinical manifestations of panarthralgia present some similarities with modern biomedically defined diseases, such as rheumatoid arthritis, Kashin-Beck disease and gout. The concepts of etiology and pathogenesis of panarthralgia can therefore be used to diagnose and explain the aforementioned conditions from a traditional Chinese perspective. Among these, the therapeutic methods for treating panarthralgia are most commonly applied to rheumatoid arthritis.

Dr. Wang[4] believes that the clinical manifestations of rheumatoid arthritis resemble those of white tiger panarthralgia, painful Wind and bone painful obstruction. The different types of etiology are Damp-Cold, Damp-Heat and Toxic Dampness. When Damp-Cold stagnates for a prolonged period, it evolves into Damp-Heat. When Damp-Heat is not transformed, it becomes Toxic Dampness. The internal causes are always either yang deficiency or an insufficiency of yin or Blood. According to Dr. Wang, the therapeutic approach falls into four different categories:

1. Heat type: This is most often seen during the exacerbation phase of the illness. Clinical signs include pain and redness of the small joints of the hand and foot, or pain with swelling of the spine. There is limitation in the range of motion of the joints. These symptoms are accompanied by fever, spontaneous sweating, irritability, thirst and difficult bowel movements. The tongue is red, the coating is thin and yellow, and the pulse is thin and rapid or slippery and rapid. The principle of treatment is to clear Heat, relieve Toxicity, dispel Blood stasis, unblock the collaterals, reduce swelling and alleviate the pain.

2. Cold type: This often corresponds to the relatively stable or latent phase. Clinical signs include deformation of the small joints of the hand and foot, which are swollen, painful and difficult to move. There is finger stiffness which is aggravated by cold. The patient also feels cold with cold limbs, and the spine is swollen and painful. The tongue is pale with a white coating, and the pulse is submerged and thin. The principle of treatment is to warm the channels, disperse Cold, invigorate the Blood and unblock the collaterals.

3. Cold and Heat complex type: Clinical signs include severe pain in the joints of the hand and foot, occasionally with very stiff or deformed fingers and toes. Pain is intermittent. There is localized burning. However, the patient is averse to cold and wind, but not to cold water. The systemic signs may or may not appear. The tongue coating is either white or thin and yellow. The pulse is slippery or rapid. The pain readily recurs. The treatment principle is to warm and cool simultaneously.

4. Moderated type: This corresponds to the stabilization phase. There may be joint deformation with no pain or swelling. There are no general signs or symptoms, and the tongue and pulse are normal. The principle of treatment is to enrich and tonify the Liver and Kidneys, nourish the Blood and expel the Wind.

Dr. Zhang[5] and colleagues used Cinnamon Twig, Peony, and Anemarrhena Decoction (*gui zhi shao yao zhi mu tang*) in treating 32 cases of rheumatoid arthritis. For fever, Gypsum (*shi gao*) and Semen Coicis Lachryma-jobi (*yi yi ren*) were added; for Blood deficiency with joint swelling, Radix et Caulis Jixueteng (*ji xue teng*), Herba Pyrolae Rotundifoliae (*lu xian cao*) and Radix Angelicae Dahuricae (*bai zhi*) were added; for excess Dampness with joint swelling, Rhizoma Dioscoreae Hypoglaucae (*bei xie*), Rhizoma Alismatis Orientalis (*ze xie*) and Radix Stephaniae Tetrandrae (*han fang ji*) were added; and for Qi deficiency, Radix Astragali Membranacei (*huang qi*) was added. If a patient presented with signs of epigastric upset after ingesting the herbs, 60g of honey were prescribed, to be taken one-half at a time mixed in with each dosage of the decoction.

Of these 32 cases, there were 14 cures (one of whom was also taking biomedical pharmaceuticals), 6 showed definite improvement, 10 had favorable responses (three of whom were also taking pharmaceuticals, including cortisone), and there were 2 failures, yielding an effectiveness rate of 95.7 percent after an average of 21.6 decoctions.

In another report, Dr. Jiao[6] cited a passage from chapter 5 in *Essentials from the Golden Cabinet*: "The various joints of the limbs are sore and painful, the body is crooked and gaunt. . ." According to him the last two words, *wāng léi* 尪羸, translated as "crooked and gaunt," mean that the joints and limbs are deformed, the body is emaciated and weak, the joints cannot move freely and gradually become disabled.

According to this author, the ancient doctors lacked a common designation for the serious joint deformation, swelling, stiffness, musculoligamentous contractions, impaired movement and alteration of bone structure described in the clinical framework of painful obstruction. Based on his study of old texts, modern research and clinical experience, Dr. Jiao arrived at his own conclusion regarding the etiology, symptomatology, pulses and treatment of this pathology which he named "crooked painful obstruction" *(wāng bì)*. He believes that from the viewpoint of clinical reality, crooked painful obstruction is not only similar to the biomedically defined disease of rheumatoid arthritis, but also to other types of disease with joint pain and deformation. However, among these, rheumatoid arthritis is the most common.

Dr. Jiao distinguishes two different etiologies and pathological mechanisms. The first is chronic Kidney deficiency with deep penetration of pathogenic Cold into the bone. The second is repeated attacks of pathogenic Wind-Damp-Cold, which settles internally in the Liver and Kidneys.

It should be noted that this is a more complex and serious disorder than most forms of painful obstruction. This is primarily because the three pathogenic influences have already deeply penetrated into the Liver, Kidneys, sinews and bones. Because the disease has been prolonged, Cold, Dampness, turbid Phlegm, Blood stasis and bandit Wind intermingle, concentrate and do not disperse; instead they obstruct the channels and collaterals, and impair the circulation of Blood and Qi. All these factors further aggravate the condition. This is the difference between crooked painful obstruction and other types of painful obstruction.

Dr. Jiao also specified that the main treatment principles must essentially be to tonify the Kidneys and expel the Cold while also transforming the Dampness, dispersing the Wind, nourishing the Liver and sinews, dispelling the stasis and unblocking the collaterals.

The prescription for crooked painful obstruction is one developed by Dr. Jiao. It is called Tonify the Kidneys, Dispel Cold, and Treat the Crooked Decoction *(bu shen qu han zhi wan tang)*. It is composed of Radix Dipsaci Asperi *(xu duan)*, Fructus Psoraleae Corylifoliae *(bu gu zhi)*, Radix Lateralis Aconiti Carmichaeli Praeparata *(fu zi)*, Radix Rehmanniae Glutinosae Conquitae *(shu di huang)*, Rhizoma Drynariae *(gu sui bu)*, Herba Epimedii *(yin yang huo)*, Ramulus Cinnamomi Cassiae *(gui zhi)*, Radix Angelicae Pubescentis *(du huo)*, Radix Paeoniae

Rubrae *(chi shao)*, Radix Paeoniae Lactiflorae *(bai shao)*, Radix Clematidis *(wei ling xian)*, Os Tigris *(hu gu)*, Herba Ephedrae *(ma huang)*, Radix Ledebouriellae Divaricatae *(fang feng)*, Herba cum Radice Lycopodii Clavati *(shen jin cao)*, Lignum Pini Nodi *(song jie)*, Rhizoma Anemarrhenae Asphodeloidis *(zhi mu)*, Squama Manitis Pentadactylae *(chuan shan jia)*, Rhizoma Atractylodis *(cang zhu)* and Radix Achyranthis Bidentatae *(niu xi)*.

Summary

Panarthralgia is characterized by deformation, impaired movement and intense pain of the joints. At the onset, only a few joints may be affected; the condition progressively affects other joints, hence the name "disease that goes through all the joints," or panarthralgia.

Etiologically there is an internal factor (Liver and Kidney deficiency) and some triggering factors (pathogenic Wind, Cold, Dampness and Heat).

Diagnosis and treatment must take the different stages of this disorder into consideration. During the onset or after the stabilization (latent) phases, the Liver and Kidneys must be tonified to prevent a new invasion of the external pathogenic influences. During exacerbation or acute phase, the focus of treatment is first to dispel and eliminate the external pathogenic influences, and then to tonify the Liver and Kidneys, and to regulate and nourish the Qi and Blood.

The very early stages of this disease, as well as its latent phase, are often marked by signs of deficiency. In the case of yang Qi deficiency and weakness, we must warm the yang and augment the Qi. If the Cold symptoms are prominent, herbs to warm the channels and disperse the Cold can be added. For severe pain, add herbs to invigorate the Blood and transform stasis. For yin Blood deficiency, the principle of treatment is to enrich the yin, clear the Heat, nourish the Blood and harmonize the Blood. For severe internal Heat, the treatment principle is to moisten the yin and direct Fire downward.

During acute crises, the usual clinical picture is pathogenic excess, which can be divided into Cold and Hot patterns. For Cold patterns, the principle of treatment is to dispel the Cold, warm the yang and alleviate the pain. For Hot patterns, the principle is to clear the Heat, relieve the Toxicity, invigorate the Blood and unblock the collaterals. In addition, if Damp-Phlegm and Blood stasis further complicate the clinical picture, the treatment principle is, according to the diagnosis, to transform the

Phlegm, eliminate the Dampness, invigorate the Blood and transform the Blood stasis. This can ameliorate the condition and raise clinical efficacy.

Panarthralgia is often stubborn, accompanied by frequent relapses, and a complete cure is difficult to obtain. Severe cases can cause permanent disability or even death. This is all the more reason to treat this condition aggressively and focus on harmonizing and regulating. The severe consequences of internal injury underscores the need to adopt preventive and protective measures, engage in physical exercise and enhance the normal Qi, in accordance with the saying, "When the normal Qi is maintained internally, pathogenic influences cannot bother [the body]."

Formulas[7]

Aconite Decoction (*wū tóu tāng*)
烏頭湯
Herba Ephedrae (*ma huang*)
Radix Paeoniae Lactiflorae (*bai shao*)
Radix Astragali Membranacei (*huang qi*)
Honey-toasted Radix Glycyrrhizae Uralensis (*zhi gan cao*)
Radix Aconiti Carmichaeli Praeparata (*zhi chuan wu*)
Honey (*feng mi*)
SOURCE: *Essentials from the Golden Cabinet*

Five-Accumulation Powder (*wǔ jī sǎn*)
五積散
Herba Ephedrae (*ma huang*)
Rhizoma Atractylodis (*cang zhu*)
Radix Angelicae Dahuricae (*bai zhi*)
Radix Angelicae Sinensis (*dang gui*)
Radix Paeoniae Lactiflorae (*bai shao yao*)
Radix Ligustici Chuanxiong (*chuan xiong*)
Fructus Citri Aurantii (*zhi ke*)
Radix Platycodi Grandiflori (*jie geng*)
Ramulus Cinnamomi Cassiae (*gui zhi*)
Rhizoma Zingiberis Officinalis (*gan jiang*)
Sclerotium Poriae Cocos (*fu ling*)
Radix Glycyrrhizae Uralensis (*gan cao*)
Cortex Magnoliae Officinalis (*hou po*)
Pericarpium Citri Reticulatae (*chen pi*)
Rhizoma Pinelliae Ternatae (*ban xia*)
Rhizoma Zingiberis Officinalis Recens (*sheng jiang*)
SOURCE: *Imperial Grace Formulary of the Tai Ping Era*

Four-Substance Decoction (*sì wù tāng*)
四物湯
Radix Rehmanniae Glutinosae Conquitae (*shu di huang*)
Radix Angelicae Sinensis (*dang gui*)
Radix Ligustici Chuanxiong (*chuan xiong*)
Radix Paeoniae Lactiflorae (*bai shao yao*)
SOURCE: *Imperial Grace Formulary of the Tai Ping Era*

Kidney Qi Pill from *Golden Cabinet*
(*jīn guì shèn qì wán*)
金櫃腎氣丸
Radix Rehmanniae Glutinosae Conquitae (*shu di huang*)
Fructus Corni Officinalis (*shan zhu yu*)
Radix Dioscoreae Oppositae (*shan yao*)
Cortex Moutan Radicis (*mu dan pi*)
Sclerotium Poriae Cocos (*fu ling*)
Rhizoma Alismatis Orientalis (*ze xie*)
Radix Lateralis Aconiti Carmichaeli Praeparata (*fu zi*)
Ramulus Cinnamomi Cassiae (*gui zhi*)
SOURCE: *Essentials from the Golden Cabinet*

Minor Prolong Life Decoction (*xiǎo xù mìng tāng*)
小續命湯
Radix Ginseng (*ren shen*)
Radix Paeoniae Lactiflorae (*bai shao*)
Radix Ligustici Chuanxiong (*chuan xiong*)
Ramulus Cinnamomi Cassiae (*gui zhi*)
Herba Ephedrae (*ma huang*)
Radix Lateralis Aconiti Carmichaeli Praeparata (*fu zi*)
Radix Ledebouriellae Divaricatae (*fang feng*)
Radix Aristolochiae Fangchi (*fang ji*)
Semen Pruni Armeniacae (*xing ren*)
Radix Glycyrrhizae Uralensis (*gan cao*)
Radix Scutellariae Baicalensis (*huang qin*)
SOURCE: *Records of Experience Past and Present*

Rhinoceros Horn Decoction (*xī jiǎo tāng*)
犀角湯
Cornu Rhinoceri (*xi jiao*)
Cornu Antelopis (*ling yang jiao*)
Radix Scutellariae Baicalensis (*huang qin*)
Fructus Gardeniae Jasminoidis (*zhi zi*)
Radix Peucedani (*qian hu*)
Rhizoma Cimicifugae (*sheng ma*)
Radix et Rhizoma Rhei (*da huang*)
Rhizoma Belamcandae Chinensis (*she gan*)
Semen Sojae Praeparatum (*dan dou chi*)
SOURCE: *Thousand Ducat Prescriptions*

Six-Ingredient Pill with Rehmannia
(liù wèi dì huáng wán)

六味地黄丸

Radix Rehmanniae Glutinosae Conquitae *(shu di huang)*
Fructus Corni Officinalis *(shan zhu yu)*
Radix Dioscoreae Oppositae *(shan yao)*
Rhizoma Alismatis Orientalis *(ze xie)*
Cortex Moutan Radicis *(mu dan pi)*
Sclerotium Poriae Cocos *(fu ling)*
SOURCE: *Craft of Medicinal Treatment for Childhood Disease Patterns*

Two-Marvel Powder *(èr miào sǎn)*

二妙散

Cortex Phellodendri *(huang bai)*
Rhizoma Atractylodis *(cang zhu)*
SOURCE: *Teachings of [Zhu] Dan-Xi*

Yang-Heartening Decoction *(yáng hé tāng)*

陽和湯

Radix Rehmanniae Glutinosae Conquitae *(shu di huang)*
Gelatinum Cornu Cervi *(lu jiao jiao)*
Quick-fried Rhizoma Zingiberis Officinalis *(pao jiang)*
Cortex Cinnamomi Cassiae *(rou gui)*
Herba Ephedrae *(ma huang)*
Semen Sinapis Albae *(bai jie zi)*
Radix Glycyrrhizae Uralensis *(gan cao)*
SOURCE: *Standards and Patterns of Treatment in External Medicine*

Chapter Notes

1. *Editors' note:* This passage is found in *Basic Questions.*, chapter 33.
2. *Editors' note:* This term usually refers to the greater yang.
3. *Editors' note:* Because all species of rhinoceros are endangered, these substitutions are highly recommended.
4. Wang Da-Jing, "Differentiation of patterns and discussion of treatment of rheumatoid arthritis," *Zhejiang Chinese Medical Journal (Zhejiang zhong yi za zhi)* 2:55, 1980.
5. Zhang Mo-Duan, "Clinical analysis of 32 cases of rheumatoid arthritis treated with cinnamon twig, peony, and anemarrhena decoction," *Journal of Traditional Chinese Medicine (Zhong yi za zhi)* 1:38, 1981.
6. Jiao Shu-De, "Personal experience in the diagnosis and treatment of rheumatoid arthritis," *Journal of Traditional Chinese Medicine (Zhong yi za zhi)* 1:16, 1982.
7. *Editors' note:* Included here are only those formulas that appear in this section of the original text, which is by no means all of the formulas noted in the chapter itself. The only change that we have made is to arrange the formulas in alphabetical order by English name. For more detailed information regarding most of these formulas, see Dan Bensky and Randall Barolet, *Chinese Herbal Medicine: Formulas & Strategies* (Seattle: Eastland Press, 1990).

7

Lower Back Pain

THERE ARE TWO expressions in Chinese for lower back pain. "Lower back pain" *(yāo tòng 腰痛)* refers to unilateral or bilateral pain in the lumbar region. "Lower back stiffness" *(yāo suān 腰痠)* refers to stiffness, soreness and discomfort in this area. Clinically, lower back pain is often accompanied by stiffness, but stiffness is not necessarily associated with lower back pain. Both have a close relationship with the Kidneys.

History

Lower back pain is first mentioned in *Yellow Emperor's Inner Classic (Huang di nei jing)*, where all of chapter 41 of *Basic Questions (Su wen)* ("On Needling Lower Back Pain") is devoted to the subject.[1] There, lower back pain is attributed to diseases of the six leg channels. Detailed description is provided of the pathological changes associated with disorders of many channels which can lead to the various symptoms of lower back pain. Needling methods for treating these problems are also noted. Among the channels discussed are the three leg yang channels, the leg lesser yin channel, the leg terminal yin channel and the yang Linking vessel.

The *Inner Classic* establishes specific distinctions about the nature and location of lower back pain, and referred lower back pain. The nature of lower back pain is categorized as follows:

- Lower back pain that feels as if something is broken. This is described in chapters 17 and 74 of *Basic Questions*.
- Lower back pain that feels as if the muscles are spasming and becoming extremely tight, especially around the lumbar spine. This is described in chapter 31 of *Basic Questions* and chapter 66 of *Divine Pivot(Ling shu)*.

The location of the pain and the areas of referred pain are categorized as follows:

- Lower and upper back pain *(yāo bēi tòng)*, which refers to lower back pain that goes up to the thoracic area. As noted in chapter 36 of *Divine Pivot*, "There is deficiency so there is pain in the lower and upper back and the shins are stiff."
- Lower back and spine pain *(yāo jǐ tòng)* refers to lower back pain that radiates to the spine. A passage in chapter 65 of *Basic Questions* observes, "In cases of Kidney disease, there is pain in the lower abdomen, lower back and spine."
- Lower back pain and vertebral pain *(yāo zhuī tòng)*, which refers to lower back pain that radiates to the buttocks. This is described in chapter 71 of *Basic Questions*: "When a patient contracts Cold, the patient's joints become prohibitively tight and the vertebrae are painful." A passage in chapter 70 of the same text elaborates that lower back and vertebral pain is due to "Damp

Qi descending and residing, with Kidney Qi ascending and following."

- Lower back and buttock pain *(yāo kāo tòng)* refers to lower back pain radiating toward the lower tip of the spine, that is, the coccyx. A passage in chapter 47 of *Divine Pivot* states, "When the Kidneys are low, there is pain in the lumbar [region] and buttocks and the patient cannot bend forward or backward. . . . When the Kidneys are slanted and skewed, the person suffers lower back and buttock pain."

- Lower back and thigh pain *(yāo gǔ tòng)*. A passage in chapter 69 of *Basic Questions* observes, "When people are sick with a sensation of fullness in the abdomen, the body is heavy and there is soft diarrhea. Cold-type ulcers weep fluid and lower back and thigh pain develops."

- Lower back and abdominal pain *(yāo fù tòng)* refers to lower back pain that radiates to the lower abdomen.

- Lower back and side pain *(yāo xié tòng)*. This refers to pain in the lower back that radiates to the ribs. A passage in chapter 41 of *Basic Questions* describes this as "lower back pain that radiates to the lower abdomen and pulls on the flanks."

Inner Classic thus provides a very detailed description of lower back pain. Its etiology can be summed up into one of three causes: deficiency, Cold and Dampness.

In chapter 6 of the late Han work *Essentials from the Golden Cabinet (Jin gui yao lue)* there is a discussion of lower back pain associated with deficiency consumption, for which Kidney Qi Pill from the *Golden Cabinet (jin gui shen qi wan)* is prescribed. Chapter 11 of that book introduces a disorder called "fixed Kidneys" *(shèn zhuó)*. This condition is found in the lower burner. It is associated with pathogenic Cold and Dampness, and manifests with "a cold and heavy sensation in the lower back and below, with heaviness in the abdomen as if carrying 5,000 gold coins." Because the disorder is treated with Licorice, Ginger, Poria, and Atractylodes Macrocephalae Decoction *(gan cao gan jiang fu ling bai zhu tang),* this formula also became known as Fixed Kidneys Decoction *(shen zhuo tang).*

In the fifth division (entitled "Various Symptoms of Upper and Lower Back Pain") of the Sui dynasty book *Discussion of the Origins of the Symptoms of Disease (Zhu bing yuan hou lun),* author Chao Yuan-Feng wrote:

> There are five types of lower back pain: one is called lesser yin . . . the second is called Wind painful obstruction . . . the third Kidney deficiency . . . the fourth involves the lower back and buttocks when falling injures the lower back and results in pain. The fifth is called residing and sleeping in a Damp environment leading to pain.

Chao emphasized the importance of pathogenic Wind in the etiology of lower back pain, but also trauma and overwork. However, in the end he believed that "When the Kidney channels are deficient, Wind-Cold takes advantage of the situation," and that "When overexertion injures the Kidneys, the channels and collaterals are perturbed and injured. If in addition Wind-Cold invades the body, the Blood and Qi struggle and therefore the lower back is painful." Given the different etiologies, Chao first divided this condition into acute and chronic types. A sudden onset of pain was called sudden lower back pain, whereas frequent relapses with no complete cure was referred to as long-standing lower back pain .

Division 19 of the Tang text *Thousand Ducat Prescriptions (Qian jin yao fang)* first provides a recapitulation of the categorization of this problem from *Discussion of the Origins of the Symptoms of Disease.* Then it adds numerous therapeutic methods for lower back pain, among which is "conducting and leading methods" *(dǎ yǐn fǎ)*, which refers to physical manipulation. Of the formulas noted, the most famous is Angelica Pubescens and Sangjisheng Decoction *(du huo ji sheng tang).*

A passage in division 17 of *Arcane Essentials from the Imperial Library (Wai tai bi yao)* states that one must also "tonify and nourish along with spreading and conducting" when treating lower back pain. This text emphasizes the importance of day-to-day care and lifestyle. A passage in *Formulas to Aid the Living (Ji sheng fang)* advises:

> Do not go to bed immediately after eating because over the course of time the Qi can become diseased, leading to the development of lower back pain. . . . Do not strain during defecation as this leads to lower back pain and rough eyes. Also too much laughter can twist and move the Kidneys, leading to lower back pain.

Division 44 of the Song compilation *Imperial Grace Formulary of the Tai Ping Era (Tai ping hui min he ji ju fang)* is an even richer source of information about lower back pain, containing more than 130 formulas for the treatment of this disorder. The most commonly cited herbs include Cortex Eucommiae Ulmoidis *(du zhong)*, Cortex Cinnamomi Cassiae *(rou gui)*, Radix Lateralis Aconiti Carmichaeli Praeparata *(fu zi)*, Gelatinum Cornu Cervi *(lu jiao jiao)*, Radix Dipsaci Asperi *(xu duan)*, Rhizoma Cibotii Barometz *(gou ji)*, Ramulus Sangjisheng *(sang ji sheng)*, Semen Cuscutae Chinensis *(tu si zi)*,

Rhizoma Dioscoreae Hypoglaucae *(bei xie)*, Cortex Acanthopanacis Gracilistylus Radicis *(wu jia pi)*, Os Tigris *(hu gu)*, and Radix Achyranthis Bidentatae *(niu xi)*.

Chen Wu-Ji, in *Discussion of Illnesses, Patterns, and Formulas Related to the Unification of the Three Etiologies (San yin ji yi bing zheng fang lun)*, wrote:

> Although lower back pain belongs to the deficient Kidney category, three causes are also worth noting. Externally, an attack of pathogenic influences on the channels and Organs; internally, the emotions of worry, rumination, fear and anger; and excessive sexual activity and trauma can all lead to this condition.

Chen introduced medicinal wines for this problem, including those which contain Radix Achyranthis Bidentatae *(niu xi)*, Cortex Eucommiae Ulmoidis *(du zhong)*, and Semen Citri Reticulatae *(ju he)*. Young Maiden Pill *(qing e wan)*, which is mentioned in this book, is still widely used today.

The chapter on lower back pain in the Yuan dynasty text *Teachings of [Zhu] Dan-Xi (Dan-Xi xin fa)* lists five etiologies for lower back pain: Damp-Heat, Kidney deficiency, Blood stasis, sprain, Phlegm accumulation. Kidney deficiency is considered the most important factor. The appended chapter on lower back pain observes:

> In case of Kidney Qi deficiency, if there is an invasion of Cold, contraction of Dampness, injury from coolness, buildup of Heat, rough flow of Blood, Qi stagnation, Water accumulation, trauma, disappointment or overexertion, the different types of lower back pain will develop.

With respect to treatment, Chen noted:

> All the various [types of] pain are categorized as Fire. Cold or cooling herbs cannot be used too harshly; it is necessary to use warming and dispersing herbs. Do not use Radix Ginseng *(ren shen)*, as tonifying the Qi will exacerbate the pain.

Exception is taken to this description in a chapter entitled "Differentiation and Treatment of Lower Back Pain" in the Ming dynasty work *Collected Treatises of [Zhang] Jing-Yue (Jing-Yue quan shu)*:

> These ideas are not entirely accurate. In the case of overwork, exhaustion, or deficiency and injury with yang insufficiency, there are often manifestations of Qi deficiency. Why not use Radix Ginseng *(ren shen)* in these cases? If, on the other hand, Fire collects in the lower burner with excruciating pain, the Fire must be cleared rapidly. Why forbid the use of cold and cool herbs? There are nevertheless complex cases of deficiency with signs of excess in which Radix Ginseng *(ren shen)* is contraindicated, and

cases of Fire without intense Heat in which it is inappropriate to use cold and cooling herbs that are to strong.

During the Qing dynasty, texts such as *Comprehensive Medicine According to Master Zhang (Zhang shi yi tong)* and *Wondrous Lantern for Peering into the Origin and Development of Miscellaneous Diseases (Za bing yuan liu xi zhu)* grouped the previous descriptions of lower back pain into different categories. These include those caused by Wind, Cold, Dampness, Phlegm, Kidney deficiency, Qi stagnation and Blood stasis. This method of classification allows for a more systematic diagnostic and therapeutic methodology.

Scope

In modern biomedicine, the symptom of lower back pain and stiffness can be treated by specialists in internal medicine, surgery, orthopedics and gynecology. In general, it can be divided into one of four categories:

- spinal conditions, including spondyloarthritis, ankylosing spondylitis and tubercular or suppurative spondylitis
- paraspinal soft tissue disorders, including lumbar muscular strain and fibromyositis
- lower back pain from stimulation of the spinal nerve roots, including spinal cord compression and acute myelitis
- visceral diseases such as renal problems (i.e., pyelonephritis, glomerular nephritis, lithiasis, tuberculosis, ptosis and hydronephrosis), acute pancreatitis, perforated ulcers, cholecystitis, cholelithiasis, retroversion of the uterus, chronic pelvic inflammatory disease and chronic prostatitis.

The last of these four categories is the one most often seen in traditional Chinese internal medicine. If, in the course of these different pathologies, lower back pain becomes the primary symptom, this chapter is an appropriate place to refer when differentiating the pattern and considering treatment.

Etiology and Pathology

Since the lower back is regarded as the residence of the Kidneys, physicians of all times have always blamed Kidney deficiency as the major factor in the genesis of lower back pain and stiffness.

During the Ming dynasty, Huang Gang-Jing wrote, in the "Lower Back Pain" chapter of his *Standards of Patterns and Treatments (Zheng zhi zhun sheng)*, that for lower back pain "there is Wind, Dampness, Cold, Heat, contusion and strain, Blood stasis, Qi stagnation and Phlegm accumulation, all of which are manifestations. Kidney deficiency is the root." This constitutes a general overview of the etiology and pathology of lower back pain. Combining the thoughts of various ancient medical writers with modern understanding of lower back pain, we can categorize its etiology as follows:

• contraction of external pathogenic influences
• overexertion and trauma
• exhausted and harmed Kidney Essence.

CONTRACTION OF EXTERNAL PATHOGENIC INFLUENCES

Pathogenic influences such as Wind, Cold, Dampness and Heat can each give rise to lower back pain. Of these the most commonly seen are Damp-Cold and Damp-Heat.

A damp house, occupational exposure to the elements, sweating, wearing wet clothes, and the invasion of pathogenic Damp-Cold can all lead to obstruction of the channels, impeding the circulation of Blood and Qi and causing lower back pain. On the other hand, during the season when Dampness and Heat steam each other, these pathogenic influences may contract, obstructing the channels and giving rise to lower back pain.

When Cold and Dampness collect and accumulate over a long period they become constrained and transform into heat, which can then turn into a Damp-Heat lower back pain pattern. The contraction of external Wind, Wind-Cold or Wind-Heat all impede the circulation in the channels and cause lower back pain.

OVEREXERTION AND TRAUMA

Overexertion, trauma, strains or injury to the lumbar musculature, spine or channels leads to impediment of the circulation of Blood and Qi. The Blood becomes static and the Qi stagnates such that the collateral vessels are obstructed, and lower back pain appears.

The "Lower Back Pain" chapter in *Collected Treatises of [Zhang] Jing-Yue* notes that, "When lower back pain is due to trauma, the injury settles in the sinews and bones, and the Blood congeals and the vessels stagnate." The "Lower Back Pain" chapter in *Appendices to the Golden Cabinet (Jin gui yi)* explains the mechanism in post-

traumatic lower back pain as follows: "The lower back represents the most important part of the body; it is called upon for all movements of forward and backward bending. If it is harmed and injured, then the pulsing movement of Blood becomes congealed and rough and the channels are clogged and obstructed."

EXHAUSTED AND HARMED KIDNEY ESSENCE

When there is a constitutional weakness, general debility after a chronic illness, exhaustion and weakening of Essence and Blood in old age, or excessive sexual activity, the Kidney Essence and Blood become exhausted and harmed. In this state they have nothing with which to nourish the channels and vessels, and lower back pain ensues. A passage in chapter 17 of *Basic Questions* notes that "The lower back area is the residence of the Kidneys; if it cannot be rotated and turned, then the Kidneys will become exhausted."

Exhaustion of Kidney Qi is also closely associated with the Liver and Spleen. Consider the following passage from the chapter entitled "On Prescriptions for Lower Back Pain" in *Straightforward Prescriptions (Zhi zhi fang)* :

If, upon examination, pain is located at the lesser yin level, the origin of the disease must be investigated in order to decide on the appropriate treatment. Although it may be one way, the ancestral sinew[2] is concentrated in the yin apparatus so the Liver is of the same system as the Kidneys. The five yin Organs get their Qi from grain, and the Spleen constitutes the Kidneys' granary. In cases of constraint or anger, the Liver is injured, and the sinews become flaccid. Sadness and rumination affect the Spleen, such that the Stomach Qi does not proceed. These two elements can act as enemies causing lower back pain, and combined, one must reach both of them.

When the Kidney Qi is exhausted and harmed it is also easy to contract external pathogenic influences, which leads to the development of disease. This process is described in the chapter from *Straightforward Prescriptions* cited above:

The lower back is the external vassal of the Kidneys, and all the movements of the body depend on it. Moreover, the different channels connect with the Kidneys and their collaterals are located in the lumbar area. When one's Kidney Qi is deficient, if one is attacked by Wind, subjected to Dampness, injured by Cold, has a buildup of Heat, stasis of Blood and stagnation of Qi, accumulation of Water, suffers traumatic injury, disappointment, or overexerts oneself physically, different types of lower back pain will appear. . . . Sadness and disappointment are harmful factors for the Kidneys; overexertion and exhaustion of the Essence aggress against the Kidneys. These can give rise to numerous patterns. People with a predisposition toward Kidney problems will contract these types of conditions. How can the lower back suffer these and not become painful?

The above discussion would indicate that the emergence of lower back pain and stiffness is caused externally by such factors as the invasion of Wind, Cold, Dampness and Heat, and by trauma. Internal factors include exhaustion and harm to the Liver, Spleen and Kidneys. In terms of etiology, Kidney deficiency is the root, whereas external pathogenic influences, trauma, overexertion and the seven emotions are the manifestations. These two elements can affect each other. For example, an invasion of pathogenic Damp-Cold can injure the Kidney yang. Pathogenic Damp-Heat can injure the Kidney yin, and deficient Kidney yang and yin can aggravate any pathological condition.

Clinical Manifestations and Differential Diagnosis

CLINICAL MANIFESTATIONS

Lower back pain and stiffness are subjective symptoms. The patient's history makes it relatively easy to establish a positive diagnosis. However, due to the wide variety of lower back pain and associated signs, and due to the nature of lower back pain, its evolution and the possibility of referred pain, a precise analysis must be undertaken in order to establish an accurate diagnosis. Three aspects must be considered: local symptoms, referred pain and general symptoms.

Local Symptoms

The condition may have a sudden onset in some patients, with severe pain radiating in a unilateral or bilateral fashion, and aggravated by the slightest movement. There will be clearly sensitive spots among the paraspinal Bladder channel points. Failing to treat the condition adequately might lead to a chronic stage, with more subdued lower back pain or latent pain and stiffness. Another type of condition may present with a more progressive onset, without acute pain, but an insidious onset of moderate, dull or stiff-type pain. The symptomatology can be aggravated by bad posture, overexertion or changes in the weather. Yet another form of lower back pain always follows a long period of inactivity or rest, such as getting up after sitting for a long time, or in the morning on awakening. All these features can help to establish the correct diagnosis for lower back pain.

Referred Pain

The most common type of referred pain affects the lower limbs. The onset can be progressive or sudden. Overexertion is often the cause. The pain travels down the leg greater yang channel into the legs, on one or both sides. If severe, the pain will be aggravated by coughing, sneezing or increased abdominal pressure, and alleviated by lying horizontally. The patient cannot raise the affected limb, and there is hypoesthesia. In the chronic stage, there may be an uneven gait and, if severe, muscular atrophy.

Lower back pain accompanied by abdominal pain is also frequently observed. The onset is usually sudden and is often due to overexertion. The pain may travel along the leg terminal yin Liver channel and radiate toward the hypogastrium, the genital area or the medial aspect of the thighs. Severe lower back pain may be accompanied by cold sweat or even hematuria.

General Symptoms

General symptoms can be divided into those from external invasion, and those from internal injury. Signs associated with external invasion are frequently seen in patients with lower back soreness and pain: fever, aversion to cold, joint and bone pain, and maybe sweating or thirst. It is not uncommon to observe such symptoms as alternating fever and chills, rather profuse sweating, and an unpleasant, full sensation in the chest and sides. This may be accompanied by dripping urination with sharp pain, or rough urination that is difficult to finish, signs of Damp-Heat in the lower burner.

Symptoms of internal injury are primarily related to the Spleen and Kidneys. These include generalized weakness, fatigue, weakness of the lower limbs, pallid complexion, poor appetite, lightheadedness, blurred vision and tinnitus. Other possible manifestations are edema, hematuria, turbid urine and retention of urine. In women such problems may manifest as irregular menstruation, leukorrhea and dysmenorrhea.

DIFFERENTIAL DIAGNOSIS

Lower back pain must be differentiated from the following conditions: lower back weakness, heaviness and fixed Kidneys.

Lower Back Weakness

Lower back weakness (*yāo ruǎn* 腰軟) involves different clinical symptomatology in which the lower back is weak and without strength, but generally without pain or stiffness. This is usually a manifestation of deficiency. Pathologically there are similarities with lower back stiffness, in that it can be due to Kidney deficiency, but can also result from Liver and Kidney deficiency with internal Heat excess, as noted in the "Lower Back Pain" chapter from *Medical Mirror of Past and Present (Gu jin yi jian)*: "Those with lower back weakness have lurking Kidney and Liver Heat."

From a clinical point of view, lower back pain and lower back weakness are two different conditions. Lower back pain affects mostly adults, whereas lower back weakness targets children and infants, and may be accompanied by weakness of the neck and limbs, delayed closure of the fontanel, and pigeon breast. When adults suffer from lower back weakness, they usually have a history of such problems as the "five retardations," "five weaknesses" or delayed closure of the fontanel.[3]

Lower Back Heaviness

Lower back heaviness (*yāo zhòng* 腰重) is a sensation in the lower back that differs from lower back pain. A passage from the chapter devoted to lower back pain in *Record of Differentiating Patterns (Bian zheng lu)* explains: "There are patients who feel that both of their loins are heavy, as if carrying 3,000 gold coins, and who find flexion and extension of the trunk to be impossible. This is different from lower back pain." To push the etiology a little further, heaviness in the lower back can be due to excessive sexual activity or physical overexertion, combined with an invasion of Wind and Dampness; this is the Kidney injury pattern.

Emaciation, abdominal distention, para-umbilical swelling, pain on urination and perineal dampness are all common symptoms of the lower back heaviness disorder. As noted in *Treasury Classic (Zhong zang jing)* in the chapter discussing Kidney deficiency:

When the Kidneys have [pathogenic] Water, then the abdomen is enlarged, the navel swollen, the lower back heavy, urination is painful and difficult, the perineal area is moist like an ox's muzzle, and the head is sweaty. This is considered rebellious Cold (*nì hán*). There is constipation yet the face is emaciated.[4]

Fixed Kidneys

The earliest description of fixed Kidney disorder (*shèn zhuó* 腎著) is in *Essentials from the Golden Cabinet*. There it is characterized by

a very heavy sensation in the body, a feeling of cold in the lumbar area as if sitting in water, lack of thirst, easy urination, a normal appetite … Below the lower back area, the patient feels a cold pain and the abdomen feels as heavy as if they were carrying 5,000 gold coins.

The most important manifestations, in terms of differential diagnosis, are cold in the lower back, pain in the lumbar area and below, and heavy sensations in the body and abdomen.

The pathological mechanism is different from that of lower back pain or stiffness. According to the commentary on this disorder in *Heart-felt Canon of Essentials from the Golden Cabinet (Jin gui yao lue xin dian)*, "The disease is not in the middle Organs of the Kidneys, but in the external Organ of the Kidneys."[5] The suggested treatment principle

is not to warm the Kidneys to disperse the Cold, but to warm the Earth in order to overcome the Water. Radix Glycyrrhizae Uralensis (*gan cao*), Rhizoma Zingiberis Officinalis (*gan jiang*), Sclerotium Poriae Cocos (*fu ling*) and Rhizoma Atractylodis Macrocephalae (*bai zhu*) are acrid, warm, sweet and neutral. They are not considered to belong to the category of Kidney herbs. However, for the disease called fixed Kidneys they are appropriate.

Although fixed Kidney disorder does have some similarities with lower back pain and stiffness, it is a separate entity and should be identified as such.

Some ancient authors believed that lower back weakness and fixed Kidney disorder were identical conditions, hence the remark made in the chapter on lumbar vertebra and lower limb pain in *Treatment Designs Arranged According to Pattern*: "Lower back weakness is due to Dampness attacking the channels and collaterals; use Fixed Kidneys Decoction (*shen zhuo tang*)." *Comprehensive Medicine According to Master Zhang* and *Encyclopedia of Chinese Medicine (Zhong guo yi xue da ci dian)* share the same view. There is, however, a clinical distinction between lower back weakness and fixed Kidney disorder. The former presents with a lack of strength in the lower back, whereas fixed Kidney disorder refers to a sensation of cold in the lower back area, pain from the lower back downward, no sensation of weakness, but a heavy sensation in the abdomen.

Some authors consider lower back heaviness and fixed Kidney disorder to be one and the same condition. In the chapter on lower back pain from *Introduction to Medicine (Yi xue ru men)* is the following passage:

> When one lives in a damp environment and is frequently exposed to rain and dampness, Dampness can become fixed in the body. The lower back becomes as heavy as stone and as cold as water. The patient likes the local application of heat, is not thirsty, has smooth urination and a normal appetite. Treatment relies on Fixed Kidneys Decoction *(shen zhuo tang)* with the addition of Radix Lateralis Aconiti Carmichaeli Praeparata *(fu zi)*.

However, the deep, heavy sensation in the lumbar area associated with lower back heaviness is different from the generalized heaviness of fixed Kidney disorder, likened to a heavy feeling in the abdomen "as if carrying 5,000 gold coins." The nature and location of these lumbar sensations are different and must be clearly differentiated.

Differentiation of Patterns

DIFFERENTIATING EXTERNALLY CONTRACTED DISEASES FROM INTERNAL INJURY

Lower back pain and stiffness fall into two main categories: external invasion and internal injury. The diagnosis must establish the nature of the lower back pain.

In the case of external invasion, the chief manifestations are a relatively sudden onset and marked lower back pain, accompanied by signs of external invasion by pathogenic influences.

Lower back pain due to Dampness is marked by a heavy and painful lower back, inability to turn over while lying down, and a heavy pain upon walking accompanied by weakness. When the problem is due to Cold, the lower back feels cold and painful but feels better when heat is applied, the limbs are tired, the feet are extremely cold and there are chills and frequent urination. When due to Damp-Heat, the lower back is hot and painful, the body is hot and sweaty, the joints are painful and swollen and urination feels hot and painful.

In the case of internal injury, the onset is slower and stiffness is the predominant complaint. Usually the lower back stiffness is accompanied by signs of deficiency and injury to the yin and yang Organs.

Characteristics associated with internal injury are described in the following passage from the chapter on lower back pain in *Precepts for Physicians (Yi men fa lü):*

When there is incessant pain, lack of strength and lower back stiffness, it is Kidney deficiency. When overexertion in labor and madly running around internally injure the basal Qi so that there is great difficulty in twisting and turning, and there is a sensation of disjointment in the spine, it is Qi deficiency. In cases where there is excessive sexual activity that exhausts the Essence and injures the marrow, movement is limited and there is a combined sensation of stiffness and pain with heaviness in the spinal area, it is Blood deficiency. Lower back pain and stiffness due to Blood stasis and Phlegm are also a problem of internal injury. If the signs are less severe during the day and more intense at night, with an inability to move at the waist, this is Blood stasis. If there are palpable [nodes] that are painful, together with dusky pale skin and flesh, it is Phlegm. If it is impossible to bend over, stand up straight or turn around, it is a lumbar sprain.

ANALYZING DEFICIENCY AND EXCESS IN THE ORGANS

The Kidneys and Bladder are coupled in an interior-exterior relationship. When the disease is located in the Bladder, the chief symptoms are those of Damp-Heat excess. There are painful back contractures accompanied by chills and fever; urination is dripping, rough and painful. Although the disease is located in the yang Organ (Bladder), there may also be signs of Kidney deficiency. It is important to differentiate the root from the manifestation, and that which is urgent from that which is not, in order to choose the proper course of therapy.

When the disease is located in an Organ, the main feature is Kidney deficiency. Consider the following passage from the chapter on lower back pain in *Collected Treatises of [Zhang] Jing-Yue:*

> As for lower back pain, eight or nine out of ten are deficiency patterns. A close analysis does not show any sign of external pathogenic influences or Damp-Heat, but points either to old age, overexertion, overconsumption of alcohol or excessive sexual activity, or to constraint and worry of the seven emotions, all of which indicate a true yin deficiency pattern.

Although the lower back is the domain of the Kidneys, the Liver and Kidneys share the same origin. The main role of the Liver is to spread and drain. If the pain is caused by frustration and anger, it is due to Liver Qi stagnation. If the lower back pain radiates toward the lower abdomen, or if it is accompanied by pain in the external genitals with swelling of the testicles and discomfort in the perineal area, it is due to Qi stagnating in the Liver channel. If the

Qi stops and the Blood stagnates, a Blood stasis-type lower back pain could develop. These are all patterns of excess. If the pain is chronic, occurs upon exertion, and the patient suffers from frequent recurrences that go away slowly, it is exhaustion of the Liver and Kidneys.

The Kidneys are the root of the congenital,[6] while the Spleen is the root of the post-natal.[7] When there is insufficiency in the Kidneys, the Spleen will not be strong. When the Kidney yang is injured, the Spleen loses its ability to transport. When lower back pain is a sign of Kidney deficiency, it is often accompanied by manifestations of Spleen deficiency. Such symptoms include lower back stiffness and weakness, fatigue and asthenia, poor appetite and a shiny, pale complexion. In addition, there may be edema, diarrhea, or a cold feeling in the extremities and epigastrium.

PAYING ATTENTION TO THE AREAS TRAVERSED BY THE CHANNELS

The various channels directly or indirectly pass through the lower back. Channel pathology may therefore generate lower back pain. A passage from the chapter on disorders of the back in *Discussion of the Origins and Symptoms of Disease* states that

> The Kidneys govern the lower back and lower limbs; the three yin and the three yang, the twelve primary channels and the eight Curious vessels all establish connecting pathways with the spine of the lower back.

If the three yang channels are affected, the lower back pain prevents the patient from bending forward; if the three yin channels are affected, he cannot bend backward. Or, as explained in another passage from the same chapter:

> Those with diseases of the yang cannot bend forward; those with diseases of the yin cannot bend backward. If both the yin and yang are affected by pathogenic Qi, there is lower back pain with inability to bend forward or backward.

When differentiating which channels are affected, it is important to pay attention to the location and nature of the pain. The three leg yang channels go from the head down to the feet, and the three leg yin channels go from the feet up to the trunk. In greater yang-type lower back pain, the pain proceeds from the cervical vertebrae to the sacrum and coccyx, the lumbar area feels heavy and stiff, and the bones and joints are painful and bothered. Chapter 71 of *Basic Questions* states, "When the greater yang is affected, there is lower back pain." Chapter 10 ("On Channels and Vessels") of *Divine Pivot* elaborates:

> As for the Bladder leg greater yang vessel . . . its straight [pathway] penetrates from the vertex and connects with the brain . . . it surrounds the spine all the way down to the lumbar region; when it is perturbed, diseases appear . . . there is pain in the spine, lower back pain, as if it were broken.

And chapter 41 of *Basic Questions* further observes, "When the leg greater yang vessel leads to lower back pain, it radiates from the back of the neck to the buttocks, and the back feels heavy." That is the reason why greater yang-type lower back pain is the most frequently encountered.

Yang brightness-type lower back pain prevents the person from looking backward, because the yang brightness channel travels alongside the throat, and penetrates deeply at ST-12 *(que pen)*. When the channels in the front are contracted, they may cause lower back pain with inability to turn around.

Lesser yang-type lower back pain feels like needles sticking into the skin of the lumbar region. Gradually it becomes impossible to bend forward or backward, or to turn to either side. This is because the leg lesser yang channel goes from the outer canthus of the eye to the shoulder.

Greater yin-type lower back pain radiates toward the lower abdomen or ribs. The person cannot bend backward because the collateral of the leg greater yin channel goes from the hips to meet with the yang brightness, connects with the sacrum and coccyx, joins with the terminal yin and the lesser yang channels in the lower burner, and internally enters the abdomen.

Lesser yin-type lower back pain goes from the spine to the posteromedial part of the thigh. This is because the leg lesser yin channel ascends the posteromedial part of the thigh to the buttock, and then follows the spine. It is also associated with the Kidneys.

In terminal yin-type lower back pain, the lumbar area is contracted like a tight bow, and often there is pain in the flanks. This is because the leg terminal yin channel reaches the hypogastrium and disperses through the sides of the rib cage.

In addition to the various types of back pain associated with the channels, if a certain channel receives a pathogenic influence or experiences pathological change, there can then be pain in any area traversed by that channel. A passage from the chapter devoted to the treatment of lower back pain in *Complete Treatises of [Zhang] Jing-Yue* notes that, "The lower back is the dwelling of the Kidneys . . . it is also the meeting place of the Penetrating,

Conception, Governing and Girdle vessels." This explains why pathology in the Penetrating, Conception, Governing and Girdle vessels can be related to lower back pain.

In Penetrating vessel-type lower back pain, there is a sensation like a piece of hard wood sitting horizontally below the lumbar area and at the level of the penis, as well as irritability and heat, and sometimes incontinence. This is because the Penetrating vessel originates at the gestation membranes *(bāo)* of the pelvis,[8] emerges at the perineum and ascends with the leg lesser yin channel, while a branch ascends along the spine. It is the sea of channels, and the origin of the twelve channels.

Conception vessel-type lower back pain is dull, constant and accompanied by sweating. This is because the Conception vessel originates in the perineum, connects with the Governing vessel, and then ascends separately. It governs the sweating of the entire body. Because sweat is a yin fluid, there is sweating when this vessel is affected.

Governing vessel-type lower back pain is accompanied by an inability to bend forward, backward or rotate the trunk, because the Governing vessel governs the yang of the whole body. It follows the spine straight up the body. It originates at the gestation membranes below the Kidneys, follows the genitals, goes around the hips to connect with the lesser yin channel, and connects with the greater yang channel.

Girdle vessel-type lower back pain is accompanied by an inability to bend the trunk, as well as Blood stasis. This is because the Girdle vessel circulates horizontally in the lumbar area. The three leg yang channels go down through the lower back, while the three leg yin channels and the Curious vessels go up through the lower back. In case of disease, the upper and lower are no longer in communication, and there is obstruction between the yin and the yang.

ANALYZING PULSE CHANGES

Pulse changes in lower back pain were described in detail as early as *Classic of the Pulse (Mai jing)*. The most important area to monitor is the proximal *(chǐ)* position of the pulse:

- If the proximal position is confined *(láo)* and long, the problem is Qi stagnation: the lower back pain radiates toward the lower abdomen.
- If the proximal position is submerged and excessive, the problem is Blood stasis: there is pain throughout the back, with an inability to bend forward or backward.

- If the proximal position is submerged, the problem is Kidney Qi deficiency: the lower back pain is indistinct.
- If the proximal position is coarse,[9] the problem is Heat in the middle: there is lower back and inguinal pain, together with dark, burning urine.
- If the pulse in the proximal and middle positions is floating and goes straight down, this signifies Governing vessel-type lower back pain with intense stiffness.

The relationships between pulse types and different kinds of lower back pain are described in the chapter on diagnosis and treatment of lower back pain in *Formulas to Aid the Living (Ji sheng fang)*:

> In general, the pulse in patients with lower back pain is submerged and wiry. When it is submerged, wiry and tight, it is Cold lower back pain; submerged, wiry with some floating aspects, [it] is Wind lower back pain; wiry, soggy and thin, [it] is Damp lower back pain; if the pain is caused by Qi and Blood stagnation subsequent to trauma, the pulse is often submerged, wiry and excessive.

A careful analysis of the pulse, clinical signs and tongue before fixing on a diagnosis ensures good therapeutic results. This is why *Formulas to Aid the Living* concludes that "discovering the cause, establishing its relationship with the pulses, and deducing the treatment principle excludes ineffectiveness."

Symptomatology

EXTERNALLY CONTRACTED LOWER BACK PAIN

Damp-Cold Lower Back Pain

Symptomatology

There is a sensation of cold, pain and heaviness in the lower back, rotation is difficult, and the pain increases progressively in intensity. Lying flat does not alleviate the pain, and may sometimes increase it. The pain is aggravated when it rains. The tongue coating is white and greasy, and the pulse is submerged, slow and lax.

Pathology

When pathogenic Damp-Cold invades the lower back, it obstructs the channels and collaterals and impairs the circulation of Blood and Qi. The nature of Cold is to congeal, and Dampness is heavy and immobile. For this reason the lower back is cold, painful and heavy, and rotation is impaired.

Dampness is a yin pathogenic influence, and its nature is sticky and stagnant. It often stagnates when the body is in a recumbent position; that is why rest does not improve the condition, and can even aggravate the lower back pain. Because darkness, rain and cold intensify Damp-Cold, under these conditions the pain worsens. Warmth can disperse Cold and overcome Dampness, thus warmth alleviates the problem. The tongue coating is white and greasy, and the pulse is submerged, thin and slow, all signs of a gathering up of Dampness and Cold.

Damp-Heat Lower Back Pain

Symptomatology

There is pain in the lower back and hips with a localized sensation of heat. The pain is aggravated by warm, rainy or heat wave conditions. The joints of the lower extremities may be swollen and red. The patient is irritable, thirsty, has scanty and dark urine, a yellow and greasy tongue coating, and a soggy and rapid pulse.

Pathology

When Dampness and Heat struggle together, they reach the lower back, collect in the greater yang level, and cause lower back pain. The greater yang governs the upper back, associated with the yang, so the pain radiates upward toward the upper back and neck, and downward toward the buttocks and hips. The rainy season is the time of year during which Damp-Heat is constrained and simmers, while late summer corresponds to Summerheat and Dampness. The lower back pain worsens during these seasons.

If there is an overconsumption of Damp-Heat-generating foods, internal and external Damp-Heat combine and can cause this type of lower back pain. Pathogenic Damp-Heat readily penetrates into the joints, which become red and swollen, and creates signs such as thirst and irritability, along with dark, scanty urine. The yellow, greasy tongue coating, as well as the soggy, rapid pulse reflect the presence of vigorous internal Damp-Heat.

When Damp-Cold lower back pain becomes chronic, the pathogenic influences can stagnate, generate Heat and transform into Damp-Heat. When Damp-Heat lower back pain is not properly treated, it can likewise transform into an atrophy or painful obstruction disorder. If Damp-Cold lower back pain is accompanied by pathogenic Wind, Wind painful obstruction with lower back pain results. Damp-Heat lower back pain accompanied by redness and swelling of the joints usually transforms into Hot painful obstruction.

Damp-Phlegm Lower Back Pain

Symptomatology

The lower back feels cold, painful and heavy. These sensations radiate toward the upper back and flanks. The condition is aggravated by wet weather, and may be accompanied by diarrhea. The tongue coating is white and greasy, and the pulse is slippery.

Pathology

If a person with a Damp-Phlegm constitution is invaded by external Dampness, the two will combine, penetrate the Kidney channel, and cause sensations of cold, pain and heaviness in the lower back. The pain extends to the upper back and flanks. Dampness is a yin pathogenic influence, and will thus become aggravated during wet weather.

The Spleen is the source for production of Phlegm. If the Spleen Qi is deficient, or if Phlegm is constantly in excess, the excess Dampness obstructs the Spleen yang, and the internal and external Dampness penetrate into the Spleen channel, which can cause diarrhea. A white, greasy tongue coating and slippery pulse indicate that the Damp-Phlegm has settled in the lower back.

If in Damp-Cold lower back pain the Cold disperses but the Dampness lingers, and if there is also underlying Damp-Phlegm, then Damp-Phlegm lower back pain can eventually develop. If Damp-Phlegm lower back pain becomes constrained, Heat may be produced, and Damp-Heat lower back pain may then develop.

Wind-Cold Lower Back Pain

Symptomatology

There is pain and spasms of the lower back, which sometimes involve the thoracic spine or lower limbs. There may be chills and feverishness. There is a sensation of cold in the lower back, and the pain is alleviated by warmth. The pulse is floating and tight, and the tongue coating is thin and white.

Pathology

When Wind and Cold invade the channels, they begin at the greater yang level. The greater yang channel follows the spine down through the lower back, and then to the knees and feet. This type of lower back pain can therefore extend to the upper and middle back, and to the knees and feet.

Cold has a contracting quality, and Wind is migratory by nature. This type of lower back pain is thus characterized by spasms, and may have no set location, sometimes appearing on the right and sometimes on the left. Cold is scattered by heat, and Wind is dispersed by heat. For this reason, the pain is alleviated by warmth. A floating, tight pulse and a thin white tongue coating are signs of an invasion by Wind-Cold.

The main feature of Wind-Cold lower back pain is its sudden onset. Wind is easily released, but Cold is hard to eliminate, and the condition may become chronic. If Dampness joins with these two pathogenic influences, the condition will transform into Damp-Cold lower back pain.

Wind-Heat Lower Back Pain

Symptomatology

The lower back is painful and feels hot. There is burning, dark urination, and the body may feel hot, with mild sweating. There is thirst, dry mouth, red and swollen throat, floating and rapid pulse, and a thin tongue coating with some red dots on the sides.

Pathology

When Wind-Heat invades the exterior it injures the greater yang. Heat is a yang pathogenic influence, thus the lower back is painful and hot. Other symptoms are classic signs of Wind-Heat attacking upward: burning, dark urine, warm body with mild sweating, dry mouth, thirst and a red, swollen throat. A floating and rapid pulse, and a thin tongue coating with red dots on the sides are indicative of exterior Wind-Heat.

Clinically speaking, Wind-Heat lower back pain is rather rarely seen, hence the adage, "In lower back pain, Cold and Dampness are common while Wind and Heat are rare." Wind-Heat lower back pain nevertheless readily transforms into Damp-Heat lower back pain, with such symptoms as painful, dripping and rough urination.

Wind-Dampness Lower Back Pain

Symptomatology

The upper and lower back is contracted, stiff, heavy and painful, and movement is restricted. There may be fever, aversion to wind, and edema of the face and limbs. The pulse is floating and choppy, and the tongue coating is thin and greasy.

Pathology

Exposure to wind and rain, as well as working in a damp environment, encourage the invasion of Wind and Dampness into the muscles and the exterior. Pathogenic Wind-Dampness settles in the lumbar region, and the lower back pain is accompanied by fever and an aversion to wind. When Wind-Dampness stagnates in the Kidney channel, it causes contraction, stiffness, heaviness and impaired movement throughout the back. In severe attacks, there is edema of the face and limbs. A floating, choppy pulse, and a thin, greasy tongue coating are signs of Wind-Dampness.

Wind-Dampness lower back pain often combines with pathogenic Cold and transforms into Damp-Cold lower back pain. Wind-Dampness lower back pain may also transform into a Wind-Water disorder.

INTERNALLY GENERATED LOWER BACK PAIN

Kidney Deficiency Lower Back Pain

Symptomatology

This type of lower back pain is defined by a sensation of soreness and weakness, with improvement upon pressure and massage. The legs and knees have no strength. The pain is aggravated by physical exertion, improves when lying down, and is marked by frequent recurrences. If the yang deficiency is predominant, there is tightness and contracture in the lower abdomen, a pallid face, cold extremities, a pale tongue, and a submerged and thin pulse. If the yin deficiency is predominant, there is irritability with insomnia, a dry mouth and throat, flushed face, hot palms and soles, a red tongue, and a wiry, thin and rapid pulse.

Pathology

The lower back is the abode of the Kidneys. Because the Kidneys govern the bones and marrow, when the Kidney Essence is exhausted and deficient, the marrow and bones are no longer nourished. This leads to lower back soreness and weakness, and lack of strength in the legs and knees. This is a pattern of deficiency, thus pressure and massage provide relief. Physical exertion depletes the Qi, which explains why the condition is aggravated by exertion and improves with rest.

When the yang is deficient it can no longer nourish the sinews, and the lower abdomen contracts and becomes tense. Deficient yang can neither warm the extremities nor nourish the limbs. The extremities are therefore cold and the face is pale. A pale tongue and a submerged and thin pulse are indicative of yang deficiency and the presence of Cold.

When the yin is deficient the Fluids are insufficient, Fire from deficiency blazes upward and there is irritability, insomnia and dryness of the mouth. A red tongue and a wiry, thin and rapid pulse are signs of yin deficiency with Heat.

Damp Spleen Lower Back Pain

Symptomatology

In this pattern, lower back pain is accompanied by sensations of heaviness and stagnation. The patient will also present with a pale complexion and poor appetite, and may experience diarrhea. The tongue coating is white and greasy, and the pulse is slippery or soggy.

Pathology

When the Spleen is deficient, Damp-Phlegm is generated internally. When Phlegm invades the lumbar area, it triggers lower back pain accompanied by a sensation of heaviness. When the Spleen is deficient, its transportive and transformative functions will diminish, reducing the appetite. Likewise, because the transformative function of the middle burner is deficient, the face will become pale. A deficient Spleen will produce Dampness, which can lead to loose stools. A white, greasy tongue coating, and a slippery or soggy pulse are indicative of Spleen deficiency with vigorous Dampness.

Liver Stagnation Lower Back Pain

Symptomatology

The lower back pain radiates toward the flanks, and the abdomen is full and distended. It feels as if there is gas inside, which can suddenly accumulate or disperse. The patient is unable to stand or walk for extended periods of time. The tongue is reddish with a thin coating, and the pulse is wiry and thin or wiry and submerged.

Pathology

When the Liver Qi does not spread freely, it stagnates in the lumbar area and the flanks. This leads to lower back pain that radiates toward the flanks, accompanied by abdominal distention. The lower abdomen is the domain of the Liver. If stagnation involves the Liver channel, the pain will radiate toward the lower abdomen. Constraint

and anger injure the Liver and cause the various sinews to become flaccid, making it difficult to stand or walk for extended periods of time. Qi-type pain is migratory, thus the pain may suddenly accumulate or disperse. A red tongue, and a wiry and thin or wiry and submerged pulse are signs of Liver yin insufficiency and Liver Qi stagnation.

Blood Stasis Lower Back Pain

Symptomatology

In this pattern, the lower back pain is stabbing and has a fixed location. If the pathology is mild, forward and backward bending of the trunk is impaired; when the condition is serious, the pain is severe and the patient cannot rotate the trunk. The painful area is very sensitive to pressure. The pain is better during the daytime and worse at night. The tongue is purple or has purple spots, and the pulse is choppy.

Pathology

When Blood stasis obstructs the channels, Qi and Blood cannot circulate freely, and the resultant lower back pain has a stabbing, fixed quality, which is aggravated by pressure. The Blood vessels are congealed and stagnant, which injures the sinews and vessels. This is why a mild condition impairs bending, and severe cases make it impossible to rotate. In the daytime the yang Qi is more vigorous and the circulation of Blood is correspondingly faster. At night the yin Qi is more vigorous and the Blood circulation is slower, which aggravates the lower back pain. A purple tongue, the presence of purple spots, and a choppy pulse all signify internal Blood stasis.

Treatment: Principles and Prescriptions

TREAT THE ROOT OF THE DISEASE

Lower back pain and stiffness are usually the consequences of other disorders. By treating the root cause of these disorders, the lower back pain symptoms will diminish or disappear of their own accord.

Emphasis on the Importance of Tonifying the Kidneys

As mentioned above, lower back pain and stiffness are often caused by Kidney deficiency. Consequently, tonification of the Kidneys should always be the foundation of treatment, whether the problem is externally contracted or internally generated. Treatment of externally contracted disorders must include herbs that expel Wind, disperse Cold, drain Dampness or purge Heat, or a combination of these. Problems related to internal injury require herbs that strengthen the Spleen, nourish the Liver, regulate the Qi and invigorate the Blood, individually or in combination.

A passage from the chapter on lower back and umbilical disorders in *Wondrous Lantern for Peering into the Origin and Development of Miscellaneous Diseases* underscores the importance of proper differentiation in selecting a remedy:

> Lower back pain signifies deficiency of the Kidney Essence and Qi, which allows the pathogenic influences to invade . . . . Kidney deficiency is the root, and Wind, Cold, Dampness, Heat, Phlegm and Congested Fluids, Qi stagnation, Blood stasis and trauma are the manifestations. Some problems come from the root; some from the manifestations. The noble [physicians] are those who never lose sight of what is appropriate.

For this reason, even though tonification of the Kidneys is the primary focus for the treatment of lower back pain, if the externally contracted problem is relatively vigorous, we must address what is most urgent first and treat the manifestation. In this case, we would first expel the pathogenic influences and then treat the root.

A passage from the chapter on lower back pain in *Comprehensive Collection of Medicine Past and Present (Gu jin yi tong da quan)* observes, "When the painful manifestation predominates, once it has been treated we must tonify and nourish to stabilize the root and avoid possible recurrences."

EXTERNALLY CONTRACTED LOWER BACK PAIN

Damp-Cold Lower Back Pain

Treatment Principle

The treatment principle is to dispel Cold, promote the movement of Dampness, warm the channels, and unblock the collaterals.

Prescriptions

Commonly used formulas are Licorice, Ginger, Poria, and Atractylodes Macrocephala Decoction *(gan cao gan jiang fu ling bai zhu tang)* and Leach Out Dampness Decoction *(shen shi tang)*. When Cold and Dampness are severe, add such herbs as Cortex Cinnamomi Cassiae *(rou gui)*, Herba Ephedrae *(ma huang)* and Radix Angelicae Dahuricae *(bai zhi)*, or prescribe Five-Accumulation Powder *(wu ji san)*.

In the chapter on lower back pain in *Teachings of [Zhu] Dan-Xi* is the following advice: "In cases of Damp-Cold lower back pain . . . it is appropriate to use Five-Accumulation Powder *(wu ji san)* with the addition of 1.5g Fructus Evodiae Rutaecarpae *(wu zhu yu)* and 3g Cortex Eucommiae Ulmoidis *(du zhong)*."

Chronic sufferers of Damp-Cold lower back pain often have Kidney deficiency. For this reason it is necessary to use herbs that tonify the Kidneys and fortify the lower back, such as Cortex Eucommiae Ulmoidis *(du zhong)*, Ramulus Sangjisheng *(sang ji sheng)* and Radix Dipsaci Asperi *(xu duan)*.

External application of herbs such as Special Pill to Massage the Lower Back *(mo yao dan)* is recommended in *Introduction to Medicine*. This formula includes 3g each of tips of Radix Lateralis Aconiti Carmichaeli Praeparata *(fu zi jian)*, tips of Radix Aconiti Carmichaeli Praeparata *(chuan wu jian)*, Rhizoma Arisaematis *(tian nan xing)*, Cinnabaris *(zhu sha)* and Rhizoma Zingiberis Officinalis *(gan jiang)*; and 1.5g each of Realgar *(xiong huang)*, Camphora *(zhang nao)*, Flos Caryophylli *(ding xiang)* and Secretio Moschus *(she xiang)*. Apply 3g of powder diluted in warm ginger juice to the lumbar area and massage until it feels hot, then bandage. This produces good results.

Pattern, Cause, Pulse, and Treatment (Zheng yin mai zhi) differentiates the treatment of Damp-Cold lower back pain as follows:

- For greater yang Damp-Cold, use Notopterygium Powder to Overcome Toxins *(qiang huo bai du san)* with the addition of Rhizoma Atractylodis *(cang zhu)*.
- For lesser yin Damp-Cold, use Angelica Pubescens and Atractylodes Decoction *(du huo cang zhu tang)*.
- For lesser yang Damp-Cold, use Bupleurum and Atractylodes Decoction *(chai hu cang zhu tang)*.
- For terminal yin Damp-Cold, use Frigid Extremities Decoction *(si ni tang)* with the addition of Radix Bupleuri *(chai hu)* and Radix Angelicae Pubescentis *(du huo)*.
- For yang brightness Damp-Cold, use Atractylodes and Angelica Dahurica Decoction *(cang zhu bai zhi tang)*.
- For greater yin Damp-Cold, use Atractylodes and Prepared Aconite Decoction to Aid the Living *(ji sheng zhu fu tang)* or Leach Out Dampness Decoction *(shen shi tang)*. If there are no results, Five-Ingredient Powder with Poria *(wu ling san)* is traditionally recommended

to promote urination; this formula should therefore be considered.

Damp-Heat Lower Back Pain

Treatment Principle

The principle of treatment is to clear Heat, drain Dampness, relax the sinews and alleviate pain.

Prescriptions

Augmented Two-Marvel Powder (*jia wei er miao san*) is often prescribed. In this formula the two herbs which transform Dampness and clear Heat, Cortex Phellodendri (*huang bai*) and Rhizoma Atractylodis (*cang zhu*), are the chief herbs. Radix Aristolochiae Fangchi (*fang ji*) and Rhizoma Dioscoreae Hypoglaucae (*bei xie*) assist them by promoting the elimination of Dampness. Radix Angelicae Sinensis (*dang gui*) and Radix Achyranthis Bidentatae (*niu xi*) invigorate the Blood, while Plastrum Testudinis (*gui ban*) nourishes the yin.

For Damp-Heat lower back pain with accompanying external pathogenic influences, add such herbs as Radix Bupleuri (*chai hu*), Radix Ledebouriellae Divaricatae (*fang feng*), Radix Angelicae Pubescentis (*du huo*) and Radix Ligustici Chuanxiong (*chuan xiong*).

For Damp-Heat lower back pain associated with Damp-Heat in the Bladder, add Major Separate the Clear Decoction (*da fen qing yin*) from *Collected Treatises of [Zhang] Jing-Yue*. In this formula, Sclerotium Poriae Cocos (*fu ling*), Rhizoma Alismatis Orientalis (*ze xie*), Caulis Mutong (*mu tong*), Sclerotium Polypori Umbellati (*zhu ling*), Fructus Gardeniae Jasminoidis (*zhi zi*) and Semen Plantaginis (*che qian zi*) act to clear and resolve Damp-Heat from the lower burner.

For Damp-Heat lower back pain associated with pain, redness, swelling and heat in the joints, prescribe Tangkuei Decoction to Draw Out Pain (*dang gui nian tong tang*) and Atractylodes Pill (*cang zhu wan*).

If the Damp-Heat lower back pain becomes chronic and is accompanied by Kidney exhaustion, prescribe Seven-Ingredient Powder with Atractylodes and Phellodendron (*qi wei cang bai san*), which clears Heat, resolves Dampness, tonifies the Kidneys and strengthens the lower back.

Damp-Phlegm Lower Back Pain

Treatment Principle

The principle of treatment is to dispel Dampness and transform Phlegm.

Prescriptions

Turtle Shell and Ailanthus Pill (*gui chu wan*) are commonly prescribed for Damp-Phlegm lower back pain. In this formula, Plastrum Testudinis (*gui ban*) tonifies the Kidneys and strengthens the Essence; Cortex Ailanthi Altissimae (*chun pi*), Rhizoma Atractylodis (*cang zhu*), and Talcum (*hua shi*) dry and resolve the Dampness; and Radix Paeoniae Lactiflorae (*bai shao*) and Rhizoma Cyperi Rotundi (*xiang fu*) harmonize the Qi and Blood.

If there is also external Dampness, add such herbs as Radix Aristolochiae Fangchi (*fang ji*), Caulis Piperis Futokadsurae (*hai feng teng*), Caulis Trachelospermi Jasminoidis (*luo shi teng*) and Ramulus Mori Albae (*sang zhi*).

For associated Dampness in the Spleen, use herbs that revive the Spleen and transform Dampness, such as Rhizoma Atractylodis Macrocephalae (*bai zhu*), Sclerotium Poriae Cocos (*fu ling*), Fructus Amomi Kravanh (*bai dou kou*) and Fructus Amomi (*sha ren*); or add herbs that warm the Spleen and dry Dampness, such as Rhizoma Atractylodis (*cang zhu*), Rhizoma Zingiberis Officinalis (*gan jiang*) and Radix Codonopsitis Pilosulae (*dang shen*).

For recalcitrant conditions, add Cortex Cinnamomi Cassiae (*rou gui*) to warm and unblock.

Wind-Cold Lower Back Pain

Treatment Principle

The treatment principle is to disperse the Wind and Cold.

Prescriptions

Ginseng Powder to Overcome Pathogenic Influences (*ren shen bai du san*) is recommended. In this formula, Radix Ginseng (*ren shen*) tonifies the Qi, strengthens the normal Qi and assists Radix et Rhizoma Notopterygii (*qiang huo*), Radix Angelicae Pubescentis (*du huo*), Radix Bupleuri (*chai hu*) and Radix Peucedani (*qian hu*) in expelling the pathogenic influences outward; Radix Platycodi Grandiflori (*jie geng*) and Fructus Citri Aurantii (*zhi ke*), one ascending and the other descending, work together to regulate and facilitate the Qi mechanism; Radix Ligustici Chuanxiong (*chuan xiong*) promotes movement in the stagnation of Qi and Blood and alleviates pain; Sclerotium Poriae Cocos (*fu ling*) leaches out Dampness; and Radix Glycyrrhizae Uralensis (*gan cao*) harmonizes the middle burner.

When the Wind-Cold is expelled externally, and the Blood and Qi are harmonized and free, the lower back pain will then go away.

Wind-Heat Lower Back Pain

Treatment Principle

The treatment principle is to disperse the Wind and Heat.

Prescriptions

The formula recommended for treating Wind-Heat lower back pain is Minor Bupleurum Decoction *(xiao chai hu tang)* minus Rhizoma Pinelliae Ternatae *(ban xia)*, but with the addition of Radix et Rhizoma Notopterygii *(qiang huo)*, Radix Dipsaci Asperi *(xu duan)* and Semen Glycines Max *(hei dou)*. In this formula, which comes from *Comprehensive Medicine According to Master Zhang*, the combination of Radix Bupleuri *(chai hu)*, Radix et Rhizoma Notopterygii *(qiang huo)* and Radix Scutellariae Baicalensis *(huang qin)* disperses the internal buildup of Wind-Heat; Radix Dipsaci Asperi *(xu duan)* tonifies the Kidneys and fortifies the lower back; and Semen Glycines Max *(hei dou)* helps the Kidneys and relieves toxicity. This prescription takes into account both the root and the manifestation.

For those with constipation, Major Bupleurum Decoction *(da chai hu tang)* can be used as a mild purgative.

Wind-Dampness Lower Back Pain

Treatment Principle

The principle of treatment is to disperse the Wind and resolve the Dampness.

Prescriptions

For Wind-Dampness lower back pain, Angelica Pubescens and Sangjisheng Decoction *(du huo ji sheng tang)* is recommended. In this formula, Cortex Eucommiae Ulmoidis *(du zhong)*, Radix Achyranthis Bidentatae *(niu xi)* and Ramulus Sangjisheng *(sang ji sheng)* tonify the Kidneys and strengthen the lower back; Radix Angelicae Sinensis *(dang gui)*, Radix Rehmanniae Glutinosae *(sheng di huang)*, Radix Paeoniae Lactiflorae *(bai shao)*, Radix Ligustici Chuanxiong *(chuan xiong)*, Radix Ginseng *(ren shen)* and Sclerotium Poriae Cocos *(fu ling)* regulate and tonify the Blood and Qi; Radix Gentianae Qinjiao *(qin jiao)*, Radix Ledebouriellae Divaricatae *(fang feng)*, Radix Angelicae Pubescentis *(du huo)*, Herba cum Radice Asari *(xi xin)* and Ramulus Cinnamomi Cassiae *(gui zhi)* expel Wind-Dampness. This prescription takes into account both the root and the manifestation and supports the normal Qi while expelling the pathogenic influences.

For those with both Liver and Kidney insufficiency, such herbs as Radix Dipsaci Asperi *(xu duan)* and Rhizoma Cibotii Barometz *(gou ji)* can be added.

For severe pathogenic Cold preventing forward and backward bending, use Aconite Decoction *(wu tou tang)*.

For lingering pathogenic Cold that has been constrained and transformed into Heat, use Cinnamon Twig, Peony, and Anemarrhena Decoction *(gui zhi shao yao zhi mu tang)*.

INTERNALLY GENERATED LOWER BACK PAIN

Kidney Deficiency Lower Back Pain

Treatment Principle

The primary treatment principle is to tonify the Kidneys. For yang deficiency, warm and tonify the Kidneys; for yin deficiency, enrich the Kidneys and augment the yin.

Prescriptions

Young Maiden Pill *(qing e wan)* is often used to warm and tonify the Kidneys. For weakness of the gate of vitality, add such substances as Cortex Cinnamomi Cassiae *(rou gui)*, Radix Lateralis Aconiti Carmichaeli Praeparata *(fu zi)*, Gelatinum Cornu Cervi *(lu jiao jiao)* and Semen Cuscutae Chinensis *(tu si zi)*. Some recommend Restore the Right [Kidney] Pill *(you gui wan)*. Often patients with weak gate of vitality fire also suffer from Kidney yin deficiency. In such cases, add Radix Rehmanniae Glutinosae Conquitae *(shu di huang)*, Fructus Corni Officinalis *(shan zhu yu)*, Radix Dioscoreae Oppositae *(shan yao)* and Fructus Lycii *(gou qi zi)*.

Tangkuei and Rehmannia Pill *(dang gui di huang wan)* may be prescribed to enrich the Kidneys and augment the yin. In this formula, Radix Rehmanniae Glutinosae Conquitae *(shu di huang)*, Fructus Corni Officinalis *(shan zhu yu)* and Radix Dioscoreae Oppositae *(shan yao)* tonify the Kidney yin; Cortex Eucommiae Ulmoidis *(du zhong)* and Radix Achyranthis Bidentatae *(niu xi)* fortify the lower back and knees; Radix Angelicae Sinensis *(dang gui)* tonifies and moves the Blood in order to help unblock the Kidney Qi. This is why the various formulas developed by Zhang Jing-Yue (also known as Zhang Jie-Bin) for tonifying the Kidneys often include Radix Angelicae Sinensis (dang gui).

For marked Kidney yin deficiency, combine Restore the Left [Kidney] Pill (zuo gui wan) with Fructus Lycii (gou qi zi) and Plastrum Testudinis (gui ban). However, patients with Kidney yin deficiency often also have Kidney yang deficiency. In such cases it is appropriate to use Gelatinum Cornu Cervi (lu jiao jiao) and Semen Cuscutae Chinensis (tu si zi) from Restore the Right [Kidney] Pill (you gui wan).

Kidney yin deficiency can also be accompanied by blazing Ministerial Fire. Use Anemarrhena, Phellodendron, and Rehmannia Pill (zhi bai di huang wan) for mild cases, and Great Tonify the Yin Pill (da bu yin wan) for severe cases of this pattern.

Lower back pain caused by deficiency consumption (xū láo) with injury to the yin and yang is a complex disorder. Eucommia Pill (du zhong wan) is generally prescribed. In this formula, Cortex Eucommiae Ulmoidis (du zhong) and Fructus Psoraleae Corylifoliae (bu gu zhi) tonify the Kidneys, and warm without drying; Fructus Lycii (gou qi zi) and Plastrum Testudinis (gui ban) enrich and moisten without being cloying; Fructus Schisandrae Chinensis (wu wei zi) and Radix Paeoniae Lactiflorae (bai shao) tonify the Liver and Kidneys; Radix Astragali Membranacei (huang qi) and Radix Angelicae Sinensis (dang gui) tonify the Qi and Blood; and Rhizoma Anemarrhenae Asphodeloidis (zhi mu) and Cortex Phellodendri (huang bai) clear the Ministerial Fire. Because it addresses all the different aspects of this disorder, Eucommia Pill (du zhong wan) is an excellent prescription for lower back pain caused by overexertion consumption.

For yang deficiency lower back pain due to excessive sexual activity, use fleshy substances to adjust and regulate. Among the recommended formulas are Great Creation Pill (da zao wan), Tonifying Extract with Ginseng and Deer Antler (shen lu bu gao) and Special Pill to Tonfiy the Marrow (bu sui dan).

Spleen Dampness Lower Back Pain

Treatment Principle

The treatment principle is to strengthen the Spleen and resolve the Dampness.

Prescriptions

Calm the Stomach Powder (ping wei san) is recommended for mild cases. When the Water-Dampness is rather severe, use Stephania and Astragalus Decoction (fang ji huang qi tang). For significant Spleen Dampness, use Bolster the Spleen Decoction (shi pi yin). Among the herbs used in these formulas, Radix Lateralis Aconiti Carmichaeli Praeparata (fu zi), Rhizoma Zingiberis Officinalis (gan jiang), Rhizoma Atractylodis Macrocephalae (bai zhu), Radix Glycyrrhizae Uralensis (gan cao), Rhizoma Zingiberis Officinalis Recens (sheng jiang) and Fructus Zizyphi Jujubae (da zao) warm the yang and bolster the Spleen. Cortex Magnoliae Officinalis (hou po), Radix Aucklandiae Lappae (mu xiang), Semen Arecae Catechu (bing lang) and Fructus Amomi Tsao-ko (cao guo) regulate the Qi and transform Dampness.

Liver Stagnation Lower Back Pain

Treatment Principle

The treatment principle is to adjust the Liver and promote the movement of Qi.

Prescriptions

Aquilaria Decoction for Directing Qi Downward (chen xiang jiang qi tang) and Top-Quality Lindera Powder (tian tai wu yao san) are recommended. Qi-regulating herbs can be added to tonify the Liver and Kidneys: Fructus Lycii (gou qi zi), Fructus Ligustri Lucidi (nu zhen zi), Herba Ecliptae Prostratae (han lian cao), Fructus Mori Albae (sang shen).

Blood Stasis Lower Back Pain

Treatment Principle

The principle of treatment is to invigorate the Blood, transform stasis, regulate the Qi and alleviate pain.

Prescriptions

Fantastically Effective Pill to Invigorate the Collaterals (huo luo xiao ling dan) is recommended. In this formula, Radix Angelicae Sinensis (dang gui) and Radix Salviae Miltiorrhizae (dan shen) nourish and invigorate the Blood; Gummi Olibanum (ru xiang) and Myrrha (mo yao) move the Qi, dispel stasis and alleviate pain. Relax the Sinews Powder (shu jin san) can also be added. For severe stasis with intense pain, Myrhh Powder to Take Advantage of Pain (ru xiang chen tong san) is recommended.

Other Therapeutic Methods

WARM HERBAL WRAPS

For Kidney deficiency lower back pain, toast, powder and then wrap in gauze Ramulus Cinnamomi Cassiae *(gui zhi)* 30g, Rhizoma Zingiberis Officinalis Recens *(sheng jiang)* 120g, Bulbus Allii Fistulosi *(cong bai)* 30g, and Fructus Zanthoxyli Bungeani *(chuan jiao)* 60g. Apply topically to the painful area and rewarm as soon as it becomes cold.

MOXIBUSTION

For cold and painful lower back pain, use indirect moxibustion either with 3-5 cones a day (placing the cones on herbal cakes) or 15-20 minutes of moxa sticks. Perform daily or every other day.

ACUPUNCTURE

For chronic lower back pain, the focus is on selecting points close to the pain. Generally, those points which are tender to the touch are used.

Primary points: BL-23 *(shen shu)*, BL-24 *(qi hai shu)*, BL-25 *(da chang shu)*

Secondary points: M-BW-35 *(hua tuo jia ji)*, M-BW-27 *(yao gen)*, BL-52 *(zhi shi)*, GV-4 *(ming men)*, GV-3 *(yao yang guan)*, and "Residing orifice *(ju qiao)*[10]

TUI-NA

The appropriate techniques for lower back pain include rolling *(gǔn)*, pushing *(tuī)*, pressing *(ān)*, softening *(róu)* and rubbing *(cā)*. These should be used on the painful points as well as on such points as BL-23 *(shen shu)*, BL-25 *(da chang shu)*, BL-31~34 *(ba liao)* and GB-29 *(ju liao)*. Start by using the rolling and pushing techniques around the painful areas, then push on BL-23 *(shen shu)*, BL-25 *(da chang shu)* and BL-31~34 *(ba liao)*. Depending on the symptomatology, add to the massage of selected areas some passive range of motion actions, followed by pressing, softening and rubbing techniques.

Prognosis

Lower back pain and stiffness may only be symptoms that can be encountered during the evolution of many diseases. When this is the case, the lower back pain will generally subside or disappear as soon as the illness is cured.

During their evolution, some types of lower back pain can become chronic. In extreme cases they can transform into atrophy disorder, paralysis or other types of disorders. The prognosis in these cases is usually less favorable.

Prevention & Care

In order to prevent lower back pain it is important to avoid damp places. People should dry themselves and change clothes after being soaked by rain or sweat due to strenuous physical activity, or drink fresh ginger tea with brown sugar to disperse Wind-Cold or Wind-Dampness. During periods of Summerheat when Damp-Heat is dense, sleeping outside, drinking cold beverages or bathing too often must be avoided.

Acute lower back pain must be treated in a timely fashion, followed by a period of rest. In addition to medication, the prevention of chronic lower back pain involves avoiding lower back strain and cold, or wearing a lumbar support belt.

When lower back pain is only the main symptom of an illness, it is important to focus treatment on the illness itself. Examples include painful urinary obstruction *(lín)*, urinary blockage *(lóng bì)*, edema and plugged and rejecting disorder *(guān gé)*.[11]

Other preventive methods are self-massage, spinal exercises, *taijiquan* and baths. If there is edema, the use of salt is proscribed.

In addition, among the special therapeutic methods mentioned in *Formulas for Nourishing Life* are:

• Going for a walk after meals, and not lying down immediately after eating. This is because the food in the Stomach needs to be warmed by the Kidneys. Appropriate exercises promote the smooth circulation of Kidney Qi and can prevent lower back pain.

• Promoting a smooth intestinal transit by having bowel movements at regular times, and refraining from straining in cases of constipation.

Modern Research

Since 1949 many studies on lower back pain have been conducted, with a rather large number of cases. Below are the results of several such studies, which can serve as references.

In Dr. Liu's[12] study of 130 cases of acute and chronic lower back pain treated with tui-na, there were 89 cures, 22 were definitely improved, and 19 were moderately improved. In another study, Dr. Zhou[13] based his approach on the idea that "long-term diseases enter the collaterals, and Blood stasis causes pain." Thus, in 337 cases of lower back pain due to trauma, overexertion and Damp-Cold, he administered daily injections for 10 days of 2 to 4ml of Radix Ligustici Chuanxiong (chuan xiong) in the painful spots or in acupuncture points. The results were 215 cures, 112 improvements and 10 failures.

Dr. Tang[14] treated 60 cases of recalcitrant lower back pain with catgut implantation at the following acupuncture points: GV-4 (ming men), GV-3 (yao yang guan), BL-24 (qi hai shu), BL-25 (da chang shu), BL-27 (xiao chang shu) and locally tender points. Of these cases, 30 were cured, 14 showed significant improvement, 13 had some improvement and 3 lacked any improvement. The points were threaded every 5 to 7 days, with three treatments constituting one course. In most cases, improvement came within one or two courses.

Dr. Wang[15] treated 90 cases of Kidney deficiency lower back pain with a formula he devised called Eucommia Decoction (du zhong tang). This is composed of Cortex Eucommiae Ulmoidis (du zhong), Radix Achyranthis Bidentatae (niu xi), Fructus Lycii (gou qi zi), Fructus Schisandrae Chinensis (wu wei zi), Radix Dioscoreae Oppositae (shan yao), Semen Cuscutae Chinensis (tu si zi), Gelatinum Cornu Cervi (lu jiao jiao), Radix Dipsaci Asperi (xu duan), Radix Rehmanniae Glutinosae Conquitae (shu di huang), Cortex Phellodendri (huang bai) and Radix Glycyrrhizae Uralensis (gan cao). The range in duration of the pain was 5 months to 10 years. There were 53 cases of Kidney yang deficiency and 37 cases of Kidney yin deficiency. After treatment, 42 cases were cured and 31 showed improvement.

Dr. Lu[16] prescribed his own Notopterygium Decoction (qiang huo tang) for externally contracted lower back pain. The basic formula is composed of Radix et Rhizoma Notopterygii (qiang huo), Radix Ledebouriellae Divaricatae (fang feng), Radix Gentianae Qinjiao (qin jiao), Cortex Acanthopanacis Gracilistylus Radicis (wu jia pi), Fructus Chaenomelis Lagenariae (mu gua), Radix Dipsaci Asperi (xu duan), Caulis Piperis Futokadsurae (hai feng teng), Radix Achyranthis Bidentatae (niu xi) and Herba cum Radice Asari (xi xin). Recommended modifications in the formula were as follows:

- For exhausted Blood and Qi leading to injury from deficiency with lower back pain, use Eight-Treasure Decoction (ba zhen tang).

- For Kidney injury with exhaustion of the Essence, use Dr. Lu's own Tonify the Lower Back Decoction (bu yao tang) made up of Radix Rehmanniae Glutinosae Conquitae (shu di huang), Radix Angelicae Sinensis (dang gui), Radix Paeoniae Lactiflorae (bai shao), Radix Dipsaci Asperi (xu duan), Radix Rehmanniae Glutinosae (sheng di huang), Rhizoma Cibotii Barometz (gou ji), Cortex Eucommiae Ulmoidis (du zhong), Fructus Psoraleae Corylifoliae (bu gu zhi), Radix Astragali Membranacei (huang qi) and Gelatinum Cornu Cervi (lu jiao jiao).

- For lower back pain due to bone consumption, use Yang-Heartening Decoction (yang he tang).

- For lower back pain associated with pregnancy, use herbs that augment the Kidneys and tonify the Blood: Radix Angelicae Sinensis (dang gui), Radix Paeoniae Lactiflorae (bai shao), Radix Dipsaci Asperi (xu duan), Cortex Eucommiae Ulmoidis (du zhong), Ramulus Sangjisheng (sang ji sheng). At the same time, use herbs that calm the fetus: Fructus Amomi (sha ren) and Ramulus Perillae Frutescentis (su geng).

- For trauma-induced lower back pain, use Dr. Lu's own Nine-Ingredient Formula for Lower Back Pain (jiu wei yao tong fang). This formula is composed of Cortex Eucommiae Ulmoidis (du zhong), Rhizoma Cibotii Barometz (gou ji), Fructus Psoraleae Corylifoliae (bu gu zhi), Radix Achyranthis Bidentatae (niu xi), Radix Angelicae Sinensis (dang gui), Radix Paeoniae Rubrae (chi shao), Radix Dipsaci Asperi (xu duan), Rhizoma Corydalis Yanhusuo (yan hu suo) and Flos Carthami Tinctorii (hong hua).

Summary

Lower back pain refers to unilateral or bilateral pain in the lumbar area. Lower back stiffness refers to an aching sensation in the same area. In fact, lower back pain and stiffness simply describe different levels of intensity of these sensations. Both share a close relationship with the Kidneys.

An entire chapter is devoted to lower back pain in *Inner Classic*, which describes it in great detail.[17] From the perspective of etiology, three main factors are noted: deficiency, Cold and Dampness. In terms of treatment, only acupuncture is used; no herbal prescriptions are noted. *Essentials from the Golden Cabinet* introduced the use of herbal formulas in the service of such strategies as warming the Kidneys, tonifying the Kidneys, dispersing Cold and resolving Dampness. *Discussion of the Origins of*

Symptoms of Disease was the first book to differentiate between acute and chronic lower back pain. *Thousand Ducat Prescriptions* recorded the use of manipulation in the treatment of lower back pain. *Formulas for Nourishing Life* emphasized the need for patients suffering from lower back pain to make changes in how they live. *Discussion of Illnesses, Patterns, and Formulas Related to the Unification of the Three Etiologies* underscored the distinction between external and internal causes. During the Ming and Qing dynasties, the systematic classification of lower back pain was further elaborated.

Lower back pain and stiffness are associated with a variety of etiologies, chief among which are invasion of Damp-Cold or Damp-Heat; injury due to overwork or trauma; or Liver, Spleen or Kidney deficiency. With respect to development of the disease mechanism, Kidney deficiency is the root, whereas the externally contracted pathogenic factors, trauma, overwork and the seven emotions are all related to the manifestations. The location of lower back pain and stiffness is at the level of the Kidneys and the channels.

When differentiating the patterns involved in lower back pain and stiffness, it is important first to differentiate between external invasion and internal injury, then to analyze the deficiency and excess of any Organ, while also paying attention to the channel pathways and monitoring changes in the pulse.

Clinically speaking, lower back pain and stiffness are classified according to their origin: external invasion (Damp-Cold, Damp-Heat, Damp-Phlegm, Wind-Heat or Wind-Dampness lower back pain) or internal injury (Kidney deficiency, Spleen Dampness or Liver stagnation lower back pain).

The main focus of treatment is to tonify the Kidneys. If the external invasion predominates, first dispel the pathogenic influence and then tonify the Kidneys. Acupuncture and massage can be used as complementary treatments.

Formulas[18]

Aconite Decoction (wū tóu tāng)
烏頭湯
Herba Ephedrae (ma huang)
Radix Paeoniae Lactiflorae (bai shao)
Radix Astragali Membranacei (huang qi)
Honey-toasted Radix Glycyrrhizae Uralensis (zhi gan cao)
Radix Aconiti Carmichaeli Praeparata (zhi chuan wu)
Honey (feng mi)

SOURCE: *Essentials from the Golden Cabinet*

Angelica Pubescens and Atractylodes Decoction
(dú huó cāng zhú tāng)
獨活蒼术湯
Radix Angelicae Pubescentis (du huo)
Radix Ligustici Chuanxiong (chuan xiong)
Rhizoma Atractylodis (cang zhu)
Radix Glycyrrhizae Uralensis (gan cao)
Radix Ledebouriellae Divaricatae (fang feng)
Herba cum Radice Asari (xi xin)
SOURCE: *Pattern, Cause, Pulse, and Treatment*

Angelica Pubescens and Sangjisheng Decoction
(dú huó jì shēng tāng)
獨活寄生湯
Ramulus Sanjisheng (sang ji sheng)
Radix Angelicae Pubescentis (du huo)
Radix Gentianae Qinjiao (qin jiao)
Radix Ledebouriellae Divaricatae (fang feng)
Herba cum Radice Asari (xi xin)
Radix Angelicae Sinensis (dang gui)
Radix Paeoniae Lactiflorae (bai shao)
Radix Ligustici Chuanxiong (chuan xiong)
Radix Rehmanniae Glutinosae (sheng di huang)
Cortex Eucommiae Ulmoidis (du zhong)
Radix Achyranthis Bidentatae (niu xi)
Radix Ginseng (ren shen)
Sclerotium Poriae Cocos (fu ling)
Radix Glycyrrhizae Uralensis (gan cao)
Cortex Cinnamomi Cassiae (rou gui)
SOURCE: *Thousand Ducat Prescriptions*

Aquilaria Decoction for Directing Qi Downward
(chén xiāng jiàng qì tāng)
沈香降氣湯
Rhizoma Cyperi Rotundi (xiang fu)
Lignum Aquilariae (chen xiang)
Fructus Amomi (sha ren)
Honey-toasted Radix Glycyrrhizae Uralensis (zhi gan cao)
SOURCE: *Imperial Grace Formulary of the Tai Ping Era*

Atractylodes and Angelica Dahurica Decoction
(cāng zhú bái zhǐ tāng)
蒼术白芷湯
Rhizoma Atractylodis (cang zhu)
Rhizoma Cimicifugae (sheng ma)

Radix Angelicae Dahuricae (bai zhi)
Rhizoma Zingiberis Officinalis (gan jiang)
Radix Ledebouriellae Divaricatae (fang feng)
Radix Glycyrrhizae Uralensis (gan cao)
Radix Angelicae Pubescentis (du huo)
Radix Puerariae (ge gen)
SOURCE: Pattern, Cause, Pulse, and Treatment

Atractylodes and Prepared Aconite Decoction to Aid the Living (jì shēng zhú fù tāng)

濟生术附湯

Rhizoma Atractylodis Macrocephalae (bai zhu)
Radix Lateralis Aconiti Carmichaeli Praeparata (fu zi)
Cortex Eucommiae Ulmoidis (du zhong)
Rhizoma Zingiberis Officinalis (gan jiang)
SOURCE: Pattern, Cause, Pulse, and Treatment

Atractylodes Pill (cāng zhú wán)

蒼术丸

Rhizoma Atractylodis (cang zhu)
Radix Aucklandiae Lappae (mu xiang)
Gummi Olibanum (ru xiang)
Myrrha (mo yao)
Radix Achyranthis Bidentatae (niu xi)
Radix Aconiti (wu tou)
Buthus Martensi (quan xie)
Rhizoma Atractylodis Macrocephalae (bai zhu)
Fructus Chaenomelis Lagenariae (mu gua)
Folium Artemisiae Argyi (ai ye)
SOURCE: Standards of Patterns and Treatments

Augmented Two-Marvel Powder (jiā wèi èr miào sǎn)

加味二妙散

Rhizoma Atractylodis (cang zhu)
Cortex Phellodendri (huang bai)
Radix Achyranthis Bidentatae (niu xi)
Extremitas Radicis Angelicae Sinensis (dang gui wei)
Radix Aristolochiae Fangchi (fang ji)
Rhizoma Dioscoreae Hypoglaucae (bei xie)
Plastrum Testudinis (gui ban)
SOURCE: Teachings of [Zhu] Dan-Xi

Bupleurum and Atractylodes Decoction (chái hú cāng zhú tāng)

柴胡蒼术湯

Radix Bupleuri (chai hu)
Rhizoma Atractylodis (cang zhu)
Radix Ligustici Chuanxiong (chuan xiong)

Radix Ledebouriellae Divaricatae (fang feng)
Radix Glycyrrhizae Uralensis (gan cao)
Radix Angelicae Pubescentis (du huo)
Pericarpium Citri Reticulatae (chen pi)
SOURCE: Pattern, Cause, Pulse, and Treatment

Cinnamon Twig, Peony, and Anemarrhena Decoction (guì zhī sháo yào zhī mǔ tāng)

桂枝芍藥知母湯

Ramulus Cinnamomi Cassiae (gui zhi)
Radix Paeoniae Lactiflorae (bai shao yao)
Rhizoma Anemarrhenae Asphodeloidis (zhi mu)
Herba Ephedrae (ma huang)
Rhizoma Atractylodis Macrocephalae (bai zhu)
Radix Ledebouriallae Divaricatae (fang feng)
Radix Lateralis Aconiti Carmichaeli Praeparata (fu zi)
Rhizoma Zingiberis Officinalis Recens (sheng jiang)
Radix Glycyrrhizae Uralensis (gan cao)
SOURCE: Essentials from the Golden Cabinet

Eucommia Pill (dù zhòng wán)

杜仲丸

Cortex Eucommiae Ulmoidis (du zhong)
Fructus Psoraleae Corylifoliae (bu gu zhi)
Fructus Lycii (gou qi zi)
Plastrum Testudinis (gui ban)
Cortex Phellodendri (huang bai)
Rhizoma Anemarrhenae Asphodeloidis (zhi mu)
Fructus Schisandrae Chinensis (wu wei zi)
Radix Paeoniae (shao yao)
Radix Angelicae Sinensis (dang gui)
Radix Astragali Membranacei (huang qi)
SOURCE: Introduction to Medicine

Five-Accumulation Powder (wǔ jī sǎn)

五積散

Herba Ephedrae (ma huang)
Rhizoma Atractylodis (cang zhu)
Radix Angelicae Dahuricae (bai zhi)
Radix Angelicae Sinensis (dang gui)
Radix Paeoniae Lactiflorae (bai shao yao)
Radix Ligustici Chuanxiong (chuan xiong)
Fructus Citri Aurantii (zhi ke)
Radix Platycodi Grandiflori (jie geng)
Ramulus Cinnamomi Cassiae (gui zhi)
Rhizoma Zingiberis Officinalis (gan jiang)
Sclerotium Poriae Cocos (fu ling)
Radix Glycyrrhizae Uralensis (gan cao)

Cortex Magnoliae Officinalis (*hou po*)
Pericarpium Citri Reticulatae (*chen pi*)
Rhizoma Pinelliae Ternatae (*ban xia*)
Rhizoma Zingiberis Officinalis Recens (sheng *jiang*)
SOURCE: *Imperial Grace Formulary of the Tai Ping Era*

Five-Ingredient Powder with Poria (*wǔ líng sǎn*)

五苓散

Sclerotium Poriae Cocos (*fu ling*)
Sclerotium Polypori Umbellati (*zhu ling*)
Rhizoma Alismatis Orientalis (*ze xie*)
Rhizoma Atractylodis Macrocephalae (*bai zhu*)
Cortex Cinnamomi Cassiae (*rou gui*)
SOURCE: *Discussion of Cold-induced Disorders*

Frigid Extremities Decoction (*sì nì tāng*)

四逆湯

Radix Lateralis Aconiti Carmichaeli Praeparata (*fu zi*)
Rhizoma Zingiberis Officinalis (*gan jiang*)
Radix Glycyrrhizae Uralensis (*gan cao*)
SOURCE: *Discussion of Cold-induced Disorders*

Leach Out Dampness Decoction (*shèn shī tāng*)

滲濕湯

Rhizoma Atractylodis (*cang zhu*)
Sclerotium Poriae Cocos (*fu ling*)
Rhizoma Atractylodis Macrocephalae (*bai zhu*)
Rhizoma Zingiberis Officinalis (*gan jiang*)
Radix Glycyrrhizae Uralensis (*gan cao*)
Pars Rubra Epicarpii Citri Erythrocarpae (*ju hong*)
Flos Caryophylli (*ding xiang*)
SOURCE: *Teachings of [Zhu] Dan-Xi*

Licorice, Ginger, Poria, and Atractylodes Decoction (*gān jiāng líng zhú tāng*)

甘薑苓朮湯

Radix Glycyrrhizae Uralensis (*gan cao*)
Rhizoma Zingiberis Officinalis (*gan jiang*)
Sclerotium Poriae Cocos (*fu ling*)
Rhizoma Atractylodis Macrocephalae (*bai zhu*)
SOURCE: *Essentials from the Golden Cabinet*

Major Separate the Clear Decoction (*dà fēn qīng yǐn*)

大分清飲

Sclerotium Poriae Cocos (*fu ling*)
Rhizoma Alismatis Orientalis (*ze xie*)

Caulis Mutong (*mu tong*)
Sclerotium Polypori Umbellati (*zhu ling*)
Fructus Gardeniae Jasminoidis (*shan zhi zi*)
Fructus Citri Aurantii (*zhi ke*)
Semen Plantaginis (*che qian zi*)
SOURCE: *Collected Treatises of [Zhang] Jing-Yue*

Myrrh Powder to Take Advantage of Pain (*rǔ xiāng chèn tòng sǎn*)

乳香趁痛散

Plastrum Testudinis (*gui ban*)
Radix Paeoniae Rubrae (*chi shao*)
Myrrha(*mo yao*)
Radix Angelicae Sinensis (*dang gui*)
Radix Ledebouriellae Divaricatae (*fang feng*)
Sanguis Draconis (*xue jie*)
Ramulus Cinnamomi Cassiae (*gui zhi*)
Radix Angelicae Dahuricae (*bai zhi*)
Radix Achyranthis Bidentatae (*niu xi*)
Rhizoma Gastrodiae Elatae (*tian ma*)
Radix et Rhizoma Notopterygii (*qiang huo*)
Semen Arecae Catechu (*bing lang*)
Gummi Olibanum (*ru xiang*)
Os Tigris (*hu gu*)
Pyritum (*zi ran tong*)
Rhizoma Typhonii Gigantei (*bai fu zi*)
Fructus Xanthii Sibirici (*cang er zi*)
Fructus Psoraleae Corylifoliae (*bu gu zhi*)
Cortex Acanthopanacis Gracilistylus Radicis (*wu jia pi*)
SOURCE: *Wondrous Lantern for Peering into the Origin and Development of Miscellaneous Diseases*

Notopterygium Powder to Overcome Toxins (*qiāng huó bài dú sǎn*)

羌活敗毒散

Radix et Rhizoma Notopterygii (*qiang huo*)
Radix Ligustici Chuanxiong (*chuan xiong*)
Rhizoma Atractylodis (*cang zhu*)
Radix Angelicae Pubescentis (*du huo*)
Radix Bupleuri (*chai hu*)
Radix Angelicae Dahuricae (*bai zhi*)
Radix Ledebouriellae Divaricatae (*fang feng*)
Radix Peucedani (*qian hu*)
Herba seu Flos Schizonepetae Tenuifoliae (*jing jie*)
Radix Glycyrrhizae Uralensis (*gan cao*)
SOURCE: *Pattern, Cause, Pulse, and Treatment*

Relax the Sinews Powder *(shū jīn sǎn)*

舒筋散

Rhizoma Corydalis Yanhusuo *(yan hu suo)*

Cortex Eucommiae Ulmoidis *(du zhong)*

Cortex Cinnamomi Cassiae Tubiformis *(guan gui)*

Radix et Rhizoma Notopterygii *(qiang huo)*

Radix Dioscoreae Oppositae *(shan yao)*

SOURCE: *Standards of Patterns and Treatments*

Restore the Left [Kidney] Pill *(zuǒ guī wán)*

左歸丸

Radix Rehmanniae Glutinosae Conquitae *(shu di huang)*

Radix Dioscoreae Oppositae *(shan yao)*

Fructus Corni Officinalis *(shan zhu yu)*

Semen Cuscutae Chinensis *(tu si zi)*

Fructus Lycii *(gou qi zi)*

Radix Achyranthis Bidentatae *(niu xi)*

Gelatinum Cornu Cervi *(lu jiao jiao)*

Gelatinum Plastri Testudinis *(gui ban jiao)*

SOURCE: *Collected Treatises of [Zhang] Jing-Yue*

Restore the Right [Kidney] Pill *(yòu guī wán)*

右歸丸

Radix Rehmanniae Glutinosae Conquitae *(shu di huang)*

Radix Dioscoreae Oppositae *(shan yao)*

Fructus Corni Officinalis *(shan zhu yu)*

Fructus Lycii *(gou qi zi)*

Cortex Eucommiae Ulmoidis *(du zhong)*

Semen Cuscutae Chinensis *(tu si zi)*

Radix Lateralis Aconiti Carmichaeli Praeparata *(fu zi)*

Cortex Cinnamomi Cassiae *(rou gui)*

Radix Angelicae Sinensis *(dang gui)*

Gelatinum Cornu Cervi *(lu jiao jiao)*

SOURCE: *Collected Treatises of [Zhang] Jing-Yue*

Seven-Ingredient Powder with Atractylodes and Phellodendron *(qī wèi cāng bái sǎn)*

七味蒼柏散

Rhizoma Atractylodis *(cang zhu)*

Cortex Phellodendri *(huang bai)*

Cortex Eucommiae Ulmoidis *(du zhong)*

Radix Angelicae Sinensis *(dang gui)*

Radix Ligustici Chuanxiong *(chuan xiong)*

Fructus Psoraleae Corylifoliae *(bu gu zhi)*

Rhizoma Atractylodis Macrocephalae *(bai zhu)*

SOURCE: *Introduction to Medicine*

Special Pill to Tonfiy the Marrow *(bǔ suǐ dān)*

補髓丹

Cornu Cervi Parvum *(lu rong)*

Cortex Eucommiae Ulmoidis *(du zhong)*

Myrrha *(mo yao)*

Semen Juglandis Regiae *(hu tao ren)*

SOURCE: *Essentials of Chinese Medical Patterns and Treatments*

Tangkuei and Rehmannia Pill *(dāng guī dì huáng wán)*

當歸地黃丸

Radix Angelicae Sinensis *(dang gui)*

Radix Rehmanniae Glutinosae Conquitae *(shu di huang)*

Radix Dioscoreae Oppositae *(shan yao)*

Cortex Eucommiae Ulmoidis *(du zhong)*

Radix Achyranthis Bidentatae *(niu xi)*

Fructus Corni Officinalis *(shan zhu yu)*

Radix Glycyrrhizae Uralensis *(gan cao)*

SOURCE: *Collected Treatises of [Zhang] Jing-Yue*

Tangkuei Decoction to Draw Out Pain
(dāng guī niān tòng tāng)

當歸拈痛湯

Radix et Rhizoma Notopterygii *(qiang huo)*

Radix Ginseng *(ren shen)*

Radix Sophorae Flavescentis *(ku shen)*

Rhizoma Cimicifugae *(sheng ma)*

Radix Puerariae *(ge gen)*

Rhizoma Atractylodis *(cang zhu)*

Honey-toasted Radix Glycyrrhizae Uralensis *(zhi gan cao)*

Radix Scutellariae Baicalensis *(huang qin)*

Herba Artemisiae Yinchenhao *(yin chen hao)*

Radix Ledebouriellae Divaricatae *(fang feng)*

Radix Angelicae Sinensis *(dang gui)*

Rhizoma Anemarrhenae Asphodeloidis *(zhi mu)*

Rhizoma Alismatis Orientalis *(ze xie)*

Sclerotium Polypori Umbellati *(zhu ling)*

Rhizoma Atractylodis Macrocephalae *(bai zhu)*

SOURCE: *Medical Innovations*

Top-Quality Lindera Powder *(tiān tái wū yào sǎn)*

天台烏藥散

Radix Linderae Strychnifoliae *(wu yao)*

Radix Aucklandiae Lappae *(mu xiang)*

Fructus Foeniculi Vulgaris *(xiao hui xiang)*

Pericarpium Citri Reticulatae Viride *(qing pi)*

Rhizoma Alpiniae Officinari *(gao liang jiang)*

Semen Arecae Catechu *(bing lang)*
Semen Croton Tiglii *(ba dou)*
Fructus Meliae Toosendan *(chuan lian zi)*
SOURCE: *Medical Innovations*

Young Maiden Pill *(qīng é wán)*

青娥丸

Fructus Psoraleae Corylifoliae *(bu gu zhi)*
Semen Juglandis Regiae *(hu tao ren)*
Cortex Eucommiae Ulmoidis *(du zhong)*
Bulbus Allii Sativi *(da suan)*
SOURCE: *Imperial Grace Formulary of the Tai Ping Era*

Chapter Notes

1. For a translation of a majority of this text, see chapter 24.
2. *Editors' note:* "Ancestral sinew" *(zóng jīn)* usually refers to the penis.
3. *Editors' note:* The "five retardations" *(wǔ chí)* refer to delayed development of the upright position, walk, hair growth, teeth growth and speech. The "five weaknesses" *(wǔ ruǎn)* relate to the head, neck, limbs, muscles and mouth. These different diagnoses are specifically associated with height underdevelopment and rickets.
4. *Editors' note:* The features of this description evoke ascites.
5. *Editors' note:* This refers to the Bladder.
6. *Editors' note:* This is also known as "before heaven" or "anterior heaven," which are literal translations of the Chinese term *xiān tiān*.
7. *Editors' note:* This is also known as "later heaven" or "posterior heaven," which are literal translations of the Chinese term *hòu tiān*.
8. See discussion of this term in chapter 8, p. 153.
9. *Editors' note:* The word *cū* is rare in pulse lore. It literally means rough or coarse.

10. *Editors' note:* We have been unable to determine which point is meant by *jū qiāo*.
11. *Editors' note:* "Plugged and rejecting disorder" is marked by blockage of urination (with or without constipation) accompanied by unremitting vomiting. It is seen in cases of injury to the Spleen yang with Kidney yang insufficiency, when the deficient yang is unable to transform the water.
12. Liu Ban-Liang, "Utilizing Tui-na as the primary treatment in 130 cases of lower back pain," *Shanghai Journal of Traditional Chinese Medicine (Shanghai zhong yi yao za zhi)* 12:36, 1964.
13. Zhou Yong-Hao, "Treatment of lower back and leg pain by invigorating the blood and transforming stasis," *New Traditional Chinese Medicine (Xin zhong yi)* 2:34, 1980.
14. Tang Tian-Lu, "Report on treating recalcitrant lower back pain by 'threading the needle'," *Jiangsu Chinese Medicine (Jiangsu zhong yi)* 6:14, 1964.
15. Wang Shen-Zhi, "Preliminary clinical observations of treating 80 cases of kidney deficiency lower back pain," *Harbin Chinese Medicine (Haerbin zhong yi)* 13:29, 1961.
16. Lu Hai-Shan, "Experience in treating lower back pain," *Zhejiang Journal of Traditional Chinese Medicine (Zhejiang zhong yi za zhi)* 11:7, 1964.
17. *Editors' note:* This is chapter 41 of *Basic Questions*, entitled "On Needling Lower Back Pain." Selections from this chapter are translated in chapter 24 below.
18. *Editors' note:* Included here are only those formulas that appear in this section of the original text, which is by no means all of the formulas noted in the chapter itself. The only change that we have made is to arrange the formulas in alphabetical order by English name. For more detailed information regarding most of these formulas, see Dan Bensky and Randall Barolet, *Chinese Herbal Medicine: Formulas & Strategies* (Seattle: Eastland Press, 1990).

PART THREE

Clinical Practice
of an Acupuncturist
in Rheumatology

Introduction

IN THIS THIRD part of the book, we propose an approach to the treatment of rheumatic diseases and osteoarticular pathologies based on our own research and experience as acupuncturists in the treatment of rheumatology. A few preliminary remarks are necessary.

The conditions in which acupuncture is practiced in China are completely different from those in the West. Although acupuncture treatment in the People's Republic of China is based on traditional data, it is nevertheless very often rigidly applied to fairly generalized pathologies. In terms of point selection, only a small minority of the over 300 points described in the traditional texts are used. It is commonly believed that their efficacy is largely due to the daily repetition of acupuncture treatments prescribed in series of ten sessions. This way of doing things is simply not practical in Western countries. Also, it is good to remember that not only are we not Chinese, we will never become Chinese. It makes sense that we use our own strengths and abilities in the practice of acupuncture.

Furthermore, acupuncture in China has, for the most part, taken a back seat to herbal medicine. This is demonstrated quite clearly in part two of this book, where herbal therapy is discussed in great detail, but only stereotyped selections of acupuncture points are provided. We believe that our work, along with the efforts of other serious practitioners in the West, will lead to an acupuncture that, while remaining true to the tradition, enriches that tradi-

tion and participates in its dissemination beyond its former frontiers.

Since we cannot replicate China's treatment modalities in our own practice, it is obvious that we must define a different approach. We need to make our own contribution to the acupuncture tradition, to customize acupuncture for our time and place without abandoning the tradition. For example, regarding the frequency of treatment, with the exception of acute pathologies that may require two or three treatments a week, acupuncture treatments are usually prescribed once a week for five or six weeks. They are then gradually spaced out according to the patient's progress. Maintenance or preventive treatments can be offered later, tailored to the patient's constitution or to the change of seasons.

This is the context in which we have selected a few examples illustrating the usefulness of acupuncture in the treatment of rheumatic diseases from the physiological, pathological, diagnostic and therapeutic viewpoints.

In other sections of this book we see how important the concept of painful obstruction is in the Chinese approach to rheumatic diseases. We have therefore chosen to present the therapeutic approach relating to painful obstruction first. The transposition of diagnostic and treatment principles to such problems as degenerative joint disease, rheumatoid arthritis and ankylosing spondylitis should be regarded as an attempt to reconcile two apparently vastly different modes of thinking.

Secondly, we will approach the pathologies from an anatomical point of view, joint by joint. Here we will deliberately adopt a different presentation and approach. This will allow the reader to adapt our ideas to his or her own methodology. This will also permit us to avoid repetitions or rigid patterns which would take us away from the reality and clinical complexity of each individual patient.

Introduction to the French Acupuncture Association Approach to Acupuncture

Before delving into the specifics of treatment it is necessary to remark on some of the basic concepts underlying the approach to acupuncture taken by the French Acupuncture Association (AFA). Under the leadership of Jean-Marc Kespi, the AFA has developed many concepts based on the traditional literature that have proven extremely effective in the clinic. As this approach may be unfamiliar to our English-speaking readers, we have added these remarks to make it easier for those totally unfamiliar with our school of acupuncture to use this book. As such, they are markedly oversimplified.[1]

Eight Diagnostic Parameters

As described above in chapter 4 ("Pain"), proper use of the eight diagnostic parameters (*bā gāng*) must be made to achieve optimal effectiveness with acupuncture. Our understanding of the local applications of this concept is rather comprehensive compared to that presented in most English-language books on Chinese medicine. For more details, please refer to that chapter. Here we would like to reiterate the salient features of the local application of these parameters.

Simply, in terms of the eight diagnostic patterns, joint pain that is ameliorated with pressure or support is deficient, while that which worsens is excessive. Pain that is relieved by warmth and aggravated by cold is due either to yang deficiency or yin excess; pain that is relieved by cold and aggravated by warmth is due either to yin deficiency or yang excess. In addition, there is an important subset of excess known as stagnation. The hallmark of pain from stagnation is that it improves with movement or massage as well as local application of warmth. Pain from stagnation is aggravated by rest and cold, and also worsens just as movement begins. This is true whether the stagnation is

of yin or yang. For example, shoulder pain due to stagnation is worse in the morning, especially if the patient has slept with the shoulder outside the blanket. While the shoulder will "catch" as soon as it starts to move, once it has been moved the pain will diminish. The only way to differentiate yin stagnation from yang stagnation is to look at the nature of the pain. Yang stagnation will lead to a yang-type pain: sharp, stabbing, paroxysmal, intense, burning, superficial and usually worse during the day. Yin stagnation leads to a yin-type pain: dull, continuous, moderate, deep and usually worse at night; moreover, it is often accompanied by a sensation of distention, numbness and localized cold.

Channels

We place very strong emphasis on the channels. Because acupuncture works through the channels, we feel it is vital to keep our focus on them. While this may seem obvious, it is an important concept that is sometimes overlooked. This is why we utilize, both in diagnosis and treatment, all aspects of the channel system. For example, we commonly use the channel sinews and channel divergences, which are relatively neglected in some other styles of acupuncture.

On one level, we believe the twelve (primary) channels are more appropriately viewed as six pairs of channels. Each pair is marked with the name of the same level. There are two greater yin channels, two lesser yang channels, and so forth. The functions of these pairs are related, and so are the symptoms or manifestations of their disharmonies. For this reason, we sometimes view the arm greater yin channel (Lung) as the Metal greater yin channel, in contrast to the Earth greater yin channel of the leg (Spleen). Both in diagnosis and treatment, this viewpoint opens up many useful possibilities.

These pairs of channels are thought to resonate with six types of cosmic energy. Viewed as units, each of these pairs is known as an axis or great channel. The constitutions and functions of each pair is related not only to their description in *Inner Classic*, but also to the schema in *Book of Changes, Discussion of Cold-induced Disorders,* and other classical sources. Over the centuries in Asia, and more recently in France, the understanding of these axes or great channels has been expanded and developed to encompass both constitutions or diatheses, as well as specific disorders.

In this section we note dysfunctions of these axes. We do this when the patient exhibits the signs and symptoms of both the leg and arm channels of the same name. Treatment often includes the stream and connecting point technique, or the root and node technique first (see below).

Although the ancient texts do not specifically note the importance of the Curious vessels in osteoarticular disorders, our clinical experience indicates that their involvement in these pathologies is significant. This is not surprising, as the Curious vessels are related to the deep levels or structures of the body, and we can describe rheumatic disorders as diseases manifesting at the level of form or structure. Is not one of the goals of energy exercises such as *taijiquan* or *qigong* to open the Curious vessels in order to remove obstacles to the free movement of Qi, especially through the joints?

Our clinical experience has therefore led us to use the Curious vessels in two different ways: first, "superficially" by using their properties of regulation to reinforce the treatment of different disorders of varying origins; and second, "fundamentally" by referring to their physiology, pathology and typology. It has helped to be creative in this. When using the Curious vessels in this manner, we analyze the symptoms that have been attributed to them in ancient Chinese texts, and then refer to their typology. This aspect has been the object of extensive research over many years by members of the AFA, and has contributed to a deeper understanding of what disruption of the various Curious vessels means.

DIALECTIC OF MOTION

The history of acupuncture in France during the last fifty years has produced many careful analyses of *Inner Classic* and other important traditional texts. Based on this work, Kespi and others have found important dialectical rules which have allowed us to understand many phenomena more clearly. This understanding, in turn, is basic to our ability to devise treatments of greater efficacy that fit our times, including the barrier point system discussed below. One way in which the dialectic is used is to further group the six axes into three sets, each of which contains a yin and a yang axis. The sets are composed of channels, the names of which include the same (or similar) qualifier:

- *Tài* 太: greatest, the first, larger, oldest, mature, supreme, extreme. This refers to the greater yin and yang.
- *Shào* 少: lesser, a little, lacking, immature, young. This refers to the lesser yin and yang.
- *Jué* 厥: to stumble, to fall, to collapse, to diminish, to exhaust, attenuated, terminal. This refers to the terminal yin and yang brightness.[2]

Using each of these qualifiers we can characterize the progression of four types of dialectics involving different aspects of life: space, time, being and transformation. Here we will discuss only the dialectics of state of being. It will serve as an example to demonstrate the thinking process that goes into this analysis. At the same time, it describes the movements of yin and yang that come into play within the system of barrier points.

Quantitatively, phenomena can be classified in terms of one of these three sets as being more or less yin or more or less yang. The most intense is *tài*, the least intense is *jué*, and the intermediate is *shào*. This relates to the meaning of the respective characters as greatest, lesser and exhausted. Qualitatively, phenomena are defined in relation to their origins. What set they belong to depends on whether they are more or less characteristic of their origin. Again, the most characteristic is *tài*, the least characteristic is *jué*, and the intermediate is *shào*. This relates to the meaning of the respective characters as supreme, exhausted or used up, and lacking (see figure below).

For example, quantitatively the head is the most yang part of the body, so it is regarded as greater yang. Qualitatively, if one looks at the yang energy that leaves the trunk for the head, it is most characteristic of its origin where it leaves the trunk. Therefore, this area is regarded as greater yang. It is less so at the neck, which is regarded, in this context, as lesser yang, and less still at the head, which is then yang brightness. This way of looking at the

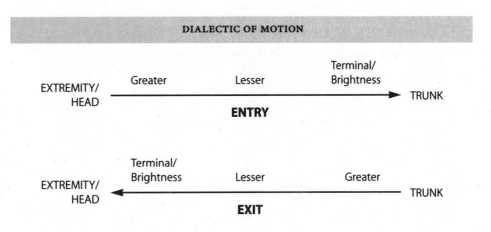

movement of yin and yang is the basis of the barrier point system. When we describe a pain in a way that helps us decide how to treat it—deficiency of yang, excess of yin—the mechanism for this description is derived from this set of concepts.

POINTS

In acupuncture as practiced by the French Acupuncture Association, there are two types of points. The first are those which have either global effects or resonate at the level of an entire channel or axis. These are referred to as command points, and include the transport points, the cleft points, the source points and the connecting points. All other points are regarded as specific, and may also be subject to grouping. Some groupings are of points with similar functions (associated points, alarm points, barrier points), and others are of points the names of which contain the same character (*huāng* "vitals," *líng* "divine," *fēng* "wind").

We believe that looking at many aspects of the traditional literature concerning specific points enables us to understand them more completely. To us, each point in some way expresses a set of local functions related to those of the entire channel. We have attempted to define the physiological and therapeutic role of each acupuncture point in the hope that this will permit us to use them in a well-reasoned and effective manner. We have based our understanding on certain criteria:

- significance of the name of the point (including alternate names)
- the channel on which the point is located
- anatomical location (including its relationship to other points at the same level)
- symptoms with which the point is traditionally associated.

In this manner we are able to define functions, properties and mechanisms for a point which are not explicitly described in Chinese texts, without in any way betraying the spirit of traditional Chinese medicine. The signs and symptoms treated by a point are regarded as manifestations of disharmonies directly related to the functioning of that point. Utilizing points in this manner has enabled us to greatly increase the efficacy of our treatments.

As an example, this is how we understand BL-11 (*da zhu*). It is the meeting point for the bones and belongs to the "sea of the twelve channels." The literal name of this point is "big shuttle." This shuttle can be regarded as the bones which tie the body together, or as the channels which do the same. We believe that this point also governs

the bones when they function as a Curious Organ. In this capacity, the bones are linked to the perineum and thereby to the perpetuation of the being or species. Looking through the major premodern texts, we find that this point is indicated for such problems as bone and joint disorders, vertebral pain, knee pain, areas of muscle contractures, difficulty in remaining still, throat problems, and even mental disorders such as dementia. Looking deeper, we read in the commentary of *Bases of Medicine* (*Yi yuan*) to the 45th difficulty of *Classic of Difficulties*, "If the shoulders can carry a heavy burden, it is due to the meeting of the bones at *da zhu.*" We extrapolate that this point is involved each time we have an excessively heavy burden (physical or psychological) to carry.

Based on various types of research, some additional categories of points have been developed in France over the last thirty years. One category, the barrier points, is extremely important in the treatment of pain and is discussed in detail below. These points will be utilized in treating many different rheumatic disorders.

There are a few sets of points that are often used to initiate the movement, or mobilize the yin or yang, of an extremity when there is local stagnation. Primary among these are a "lesser" (*shào*) set of barrier points used for the general mobilization of the yin and yang of the extremities. We have chosen "lesser" yin or yang channel points as we believe that the lesser yin is the hinge of the yin and the lesser yang the hinge of the yang. Thus, to mobilize the yang of the upper extremities, we use TB-14 (*jian liao);* for the yang of the lower extremities, GB-30 (*huan tiao);* for the yin of the upper extremities, HT-1 (*ji quan);* and for the yin of the lower extremities, KI-8 (*jiao xin).* This process is aided by the four connecting points of the extremities: TB-8 (*san yang luo*) for the yang of the upper extremities; PC-5 (*jian shi*) for the yin of the upper extremities; GB-39 (*xuan zhong*) for the yang of the lower extremities; and SP-6 (*san yin jiao*) for the yin of the lower extremities.

Also of particular importance in this regard are the wind points. As noted earlier, these are points that contain the word wind (*fēng*) in their names. There are two wind points that are especially important in helping to mobilize the various energies of the extremities. These are GB-31 (*feng shi*) for the lower extremities, and SI-12 (*bing feng*) for the upper extremities.

A final category that is occasionally mentioned in this text are the visceral points.[3] We have found that specific points are related to the functions of the different viscera when they are considered from the standpoint of biomedical physiology. The points for the viscera related to the yin Organs are located on the leg lesser yin (Kidney) channel:[4]

- Kidneys: KI-14 *(si man)*
- Spleen: KI-17 *(shang qu)*
- Liver: KI-21 *(you men)*
- Lungs: KI-22 *(bu lang)*
- Heart: KI-23 *(shen feng)*

The points for those viscera related to the yang Organs are located on the leg yang brightness (Stomach) channel:

- Stomach: ST-21 *(liang men)*
- Gallbladder: ST-22 *(guan men)*
- Small Intestine: ST-24 *(hua rou men)*
- Large Intestine: ST-26 *(wai ling)*
- Bladder: ST-28 *(shui dao)*

Relationship Between Biomedicine and Acupuncture

It would add unnecessarily to the bulk of this book if we presented information about the biomedical understanding and diagnoses of these diseases. If you are treating these patients that is information you should already know. In any case, we could not describe them any better than the standard biomedical literature. This applies equally to the physical examination and various imaging and biochemical tests. All the prerequisite work must be done before any patient is given a diagnosis or offered treatment.

Our therapeutic suggestions are to be viewed as guidelines, which must always accommodate the patient's individual reality. They are in no way recipes to be followed blindly.

One of the special features of acupuncture is that it provides the practitioner, through questioning and examination, with a guiding pathogenic energetic principle, allowing the practitioner to connect all of the patient's pathological events (present and past), thereby creating a unique reality which can only lead to a customized treatment. This approach pointedly raises all the methodological issues regarding the assessment of the effects of acupuncture. Studies to test this can in no way be molded after the Western biomedical model, which is, after all, designed to evaluate drugs, not acupuncture.

Illustrative Case Histories

To illustrate the complexity of the matter, we would like to present two cases of cervicobrachial neuralgia corresponding to classical neuralgia of the C7 nerve roots.

Case One is a 35-year-old male who has been seen by the hospital neurology department for a C7 type cervicobrachial neuralgia on the right side. After failure of both drug and physical therapies, and with x-rays indicating the possibility of a radiculopathy secondary to disc disease, surgical intervention was suggested. Surgery was postponed for a few days due to the New Year holiday. In the meantime, the patient came to see us. A detailed questionnaire revealed that two days before the occurrence of this neuralgia, the patient (a physical education coach) had attended a canoeing competition and spent many hours stationed by the river. He felt the effects of cold and dampness, as well as drafts of wind, which he described as feeling like a "heavy cloak weighing on my shoulders." These symptoms were not alleviated by attempts to warm up. The pain peaked two days after this incident.

Based on the information provided by the patient, we can diagnose a yang-type stagnation: stabbing pain aggravated by rest and alleviated by warmth, improved by gentle range of motion and massage, and radiating along the arm greater yang pathway corresponding to the seventh cervical nerve dermatome. Diagnosis points to an exterior problem secondary to an attack of external origin, in this case Wind-Damp-Cold, and manifesting on the greater yang level. Treatment consisted of acupuncture and moxibustion at BL-12 *(feng men)* and SI-12 *(bing feng)*, two points related to the invasion of Wind, which brought instant relief from pain. All the associated symptoms disappeared in that session.

Can we infer from this case study that acupuncture is capable of instantly curing any neuralgia resulting from a disc disorder? Certainly not. However, it demonstrates the important role played by the external pathogenic factors, which was not addressed in the biomedical concept of etiology.

Case Two is a 30-year-old woman with a history of hepatitis, leading us at first to fear an active chronic hepatitis, who was seen on an emergency basis for a C7 type cervicobrachial neuralgia on the left side. She was given a first session of acupuncture with a classic combination of points including BL-12 *(feng men)* and SI-12 *(bing feng)*. This first session brought absolutely no results. The pain continued to increase, and such was the functional disability that the patient had to wear an orthopedic collar for relief. After four days, and with no sign of significant improvement, we saw the patient again. She then revealed that this cervicobrachial neuralgia started after she underwent surgery for an inguinal hernia on the right side. The pain, as described by the patient, followed the arm greater yang pathway and corresponded to a yang deficiency, relieved by warmth and pressure, which explains the slight improvement provided by wearing the collar.

The hypothesis of a minor vertebral dislocation due to an untimely movement during the operation was rejected. Our final diagnosis was deficiency of the arm greater yang on the left side, due to an obstruction in the circulation of the leg terminal yin channel on the right side, resulting from the surgical intervention located precisely on its pathway. The midday-midnight relationship between arm greater yang and leg terminal yin provides the basis for our hypothesis. Needling LR-6 *(zhong du)*, the cleft point of the leg terminal yin, brought instant and permanent relief of the neuralgia, enabling the patient to go home without her collar.

If such proof is still needed, this demonstrates once again that the effect of acupuncture cannot be ascribed to a simple neurological reflex action brought about by needling.

These two clinical observations illustrate the fact that when different energetic pathogenic mechanisms yield a similar biomedical diagnosis, they nonetheless call for different treatment plans. Today, with an ever-increasing need to effectively monitor the therapeutic efficacy of acupuncture, it becomes quite clear that biomedical diagnostic criteria and the conventional methodology used for drug testing do not apply, and should not be used, for evaluating acupuncture. Likewise, adapting standardized acupuncture protocols to a biomedical nosology would equally fail to assess acupuncture accurately, or to meet the requirements of acupuncture practitioners.

Therefore, if we are to retain our professional credibility, we must search for and establish, as soon as possible, an evaluation methodology that meets scientific criteria and also preserves the specificity of established acupuncture theory.

Notes

1. *Editors' note:* This additional information is primarily taken from Kespi (1982), which is by far the most comprehensive source for this approach to acupuncture. At present, information in English about the French traditions of acupuncture is scanty, but that is beginning to change. For more in-depth views, see Joseph Helms, *Acupuncture Energetics: A Clinical Approach for Physicians* (Berkeley: Medical Acupuncture Publishers, 1995), and George Soulié de Morant, *Chinese Acupuncture (L'Acuponcture Chinoise)*, translated by Lawrence Grinnell, Claudy Jeanmougin, Maurice Leveque, and edited by Paul Zmiewski (Brookline, MA: Paradigm, 1994).

2. We consider yang brightness to be the "terminal yang" for a variety of reasons. The yang brightness channels are the only yang channels that traverse the face and anterior of the body. On the one hand, this confirms its status as the terminal or exhausted yang. On the other hand, because the face and anterior surface of the body are what people use to face the sun and the world, this explains its appellation as "yang brightness." In addition, a passage in chapter 5 of *Divine Pivot* states that the greater yang serves as an opening, the yang brightness serves as a closure (literally "door leaf"), and the lesser yang serves as a hinge. Later in the same chapter the terminal yin is also referred to as a closure.

3. For more information on this point category, see Kespi (1982), pp. 542-45.

4. There is some variation to this scheme among practitioners. Some think that KI-25 *(shen cang)* is the point for the Lungs and that KI-14 *(si man)* relates only to the Kidneys' urinary function, while KI-11 *(heng gu)* relates to the genital functions.

CHAPTER EIGHT

Painful Obstruction Disorders

General Treatment Principles for Painful Obstruction

The goals of treatment are to alleviate pain, eliminate the pathogenic factors, harmonize the nutritive and protective Qi, and prevent relapse. The achievement of these goals depends on a precise diagnosis relating to both etiology and pathogenesis.

Three phases can be isolated within the treatment: symptomatic, etiologic and preventive. Any one of these three phases can become a priority, according to the clinical condition and the urgency of the situation; it is essentially a question of common sense, but the treatment should in no way be limited to symptomatic intervention. Treatment by acupuncture alone is not always enough; it must be complemented with herbs, appropriate diet, physical exercise or physical therapy.

Combination of acupuncture with conventional medical therapy is sometimes necessary, either because the patient is already undergoing pharmaceutical treatment which cannot be safely discontinued, or because the urgency or severity of the condition warrants it. This observation in itself justifies that the practice of acupuncture in the West should not be totally divorced from mainstream medicine. In such a situation, acupuncture demonstrates its usefulness as an alternative, transitory or complementary form of treatment to conventional phar-maceuticals. This may allow for a reduction in dosage as well as fewer side effects.

Acupuncture Treatment

The selection and combination of points play a critical role in the treatment plan; they are to be selected according to the theory of channels and collaterals. There is no standard recipe, and we can only provide general guidelines, as each clinical case is different.

Local and regional treatment is one of the cornerstones of acupuncture treatment of rheumatic diseases. Its purpose is to relax the muscles, loosen the joints, eliminate pain, activate the collaterals, harmonize the Qi and Blood locally, and expel the pathogenic influences.

Several modalities can guide the selection of acupuncture points:

• traditional local points
• barrier points
• *ashi* points
• trigger points.

TRADITIONAL LOCAL POINTS

In the classical medical literature there are a great number of points which are noted to affect various joints. The indications listed for these points are not always very precise. This can make the point selection process difficult. Point selection becomes even more complicated if we consult other source texts which increase the number of possible points. The practitioner's clinical experience is therefore invaluable.

BARRIER POINTS

Among local points the most interesting ones for rheumatology are, in our opinion and practice, the so-called "barrier" or "gate" points. Under the direction of J.-M. Kespi, this approach has been the subject of specific study at the French Acupuncture Association for more than twenty years. We will simply review the conclusions here, which have been verified in daily practice.[1]

The idea of barrier comes from the Chinese word *guān* 關, often translated as barrier or gate. Dr. Kespi and his associates were struck by the number of points that have this word in their names (either primary or alternate). They also noted the importance of the concept of barriers or gates in the discussion of joint problems in chapter 60 of *Basic Questions*.[2]

Each joint is thought to be a place through which physiologic energies pass and which, under certain pathological circumstances, can turn into a barrier that obstructs the circulation of these energies. The yin and yang Qi enter and exit the joints according to a centripetal and centrifugal pattern. From this particular perspective, the Qi is described in relation to its origin: greater (yang or yin) when it is closest to its origin, yang brightness or terminal yin when it is farthest from its origin, and lesser (yang or yin) when it is in between. This idea comes from our understanding of the qualitative dialectic of state of being discussed above, and is also buttressed by our reading of the following passage in chapter 71 of *Divine Pivot*:

> The Yellow Emperor asked Qi Bo, "People have eight concavities.[3] Each of them is an indicator of what?"
>
> Qi Bo replied, "They serve as indicators for the five yin Organs."
>
> The Yellow Emperor said, "How do they serve as indicators for them?"
>
> Qi Bo said, "When there is a pathogenic influence in the Lungs and Heart, its Qi resides in the two elbows. When there is a pathogenic influence in the Liver, its Qi flows in the two axillae. When there is a pathogenic influence in the Spleen, its Qi resides in the two hips. When there is a pathogenic influence in the Kidneys, its Qi resides in the two popliteal fossae. These eight concavities all relate to the chambers of joints through which the true Qi passes, and over which the Blood collaterals flow. Thus pathogenic Qi and bad Blood should not be allowed to lodge there. If they

do lodge there then there is injury to the sinews, collaterals, bones and articulations. The joints cannot flex or extend and so they become rigid and spasmodic."

Taking all the above together we can, for example, describe the Qi circulation between the trunk and the limbs as follows (SEE ALSO FIG. 8-1).

The yang Qi that emerges from the trunk is:

- greater yang at the shoulders and hips
- lesser yang at the elbows and knees
- yang brightness at the wrists and ankles.

The yang Qi that enters the trunk is:

- greater yang at the wrists and ankles
- lesser yang at the elbows and knees
- yang brightness at the shoulders and hips.

The yin Qi that emerges from the trunk is:

- greater yin at the shoulders and hips
- lesser yin at the elbows and knees
- terminal yin at the wrists and ankles.

The yin Qi that enters the trunk is:

- greater yin at the wrists and ankles
- lesser yin at the elbows and knees
- terminal yin at the shoulders and hips.

In the barrier point system, the flow of yin or yang Qi is always looked at from a perspective outside the body. Blockage of the Qi in its outward movement from the trunk to the extremities causes excess upstream (proximal) from the pathological joint, and deficiency downstream (distal). An obstruction of the Qi in its inward movement from the extremity toward the trunk creates excess upstream (distal) from the joint, and deficiency downstream. For example, if there is a blockage of the yang Qi going from the trunk toward the upper extremity it will manifest at the level of the shoulder with yang excess upstream (at the scapular region), and yang deficiency downstream (in the arm). Conversely, if there is a problem with the entry of yang from the upper extremity to the trunk, it will manifest as deficiency pain in the scapular region and excess pain in the arm. In any given patient, determining the direction in which the circulation is impaired can only be achieved through an analysis of pain according to the eight parameters (see chapter 3).

Barrier points govern the inward and outward movement of the yin and yang at the level of each joint, and are located on their related primary channels. These points were initially chosen on the basis of the indications attributed to them in traditional texts, as well as their primary or secondary names. They were then used clinically to test their utility.

In general, when one wishes to facilitate a centripetal movement, use a point distal to the articulation; conversely, use a proximal point to promote centrifugal movement. For example, to facilitate the exit of yang from the trunk toward the upper extremity, the review of traditional point indications and names indicated that the barrier point should be one of the following: SI-9 *(jian zhen)*, SI-10 *(nao shu)* or SI-11 *(tian zong)*. Further research led to SI-11 *(tian zong)* being considered the most probable point, and this was confirmed by experience. To facilitate the entry of yin to the trunk at the hip from the lower extremity, the barrier point is found on the leg terminal yin Liver channel. After research and analysis of the point properties, the choice came down to LR-10 *(zu wu li)* and LR-11 *(yin lian)*. For a long time we thought that it should be LR-10 *(zu wu li)*, but practice revealed that LR-11 *(yin lian)* was more effective and therefore a better choice. When there is no specific barrier point, use the cleft point to clear the obstruction in the corresponding channel (TABLE 8-1).

From a mnemonic point of view, it is sometimes easier to look upon this system as describing resonances, rather than actual circulation. That is, problems of a "greater" level, yin or yang, looked at from the perspective of Qi

going from the trunk to the extremities, resonate at the shoulders and hips. This way of looking at the barrier point system is reinforced when we realize that many of the points are "downstream" from joints they unblock. For example, HT-6 *(yin xi)* is used for elbow problems, whether it be with yin emerging from the trunk or entering it. In fact, most of the yin barrier points are cleft points. Another way of looking at this is that when a barrier is blocked, the obstruction manifests on the channel that carries the same name as the corresponding Qi. Therefore, when there is an obstruction to the exit of yang Qi from the shoulder, where it is closest to its origin, it manifests on the greater yang channel of the arm, the Small Intestine channel.

The utility of the barrier point system is not limited to the peripheral joints. There are also barrier points identified between the trunk and head, and between the skull and face. We will discuss the former here. The "windows of the sky" points, described in chapter 2 of *Divine Pivot*, allow the Qi to circulate between the trunk and the head. They include BL-10 *(tian zhu)*, ST-9 *(ren ying)*, SI-17 *(tian rong)*, SI-16 *(tian chuang)*, TB-16 *(tian you)* and LI-17 *(tian ding)*. These are discussed at greater length in chapter 17 below ("Neck Pain"). In addition, there are barrier points in this area. One set promotes the downward movement of yang Qi from the head to the trunk. This follows the progression of greater yang close to the origin, lesser yang at the intermediate stage, and yang brightness farthest from the origin. The points are BL-10 *(tian zhu)* on the leg greater yang, GB-21 *(jian jing)* on the leg lesser yang, and ST-11 *(qi she)* on the leg yang brightness. The other set promotes the upward movement of yang Qi from the trunk to the head: SI-14 *(jian wai shu)* on the arm greater yang, TB-15 *(tian liao)* on the arm lesser yang, and ST-3 *(ju liao)* on the leg yang brightness.

While not directly relevant to rheumatology, we would like to mention the more important barrier and related points for the cranium and face. As this is the most yang aspect of the body, we will limit our discussion here to the yang level. The temporomandibular joint is an important link between the cranium and the face. The yang Qi that descends from the cranium is greater yang at its source and relates to BL-6 *(cheng guang)*; lesser yang at its intermediate level, relating to GB-3 *(shang guan)*; and yang brightness at its terminus, relating to ST-7 *(xia guan)*. Another barrier system exists between the face and the cranium anteriorly over the frontal region. It is greater yang at its lower origin, relating to BL-2 *(zan zhu)*; lesser

TABLE 8-1 BARRIER POINTS

	Yang Exiting	Yang Entering	Yin Exiting	Yin Entering
Shoulder	Greater Yang SI-11	Yang Brightness LI-15	Greater Yin LU-2	Terminal Yin PC-2
Elbow	Lesser Yang TB-13	Lesser Yang TB-7	Lesser Yin HT-6	Lesser Yin HT-6
Wrist	Yang Brightness LI-9	Greater Yang SI-6	Terminal Yin PC-4	Greater Yin LU-6
Hip	Greater Yang BL-29	Yang Brightness ST-31	Greater Yin SP-12	Terminal Yin LR-11
Knee	Lesser Yang GB-33	Lesser Yang GB-36	Lesser Yin KI-5	Lesser Yin KI-5
Ankle	Yang Brightness ST-37	Greater Yang BL-63	Terminal Yin LR-6	Greater Yin SP-8

yang at its intermediate level, relating to GB-14 (*yang bai*); and ends at the yang brightness level, relating to ST-8 (*tou wei*). When we want to mobilize the yang Qi of any part of the cranium or face, we rely on the lesser yang channels. At the level of the occiput and posterior neck we use the lesser yang point GB-20 (*feng chi*), and possibly the wind point for this region, BL-12 (*feng men*). For the face in an anteroposterior direction we use GB-1 (*tong zi liao*); in a posteroanterior direction we use GB-2 (*ting hui*). Between the face and cranium generally, we use TB-23 (*si zhu kong*).

When we examine the diagnostic and therapeutic approach for each area in the following chapters, we will review the different barrier points and their applications. Here we have provided just an outline of their use in diagnosis and treatment (FIG. 8-1). One remarkable characteristic of the barrier points is that, when correctly chosen, their use can lead to almost immediate disappearance of pain. Of course, long-lasting relief depends on a treatment which includes addressing the underlying disharmonies.

Using the barrier system for the extremities requires

FIG. 8-1 OVERVIEW OF BARRIER AND MOBILIZING POINTS BETWEEN THE TRUNK & EXTREMITIES

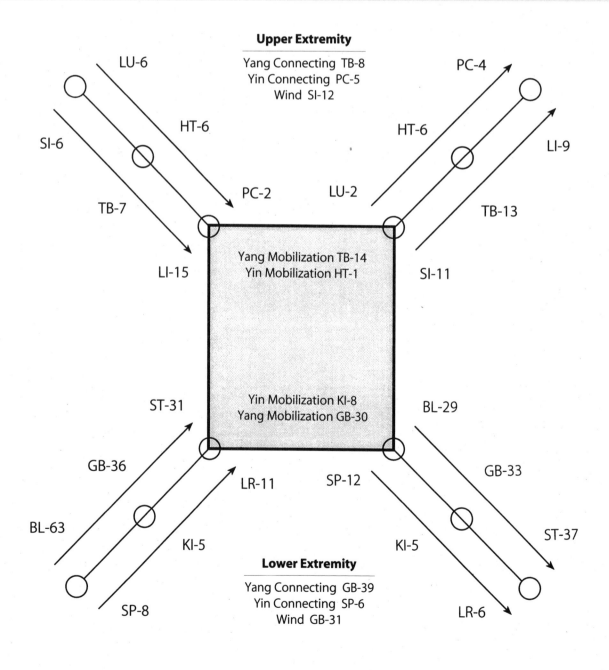

an understanding of the local application of the eight diagnostic parameters. This understanding is based on the following premises:

- Excess is defined as the Qi not entering into the trunk (also called nonentry).
- Deficiency is defined as the Qi not exiting from the trunk (also called nonexit).

Thus, viewed from the perspective of the outside, if the yang or yin cannot gain entry to the trunk, the extremities, which are distal or "upstream" from the trunk, become excessive (while deficiency may develop in the trunk). Similarly, when there is a problem with the exit of yin or yang from the trunk, there is deficiency in the extremities (while there may be excess in the trunk).

Based on these premises we can set forth a simple scheme for treating different types of shoulder pain:

- For yin excess pain, use the terminal yin point PC-2 *(tian quan),* as this is due to the yin not entering into the trunk from the extremities, and backing up in the shoulder.
- For yin deficiency pain, use the greater yin point LU-2 *(yun men),* as the yin is not exiting from the trunk to the arm.
- For yang excess pain, use the yang brightness point LI-15 *(jian yu),* as this results from the yang not entering into the trunk from the arm.
- For yang deficiency pain, use the greater yang point SI-11 *(tian zong),* as this is a problem of the yang not exiting from the trunk to the arm.

Whenever stagnation plays a major part in an illness, it must be addressed. This involves a set of points related to, but different from, the barrier points. We feel that the *shào* or lesser level of the channels can be used to activate or mobilize areas that are stagnant. For this reason we use lesser yin points to activate the yin, and lesser yang points to activate the yin and yang (as yang can mobilize yin). In addition, wind points (i.e., points with the word "wind" [*fēng*] in their names) can also be used to activate areas of stagnation.

Let us briefly walk through a few clinical examples to demonstrate how the local application of the eight diagnostic parameters and the concept of barrier points are used in practice.

A patient presents with right knee pain. The pain worsens with activity, but also at night: these are signs of deficiency. Cool compresses help relieve the pain, which worsens in hot weather: this suggests the presence of local Heat. It feels good to rub the knee and the patient always wears an elastic brace when running or playing sports. This improvement with local support is another sign of deficiency. At the same time, the patient has abdominal distention, a sign of lesser yin excess. The diagnosis would be a nonexit of yin from the trunk to the lower extremities at the level of the lesser yin, leading to yin excess in the abdomen and a yin deficiency type of knee pain. For this type of knee pain, the appropriate barrier point would be KI-5 *(shui quan).*

Another, slightly more complicated example would be a patient with right shoulder and neck pain. The neck pain is related to his work as a telephone operator, where he cradles the phone between his right neck and shoulder. Both pains worsen when he raises his hands to adjust the equipment. One pain goes from the base of the neck and upper back up to the right mastoid area. The shoulder pain involves both anterior and posterior aspects, but seems to come from beneath the scapula. The pain is dull, achy and deep. Heat and massage give temporary relief, and the patient prefers to lie on the affected side. In addition, there is occasional numbness along the lateral aspect of the arm. The primary factor in this disorder is stagnation of yin in the shoulder. One marker of this is that when the arms are raised, the pain increases. Raising the arms encourages the flow of yin (which is heavy) toward the shoulders, which exacerbates yin stagnation. This stagnation leads to a nonexit of yang from the trunk to the head and arms. This manifests as deficiency of yang in the arms (numbness). The initial treatment would be HT-1 *(ji quan)* to mobilize stagnation of yin in the shoulder, and SI-14 *(jian wai shu)* to induce the exit of yang from the shoulder.

INSERTION POINTS

When musculoskeletal structures are involved in pain, it is often very helpful to treat the insertion points. These are anatomically defined local points in one or another part of the painful area where there are muscle attachments (either origins or insertions). It is important to note that these insertion points will not necessarily be tender on palpation. Needling these points is an important way to avoid the spread of pain.

ASHI POINTS

First described by Sun Si-Miao in the Tang dynasty, these points are different from traditional points. They do not have fixed locations but are found by palpation. When these points are pressed, they elicit an exclamation of "Ah *shì* 阿是 (Chinese for "Oh, that's it!") from the patient, hence the name. Stimulation of these points of variable location complement the classic treatment methods. Their sensitivity disappears when the treated symptom is alleviated. These features are similar to those of the "trigger" points.

Trigger Points

Trigger points were described by Janet Travell, M.D., as early as 1952. The patient is unaware of these points, and they are usually located outside the area of reported pain. Indeed, we can say that all trigger points are painful, but the reverse is not true. They correspond to a precise myofascial symptomatology. Elicited by pressure, trigger points are characterized not only by local pain, but also by referred pain which replicates the original pain. The identification of trigger points requires a good knowledge of muscular anatomy and relies on a careful and systematic physical examination, which may also point to a local induration. The charts published by Travell are most useful in this respect. We will go over the description of these points in our systematic study of each joint. The relationship between the trigger points and acupuncture points has been studied by C. Chung in Taipei, P. E. Baldry in Great Britain, J. Taillandier and the AFERA (Association Française pour l'Étude des Réflexothérapies et de l'Acupuncture) team in France, as well as the authors. All trigger point locations in this book are based on those of Travell and Simmons (1984 and 1992), except those for the lumbar and pelvic ligaments, which are derived from those of Hackett (1958).

Meeting and Command Points

The idea of meeting (*huì* 會) points for specific tissues or areas of the body can be traced back to many of the classical acupuncture texts. The most important of these points are:

- BL-11 (*da zhu*): meeting point for the bones
- GB-34 (*yang ling quan*): meeting point for the sinews
- GB-39 (*xuan zhong*): meeting point for the marrow
- LU-9 (*tai yuan*): meeting point for the vessels
- BL-17 (*ge shu*): meeting point for the Blood
- CV-17 (*shan zhong*): meeting point for the Qi.

Based on the same principles, we have developed our own understanding of key focused points. Using them allows us to intervene in many of the important functions of the organism. The most commonly used of these points are:

- CV-3 (*zhong ji*). This is the alarm point for the Bladder, and is related to the Water phase and to winter. Winter is the season characterized by the withdrawal of energy toward the interior. As such, this point governs the movement of Qi toward the interior, thereby influencing the entire bone structure.
- BL-57 (*cheng shan*). This is the command point for the muscle structure.
- ST-38 (*tiao kou*). In our opinion, this point governs all motor and gestural expression in humans. It influences all the joints and sums up the action of the following points:

  LI-14 (*bi nao*): command point for the shoulders
  LI-12 (*zhou liao*): command point for the elbows
  ST-31 (*bi guan*): command point for the hips
  ST-35 (*du bi*): command point for the knees
  LU-7 (*lie que*): command point for the hand
  GB-37 (*guang ming*): command point for the foot.

Treatment Based on Etiology and Pathogenesis

The purpose of this essential aspect of treatment is to establish communication between the channels and collaterals, to eliminate the pathogenic influences, and to harmonize the nutritive Qi and defensive Qi. Since this aspect of treatment is tailored to the individual case, we can only provide general guidelines.

It is always important to include treatment which addresses the root cause of a disorder. When dealing with rheumatic diseases, this aspect of treatment addresses the following goals:

- elimination of the painful obstruction
- tonification of the true Qi
- harmonization of the nutritive and protective Qi
- promotion of the circulation of Blood and Qi
- unblocking of the channels
- strengthening of the affected anatomico-energetic structure
- restoration, if necessary, of the energetic balance of the Qi in the pelvis
- support of the innate Qi, particularly the source Qi.

For example, tonification of the true Qi involves tonification of the essential Qi. This includes both the prenatal aspects (Kidney) by utilizing such points as BL-23 (*shen shu*) and BL-52 (*zhi shi*), together with the postnatal aspects (Spleen/Stomach) at such points as BL-20 (*pi shu*), CV-12 (*zhong wan*) and ST-36 (*zu san li*). We have found, particularly in women, that problems with the energetic balance of the pelvis can often be part of the pathogenesis of rheumatic disorders. When this occurs, it is common for the various signs and symptoms to be affected by changes in the hormonal milieu, that is, they may worsen before menstruation, be ameliorated during pregnancy only to be reactivated after delivery, and so on. Depending on the presentation, it may be necessary to tonify the Blood at a point such as BL-53 *(bao huang)*; mobilize the Blood at a Girdle vessel point like GB-28 *(wei dao)* or a sacral point such as BL-34 *(xia liao)*; or tonify the Qi at CV-6 *(qi hai)*.

The following are important treatment principles for the specific pathological aspects of painful obstruction:

- Expel the Wind for Wind-predominant painful obstruction; needles are recommended in these cases.
- Dissipate the Cold for Cold-predominant painful obstruction; in these cases, use fewer needles and a greater amount of moxa to fight the Cold with warmth.
- Transform Dampness for Dampness-predominant painful obstruction; combine Dampness-transforming moxa with Qi-invigorating needles. The use of the warm needle technique is also appropriate in such cases.

Regulating Points of the Axes: Roots and Nodes

The roots and nodes *(gēn jié* 根節*)*, also translated as origins and ends (or terminations), were first mentioned in chapter 5 of *Divine Pivot*. It is interesting to note that in that text some of the nodes were identified as areas rather than points. They have since been associated with specific points:

Greater yang: root — BL-67 *(zhi yin)*;
   node — BL-1 *(jing ming)*
Lesser yang: root — GB-44 *(zu qiao yin)*;
   nodes — TB-22 *(er he liao)* & TB-23 *(si zhu kong)*
Yang brightness: root — ST-45 *(li dui)*;
   nodes — ST-3 *(ju liao)* & LI-19 *(kou he liao)*
Greater yin: root — SP-1 *(yin bai)*;
   node — CV-12 *(zhong wan)*
Lesser yin: root — KI-1 *(yong quan)*;
   node — CV-23 *(lian quan)*
Terminal yin: root — LR-1 *(da dun)*;
   node — CV-18 *(yu tang)*

The roots and nodes are often used as coupled points for supporting the involved axis. The metaphor is that the root is on the earth, and the node in the trunk or on the head. The root points thus represent the nourishing or yin functions while the node points express the circulating and moving or yang functions of the axis.

Regulating Points of the Channels: Transport Points

The transport *(shū)* points provide the means to intervene in all the physiological functions regulated by the channels and the Five Phases. Their range of application includes the elimination of pathogenic influences, regulation of anatomical layers, and adjustment to the change of seasons. Their ability to regulate the Five Phases makes them very useful in prevention.

These points are divided into groups of five for each of the twelve primary channels, and are located between the limb extremities and the knees or the elbows. Each of these points has a specific function defined by its Chinese character. They are listed in distal to proximal order:

- the well *(jǐng* 井*)* point from which the Qi emerges
- the spring *(yíng* or *róng* 滎*)* or gushing point where it seeps out
- the stream *(shū* 輸*)* or transporting point where it flows
- the river *(jīng* 經*)* or traversing point where it circulates
- the sea *(hé* 合*)* or uniting point where it enters (or gathers).

The five transport points are related to the Five Phases and affect their regulation, as shown (TABLE 8-2).

The well points on the yin channels correspond to Wood, and to Metal on the yang channels. The well points treat fullness below the Heart *(Classic of Difficulties,* 68th difficulty). The yang well points cool, cause the Qi to descend, and treat Dampness. The yin well points spread the Liver Qi, regulate the Qi, drain Heat, cool the Blood, open the orifices, and awaken the brain.

The spring points on the yin channels correspond to Fire, and to Water on the yang channels. The spring points treat body Heat *(Classic of Difficulties,* 68th difficulty). Drain the yin spring points to eliminate Heat, and tonify the yang spring points to control Fire with Water.

The stream points on the yin channels correspond to Earth, and to Wood on the yang channels. The stream points treat sensations of heaviness in the body and pain in the joints *(Classic of Difficulties,* 68th difficulty). According to a passage in chapter 43 of *Basic Questions*, the yin stream points and yang sea points are used together to treat painful obstruction.

The river points on the yin channels correspond to Metal, and to Fire on the yang channels. The river points treat dyspnea, coughing, and alternating chills and fevers *(Classic of Difficulties,* 68th difficulty).

TABLE 8-2 TRANSPORT POINTS

Yin Channel	Phase	Well	Spring	Stream	River	Sea
Arm Greater Yin Lung	Metal	LU-11	LU-10	LU-9	LU-8	LU-5
Leg Greater Yin Spleen	Earth	SP-1	SP-2	SP-3	SP-5	SP-9
Arm Lesser Yin Heart	Fire	HT-9	HT-8	HT-7	HT-4	HT-3
Leg Lesser Yin Kidney	Water	KI-1	KI-2	KI-3	KI-7	KI-10
Arm Terminal Yin Pericardium	Fire	PC-9	PC-8	PC-7	PC-5	PC-3
Leg Terminal Yin Liver	Wood	LR-1	LR-2	LR-3	LR-4	LR-8

Yang Channel	Phase	Well	Spring	Stream	River	Sea
Arm Yang Brightness Large Intestine	Metal	LI-1	LI-2	LI-3	LI-5	LI-11
Leg Yang Brightness Stomach	Earth	ST-45	ST-44	ST-43	ST-41	ST-36
Arm Greater Yang Small Intestine	Fire	SI-1	SI-2	SI-3	SI-5	SI-8
Leg Greater Yang Bladder	Water	BL-67	BL-66	BL-65	BL-60	BL-40
Arm Lesser Yang Triple Burner	Fire	TB-1	TB-2	TB-3	TB-4	TB-10
Leg Lesser Yang Gallbladder	Wood	GB-44	GB-43	GB-41	GB-38	GB-34

The sea points on the yin channels correspond to Water, and to Earth on the yang channels. The sea points control upward rebellious Qi and downward leakages (diarrhea) (*Classic of Difficulties*, 68th difficulty).

On the yang channels, the source (*yuán* 原) points are a separate point grouping. Usually they are proximal to the stream points (TABLE 8-3). They are linked to the six yang Organs, affect the physiology of the three burners, and have a relationship with the ancestral Qi. On the yin channels, the stream points serve as the source points.

TABLE 8-3 YANG CHANNEL SOURCE POINTS

Phase	Yang Organ	Source Point
Wood	Gallbaldder	GB-40
Fire	Small Intestine	SI-4
Fire	Triple Burner	TB-4
Earth	Stomach	ST-42
Metal	Large Intestine	LI-4
Water	Bladder	BL-64

Using the Transport Points

According to the Tonification and Drainage Methods

The rules of the Five Phases are used to determine the tonification and drainage points in accordance with the "mother-child" relationship: when a particular phase is deficient, its mother should be tonified; when a phase is excessive, its child should be drained (TABLE 8-4).

The tonification and drainage methods can be used for the change of seasons, the circadian rhythms of the channels, and the opening and closing times of the points according to the "stem and branch" theory.

According to the Location of the Disease

Chapters 4 and 5 of *Divine Pivot* set forth other rules for using the transport points:

- When the disease affects the yin of yin (yin Organs), needle the spring and stream points on the yin channels.
- When the disease affects the yang of yin (yang Organs), needle the sea points on the yang channels.
- When the disease affects the yin of yang (sinews, bones), needle the river points on the yin channels.
- When the disease affects the yang of yang (skin, flesh), needle points on the collateral vessels.

According to the Season

SPRING: "In spring, heaven Qi starts to open, earth Qi starts to vent, the cold and frozen thaw out, the waters [Fluids] move and the channels are unobstructed, so the Qi of humans resides in the vessels." (*Basic Questions*, chapter 64)

TABLE 8-4 TONIFICATION & DRAINAGE WITH TRANSPORT POINTS

Phase	Yin Organ	Tonification Point	Drainage Point
Wood	Liver	LR-8 (sea)	LR-2 (spring)
Fire	Heart	HT-9 (well)	HT-7 (stream)
Fire	Pericardium	PC-9 (well)	PC-7 (stream)
Earth	Spleen	SP-2 (spring)	SP-5 (river)
Metal	Lung	LU-9 (stream)	LU-5 (sea)
Water	Kidneys	KI-7 (river)	KI-1 (well)

Phase	Yang Organ	Tonification Point	Drainage Point
Wood	Gallbladder	GB-43 (spring)	GB-38 (river)
Fire	Small Intestine	SI-3 (stream)	SI-8 (sea)
Fire	Triple Burner	TB-3 (stream)	TB-10 (sea)
Earth	Stomach	ST-41 (river)	ST-45 (well)
Metal	Large Intestine	LI-9 (sea)	LI-2 (spring)
Water	Bladder	BL-67 (well)	BL-65 (stream)

"In spring, needle the dispersed points[4] until you come to the division. When blood emerges, stop. In severe cases, transmit the Qi [to different levels]; simple cases will be alleviated." (*Basic Questions*, chapter 16)

"In spring, needle the connecting points." (*Basic Questions*, chapter 28)

"In spring, choose the collaterals in the flesh interstices." (*Basic Questions*, chapter 61)

"In spring, choose the collaterals, the various spring points, and [those] in the midst of the divisions of the flesh of the major channels. For severe cases, go deeply; for more superficial cases, needle superficially." (*Divine Pivot*, chapter 2)

"In spring, choose the points that are located at the level of the channels, Blood vessels and muscle interstices. Needle deeply for severe cases, and more superficially for mild cases." (*Divine Pivot*, chapter 19)

"In spring, choose the collaterals. . . . The collaterals treat the skin." (*Divine Pivot*, chapter 21)

"Colors and appearances correspond to spring. In spring, needle the spring points." (*Divine Pivot*, chapter 44)

"In spring, one needles the well points when the pathogenic [Qi] resides in the Liver." (*Classic of Difficulties*, 74th difficulty)

SUMMER: "In summer, the channels are full and the Qi spills over. The minute vessels and collaterals receive Blood. The skin and flesh are substantial and full." (*Basic Questions*, chapter 64)

"In summer, needle the connecting points and stop when you see blood. If you slow the Qi and close the holes, painful diseases will certainly be purged." (*Basic Questions*, chapter 16)

"In summer, treat the stream points." (*Basic Questions*, chapter 28)

"In summer, choose the pores and interstices of the brimming channels." (*Basic Questions*, chapter 61)

"In summer, choose the various stream points, the minute [vessels] and the surface of the flesh and skin." (*Divine Pivot*, chapter 2)

"In summer, treat the channels with abundance[5] and the minute [vessels]; choose [to needle] between the divisions just underneath the skin." (*Divine Pivot*, chapter 19)

"In summer, choose the divisional interstices (*fèn ròu*).[6] The divisional interstices treat the flesh." (*Divine Pivot*, chapter 21)

"Periods of time correspond to summer. In summer, needle the stream points." (*Divine Pivot*, chapter 44)

"Sounds correspond to late summer. In late summer, needle the river points." (*Divine Pivot*, chapter 44)

"In summer, one needles the spring points when the pathogenic [Qi] resides in the Heart." (*Classic of Difficulties*, 74th difficulty)

FALL: "In fall, the heaven Qi starts to recede, the skin interstices close up and the skin becomes tight." (*Basic Questions*, chapter 64)

"In fall, needle the skin while following the fibers. Do above and below in the same manner and stop when the spirit changes." (*Basic Questions*, chapter 16)

"In fall, treat the six yang Organs' sea points." (*Basic Questions*, chapter 28)

"In fall, choose the channels' stream points." (*Basic Questions*, chapter 61)

"In fall, choose the different sea points, and otherwise use the same methods as in spring." (*Divine Pivot*, chapter 2)

"In fall, choose the river and stream points; if the pathogenic influences are located in the yang Organs, choose the sea points." (*Divine Pivot*, chapter 19)

"In fall, treat the Qi openings. . . . The Qi openings treat the sinew vessels." (*Divine Pivot*, chapter 21)

"Tastes correspond to fall. In fall, needle the sea points." (*Divine Pivot*, chapter 44)

"In fall, one needles the river points when the pathogenic [Qi] resides in the Lungs." (*Classic of Difficulties*, 74th difficulty)

WINTER: "Winter [is a time of] burying and storage. The Blood and Qi reside in the center [of the body] to make contact with the bones and marrow and flow through the five yin Organs." (*Basic Questions*, chapter 64)

"In winter, needle hollows and points [of the bone and marrow] to the division. In severe cases, needle directly. For mild cases, spread the needling [over a wide area]." (*Basic Questions*, chapter 16)

"In winter, [the Qi] is closed and obstructed. For those who are closed and obstructed use herbs and less needles and stones." (*Basic Questions*, chapter 28)

"In winter, treat the well and spring points." (*Basic Questions*, chapter 61)

"In winter, choose the various well points and stream points, leaving the needle in place for a long period of time." (*Divine Pivot*, chapter 2)

"In winter, needle the well and spring points; needles must be inserted deeply and retained." (*Divine Pivot*, chapter 19)

"In winter, treat the channel points.[7] . . . The channel points treat the bones, marrow and the five Organs." (*Divine Pivot*, chapter 21)

"The yin Organs correspond to winter. In winter, needle the well points." (*Divine Pivot*, chapter 44)

"In winter, one needles the sea points when the pathogenic [Qi] resides in the Kidneys." (*Classic of Difficulties*, 74th difficulty)

Treatment According to the Different Aspects of Painful Obstruction

WIND-PREDOMINANT PAINFUL OBSTRUCTION

Treatment Principle

Expel the Wind and unblock the channels.

Methods

The main rule when expelling Wind is to tonify the Blood by using BL-17 (*ge shu*) and SP-10 (*xue hai*). Wind can also be dispersed by using points for Wind invasion, according to its location: GV-16 (*feng fu*), GB-20 (*feng chi*), BL-12 (*feng men*), TB-17 (*yi feng*), SI-12 (*bing feng*), GB-31 (*feng shi*). Note that all of these points have the word "wind" (*fēng*) in their names.

Regulating the five transport points in accordance with the methods explained above is sometimes the appropriate course of treatment.

General Treatise on Acupuncture, quoted by Dr. Chamfrault, recommends using GB-41 (*zu lin qi*), TB-5 (*wai guan*), GV-1 (*chang qiang*), LI-11 (*qu chi*), ST-36 (*zu san li*) and BL-40 (*wei zhong*).

Collection on Chinese Medicine, also quoted by Dr. Chamfrault, prescribes GV-20 (*bai hui*), GB-20 (*feng chi*) and GB-30 (*huan tiao*).

COLD-PREDOMINANT PAINFUL OBSTRUCTION

Treatment Principle

Disperse the Cold and restore communication between the channels.

Methods

When Cold lingers inside the body, the yang becomes weak. It is therefore necessary to tonify the source Qi to eliminate the Cold by using mild and long sessions of moxa at BL-23 (*shen shu*) and CV-4 (*guan yuan*); GB-39 (*xuan zhong*) can be a useful complement.

Regulating the five transport points in accordance with the methods explained above reinforces the treatment.

DAMPNESS-PREDOMINANT PAINFUL OBSTRUCTION

Treatment Principle

Drain the Dampness and unblock the channels.

Methods

Eliminating Dampness is always a long process; using the warm needle technique yields the most satisfactory results. The most commonly used points are: SP-5 (*shang qiu*), the Dryness point (river point) of the leg greater yin; ST-38 (*tiao kou*), a classical point for Damp painful obstruction; and ST-36 (*zu san li*). A passage in chapter 19 of *Divine Pivot* notes, "For fixed painful obstruction that does not leave, with long-term Cold that has no end, quickly choose ST-36 (*zu san li*)."

Other possible points: LI-13 (*shou wu li*), ST-32 (*fu tu*), BL-38 (*fu xi*), and, according to *Introduction to Medicine*, GB-30 (*huan tiao*), GB-34 (*yang ling quan*), TB-8 (*san yang luo*) and GV-1 (*chang qiang*).

Tonifying the Spleen by applying moxa at BL-20 (*pi shu*) in combination with SP-9 (*yin ling quan*) promotes the metabolization of Dampness.

When the rheumatism is affected by changes in the weather, one should regulate the yang Linking vessel by using TB-5 *(wai guan)* and BL-35 *(yang jiao)*.

HEAT-PREDOMINANT PAINFUL OBSTRUCTION

Treatment Principle

Clear the Heat, disperse the Wind and Dampness, invigorate the Blood and unblock the channels.

Methods

When Heat is present it should be cleared at the level of the yang brightness channel and Governing vessel. This is accomplished with such points as LI-4 *(he gu)*, LI-11 *(qu chi)* and GV-14 *(da zhui)*, as well as GV-8 *(jin suo)*, GV-9 *(zhi yang)*, GV-11 *(shen dao)* and GV-12 *(shen zhu)*. All points should be drained.

Excess Heat injures the Fluids, which should then be tonified by stimulation of the Spleen, Lungs or Kidneys, according to the symptomatology. In severe cases, we should cool the Blood and eliminate the Toxins. Use SP-10 *(xue hai)* and LR-2 *(xing jian)* to cool the Blood. It is best to eliminate Toxins with herbs.

STUBBORN PAINFUL OBSTRUCTION

Treatment Principle

Clear the Heat, disperse the Wind and Dampness, invigorate the Blood and unblock the channels.

Methods

For this type of painful obstruction we should expel the Wind, invigorate the Blood, disperse the Cold, clear the Heat and support the normal Qi. It is also important to transform the Phlegm and invigorate the Blood. In any case, treatment is difficult and generally relies on herbs, either alone or in combination with acupuncture.

BLOOD AND QI DEFICIENT PAINFUL OBSTRUCTION

Treatment Principle

Tonify and harmonize the Blood and Qi. It will also be necessary to tonify the Kidney and Spleen yang.

Methods

Use moxa rather than needles at points influencing these general functions.

YANG DEFICIENT PAINFUL OBSTRUCTION

Treatment Principle

Warm the yang and strengthen the Qi by tonifying the Kidney, Liver and Spleen yang.

Methods

Focus the tonification effect by using moxa at such points as GV-4 *(ming men)*, BL-23 *(shen shu)*, BL-18 *(gan shu)*, CV-6 *(qi hai)*, CV-17 *(shan zhong)* and CV-12 *(zhong wan)*.

YIN DEFICIENT PAINFUL OBSTRUCTION

Treatment Principle

Tonifying the Kidney yin and nourishing the Liver yin are the basis of treatment.

Methods

While herbal therapy is usually the primary treatment of choice, the following acupuncture points can also be of use: BL-23 *(shen shu)*, KI-3 *(tai xi)*, KI-15 *(zhong zhu)*, KI-21 *(you men)*, and lastly LR-3 *(tai chong)* to nourish the Liver yin as a means of supporting the Kidney yin.

Treatment of Complications

One of the prominent features of Chinese energetic physiology is the relationship established between Organs and tissues: Liver with the sinews, Heart with the vessels, Spleen with muscle mass (i.e., the flesh), Lungs with the skin, and Kidneys with the bones. This relationship explains possible complications when the pathogenic influences spread toward the interior. When a disease affecting a particular tissue lingers on, it propagates toward the inside and settles in its associated Organ, where it causes painful obstruction. Thus, painful obstruction of the skin affects the Lungs; painful obstruction of the vessels affects the Heart; painful obstruction of the sinews affects the Liver; painful obstruction of the bones affects the Kidneys; and painful obstruction of the flesh affects the Spleen. "As for those things that are considered painful obstruction, each occurs when a person severely contracts Wind, Cold or Dampness in its particular season." (*Basic Questions*, chapter 43)

Basic Questions calls on the transportive and distributive functions of the stream points to treat the yin Organs, and designates the sea points for treatment of the yang Organs. According to contemporary Chinese authors, however, it is preferable to use the Organs' associated and alarm points.

LUNG PAINFUL OBSTRUCTION

Symptomatology

When skin painful obstruction remains unresolved and there are repeated attacks by pathogenic influences, the Lungs are affected with the following symptoms: fever, aversion to cold, cough, shortness of breath, a sense of fullness in the chest, vomiting, anxiety and restlessness. This pattern sometimes results from the direct invasion of pathogenic influences obstructing the circulation of Lung Qi.

Treatment

In *Basic Questions,* LU-9 *(tai yuan)* is the recommended point. Modern texts suggest the associated and alarm points of the Lungs, BL-13 *(fei shu)* and LU-1 *(zhong fu).*

HEART PAINFUL OBSTRUCTION

Symptomatology

When painful obstruction in a vessel lingers on and is subjected to the repeated invasion of pathogenic influences, it affects the Heart. Symptoms include the following: palpitations, heart "beating like a drum," sensation of precordial swelling, shortness of breath, dry throat, frequent sighs, anxiety and fear. This pattern is sometimes caused by overworry and anxiety, which weaken the Heart Blood and promote the invasion of pathogenic influences that accumulate in the chest.

Treatment

In *Basic Questions,* HT-7 *(shen men)* is the recommended point. Modern texts recommend PC-4 *(xi men),* PC-6 *(nei guan)* and HT-7 *(shen men).*

LIVER PAINFUL OBSTRUCTION

Symptomatology

When painful obstruction in the sinews does not heal and there are repeated invasions of pathogenic influences,

it affects the Liver, giving rise to the following pattern: headaches, restless sleep, nightmares, excessive thirst, frequent urination, abdominal distention, flank, thoracic and costal pain, lower back pain and cold legs and feet. This pattern can also follow upon great anger or emotional pain, which leaves the Liver open to the invasion of pathogenic influences.

Treatment

In *Basic Questions,* LR-3 *(tai chong)* is the preferred point. Modern texts recommend BL-18 *(gan shu),* LR-14 *(qi men)* and LR-3 *(tai chong).*

KIDNEY PAINFUL OBSTRUCTION

Symptomatology

Under repeated attack by pathogenic influences, painful obstruction in the bones that does not heal can progress toward the Kidneys and give rise to the following symptoms: weak sensation in the bones with great difficulty in walking; the back is bent forward and the patient cannot straighten up; and the joints are swollen, stiff and difficult to move. In some cases this pattern is linked to an accumulation of pathogenic influences in the pelvis and external genitalia, where they injure the Kidney Qi; this is Kidney painful obstruction, attributed in *Basic Questions,* chapter 10 to falling asleep after a cold bath.

Treatment

In *Basic Questions,* KI-3 *(tai xi)* is the preferred point. Modern texts recommend BL-23 *(shen shu)* and GB-25 *(jing men).*

SPLEEN PAINFUL OBSTRUCTION

Symptomatology

Lingering painful obstruction in the flesh, under constant attack by pathogenic influences, will affect the Spleen. The chief clinical signs include weariness of the limbs, sensation of fullness in the chest, cough, and vomiting and regurgitation of clear liquids.

Treatment

In *Basic Questions,* SP-3 *(tai bai)* is the preferred point. Modern texts recommend BL-20 *(pi shu)* and LR-13 *(zhang men).*

The concept of internal propagation of painful obstruction disorders toward the Organs underscores the fact that the framework of painful obstruction goes beyond the biomedical understanding of rheumatism. From the biomedical perspective, Kidney painful obstruction can be seen as a form of rheumatism, Heart painful obstruction as certain types of cardiovascular complications, and conditions affecting other Organs as various systemic diseases. Two other clinical aspects are described in *Basic Questions*: painful obstruction of the Intestines and painful obstruction of the gestation membranes.

INTESTINES PAINFUL OBSTRUCTION

Symptomatology

In this pattern the pathogenic influence obstructs the circulation of Qi in the Intestines, which are then unable to perform their function of separating the pure from the turbid. The chief signs are excessive thirst, oliguria or inability to urinate, abdominal swelling, diarrhea and a stifling sensation in the chest.

Treatment

In *Basic Questions*, LI-11 *(qu chi)* and SI-8 *(xiao hai)* are the preferred points. Modern texts recommend BL-25 *(da chang shu)*, ST-25 *(tian shu)*, BL-27 *(xiao chang shu)* and CV-4 *(guan yuan)*.

GESTATION MEMBRANES OR BLADDER PAINFUL OBSTRUCTION

Symptomatology

The word *bāo* 胞, which we have translated as gestation membranes, has been the subject of discussion for thousands of years. It has several different meanings: Womb (when viewed as one of the Curious Organs), Bladder, the primordial area located between the Kidneys where the Curious vessels emerge, and even the Pericardium. According to Elizabeth Rochat de la Vallée, it is always used to describe an intimate wrapping designed to preserve and protect vital transformations. In this sense, when it refers to the Bladder it describes the deep mechanism of Qi transformation at the level of the Bladder. Ma Shi, one of the great *Inner Classic* commentators, put it this way: "The Bladder is located inside the lower abdomen and the *bāo* is found inside the Bladder."

According to most sources, this pattern corresponds to Bladder painful obstruction, where pathogenic Wind and Cold invade the Bladder and obstruct the Qi transformations which normally occur at this level. The lower abdomen and bladder are painful to the touch, urination is difficult, and the patient suffers from symptoms of a common cold due to the uprising of Qi.

Treatment

In *Basic Questions*, BL-40 *(wei zhong)* is the preferred point. Modern texts recommend BL-28 *(pang guang shu)* and CV-3 *(zhong ji)*.

PREVENTIVE TREATMENT

Basic prevention of relapses relies on the regulation of the Five Phases. The many different therapeutic methods at our disposal all involve use of the transport points, which presupposes that we have identified with great accuracy the unbalanced phase; in this respect, the energetic pattern prevailing at the time of birth of the patient can prove extremely useful. These methods are very easy to implement if we address only the mother-child relationship, a little more complex if we take into account seasonal variations, and extremely complex if we include the concept of "open" points according to the stem and branch theory. Although tables are available to guide us in our decisions, the issue is far from resolved since opinions vary widely on this matter. At this point we lack convincing evidence to enable us to take sides, and various meetings and research projects in China have been unable to shed much light on our initial questions.

Herewith is an example of regulation of a deficient phase: if the yin correspondences are affected, focus on the channel that has the most Qi, and if the yang correspondences are affected, focus on the channel that has the most Blood, either by needling the open point, or by selecting the tonifying point and the sprin—*yíng*, literally "flourishing"—point.

Another method utilizes the four-needle technique according to the mother-child rule: on the left, tonify in the deficient phase the point sharing the same nature as that phase's mother, and reinforce this action by tonifying the "mother" phase's intrinsic or phasic point[8] (i.e., the point that corresponds to the same phase as the particular channel, e.g., the Wood point on a Wood channel). On the right, drain in the deficient phase the point sharing the same nature as the controlling phase, and reinforce this action by draining the controlling phase's intrinsic or phasic point. Thus, in the case of a deficient Wood phase affecting the yang correspondences, the terminal yin channel (which has the most Blood) should be treated by needling LR-8 *(qu quan)* and LR-2 *(xing jian)*.

As another example, on the left we should tonify such points as LR-8 *(qu quan)* (Water point on the terminal yin channel) and KI-10 *(yin gu)* (Water point of the Water phase's yin channel), and on the right we should drain LR-4 *(zhong feng)* (Metal point on the terminal yin channel) and LU-8 *(jing qu)* (Metal point of the Metal phase's yin channel).

To be complete, prevention requires that patients protect themselves from the pathogenic influences associated with the weather, especially Dampness, and that they modify their diets.

Phytotherapy

Although not as diverse in its range nor as precise in its indications as traditional Chinese medicine, the Western materia medica boasts a long tradition of treating osteoarticular disorders with a variety of medicinal herbs. To date, the efficacy of these herbs has rarely been validated scientifically, and their prescription relies largely on empirical data. No detailed data have been recorded regarding the nature and type of "rheumatisms" for which they are prescribed.

The herbs are presented below in the following order: botanical name, common English name, and then family name in brackets.

ANTIRHEUMATIC AND ANALGESIC HERBS

Betula Alba L. - Birch [Betulacea]

The medicinal properties of birch are not mentioned before the Middle Ages. Hildegarde, in the twelfth century, was the first to mention the healing action of its flowers. The leaves are mostly used at present, as well as the bark, buds and sap. The leaves have a diuretic effect due to their flavonoid content, mostly in the form of hyperoside or quercetol-3 galactoside. The antipyretic properties of the bark are due to a triterpenic alcohol, betulinol.

Birch is classically described as having diuretic, purifying, antirheumatic, antipyretic and vulnerary (useful in healing wounds) properties. An infusion of birch leaves could eliminate edema due to cardiorenal complications. In the old days, country people affected by rheumatic pain used to lie in a bed filled with birch leaves in order to induce sweating.

Although its diuretic properties are useful in the treatment of gout, its antirheumatic action has yet to be proven scientifically.

Birch sap is used in folk medicine for urinary tract disorders, gout and rheumatism: take one teaspoon 3 to 4 times daily.

An infusion of the leaves is the traditional mode of preparation: add 10 to 50g per liter of boiling water, let it boil for one or two seconds, then let it steep for one to two hours. You may add 1g of bicarbonate of soda when the temperature has gone down to 40°C (104°F) to assist the dissolution of the resin content. Take 3 cups a day, a half-hour before, or two to three hours after each meal.

To prepare a bud infusion, add 150 to 200g of buds per liter of water, and boil it down to one-fifth of its volume; drink 2 cups daily.

Other modes of preparation include:

- fluid extract: 1 to 3g/day
- aerosol: 600 to 900mg/day
- powder: 3g/day
- glycerin maceration of the buds: 50 drops 3 times/day

No toxicity or side effects have been reported at the recommended dosage.

Colchicum Automnale L. - Autumn Crocus [Liliacea]

We only mention the autumn crocus for reference; all of its parts are extremely toxic. The function of this herb is largely due to its alkaloid content, primarily colchicine. Other chemical constituents are demecolcine and colchicoside. The diuretic, analgesic, anti-inflammatory and sedative properties of the herb are used to treat joint pain. Colchicine is one of the chief remedies for gout pain.

Only one form of medicinal preparation is still in use today: Colcheux tincture, which is an alcohol-based tincture of autumn crocus bulbs, deprived of their purging action, containing 5mg of total alkaloids. The toxicity of the plant manifests as irritation of the digestive tract with nausea, vomiting, visceral pain, cardiovascular disorders with hypotension, paralysis- and paresthesia-type nervous disorders, and breathing disorders which can lead to suffocation.

Erigeron Canadensis L. - Canadian Vergerette [Compositae]

Originally from North America, vergerette was introduced to Europe in 1655.

The whole plant is used, especially the leaves, for its tonic, diuretic, astringent and hemostatic effects. Leclerc (1976) reported a high efficacy rate in the treatment of rheumatism and gout, with a marked increase in the elimination of uric acid. Its principal chemical ingredients are flavones (polyenes, polyines), tannins, an essential oil made of terpenic ingredients, and gallic acid.

An infusion of the leaves is the traditional mode of preparation: add 30g per liter of water, and take 3 to 4 cups a day.

Other modes of preparation:

• fluid extract: 3g/day
• aerosol: up to 3g/day

No intolerance or side effects have been reported at the recommended dosage.

Fraxinus Excelsior L. - Ash Tree [Oleacea]

The properties of ash have been known in Europe since earliest times. Hippocrates and Theophrastus (fourth century B.C.) prescribed its leaves as a diuretic and laxative to treat rheumatism and gout.

Although the leaves, bark and sap all possess medicinal properties, we will focus our attention on the leaves alone. They are harvested when young, in May and June, when they are still covered with a viscous coating. After removing their petioles, they are laid to dry in the shade in thin layers on cloth or a grid.

The leaves have diuretic, antirheumatic, antigout, diaphoretic, slightly tonic and laxative properties. They have a bitter, acrid and astringent taste. We may infer from their properties that they act on the leg lesser yin Kidney and arm yang brightness Large Intestine channels. Today, ash is still a popular folk remedy for the treatment of rheumatism and gout.

None of the chemical ingredients explains the traditional use of ash leaves in the treatment of rheumatism and gout: flavonoids, mannitol, rutoside, fraxoside, gallic and catechic tannins.

Infusion is the traditional mode of preparation, either by itself (add 30 to 60g per liter of water), or in combination with spirae ulmaire and blackcurrant leaves.

Other modes of preparation:

• dry extracts and aerosol: 300 to 800mg/day
• fluid extract: 1 to 3ml/day
• mother tincture: 5 to 10ml/day
• glycerin maceration of the buds: 30 to 50 drops/day

No toxicity or side effects have been reported in using these different ash preparations.

Harpagophytum Procumbens D.C. - Devil's Claw [Pedaliacea]

This plant comes from Namibia, the capital of which is Windhoeck, hence one of its common names: Windhoeck root. It was traditionally used by the Bantus as a bitter tonic, for fever, digestive disorders and labor pains. The parts used are the secondary roots, cut in slices, dried in an airy place, in the sun or in the shade.

The dried root contains sugars (glucose, fructose, saccharose, raffinose, stachyose), triterpenic acids (ursolic and oleanolic), flavonic aglycones, but most of all heterosides (harpagoside, harpagide, procumbide) and betasitosterols. Harpagoside has analgesic, anti-inflammatory and spasmolytic properties; betasitosterols inhibit the formation of prostaglandin-synthetase.

An infusion of the roots has an anti-inflammatory and anti-arthritic action. Numerous recent writings have underscored the beneficial properties of harpagophytum in the treatment of arthritic or inflammatory rheumatism.

Traditional modes of preparation include:

• decoction: add 15g to 750g of water, boil for a few minutes and macerate overnight; drink it cold the next day without sugar
• aerosol with a minimum of 3 percent iridoides
• gelatin capsules: 1 to 3g/day, up to 9 to 12g
• suppositories: 0.5 to 1.5g/suppository
• suspension: gastric-coated capsules, up to 1.5g/day

Precautions should be taken in cases of high blood pressure, colitis, diarrhea and gastritis; the LD50 given intraperitoneally for rats and mice is 10g/kg in aerosol.

Ribes Nigrum L. - Blackcurrant [Saxifragacea]

The medicinal properties of the leaves and fruits of the blackcurrant bush were not mentioned before the seventeenth century. An infusion of the leaves and heads is diuretic and anti-rheumatic, and has a slightly tonic, astringent and diaphoretic action.

The main chemical ingredients of the leaves are flavonoids (3 flavonic aglycones, 5 flavonic heterosides), which inhibit the synthesis and release of prostaglandins, tannins, phenol acids, amino acids including arginin and prolin, quinic and ascorbic acid, and an essential oil. The buds exhibit an anti-inflammatory and cortisone-like effect.

Infusion is the traditional mode of preparation, either by itself (add 50g per liter of water, 500ml per day), or in combination with ash and ulmaire:

- blackcurrant leaves: 100g
- ash leaves: 50g
- ulmaire flowering heads: 50g

Other modes of preparation:

- M.D.E.[9]: 20ml/day
- S.I.P.F[10]: 10ml/day
- aerosol: 2g/day
- fluid extract: 2 to 4ml/day
- glycerin maceration of the buds: 50 drops, 3 times/day
- mother tincture: 2 to 4ml/day

No toxicity or side effects have been reported in using these different preparations at the recommended dosage.

Salix Alba L. - White Willow [Salicacea]

White willow is traditionally classified as a tonic, astringent and antipyretic, but it has been used mostly for its sedative and calming action on the nerves, and for uterine pain; this last property may have something to do with the presence of estrogen-like substances (such as estriol) in the pussy willows.

The bark, very bitter to the taste, has an antirheumatic effect due to the presence of a glucoside—salicine or salicoside. For medicinal purposes, the bark is harvested from 2- to 3-year-old shoots. A decoction of bark is the traditional mode of preparation: add 30 to 60g per liter of water, and drink one cup before each meal.

Other modes of preparation:

- fluid extract: 75 drops, 3 times/day
- aerosol: 0.3 to 3g/day
- powdered bark: 4 to 6g/day

No toxicity or side effects have been reported at the recommended dosage.

Spirae Ulmaria L. - Meadowsweet [Rosacea]

Nowhere in ancient Western texts is meadowsweet mentioned, which is not surprising since it is rarely found in the Mediterranean region. Its medicinal properties were discovered during the Renaissance era. At the turn of the nineteenth century, the priest of Tremilly brought it out of a long period of oblivion when he mentioned its action on anasarca. Later on, this rosacea was known for its diuretic, diaphoretic, slightly astringent and tonic properties, as an antiphlogistic and sedative, for healing

and cleansing of wounds, and for its cardiotonic actions. Its numerous properties qualify it as one of the remedies used to treat cellulitis and adiposis. Leclerc regarded this herb as an excellent auxiliary remedy for the treatment of acute joint rheumatism.

Its chemical ingredients account for its antirheumatic and analgesic actions:

- heterosides: monotropitoside which releases methylsalicylate by hydrolysis
- flavonoids: spireoside, isoquercitrine, and astragaline in the flowers; avicularine and hyperoside in the leaves

The flowering heads or hulled flowers are used. Since the flowering season is rather short, harvesting must be done before the flowers are fully in bloom.

An infusion of 50g of flowers or flowering heads per liter of boiling water is the traditional mode of preparation, but you must wait for the water to cool down to 90°C (194°F) before pouring it onto the flowers. Allow it to infuse for 12 hours in a closed container; drink 3 to 5 cups per day between meals.

Other modes of preparation:

- M.D.E.: 20ml/day
- S.I.P.F.: 10ml/day
- fluid extract: 5ml/day
- aerosol: 800mg/day

No toxicity or side effects have been reported at the recommended dosage.

An infusion of the leaves is the traditional mode of preparation: add 30g per liter of water, and take 3 to 4 cups a day.

Other modes of preparation:

- fluid extract: 3g/day
- aerosol: up to 3g/day

No intolerance or side effects have been reported at the recommended dosage.

REMINERALIZING HERBS

Equisetum Arvense L. - Prele Des Champs [Equisetacea]

Known since antiquity, prele was not always clearly differentiated from other plants that were similar to it. In the Middle Ages, the hemostatic action of preles is mostly attributed to prele des champs. Prele is diuretic, hemostatic and remineralizing.

In the Chinese materia medica, prele is classified as a Heat-clearing herb. It is bitter and cool. The channels it goes to are not specified, but we can infer from its indications that it would have an effect on the leg lesser yin Kidney, leg greater yang Bladder, and arm greater yin Lung channels. It expels Heat, cools the Blood, alleviates cough and promotes urination.

The part of the plant used is the sterile dried stem, which is very rich in minerals (15 to 18 percent): potassium, calcium, manganese and especially silica (5.2 to 7.8 percent). It contains flavonoids: quercetol, kamferol and apigenine heterosides; saponosides: equisetonoside; organic acids: citric acid, glyceric acid; phenol acids: cafeic, ferulic; and indanone derivatives.

A decoction of 30 to 50g of dry herbs per half-liter of water is the traditional mode of preparation. Boil for a half hour and drink in three doses over a 24-hour period.

Other modes of preparation:

• M.D.E.: 10ml/day
• S.I.P.F.: 1 measure 3 times/day
• fluid extract: 2g/day
• aerosol: 2g/day
• powder: 4g/day

Galeopsis Dubia L. - Galeopsis Douteux [Labiatae]

Galeopsis is not mentioned in any of the ancient Western texts. In fact, not until the nineteenth century did some German doctors mention its effect in the treatment of pulmonary catarrh and phthisis. This plant has expectorant, remineralizing, astringent and anti-anemia properties. Rich in silica (0.7 to 0.9 percent), it also contains phenol acids (cafeic, chlorogenic), flavonoids, a tannin and saponosides.

Galeopsis is harvested during flowering time, between July and September. The part used is the flowering plant.

It is traditionally prescribed as an infusion: 30g/liter of water to be taken during the day, or as part of the Siliceous Tea formula:

• galeopsis: 50 parts
• prele: 75 parts
• knotweed: 150 parts

A 10 to 20g/liter of water decoction has an expectorant action.

Polygonum Aviculare L. - Knotweed [Polygonacea]

In ancient times, knotweed was known to be a hemostatic remedy. Dioscorides prescribed it for spitting blood and hemorrhage, cholera, diarrhea and urine retention. Due to its hemostatic qualities, the Latins called this plant

Herba Sanguinalis or sanguinaria. Its indications remained the same until the sixteenth century, after which it gradually fell into oblivion. Around 1840, physicians started to recognize its powerful astringent properties, which were particularly indicated in the treatment of such problems as diarrhea, dysenteric disorders and colitis. This plant is also a tonic, diuretic and healing agent for wounds. Its hemostatic properties are solely based on a long tradition. It is also used to quench the thirst of diabetic patients.

The entire plant is used in China as a diuretic, to expel Water and Dampness. Being bitter and cold, it goes to the leg greater yang Bladder channel, and expels Heat.

The entire plant is used: rich in silica, it also contains a tannin, flavonic pigments, a resin and an essential oil. Despite its rich silica content, it was never indicated in Chinese or European literature for any osteoarticular pathology (except for gout).

Knotweed is rarely used in France, but more so in Germany; it is a part of the Siliceous Tea formula given above. It is prescribed as an astringent in a decoction form: add 25 to 30g of leaves or the entire plant with the rhizome per liter of water.

Urtica Dioica L., *Urtica Urens* L. - Big and Small Stinging Nettle [Urticacea]

A universal weed, nettle has been used as a vegetable since prehistoric times. Its medicinal properties were described by Dioscorides, and later by Galen. Throughout history the stinging nettle has been regarded as one of the most precious plants. Fournier describes it as follows:

> It activates digestive functions, it nourishes, it has diuretic, antidiarrheic, hemostatic, antidiabetic, probably lactagogue and emmenagogue, purifying and tonic properties. It has a definite effect on the skin and helps skin conditions. Used externally, it exhibits astringent, resolvent and cleansing actions, and, as an urtication, it proves to be powerfully cleansing. The seeds are said to be diuretic, purgative, emmenagogue, vermifugal and even more or less antipyretic, but allegedly could become drastic and dangerous at over 15g a day.

The leaves are rich in chlorophyll, and contain carotenes, some minerals (potassium, calcium, magnesium salts), glycolic and glyceric acids, and, in its stinging hairs, histamine- and acetylcholine-like substances.

Nettle promotes the elimination of uric acid; it is used to treat gout, and its hypoglycemiative and diuretic effects justify its use in purifying the Blood according to the traditional terminology.

Nettle is traditionally prescribed as an infusion or a decoction: 30 to 60g/liter of water, to be taken between or before meals, 3 cups a day.

Other modes of preparation:

- nettle juice: 1 Tbsp/day
- M.D.E.: 20ml/day
- S.I.P.F.: 1 measure 3 times/day
- aerosol: 2g/day
- fluid extract: 10ml/day

No adverse reactions have been reported at the recommended dosage.

OTHER HERBS

A few words about aconite. As we have seen, aconite has become an extremely important herb in the treatment of rheumatic disorders in China. The Western variety (*Aconitum napellus* L.) possesses similar properties and indications, but its extreme toxicity excludes it from the traditional materia medica.

Other herbs are prescribed whose indications are not consistently supported by traditional use and whose modes of action are yet to be scientifically validated, such as *Glechoma hederacea* (ivy), *Ulmus campestris* L. (elm), *Sequoia gigantea* (Lindl.) (giant sequoia), *Physalis alkekengi* L. (alkekenge), *Pinus montana* L. (pine) and *Populus nigra* (black poplar).

Western herbs often perform a draining action on the body, focusing, according to circumstances, on the hepatobiliary, renal, intestinal or pancreatic systems. Although this therapeutic approach deserves much attention, we can only make a brief note of it here, as this topic does not fit within our discussion.

HERBS FOR EXTERNAL USE

There are many herbs in the Western materia medica that are used externally for rheumatic disorders. The following are among the most common:

Arnica montana L. (arnica): in tincture form, diluted with at least an equal volume of water

Brassica oleracea L. (cabbage): topical application of the fresh leaf

Brassica nigra (Koch) (black mustard): ointment with essential oil

Juniperus communis L. (juniper): essential oil

Hedera helix L. (ivy): leaf extract ointment

Rosmarinus officinalis L. (rosemary): liniment with rosemary alcoholate

Larix decidua L. or *Pinus pinaster* Ait.: turpentine essential oil, as a rubbing oil, liniment, ointment

Gaultheria procumbens: wintergreen essential oil

Eucalyptus citriodora: essential oil as a rubbing oil, liniment, ointment

Helichrysum italicum: essential oil as a rubbing oil, liniment, ointment

Chapter Notes

1. *Editors' note:* For more information about this in English, see the video series on barrier points by Peter Eckman, M.D., Claude Roustan, M.D., and Gerard Guillaume, available from the Medical Acupuncture Video Library (Berkeley: Medical Acupuncture Publishers).

2. Portions of this chapter are translated in chapter 24 below.

3. Note that the word for concavity, *xū*, is the same as that for deficiency.

4. Modern commentators (see Bibliography) interpret this to mean the transport points.

5. Modern commentators interpret this to mean the yang channels.

6. Modern commentators interpret this to mean the interstices and pores.

7. Modern commentators interpret this to mean points on channels that do not belong to any of the special categories of points.

8. Because these points are often used in correlation with the two-hour periods associated with the various channels, they are sometimes known as "hoary" points.

9. M.D.E.: This is a standard abbreviation for "medical drug extracts." These preparations are obtained by reverse osmosis at ambient temperature.

10. S.I.P.F.: This is a standard abbreviation for what in English would be "suspension of whole plant." These micro-suspensions are prepared within 24 hours after harvesting by washing, freezing (cryogenesis), grinding into particles, placing the particles in suspension (30 percent solution of water/alcohol), and concentration under high pressure.

CHAPTER NINE

Polyarticular Painful Syndromes[1]

Introduction

What we are presenting here is theoretical and practical research of our own, which aims at identifying the fundamental mechanisms responsible for polyarticular painful syndromes, particularly chronic ones.

We, like all responsible acupuncturists, get involved in treating the symptoms affecting the Qi, Blood and Fluids, tonifying the normal Qi and eliminating the external pathogenic Qi. In addition, in order to ensure lasting results, we set out to discover each patient's two or three triggering mechanisms. These mechanisms, whether innate or acquired, can combine to create a vicious circle, which is the source of the chronicity of the condition. It is up to us to diagnose and differentiate these interconnected mechanisms. Once we accomplish that we can treat the patient in such a way that they develop better health, instead of just temporarily improving their symptoms.

In the presence of acute pain, we favor first a symptomatic treatment. In addition, or soon after instituting treatment, we recommend any one of a few basic approaches. These include: tonification of the Qi, Blood or Fluids, which constitutes an essential preliminary to any etiological treatment; elimination of the pathogenic influences while strengthening the body's Qi, if the pathogenic invasion appears to be severe in terms of the involved

mechanisms or symptoms; or, finally, an etiological treatment of the two or three mechanisms involved. This last treatment, whether applied right away or after another course of action, is of paramount importance to achieving profound and lasting results.

Of course, intervention with acupuncture does not preclude the use of other therapeutic modalities. On the contrary, combining different therapies for stubbornly recurrent or chronic conditions is advisable in most cases.

Acupuncture treatment of the underlying cause and its unfolding is unavoidably a long-term process. As such, the frequency of treatments will change over time. We needle our patients every one or two weeks in the beginning, and later, when some improvement appears, we progressively space out our sessions to once a month, every two months, every trimester, and finally a biannual maintenance regimen, usually at the time of the equinoxes.

The correct needling of the points, whether superficially or deeply, is of utmost importance in effective treatment, especially of chronic disorders. What is necessary, when needling any acupuncture point, is that the patient experience the *deqi* ("obtaining Qi") sensation, and that the practitioner experience the feeling of having reached the bottom of a well. This, in our opinion, is even more important than any traditional needling manipulation for tonification or draining.

For the sake of clarity, we shall classify the involved mechanisms for polyarticular painful syndromes into five categories:

- direct invasion of the joints
- disruptions in the movement of Qi
- channel disorders
- Organ pathologies
- disruption in one of the Five Revolutions (wǔ yùn).

We have elected not to classify these polyarticular conditions as acute, chronic, or chronic with progressive flare-ups; these categories lack clear and definite distinctions for our research into the mechanisms of acupuncture treatment of different etiologies.

Please note that we have developed a view of the properties, and sometimes even the locations, of acupuncture points that is quite different from traditional viewpoints. Anything like a complete description of our ideas is beyond the scope of this book. Still, in the introductory sections of chapter 8, some of our basic ideas are presented.

DIRECT INVASION OF THE JOINTS

Two mechanisms fall within this category, corresponding to BL-11 (da zhu) and ST-38 (tiao kou) respectively.

BL-11 (da zhu)

This point is located 1.5 unit lateral to GV-13 (tao dao) below the spinal process of the first thoracic vertebra. It is the meeting point for the bones and belongs to the "sea of the twelve channels." The word zhù in its name refers to "the weaver's shuttle." This analogy refers to the warp of a loom, considered at two different levels of interpretation: (1) materially, i.e., the bones, and (2) energetically, i.e., the channels. Through its influence on the bones, BL-11 (da zhu) has a relationship with the joints' marrow.

We believe that this point also governs the bones when they function as a Curious Organ. In this capacity the bones are linked to the perineum, and thereby to the perpetuation of the being or species. In this context, it is related to the energetic Blood vessels.

From a symptomatological point of view, we observe:

- bone and joint disorders
- vertebral pain, knee pain
- local, spinal or generalized muscle contractures
- nervousness, inability to remain still, or to rest in bed
- ocular symptoms, and conditions involving the throat
- pulmonary and abdominal disorders
- mental disorders (such as dementia), convulsions.

Patients for whom this point is indicated often have muscle contractures, and may also have dementia, epilepsy, joint syndromes and vertebral pain.

This point seems to be indicated for chronic polyarticular syndromes involving vertebral complications and knee pain, which is accompanied by muscle contractures causing stiffness and discomfort during activity.

As noted in the commentary to the 45th difficulty of Classic of Difficulties found in Bases of Medicine (Yi yuan), "If the shoulders can carry a heavy burden, it is due to the meeting of the bones at da zhu." We can extrapolate from this statement that BL-11 (da zhu) is involved each time we have an excessively heavy burden (physical or psychological) to carry. For some people, this burden is too heavy or difficult to carry due to a deficiency in the "warp" of the loom, hence the involvement of this point. According to Soulié de Morant, it is the meeting point of the Governing and Conception vessels.

ST-38 (tiao kou)

This point is located halfway between the tip of the lateral malleolus and the depression formed by the lateral foramen of the patella on the leg yang brightness channel. To needle it correctly the patient must dorsiflex the foot; depending on which source you use, it is either the entire foot or just the big toe which must be dorsiflexed.

Its symptomatology involves:

- rheumatism due to Dampness
- at the level of the lower limbs: paralysis, paresthesia with sensations of cold or heat, pain with functional disability, cold and swelling. All of these symptoms correspond to a pattern of Dampness, which is a heavy and stagnant pathogenic influence.
- the shoulders and knees are especially affected.

This point seems to govern the mobility of the entire body, summing up the actions of points governing the mobility of the shoulders—LI-14 (bi nao); elbows—LI-12 (zhou liao); hips—ST-31 (bi guan); and knees—ST-35 (du bi); as well as all the other joints.

This point is indicated for chronic polyarticular syndromes with severe limitation in the range of motion (which cannot be explained by anatomical lesions), aggravated by damp conditions, accompanied by paresthesia, local edema, and always involving the shoulders and knees. This condition implies difficulty in gestural expression. By gestural expression we are referring to how comfortable a person is with their body in space, and how smoothly they move. People with poor gestural expression are out of touch with themselves in space and move awkwardly. The origins of difficulties in gestural expression are to be found in the history. We need to understand why there is a blockage and why it affects their gestural expression.

DISRUPTION IN THE DEEP CIRCULATION OF QI

In the "skin, flesh, muscles and bones" family, the bones and joints represent the deepest structure. They are therefore related to the deep circulation of Qi. Disruption of this circulation can contribute to the emergence of chronic polyarticular syndromes. Two particular types of circulation seem to be involved, corresponding to CV-3 (*zhong ji*) and GB-39 (*xuan zhong*).

CV-3 (*zhong ji*)

This point is located one unit above the superior border of the pubic bone, on the midline. It is the alarm point for the Bladder, and the meeting point of the three leg yin channels. It regulates menstruation, promotes the circulation of Blood when there is stasis (with the use of moxa), promotes movement in the Bladder, regulates the lower burner, and tonifies the nutritive Qi (Auteroche, 1983).

In our opinion, CV-3 (*zhong ji*) has two functions as an alarm point: a seasonal action and a visceral action. From a seasonal point of view, it corresponds to the winter retreat of the various energies toward the interior (yin) of the body. That is, these energies retreat from the trunk (pelvis) and the limbs (bones and joints), particularly the lower limbs. From a visceral perspective, this point is related to the Bladder, which organizes and defines the territory to allow life to manifest, and which preserves, transforms and distributes the Fluids.

This point therefore sends the Qi underground (toward the interior) from where life sprouts outwardly, in order to define the territory where it will manifest, and to organize its irrigation.

The symptomatology of CV-3 (*zhong ji*) indicates an obstruction of these two actions:

• failure of the energies to retreat toward the interior with joint pain (due to deficiency) and Qi insufficiency in the pelvic area, leading either to some form of stagnation (e.g., constipation, delayed menstruation), or to leakage (incontinence, repeated miscarriage, premature labor), or to problems with becoming pregnant (infertility, male and female)

• dysfunction of the Bladder, which influences the transformation, conservation and distribution of the Fluids.

We therefore observe:

• general lassitude with night sweats
• edema
• "accumulation of Cold in the lower part of the body, which aggresses against the Heart from time to time"[2]
• pelvic accumulation: either of an energetic type (Cold, Heat) with distention, genital pruritus, sensation of a hard mass below the umbilicus; or material, particularly of the gynecological system
• pelvic stagnation (constipation, irregular or absent menstruation, inability to expel the placenta)
• leakage (incontinence, repeated miscarriages, premature labor, leukorrhea)
• joint pain with cramps, muscle spasms, and weariness of the lower limbs.

This point is therefore prescribed for chronic polyarticular syndromes:

• with general fatigue and, often, weariness of the lower limbs
• with urinary dysfunctions: rarely with edema and incontinence, most often with pollakiuria, and urinary urgency
• with subumbilical pelvic signs: sensation of cold, heat or a hard mass
• with infertility, menstrual dysfunctions, or difficult pregnancies
• with the pulses of both feet usually deficient.

We must now try to understand why a being cannot retreat to his innermost interior, where life sprouts and is organized, and where its place of manifestation (the body) is defined. We cannot analyze the body, mind and energy separately. The same knots, stresses and conflicts are simultaneously recorded at the level of the brain cortex and in certain areas of the body, generating the same blockages, whether at a somatic, psychological or energetic level: in this case, an inability to retreat toward the germinative interior. One of the most important effects of acupuncture occurs at this level of cellular memory.

GB-39 (*xuan zhong*)

Located three units above the lateral malleolus, on the anterior border of the fibula "where the bone can no longer be felt," it is the meeting point for the marrow. "The eight meetings are points which communicate with the beginning and the end of the Curious vessels, and represent the supreme principle of human life."

This point is also the group connecting point of the three leg yang channels. According to Duron (1978), it governs the Fluids. According to Schnorenberger (1990-1), "It promotes a downward movement when the Liver yang ascends, clears Heat and expels Wind."

Its symptomatology describes:

- rebellious Qi
- in the upper body: sensation of burning head, epistaxis, stuffy nose, dry nose
- mentally: dementia, constant low-grade anger or bad mood, overexcitement, indignation, nervousness, worry, short temper
- stroke due to indignation or rage; convulsive epilepsy; mobility disorders of the limbs due to a direct attack of Wind; brain and spinal cord diseases
- on the skin: abscesses, furuncles
- at the level of the Organs: cough, dyspnea, pain in the area of the heart when coughing, swelling sensation in the chest; abdominal distention, heat in the epigastrium, constipation and anuria, hemorrhoids, anorexia; anuria, dysuria; cramps in the genital region, vaginal dryness
- edema: edema and pain in the joints; retention of fluids
- aversion to coitus
- rheumatism due to Dampness, with swelling, that moves from one joint to another; pain in the bones and muscles with sensation of contractures and cramps; pain in various joints with no apparent etiology; moving pain in all the joints
- all bone disorders: according to Soulié de Morant, this point shortens the healing time for all fractures.

From our perspective, the functions of this lesser yang point are as follows:

- As the group connecting point of the three leg yang channels, it causes the Liver yang to descend, treats rebellious Qi, clears Heat and disperses Wind. It describes yang or Heat symptoms (cephalic, mental, cutaneous disorders) and Wind symptoms (mobility disorders of the limbs, contractures, cramps, moving pain in all the joints).
- As the meeting point of the marrow (just as BL-11 *[da zhu]* is the meeting point of the bones), it can contribute to the treatment of brain and marrow diseases, and has an effect on the metabolization of the Fluids (dryness signs, edema) and includes abdominal, intestinal, gastric, and pulmonary indications.

- From a basic point of view, it promotes the penetration of Heat-yang in excess at the top and on the surface toward the interior-yin. Furthermore, it brings down the upward rebelling Liver Wind-yang.
- On a deeper level, it acts on the bones, marrow and Fluids, maybe even on the Kidneys, which govern them and nourish the Liver yin.

This point is indicated in the following chronic polyarticular syndromes:

- moving pain in all the joints, with no apparent etiology, with cramps and contractures
- for people who are nervous, overexcited, short tempered, angry, in a bad mood, who easily become indignant or enraged, worried or anxious
- with a sensation of swelling in the chest and abdomen, disorders of the Fluids (dryness of the mucous membranes or edema), urinary dysfunctions (dysuria), digestive and respiratory disorders, and, therefore, different Organ diseases.

Channel Disorders

Here we are concerned with channels that, if disrupted, can generate an acute or chronic polyarticular painful syndrome, or contribute to its emergence:

- among the great channels or axes: greater yang
- among the primary channels: leg lesser yang, leg terminal yin, and arm yang brightness
- among the Curious vessels: both Heel vessels, the Girdle and yang Linking vessels
- the great Spleen collateral, governed by SP-21 *(da bao)*.

In each case, diagnosis is based on the simultaneous presence of symptoms of the involved channel and of a polyarticular syndrome.

GREATER YANG AXIS

Symptomatology includes "painful joints due to pathogenic Cold." It can generate acute or chronic syndromes, or even acute flare-ups within a chronic pattern.

Greater yang is related to the skin, the surface of the body, muscles, the Small Intestine and the Bladder. Muscle involvement (contractures and cramps) is significant in this case: it is not necessarily limited to the greater yang area. A useful point in this case is BL-57 *(cheng shan)*. This point is located on the posterior aspect of the calf, in the middle, just below the belly of the gastrocnemius muscle, eight units below the popliteal crease. Its symptomatology includes myalgia, muscle spasms and cramps, as well as tight, painful tendons. It is an excellent point for traumatic contusions, and is also indicated for some lower back pain related to the yang Linking vessel. It relaxes the sinews and is prescribed for the greater yang pattern with significant muscle involvement.

A greater yang axis diagnosis is established by the presence of:

- signs or syndromes along its pathway (e.g., frontal sinusitis)
- muscle symptoms
- discrete intestinal or urinary disorders
- invasion of Wind-Cold
- occasionally skin diseases.

The greater yang axis is connected to the integration of the "celestial rule" in man. This rule ideally corresponds to a natural order of life, a cosmic order of all living beings in the same universal time, and specific to each being. It does not correspond to an artificial order. Because it is a celestial rule, it corresponds to the father, representative and mediator of the order, or of an order. Whatever the case, each one of us, after having been subjected until adolescence to an external order (usually paternal), needs to find in himself his own order in life. Most of the time, people with problems relating to these matters develop a greater yang pathology.

Treatments differ depending on whether it is an acute or chronic polyarticular painful syndrome.

- For acute disorders, *Great Compendium of Acupuncture (Zhen jiu da cheng)* recommends needling the sea point BL-40 *(wei zhong)*, which is indicated for moving pain and Wind painful obstruction, along with the connecting point BL-58 *(fei yang)*, which is indicated for joint Wind and panarthralgia.
- For chronic disorders, we prefer needling the sea point BL-40 *(wei zhong)* as well as SI-9 *(jian zhen),* which is indicated for Wind painful obstruction with paresthesia of the limbs. SI-9 *(jian zhen)* is also said to be the originating point of the greater yang energy. We might also treat other points depending on the symptomatology and typology of the patient.

PRIMARY CHANNELS

Leg Lesser Yang

The leg lesser yang governs the bones *(Divine Pivot,* chapter 10). It is involved in such problems as stiff joints, generalized painful joints, and acute and chronic inflammation of the joints. The pain it causes is often aggravated by rotation as well as dampness.

In addition to signs manifesting along its pathway (e.g., headaches), the diagnosis will be supported by the presence of Gallbladder disorders such as vertigo, bitter taste, sighs and a lusterless complexion. A primary Gallbladder disorder affecting its channel, or an invasion of the yang Linking or Girdle vessels, must be ruled out.

The most commonly used points are GB-11 *(tou qiao yin)*, GB-30 *(huan tiao)*, GB-38 *(yang fu)*, GB-41 *(zu lin qi)* and GB-43 *(xia xi)*. GB-39 *(xuan zhong)* can also be used, as was discussed above.

- GB-11 *(tou qiao yin)* is indicated for muscle contractures of the limbs; it is located in the hollow posterior to the mastoid process, above GB-12 *(wan gu)*. It is said to be the quintessential point of the leg lesser yang energy. We often treat GB-11 *(tou qiao yin)* and GB-44 *(zu qiao yin)* together for chronic disorders due to direct invasion of this channel.
- GB-30 *(huan tiao)* is located at the posterosuperior angle of the greater trochanter, with the patient lying in a lateral recumbent position, top leg bent. It is indicated for Wind-Damp painful obstruction with impairment in function or disability. It is often needled in association with LI-18 *(fu tu)* and ST-39 *(xia ju xu)* for Wind-Damp-Cold painful obstruction, to fight these three pathogenic energies. We tonify this point for pathogenic invasion of the leg lesser yang channel.
- GB-38 *(yang fu)*, GB-41 *(zu lin qi)* and GB-43 *(xia xi)* are specifically indicated for moving joint pain. GB-38 *(yang fu)* is the river or "unloading" point of the channel Qi. GB-41 *(zu lin qi)* is a stream point and the confluent point communicating with the Girdle channel; we will discuss it further when we talk about this vessel. GB-43 *(xia xi)* tonifies the Wood phase, and will be discussed when we study this phase. For now, what is important to know is that GB-38 *(yang fu)* is indicated for acute or chronic generalized joint pain with no specific location. It can also be used to drain an excess of Wood when this process does not generate any joint manifestations.
- It is worth mentioning that GB-4 *(han yan)* is indicated for acute joint disorders with sweating.
- Other points on the leg lesser yang channel may be needled according to the other presenting symptoms.

Leg Terminal Yin

This channel is involved in either acute or chronic

polyarticular syndromes. The diagnosis will be determined by the presence of associated lower back pain with inability to bend forward or backward, an effect on the external genitals, inguinal or scrotal hernia, vomiting with a stifling sensation in the chest, and urinary dysfunctions (retention or incontinence).

The most frequently prescribed points are LR-2 *(xing jian)*, LR-4 *(zhong feng)*, LR-6 *(zhong du)* and LR-7 *(xi guan)*.

- LR-2 *(xing jian)*, which also drains the Wood phase, is used for acute syndromes.
- LR-4 *(zhong feng)* is the river or "unloading" point. It is indicated when all the joints are painful and walking is difficult. In our opinion, it is best used for treating chronic conditions.
- LR-6 *(zhong du)*, cleft point of "disobstruction," is more appropriate for disorders of recent origin, as are all cleft points. It is especially useful when the obstruction is traumatic, psychological or secondary to the invasion of a pathogenic influence.
- LR-7 *(xi guan)* is located three units below the medial crease of the popliteal fossa. Its symptomatology includes painful joints and rheumatism of the joints. The knee problem is constant in this case, and walking is impossible.

Arm Yang Brightness

This channel is involved in polyarthralgia related to Heat or Intestinal pathology. For Hot disorders the most efficient point is LI-11 *(qu chi)*, a sea point that "expels or cools Heat and makes the joints flexible." It is used whether the Heat is of internal origin or is due to poor ventilation of the Fluids by the Lungs (see "Disruption of the Lungs" below).

Some rheumatism seems to be linked to an Intestinal pathology, which is definitely improved by focusing the therapy on this Organ. Three points are especially useful in this respect: LI-8 *(xia lian)*, LI-13 *(shou wu li)* and GV-3 *(yao yang guan)*.

- LI-8 *(xia lian)* is indicated for all types of rheumatism, Wind-Damp-Cold painful obstruction, and painful obstruction with anxiety.
- LI-13 *(shou wu li)* is involved in Wind- and Dampness-induced joint rheumatism. It is an important point for vitality, as noted in chapter 3 of *Divine Pivot*.
- GV-3 *(yao yang guan)*, located below the spinal process of L4, between the two BL-25 *(da chang shu)* associated points of the Large Intestine, corresponds from our

perspective to the Large Intestine as "the ground of the Lungs." It receives, transports and coordinates the Qi sent down by the latter Organ. *Great Compendium of Acupuncture* prescribes this point for Wind painful obstruction with functional disability.

CURIOUS VESSELS

Both Heel vessels, together with the Girdle and yang Linking vessels, are often involved in chronic polyarticular painful syndromes. They should be thoroughly investigated.

Heel Vessels

The Heel vessels are responsible for moving (migratory) joint pain which becomes aggravated at night (yin Heel) or during the day (yang Heel). In such cases, general muscle stiffness is virtually a constant feature.

In addition, typical symptoms of the Heel vessels are present. For the yin Heel vessel these would include sleep disorders and pelvic signs (constipation, delayed menstruation, dysmenorrhea, infertility), and for the yang Heel vessel, acne and cutaneous suppurations. Teary eyes and conjunctivitis relating to BL-1 *(jing ming)* are manifestations of problems with either Heel vessel.

Needle KI-6 *(zhao hai)* and KI-8 *(jiao xin)* for the yin Heel, and BL-59 *(fu yang)* and BL-62 *(shen mai)* for the yang Heel. KI-6 *(zhao hai)*, located one unit below the tip of the medial malleolus, and BL-62 *(shen mai)*, located 0.5 unit below the tip of the lateral malleolus, are the confluent points for these two vessels. KI-8 *(jiao xin)*, located two units above the most prominent part of the medial malleolus, posterior to the medial border of the tibia, and BL-59 *(fu yang)*, located at the same level between the fibula and the Achilles tendon, are their "disobstruction" cleft points.

The Heel vessels harmonize the yin and the yang; they ground us and rule temporality, particularly diurnal and nocturnal temporality. Once the diagnosis of a Heel vessel disorder has been established, the practitioner will be able to find the origin by examining the areas encompassed by their functions: harmony within oneself (e.g., between the masculine and the feminine), or with significant others (marriage), or with inner, family or geographical roots.

Girdle Vessel

Problems with the Girdle vessel can lead to pain in all the joints, most often accompanied by lower back pain radiating toward the abdomen. Besides the pain, other

Girdle vessel signs are present: pelvic heaviness, cystitis, tenesmus or colic, painful uterine contractions, endometriosis, dysmenorrhea, irregular menstruation, leukorrhea, lower abdomen spasms, and in men, testicular inflammation or pain.

For polyarticular painful syndromes originating from the Girdle vessel, tonify GB-26 *(dai mai)* and GB-41 *(zu lin qi)*.

• GB-26 *(dai mai)*, located on the axillary line, level with the umbilicus, is the representative of this vessel: its name means Girdle vessel.
• GB-41 *(zu lin qi)*, located between the fourth and fifth metatarsals, distal to their junction, is the confluent point of this vessel. It is indicated for moving painful obstruction and moving joint pain. It reinforces the action of BL-62 *(shen mai)*, which, as the confluent point of the yang Heel vessel, is one of the important points for erratic pain.

Patients with Girdle vessel dysfunction are disoriented, scattered, go in different directions simultaneously, and do a thousand things at the same time, without any particular purpose. This scatteredness is sustained by a considerable energy that overrides all signs of fatigue.

Yang Linking Vessel

Dysfunctions of the yang Linking vessel cause pain in the muscles, joints and even the bones (at the site of fractures). This pain is highly sensitive to variations in the weather and even barometric pressure. These are the patients who can anticipate changes in the weather.

The yang Linking vessel has many different functions. The one that is altered in these cases is the regulation of the body's yang (lateral and superficial) areas. This disruption often corresponds to a need for protection against the external environment (because of the aggressive nature of the environment or the patient's sensitive nature), or is a result of being confined or imprisoned.

For this type of pain needle TB-5 *(wai guan)*, the confluent point of the yang Linking vessel. Add GB-41 *(zu lin qi)*, its paired confluent point, if there is moving pain. GB-35 *(yang jiao)*, the cleft point of the yang Linking vessel, is added in cases of Wind-predominant painful obstruction.

Great Spleen Collateral

The symptomatology of disturbances in the great Spleen collateral is summarized in chapter 10 of *Divine Pivot*: "If excess, the whole body is painful; if deficiency, the joints are flaccid." Its command point, SP-21 *(da bao)*, is located in the sixth intercostal space on the anterior axillary line. This point is indicated for the following symptoms: "general stiffness, whole body pain, muscle pain, asthenia of the limbs." According to *Divine Pivot* (chapter 10), it allows "the Fluids originating from the Stomach to nourish all the different parts of the body. . . . This vessel is like the reticular mesh in relation to the Blood." This has been interpreted to mean that it is a good point for treating Blood stasis.

We use this point to treat chronic polyarticular painful syndromes with paresthesia or a poor distribution of Fluids to the joints (atrophic disorders and Heat signs).

Organ Pathologies

Three Organs are involved: the Kidneys (more specifically the Kidney yang), the Liver in relation to the etheric soul *(hún)*, and the Lungs.

Kidney Yang Deficiency

Kidney yang corresponds first and foremost to GV-4 *(ming men)*, which is located below the spinal process of the second lumbar vertebra. According to several ancient texts, including *Great Compendium of Acupuncture and Moxibustion* and *Classified Classic (Lei jing)* , it should be tonified in treating such problems as steaming bone disorder, moving pain in the limbs, as well as stabbing and generalized joint pain.

The diagnosis is determined by the presence of physical, mental and sexual fatigue, with chills, accompanied by a false sensation of fever, and deep internal cold in the lumbar area extending to the lower limbs. Obesity is a telltale sign, as is rectal prolapse, frequent urination, or urinary incontinence. This deficiency can either be constitutional or acquired through overwork or excessive sexual activity.

Liver Disorders Treated with BL-47 *(hun men)*

BL-47 *(hun men)*, located on the lateral branch of the Bladder channel, level with GV-8 *(jin suo)* and BL-18 *(gan shu)*, corresponds to the *hún* which rules the somatic or psychological "comings and goings" during wakefulness or sleep. Its symptomatology includes chronic rheumatism, contracture of the sinews, bone pain, muscle spasms and polyarticular pain.

Diagnosis is determined by a history of fainting or sleep-walking, pain in the heart area radiating toward the back and the chest, and various hepatic-generated digestive disorders.

Its disruption always corresponds to a limitation of the "comings and goings" mechanisms. The origin of these should be discovered through the history within the life of the patient.

DISRUPTION OF THE LUNGS

The Lungs are involved in the functioning of the joints at two different levels:

- by their action on the ventilation and distribution of the Fluids
- by their "rulings and joints" function, as noted in *Basic Questions,* chapter 8.[3]

When the distribution of Fluids to the joints is obstructed, Heat-type chronic rheumatism is generated with joint swelling, redness, heat and pain. We do not know to what type of disorder we can attribute the impairment of the "rulings and joints" function.

Besides LI-11 *(qu chi),* which was discussed previously, three other points, all located on the arm greater yin channel, are involved: LU-3 *(tian fu),* LU-8 *(jing qu)* and LU-10 *(yu ji).*

- LU-3 *(tian fu)* is located on the radial side of the biceps muscle, three units below the end of the axillary fold, where the nose touches the biceps when one lifts the arm. In our opinion this point is the most important one for the upward rebellion of Lung Qi. It is indicated for chronic rheumatism and for "sudden" painful obstruction. Its symptomatology includes excess energy in the head due to the upward rebellion of Lung Qi (memory loss and cephalic, ocular or nasal congestion) as well as pulmonary signs.
- LU-8 *(jing qu),* river-Dryness point, is indicated for severe rheumatism, and sudden painful obstruction with dyspnea.
- LU-10 *(yu ji),* spring-Heat point, is indicated for generalized or moving rheumatism. It is said to cool Lung Heat.

We therefore tonify LU-8 *(jing qu)* and LU-10 *(yu ji)* with LI-11 *(qu chi)* for Heat disorders due to poor distribution of the Fluids by the Lungs. We tonify LU-3 *(tian fu)* when excess energy in the head and pulmonary signs point to an upward rebellion of Lung Qi.

Finally, we have to determine why the Lungs have been affected. This can be a laborious process, but it is necessary to differentiate what is hereditary from what is acquired, and the origins and methods of the acquired etiology.

Disruption in One of the Five Revolutions

This subject does not concern the Five Phases, but rather the Five Revolutions *(wǔ yùn)* which, along with the Six Qi, the Ten Celestial Stems, and the Twelve Earthly Branches, energetically qualify each moment in time. All of this is analyzed in detail in *Basic Questions* (chapters 66~74).

To us the Five Revolutions are an aspect of the synchronization between the energies of humans and those of the cosmos. The cosmic energies regulate all activities on earth. When there is a disharmony between the cosmos and earth, pathologies can occur that are characteristically unexpected, sudden and intense, without obvious precipitants.

The occurrence of polyarticular pain is mentioned in the four possible instances described immediately below. Most of the time the symptoms are acute, recurrent and apparently spontaneous; besides joint pain, they involve the channels as well as (more discretely) their paired Organs. A disruption in the Five Revolutions can contribute to the emergence of chronic disorders.

DEFICIENCY OF THE FIRE PHASE

Deficiency of the Fire phase causes "rheumatoid pain." We suggest treating it by tonifying TB-2 *(ye men)* and TB-3 *(zhong zhu).* The latter is the tonification point of the Fire Phase.

DEFICIENCY OF THE WOOD PHASE

Deficiency of the Wood phase generates pain "outside the joints." We address it by tonifying LR-3 *(tai chong),* the stream and source point, and GB-43 *(xia xi),* a tonification point often prescribed for moving joint pain.

EASING OF THE FIRE PHASE

Easing or slackening of the Fire phase is always a consequence of a deficiency in another phase. This easing generates "moving joint pain." Draining TB-10 *(tian jing),* the sea point indicated for Wind painful obstruction, can correct the effects of this imbalance.

GREATER YIN RULING IN HEAVEN

When the greater yin rules in Heaven, Dampness dominates and polyarticular syndromes may appear. SP-5 *(shang qiu)*, the draining river-Dryness point, is indicated for painful joints and bones, and to remove Dampness. This point corrects the symptoms generated by this ruling in Heaven.

We have reviewed the most frequently encountered patterns responsible for polyarticular painful syndromes. The practitioner must determine which two or three patterns are involved for each patient. After doing so, and depending on the intensity of the symptoms, the presence of pathogenic Qi, the status of the Qi, Blood and Fluids, as well as the physical and mental constitution of each patient—we must then establish an acupuncture treatment protocol.

Sometimes other therapeutic modalities are deemed necessary, but we recommend that they not be implemented or modified when acupuncture treatment is initiated, so as not to introduce other variables.

Chapter Notes

1. We have asked J.-M. Kespi, M.D., to write this chapter, which reflects specific research and experience conducted by the French Acupuncture Association, of which he is the president.
2. All of the quoted material in this chapter comes from Soulié de Morant (1972), unless otherwise noted.
3. Note that some believe that the phrase *zhì jié* 治節 should more properly be translated as "control and restraint."

CHAPTER TEN

Degenerative Joint Disease

THIS CHRONIC NONINFLAMMATORY arthropathy, also known as osteoarthritis, combines destructive alterations of the joint cartilage with epiphyseal bone modifications. It is a particularly good indication for acupuncture, both to alleviate the painful flare-ups and to treat the chronic condition, especially when used in combination with other traditional Chinese medical modalities. In modern Chinese this disease is called *guān jié bìng*, which simply means joint disease.

In addition to purely mechanical causes, this so-called primary degenerative joint disease involves partly, or in their entirety, several interlocking and mutually supporting energetic mechanisms. These mechanisms contribute to the chronic progressive and degenerative nature of the disorder.

INNATE ENERGIES

Innate energies are those which underlie certain familiar genetic predispositions over which we have no control. Tonifying the source Qi is recommended in all patients by applying moxa at BL-23 *(shen shu)*, GV-4 *(ming men)* and CV-4 *(guan yuan)*.

PATHOGENIC INFLUENCES

Cold and Dampness predominate within the painful obstruction framework. Besides traditional diagnosis, a radiological examination adds, in our experience, a very useful investigational tool to identify the involved pathogenic Qi. X-rays showing different degrees of pinching in the joint structure, marginal osteophytosis and subchondral densification of the bone with synovial cysts (geodes) point to the presence of Cold when they are well-defined and their shapes are clearly visible, whereas prevalent Dampness makes the contours blurry, dappled and irregular. Treatment of these pathogenic influences follows the principles previously discussed.

FLUIDS

As we have seen in part one, the *yè* portion of the Fluids drain and nourish the joints, bones, brain and marrow. A passage in chapter 36 of *Divine Pivot* describes what happens when this function is disrupted:

> When the yin and yang are not harmonized, the *yè* deviate and drain into the yin [lower orifices]. The marrow *yè* decrease on the whole and go down; when they drop too low, deficiency occurs. Due to this deficiency, the hips and lower back hurt and the neck is painful.

Similarly, a passage in chapter 29 of *Basic Questions* explains the role of the Spleen in this pathology:

> If the limbs cannot receive the Qi from food and water, they become weaker and weaker every day. The yin pathways close down, the vessel pathways are not open, and the

sinews, bones and flesh, deprived of their life-giving Qi, become disabled.

Another passage in chapter 30 of *Divine Pivot* notes that, "When the *yè* Fluids are exhausted, the bones [joints] have difficulty flexing and extending."

Kidneys

The Kidneys, "governor of the bones" and preserver of the Essence, can only weaken with age, while degenerative joint disease often progresses.

Local Factors

There are local factors that will, for various reasons, transform a joint into a real energetic barrier, obstructing the free circulation of Qi. These give focus to the arthritic location and generate painful flare-ups. To alleviate these painful episodes, we need to restore the free circulation of Qi locally by regulating the channels, the barriers and the local "disobstruction" points, in accordance with the characteristic symptoms of the condition. If Dampness predominates, we can follow the method prescribed in chapter 43 of *Basic Questions*: needle the yang sea points and yin stream points, or use warm needles.

Treatment of the root cause depends on the pathogenic mechanisms involved in each individual case. The efficacy of acupuncture is such, particularly in the successful management of acute flare-ups, that it should be an integral part of the therapeutic tools used today to treat degenerative joint disease. Massage and herbs are useful adjuncts.

Chapters 17 through 23 below discuss the treatment of pain in various parts of the body. When degenerative joint disease occurs in a particular area, it will be useful to read the appropriate chapter.

CHAPTER ELEVEN

Rheumatoid Arthritis

C ONTEMPORARY RHEUMATOLOGY IS undergoing transformations which subtly yet continually modify its framework. It is shifting progressively from Laennec's method of clinical examination, and from a radiological description, to a pathophysiological approach combining different aspects of immunology, and leading us to the frontier of systemic diseases. Rheumatoid arthritis is a typical example. We believe that it will be useful to compare the biomedical approach to these problems with that of traditional Chinese medicine, which early on developed its own methodology regarding osteoarticular disorders.

Background

Rheumatoid arthritis (RA) is a disabling inflammatory disease, with joint lesions secondary to a chronic synovitis responsible for the formation of pannus, a true localized malignant inflammatory proliferation, as well as chondrocyte diseases. It has an immunological origin, under the dual action of humoral immunity (immune complex) and cell-mediated immunity. It is self-sustained. Extra-articular conditions characterize the systemic rheumatoid disease: rheumatoid nodules, pleuropulmonary, vascular and pericardial manifestations, along with fever. These often alternate with articular manifestations.

From a pathogenic point of view, it appears to be a multiple factor condition.

Genetic factors: These include excessive expression of class II HLA antigens:
- DR4 (DW4, DW14): over 60 percent of Caucasians
- DR1: significant among Jews
- DR3: promotes intolerance to gold salts or D-penicillamine

Environmental factors: The most important of these are infections. Among those implicated in RA are Epstein-Barr virus (EBV) and cytomegalovirus (CMV).

Hormonal factors: There is a preponderance of women among those who develop RA (three women to every man). This proportion decreases after menopause, and pregnancy is a favorable factor. The effects of female hormonal therapy are controversial.

Because the viral induction of RA theory is today gaining more and more credibility, the Chinese concept of linking rheumatic disorders to exogenous pathologies demonstrates a high level of insight.

The presence in RA of common epitopes between inducting germs and the HLA groups was validated in 1988 with the discovery of a six-amino-acid polypeptide (gp 110) common between the Epstein-Barr virus capsid and a DR4, DR1 and DW14 antigenic subunit (Roudier, 1988). Thus, when a viral agent possesses a common antigen with the "biological self," the antibody produced by the threatened body to protect itself attacks, through the common marker, the "biological self."

In light of this modern research, the response given by Qi Bo to the Yellow Emperor in chapter 27 of *Divine Pivot* when asked about fixed painful obstruction is most interesting:

> Wind, Cold and Damp [pathogenic] Qi settle externally in the intramuscular spaces. Their attack produces a humor *(mò)* [from the Fluids]. Under the influence of Cold, the humor clusters. This clustering separates the muscular layers, which split up. With this splitting there is pain. With the pain the spirit [protective Qi] returns there. When the spirit returns there is heat. With heat the pain is relieved. When the pain is relieved there is inversion *(jué)* [cooling down]. With this inversion other [areas of] painful obstruction develop. When they develop, they have similar features.

Rheumatoid Arthritis in Traditional Chinese Medicine

In modern Chinese this disease is called *lèi fēng shī xìng guān jié bìng*, which literally means "Wind-Dampness-like type of joint disease." This appellation clearly situates RA within the exogenous disease *(wài gǎn)* group.

Generally speaking, RA is considered to be part of the painful obstruction clinical framework. Some authors are more inclined to put it in the panarthralgia *(lì jié bìng)* category, due to the bone and joint involvement, and the importance of joint deformations. Other authors disagree with this classification, claiming that panarthralgia is but one aspect of painful obstruction disorder. From a factual perspective, RA presents with different stages of evolution, which can be identified.

BEGINNING STAGE

At the onset, RA may pass for an externally contracted invasion of Wind, or can go completely undetected. When it is the former, it is usually due to Cold and Damp pathogenic influences. At this stage the pathogenic Qi obstructs the circulation of (normal) Qi and congeals in the channels and collaterals. This causes the protective and nutritive Qi to stagnate, and there is no longer communication between them.

A predominance of Cold is characterized by intense pain, which is aggravated by cold and alleviated by warmth. It is often more intense at night than during the day. There are no local signs of inflammation, and the pain may actually be accompanied by a sensation of cold.

Typically, the tongue coating is white and thin, and the pulse is submerged and wiry.

A predominance of Dampness manifests as heaviness of the body, fixed joint pain, sensitivity to the weather, especially dampness, which can trigger painful crises. These symptoms are accompanied by numbness and paresthesia, swelling and a progressive deformation of the joints. The tongue coating is white and greasy, and the pulse is submerged and choppy.

The condition may progress according to a Heat pattern, which will occur when latent Heat, from a latent pathogenic influence, is reactivated by a new external pathogenic invasion, or when Wind-Damp-Cold stagnation in the channels progressively transforms into Heat.

The ensuing pattern is an inflammatory condition with its traditional assorted symptoms: localized pain, redness, heat and swelling, which can be accompanied by fever during crises. Patients describe the pain as hot, burning and as a shooting sensation. The intensity of pain is high, and is more pronounced during the later hours of the night. Pain persists in the morning and is accompanied by a sensation of stiffening, which prevents the patient from freely moving the joints. The tongue coating is yellow, and the pulse is wiry and fast.

CHRONIC STAGE

The beginning stage described above may last several months or years. Sometimes it does not progress beyond that point. But more often the condition progresses, even if on an intermittent basis, toward an aggravation which manifests as a worsening of the joints already affected or an invasion of other joints, and more rarely, as a condition which affects the viscera.

At this stage the circulation of Qi and Blood in the channels is markedly slowed, and the Blood and turbid Phlegm stagnate at the level of the joints; this condition is called stubborn painful obstruction *(wán bì)*. The affected joints exhibit signs of chronic inflammation, the pain occurs spontaneously, under pressure, or with movement. Pain and stiffness are particularly acute during the second half of the night and on awakening, and disappear later in the morning or during the day, after a more or less long period of warming up. They are sensitive to the weather. The locations of the deformation depend on the antalgic attitude adopted by the patients. A deep red color of the joints, purple spots on the tongue and a thin, choppy pulse point to Blood stasis. Redness of the joints, fever, a greasy tongue coating and rapid pulse indicate that Damp-Heat has combined with Blood stasis.

If the pain is aggravated by cold and alleviated by warmth, the tongue coating is white and the pulse is slow, then the Wind-Damp-Cold pathogenic influences have penetrated more deeply into the sinews and bones, and have combined with Blood stasis and Phlegm.

This stage in the evolution of rheumatoid arthritis may correspond to panarthralgia, especially if the pain is very severe. This indicates a pre-existing deficiency in the Liver and of the Kidney Essence, inducing stagnation of the Qi and Blood in the joints, which transform into Heat and give rise to Phlegm and Blood stasis. The presence of Phlegm and static Blood causes the joints to swell up and gradually deform.

Depending on the nature of the pathogenic influence involved, the condition can then progress according to a pattern of Cold or Heat:

• Cold pattern: severe arthralgia which affects several joints successively and impairs their range of motion, and which is aggravated by cold and alleviated by warmth
• Heat pattern: the joints are very inflamed, accompanied by typical symptoms of Heat.

EXTRA-ARTICULAR MANIFESTATIONS

Fever

There is often no fever between crises, but the fever can be quite high during flare-ups. The nature of the fever can indicate which pathogenic influence is involved:

• high fever with aversion to cold and absence of sweating indicates Wind-Cold
• moderate fever that is not abated by sweating indicates Wind-Dampness
• high fever with aversion to wind that is not abated by sweating indicates Heat
• fever at night indicates yin deficiency.

Subcutaneous Nodules

The presence of freely movable, painless nodules over bony prominences is considered by some to be virtually a pathognomonic sign of rheumatoid arthritis, and certainly does usually indicate a positive rheumatoid factor. They occur in 10 to 20 percent of the cases and are located on the posterior aspect of the forearms, along the ulnar crest, near the elbows or on the dorsal aspect of the fingers. In Chinese medicine they indicate a knotting of turbid Phlegm in the collaterals.

Visceral Disorders

Pleuropulmonary, pericardial, splenic and renal disorders can be interpreted as a spreading of the painful obstruction internally, as described in chapter 43 of *Basic Questions* (translated below in chapter 24). Rheumatoid vasculitis corresponds to vessel painful obstruction. Ocular disorders can result from several mechanisms, such as the localization of anatomical correspondences of the Wood or Fire phase, or the involvement of the yang or yin Heel vessels. Sjögren's syndrome indicates that the Fluids have been affected.

EVOLUTION

The severe and malignant forms of this disorder, characterized by rapid progression of the articular lesions and the emergence of a necrotic angiitis, are related to Toxic Heat.

After several years of evolution, rheumatoid arthritis may gradually disappear, leaving residual Qi and Blood deficiency, yang deficiency or yin deficiency, depending on the case.

Treatment Principles

The treatment of rheumatoid arthritis is especially complex. It involves different stages which, according to the circumstances, focus on either treating the root cause or the symptoms. Acupuncture is very often used as merely an adjunct to conventional medical treatment, permitting a lower dosage of drugs, and thereby limiting their toxicity and side effects.

Treatment of the root cause addresses the following goals:

• elimination of the painful obstruction
• tonification of the true Qi
• harmonization of the nutritive and protective Qi
• promotion of the circulation of Blood and Qi
• opening of the channels
• strengthening of the affected anatomico-energetic structure
• restoration, if necessary, of the energetic balance of the pelvic Qi
• support of the innate Qi, particularly the source Qi.

The symptomatic treatment:

• eliminates the external pathogenic influences
• restores the free circulation of Qi at the level of the joints
• alleviates pain.

The selection of points corresponding to these mechanisms has already been addressed, and the approach to treatment of specific areas is discussed in chapters 17~23. Whatever the circumstances, acupuncture must be combined with herbs and modifications in the diet; its therapeutic efficacy is then quite significant, which allows it to be integrated with conventional therapies.

12

Ankylosing Spondylitis

In modern Chinese the name of this disease is *fēng shī xìng jǐ zhù yán,* or literally "Wind-Dampness-type spinal column inflammation." It is thus considered to have a direct connection with exogenous diseases such as rheumatoid arthritis.

Ankylosing spondylitis is particularly interesting from the perspective of acupuncture because it combines several symptoms which are easy to identify on an energetic level. Indeed, we observe:

• a pelvic syndrome affecting particularly the sacroiliac joints, with a typical pain pattern that is located in the buttocks, occurs in the morning, and diminishes as one warms up

• a spinal syndrome characterized by stiffness which progresses upward, accompanied by night or morning pain, and which diminishes after one warms up. This stage precedes the deformation stage.

• an articular syndrome which generates peripheral arthritis mostly affecting the lower limbs. There is also arthritis of the proximal joints of the extremities, primarily the hips, but sometimes the shoulders.

• inflammation at the insertion of ligaments, tendons and capsules with the bones, known as enthesitis. This most commonly affects the heel, spinous processes and greater trochanter.

• extra-articular complications, which include such problems as iridocyclitis or anterior uveitis, a cardiac condition characterized by aortic insufficiency, uremia from amyloidosis, or upper lobe fibrosis of the lungs that can mimic tuberculosis.

This disease targets young men between the age of twenty and thirty; there is a hereditary predisposition component, confirmed by the presence of the HLA B27 antigen.

This brief overview enables us to consider several possible interlocking energetic mechanisms, all contributing to the chronic aspect of this disorder.

Importance of the Prenatal Qi

The prenatal Qi governs a person's organization, creation and continual re-creation. It is concentrated in the area located below, anterior to and between the Kidneys, below the umbilicus in the pelvis. The gate of vitality *(mìng mén)* is its gateway. It is transported by the Curious vessels, which originate in the Kidneys and in the heel of the foot, and is transmitted to the Curious Organs, especially the bones. The circumstances surrounding this disease, its hereditary nature, the age of onset and the location of symptoms all coalesce to substantiate the hypothesis that disturbances of the prenatal Qi are involved in the genesis of this disorder.

The prenatal Qi promotes proper function in:

- the pelvis, reservoir of the prenatal Qi, through the following points: GV-4 *(ming men)*, CV-8 *(shen qu)*, CV-4 *(guan yuan)* and BL-23 *(shen shu)*
- the Governing vessel, sea of the yang, which gathers all the body's yang and supports life itself. Its pathway establishes an intimate link with the spine-tree of life, representing the being's vertical axis and meeting place of dualities, through the following points: GV-1 *(chang qiang)* and BL-11 *(da zhu)*.
- the yin and yang Heel vessels, which ground life in its yin and yang aspects, and which account (when in a state of imbalance) for predominant symptoms such as rigidity and stiffness, morning pain, with a localization centered around the "hips' barrier," the "heels' barrier," the shoulders and the eyes. Regulation of these vessels is achieved by needling their confluent and cleft points, BL-62 *(shen mai)*, BL-59 *(fu yang)*, KI-6 *(zhao hai)* and KI-8 *(jiao xin)*, as well as the command points of the heels' and hips' barriers, BL-61 *(pu shen)* and GB-29 *(ju liao)* respectively.

GENERAL DISRUPTION OF THE QI'S MOVEMENT

A yin-type stagnation due to sluggish or deficient yang is indicated by such signs as increased severity of symptoms at night or in the early morning, which is ameliorated by mild movement; progression toward stiffness and kyphosis due to yin accumulation; and improvement with the application of warmth, massage or movement. The causative factors can only be identified by an eight-parameter analysis; the lesser yang level is frequently involved, as well as a point such as BL-31 *(shang liao)*, which promotes movement to disperse pelvic yin stagnation.

DAMP-COLD PATHOGENIC INFLUENCES

Dampness and Cold are triggering or aggravating factors for crises. Their elimination is achieved by following the previously discussed principles.

To be effective, treatment must take these different elements into account by emphasizing slow, prolonged and deeply penetrating moxibustion. Combined with Chinese-style massage and body-centered techniques to promote the movement of Qi, the patient's comfort will be significantly increased.

DISRUPTION OF THE YANG ORGANS

In our experience, it is always important to check the functions of the Large Intestine and/or Gallbladder, which should be regulated if found to be imbalanced.

CHAPTER THIRTEEN

Postmenopausal Osteoporosis[1]

THE CONSEQUENCES OF postmenopausal osteo-porosis and associated fractures involve enor-mous financial costs as well as considerable physical disability and many premature deaths. Consequently, the public, health professionals and policy makers have become increasingly concerned with the prevention of this disease.

Can acupuncture and herbal therapy provide a viable preventive measure, particularly for people who cannot take hormonal medication? Such is the issue raised in this chapter. An understanding of the energetic mechanisms of osteoporosis according to Chinese medicine may offer a possible component in its prevention and treatment. Only a long-term prospective study can possibly provide confirmation.

Menopause and Modern Biomedicine

According to the Group for Research and Information on Osteoporosis (GRIO, France 1990), osteoporosis is de-fined as bone depletion, whereby the bone's mechanical resistance is compromised during normal daily activities.

PATHOGENESIS

Bone tissue depletion is the result of an imbalance between the osteoclasts, which activate bone resorption, and the osteoblasts, which activate bone formation. The deficit can be the result of either an acceleration in cellular changes, resorption overtaking formation, or a marked depression of bone formation.

Reduction in bone mass explains the occurrence of spontaneous fractures, or those due to minimal trauma, including the hip, distal forearm, vertebrae and other bones. The breaking point is reached when the bone mass has diminished to a value below which the bone's physio-logical mechanical resistance is compromised.

EPIDEMIOLOGY

The amount of bone mass is related to important ethnic variations in a descending scale: African-Americans > Polynesians > Hispanics > Caucasians > Asians, respec-tively. According to S. R. Cummings (1985), the incidence of hip fractures doubles every ten years after age 70. In a 50-year-old woman, the risk of such a fracture represents a higher mortality risk than does breast cancer. Furthermore, the overall risk of hip fracture during a Caucasian woman's life is 30 percent, compared to a 9 percent risk for breast cancer. This frequency varies from one country to another, with the highest ratios found in developed countries.

Risk Factors

Epidemiological surveys have helped identify certain risk factors associated with bone mass deficiency:

• Caucasian or Asian descent
• female
• below average height and weight
• low calcium intake, especially during adolescence and after menopause
• early menopause and long periods of amenorrhea
• immobilization for several months
• anorexia
• sedentary life style and lack of physical activity
• prolonged steroid therapy
• certain endocrine dysfunctions: hyperthyroidism, diabetes
• nicotine addiction
• alcoholism.

Conversely, obesity seems to play a protective role.

Preventive Treatment

The only recommended preventive treatment is estrogen-progesterone or simply estrogen therapy. In France only 4 to 5 percent of menopausal women receive hormone replacement therapy, although more than eight million women are affected. Can Chinese medicine offer an alternative?

Menopause in Chinese Medicine

Both the male and female climacteric are physiological stages described in the first chapter of *Basic Questions* : "In a seven times seven [49-year-old woman], the Conception vessel is deficient, the Penetrating vessel becomes weak and meager, the heavenly dew [sexual energy] is exhausted, the earth passageways [of the menstrual period] are blocked, so the form is wasted and there is infertility." For men the process starts at seven times eight years and ends at eight times eight years. During this time, the Liver Qi weakens, the sinews can no longer move, the heavenly dew is exhausted, the Essence diminishes, the body passes its limit, and the teeth and hair fall out.

The contemporary term for menopause in Chinese is *gēng nián qī*. The word *gēng* means to change, to modify, to take the place of, to replace, to alternate; *nían* means year or age; and *qī* means time, period, phase or fixed period of time.

Deficiency of Kidney Qi, manifested when the Essence begins to diminish at 49 years of age, is therefore the root cause of menopause. Because of this, the Penetrating and Conception vessels lack adequate nourishment, the Blood and Essence are insufficient, and the yin and yang are imbalanced. Consequently, women may develop symptoms arising from deficiency of Kidney yin or yang. Those symptoms can eventually disturb the function of the other Organs, especially deficiency of the Heart and the Spleen, which then leads to an imbalance of the Qi and Blood.

Contemporary Chinese describe the following patterns:

Deficiency of Kidney and Liver Yin

Due to the weakening of the Kidneys and depletion of yin, the Liver becomes malnourished and the Liver yang Qi rises, accentuating the imbalance of yin and yang.

Excess or blazing Fire due to Water deficiency manifests in the following symptoms: profuse sweating and intermittent low fever, irritability, anxiety, emotional lability, sensation of heat in the five centers (palms of the hands, soles of the feet, and midsternal region), a sense of pressure in the rib cage, distention of the hypochondrium, heartburn, vertigo, headache, dizziness, palpitations, insomnia, intense dream activity, tinnitus, weakness of the lower back and knees, thirst, dryness of the mouth, redness of the cheeks and constipation. The tip of the tongue is red with a thin coating. The pulse is wiry, thin and rapid. Treatment is directed at bringing down the Fire by nourishing the yin, and augmenting the Kidneys in order to control Liver yang.

When emotional symptoms predominate, for example, sleep disturbances and palpitations, the Heart and Kidneys are no longer in harmony. It is then appropriate to augment the Kidneys, calm the Heart and quiet the Spirit.

When psychological symptoms occur, including depression or melancholy, or there is sighing and yawning, this signifies deficiency of yin and Blood in the Five Organs, which are malnourished. These symptoms are related to an internal stirring of Fire associated with restless Organ disorder (*zàng zào*).

Deficiency of Kidney Yang

When the Kidney yang is deficient, its storing function is deficient. There is a disturbance in the menstrual pattern, including irregularity of menses and either increased or decreased flow. Since the Kidney yang can no longer warm the yin and yang Organs, the following symptoms may appear: pallid complexion, aversion to cold and need for warmth, cold limbs and abdomen, general lassitude, weariness of the lower limbs and lower back pain. The closing function of the Bladder is disturbed, the urine may be clear and abundant, or reduced with signs of incomplete emptying. The tongue is pale with a thin white coating, and the pulse is submerged, thin and weak. The treatment principle is to tonify the Kidneys and warm the yang.

When the Kidney yang is unable to warm the Spleen yang, described as Spleen and Kidney deficiency, the menses are at first irregular and then the signs of Spleen deficiency become evident, including sallow complexion, pasty stool, loss of appetite, loss of taste, asthenia and poor memory. The tongue is pale with a white coating, and the pulse is submerged, thin and weak. It is advisable in this situation to tonify the Spleen and Kidneys and nourish the yang.

DEFICIENCY OF KIDNEY YIN AND YANG

Symptoms of this pattern include vertigo, dizziness, tinnitus, weak lower back, cold limbs, or alternating sensations of cold and heat. The tongue is pale, and the pulse is submerged, thin and weak. In this case it is important to tonify the Kidney yin and yang.

In addition to the patterns described by contemporary Chinese, we think that the menopause process encompasses a sociocultural dimension that should be considered, and which may partly explain the presence or absence of pathology during menopause in the individual.

Menopause, as well as andropause, represents the passage from one stage of life into another, for women the loss of ability to procreate, and the return to a primordial androgyny. It provides the individual with an opportunity for self-realization at another level and on another plane. As a woman becomes acyclical, she enters another phase, one of spiritual realization, accomplishment and preparation for death. From a channel/stage perspective, women are considered to be lesser yin before puberty and greater yin during the child-bearing years. After menopause they are considered to be terminal yin.

When menopause is well-accepted, the woman reaches a state of inner fulfillment, a serenity that prepares her to assume her own mortality. When menopause is resisted or rejected, it can initiate a whole chain of symp-

toms. Perhaps one can see here a basis for the frequent problems linked to menopause, especially in Western societies which reject the signs of aging. This dimension of menopause should lead us to consider that its treatment should not be reduced to medical therapy only, whatever that might be, and that through menopause there is the possibility for reflection on life.

Osteoporosis in Chinese Medicine

The modern concept of the pathology of osteoporosis is not described in traditional Chinese literature. However, we can attempt to describe it from a traditional perspective. We saw that, from a physiological point of view, menopause is defined as deficiency of Blood and Essence, which weakens the internal Organs, along with pelvic yin deficiency, which allows the yang to rise; together they cause the classic hot flashes and other well-known symptoms to appear. As this progresses, the Kidney yin becomes exhausted, and the Essence and *yè* portion of the Fluids diminish. This means that the bone marrow is no longer nourished, resulting in the pathological phenomena of osteoporosis.

Therapeutics

ACUPUNCTURE

Following are general principles regarding the treatment of menopausal disorders. However, as always, each case requires an individualized approach. An energetic concept of menopause provides the framework for preventive treatment which can facilitate changes integral to this transitional time. This shift in time to terminal yin is facilitated by LR-14 *(qi men)*,[2] which regulates the third stage of a woman's life. The preservation of the energetic balance of the pelvis is facilitated through CV-4 *(guan yuan)*, which responds to the source Qi, and KI-4 *(da zhong)*, influential point of the lower burner, as well as CV-7 *(yin jiao)*, which further promotes the movement of the Essence.

To restore the balance of yin and yang by eliminating Heat, use BL-43 *(gao huang shu)*, which regulates and tonifies the Qi and Blood at the level of the Pericardium. According to *Volume Investigating the Points by Following the Channels (Xun jing kao xue)*, this point can affect spontaneous sweating, steaming bone disorder and the Five Consumptions. It can also influence the storage of the *yè* portion of the Fluids. According to the same text,

KI-27 *(shu fu)* treats steaming bone disorder and the "reckless" circulation due to Heat in the Blood in women.

Steaming bone disorder is characterized by Heat generated by dysfunction at the level of the marrow. It relates to consumption and fatigue and is generated by yin deficiency with internal Heat. Steaming bone disorder is marked by "tidal" or intermittent fevers, spontaneous sweating, dyspnea, lack of strength, irritability, light sleeping, heat in the palms of the hands and dark urine. The points for treatment include BL-17 *(ge shu)*, HT-6 *(yin xi)*, BL-13 *(fei shu)*, BL-19 *(dan shu)* and KI-7 *(fu liu)*.

When pathological signs appear, it is important to tonify the Kidney yin with BL-23 *(shen shu)*, BL-52 *(zhi shi)*, KI-15 *(zhong zhu)* and KI-2 *(ran gu)*, as well as the sea of marrow with BL-11 *(da zhu)* and GB-39 *(xuan zhong)*. Addressing any imbalance between the Spleen and Stomach as well as problems involving the Large and Small Intestines can, in some cases, be an essential aspect of the treatment.

PHYTOTHERAPY

Herbal formulas can be useful as part of a program for preventing difficult symptoms of menopause. For patients experiencing a difficult or pathological menopause, herbal treatment should prevent some of the associated consequences. And, for the patient with advanced osteoporosis, although conventional treatment may still be necessary, herbal treatment can be an important adjunct.

Postmenopausal osteoporosis is the result of two concurring phenomena: loss of bone mass linked to age, and the acceleration of the process as a result of menopausal estrogen deficiency.

Preventive treatment should consist of a combination of modalities, including:

• plants known to be estrogen stimulants, which usually correspond to Blood tonics in Chinese medicine
• remineralizing plants, which can nourish the tissues, and which usually correspond to Kidney yin tonics in Chinese medicine.

In the absence of major risk factors, we feel that herbal treatment can constitute an excellent alternative in the prevention of osteoporosis for women undergoing menopause who either do not tolerate or are opposed to hormone replacement therapy. From this perspective, it is not necessary to resort to Chinese plants only, since the Western materia medica offers a wide variety of plants.[3] As our own experience is weighted toward Western phytotherapy, that is what we will discuss below.

Estrogen-stimulating Plants

There are many estrogen-stimulating plants among the Western materia medica. Among these are *Cimicifuga racemosa* (black cohosh), *Angelica archangelica* (angelica), *Cupressus sempervirens* (cypress), *Humulus lupulus* (hops), *Punica granatum* (pomegranate), *Salvia officinalis* (sage), *Panax ginseng* (ginseng) and *Glycyrrhizia glabra* (licorice).

Sample prescriptions:

Sage: 400mg
Sage essential oil: 4mg
Colloidal gel of silica: 20mg
METHOD: One capsule two to three times daily.

or

Angelica M.D.E.[4]: 125ml
Cypress M.D.E: 125ml
METHOD: One tablespoon morning and evening in water.

or

Sage essential oil: 0.03g
Cypress essential oil: 0.02g
Tixosil (or other neutral base in a quantity sufficient to fill an enteric-coated size): no. 2 capsule
METHOD: One to two capsules, morning and evening.

Progesterone-stimulating Plants

The category of progesterone-stimulating plants includes *Alchemilla vulgaris* (lady's mantle), *Vitex agnus castus* (chaste tree) and *Lithospermum officinale* [also *L. erythrorhizon*] (gromwell root).

Sample prescription:

Lady's mantle: 0.15gm dry extract[5]
Chaste tree: 0.10mg dry extract
Gromwell root: 0.05gm dry extract
METHOD: Combine in one capsule. Take one capsule morning and evening, 15 days per month, together with one of the preceding estrogen-stimulating herbal prescriptions.

Remineralizing Plants

Among the plants known to have a remineralizing property, a useful choice would be *Equisetum arvense* (horsetail). Its sterile stem contains between 5.2 and 7.8 percent silica, calcium, potassium and manganese.

According to the Chinese, it is bitter and slightly cold, cools the Blood, eliminates Heat, and stimulates the Kidneys and the Lungs. *Urtica dioica* (stinging nettle) also contains potassium salts, calcium and magnesium. Other plants that fall into this category include *Polygonum aviculare* (knotweed), rich in silica, *Galeopsis dubia* [also *Galeopsis ochroleuca*] (hemp nettle) and *Lithothamnium calcareum*, a seaweed rich in calcium.

Sample prescription:

Horsetail S.I.P.F.[6]: 125ml
Stinging nettle S.I.P.F.: 125ml
METHOD: One tablespoon in water, morning and evening. Stinging nettle can also be prescribed as nettle juice, one tablespoon taken daily.

Calcium Supply

The daily calcium requirement is 700mg for adults age 30 to 55, and 1000mg for those over 55. After age 55 the ratio of calcium absorption by the intestines diminishes. An average meal provides between 150 and 200mg of calcium acquired from bread, vegetables and fruits, meat or fish and liquids. It is desirable to spread the daily calcium intake over three meals so that the body does not exceed 12 hours without replenishment of its calcium.

Drainage

Carex arenaria (sand sedge), high in silica, is recommended as a maintenance treatment. It potentiates treatment through its silica content together with efficient drainage from its diuretic, choleretic and gentle laxative properties, as well as the sudorific action of the saponosides. A mother tincture should be prescribed, 50 drops three times daily.

COMPLEMENTARY TREATMENTS

Autonomic Disturbances

Disturbances of the autonomic nervous system are often ranked first among the problems linked to menopause. They respond well to sedative and anti-spasmodic plants. Useful herbs include *Ballota nigra* (black horehound), *Melissa officinalis* (lemon balm) and *Crataegus oxyacantha* (hawthorn berry).

Sample prescriptions:

Black horehound M.D.E.

METHOD: One tablespoon at night.

or

Lemon balm S.I.P.F.: 60ml
Hawthorn berry S.I.P.F.: 60ml
METHOD: One tablespoon morning, midday and evening.

Water Retention

Symptoms related to water retention are common complaints in menopausal women and are often caused by conventional hormone replacement therapy. To improve venous circulation, and to insure adequate diuresis, we can select plants with proven efficacy in those areas. Useful herbs include horse chestnut (S.I.P.F. and dry extract), grape vine leaf (M.D.E. and dry extract) and witch hazel (fluid extract and dry extract).

Diuresis can be induced by plants such as orthosiphon (fluid extract), meadowsweet (S.I.P.F. or M.D.E.) and fennel (M.D.E.).

Thyroid stimulation with a S.I.P.F. of *Fucus vesiculosis* (bladder wrack, kelp) can be a valid complement to the treatment.

Physical Activity

There are numerous studies showing that an improvement in muscle tone through physical exercise indirectly increases bone mass. We believe that exercise, based on techniques like *qigong* and practiced before and during menopause, should have a beneficial effect by stabilizing energy in the pelvis and tonifying the Kidneys.

Conclusion

Experience has shown that acupuncture is a therapeutic method which has a definite effect on the regulation of menopausal problems. Its effect on the prevention of osteoporosis remains to be proven. A prospective study by acupuncturists would be very useful and needs to be done.

Chapter Notes

1. *Editors' note:* This is an edited version of an article by Gérard Guillaume, translated by Monique Fay, which appeared in *American Journal of Acupuncture* 20(2): 105-11 (1992). Permission to reprint is gratefully acknowledged.

2. LR-14 *(qi men)*: The name of this point is very relevant to this function. The word *qī* means time, period, phase, agreed date or fixed term. *Mén* is a door, portal or opening.

3. Several of the following prescriptions utilize herbs which have been specially processed by herbal laboratories in France. Equivalent ingredients are recommended.

4. M.D.E.: A standard abbreviation for "medical drug extracts." These preparations are obtained by reverse osmosis at ambient temperature.

5. "Dry extracts" are obtained by rapid desiccation of herbs. Clouds of particles are dry extracted into a drying chamber; circulating warm currents remove the moisture. This process is not patented by any specific laboratory in France.

6. S.I.P.F.: A standard French abbreviation for what in English would be "suspension of whole plant." These micro-suspensions are prepared within 24 hours after harvesting by washing, freezing (cryogenesis), grinding into particles, placing particles in suspension (30 percent solution of water/alcohol), and concentrating under high molecular pressure.

CHAPTER FOURTEEN

Gout

Because gout is a problem that is usually directly related to an overconsumption of protein, this pathology has never been as important in China as in Western societies. In our opinion, it is not a clearly defined disorder in traditional texts. This example, which has been the object of our personal research, provides a good illustration of how Chinese pathophysiology can be used to interpret a well-defined biomedical syndrome.

Gout corresponds to a disruption of fluid metabolism which involves the following systems: Spleen, Lungs, Kidneys and Triple Burner. In its primary form, gout occurs as a result of a constitutional or acquired yang deficiency, with yin excess affecting the transportive and transformative functions. Most of the time, secondary gout is consecutive to a dysfunction of the Spleen (hemopathies) or Kidneys (nephropathies).

Painful joint flare-ups occurring at night are an illustration of the most typical pattern: the joints are red, hot, swollen and extremely painful. These are all symptoms of Damp-Heat stagnation. These acute flare-ups are triggered by an excessive intake of Dampness through diet, or are the result of yang-depleting circumstances such as overexertion, recurrent infections, trauma or surgical interventions. The predominant location of these inflammatory crises is in the Spleen channel at the level of the big toe, and is due to an accumulation of Damp-Heat or a discharge of Phlegm-Heat. Although some cases simply involve a few acute attacks spaced out over time in various ways, most cases are accompanied by frequent relapses which may follow the spring and fall cycles.

Tophi, also known as "chalkstone" deposits, among other complications, corresponds to an accumulation of Phlegm-Cold at the level of the collaterals in the subcutaneous tissue, which is governed by the Lungs. Uremic arthropathies indicate a dysfunction of the Spleen, which governs the circulation of Fluids in the joints. Uremic nephropathies are a consequence of Kidney dysfunction.

Modern therapies are in general able to prevent the recurrence of crises and, to a certain degree, the development of chronic gout. Acupuncture, based on the above-mentioned understanding of pathophysiology, represents a supplemental treatment modality. In many cases it is sufficient in itself. The selection and combination of points depend on the individual circumstances of each case.

Which are these points? We need to:

- tonify the Spleen to eliminate excess Damp-Heat by applying moxa at both BL-20 (*pi shu*) and KI-17 (*shang qu*), a point which we feel is specific to the anatomical spleen, and also treats Spleen disorders

- assist the Spleen's transportive and transformative functions by needling SP-17 (*shi dou*), which promotes the upward movement of the Fluids toward the Lungs

- cause the Fluids to descend and become clearer by needling LU-1 *(zhong fu)*, a point that lowers uricemia according to Soulié de Morant (this claim still awaits systematic study to be verified)
- tonify the yang by needling CV-6 *(qi hai)* to promote the circulation of Fluids and correct the yang deficiency
- promote the circulation of Fluids in the joints by needling SP-21 *(da bao)*, the point on the great collateral of the Spleen, which is a command point for the joints[1]
- transform Phlegm by needling ST-40 *(feng long)*
- regulate the opening and closing functions of the Kidneys by needling BL-23 *(shen shu)* and KI-3 *(tai xi)* or KI-6 *(zhao hai)*.

Acute crises affecting the big toe can be alleviated by combining ST-40 *(feng long)*, which transforms Phlegm, BL-40 *(wei zhong)*, which promotes Blood circulation, and LR-3 *(tai chong)*, the Dampness point of the leg terminal yin channel.

Avoidance of all Damp-Heat generating foods must be added to the classical dietary recommendations. These include all greasy, rich and fried foods as well as alcoholic beverages.

Chapter Notes

1. It is said that this point should be used in cases of deficiency of the joints. In our study of various important premodern texts, we have found that the indications for this point specify that it consolidates the sinews and bones, while GB-34 *(yang ling quan)*, the meeting point of the sinews *(jīn)*, governs the sinews as a contractile force located primarily in the muscles and ligaments.

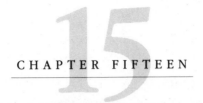

CHAPTER FIFTEEN

Lower Back Pain

Energetic Relationships of the Spine and Channel System

The trunk is the permanent seat of the Qi movements which communicate with the top, the bottom, the interior, the exterior, the right and the left. The spine can be particularly involved in the energetic exchanges between the trunk, the shoulder and pelvic girdles, and the limbs, by blocking the entry or exit of the yin and yang. This is one reason why back pain is so prevalent. It is also important to remember that the spine is located in the deepest part of the trunk (greater yin). Thus, disorders of an extremely yin nature in the thorax or abdomen can affect this level.

VERTEBRAL COLUMN

The spine is governed by three Curious vessels: the Penetrating vessel (FIG. 15-1), the Conception vessel (FIG. 15-2) and the Governing vessel (FIG. 15-3). The leg lesser yin (Kidney) primary channel (FIG. 15-4) is also important in spinal function.

The Penetrating vessel includes in its pathway a branch that "originates in the lower abdomen, goes inward toward the spine, which it penetrates, and follows up to the back."[1]

The Conception vessel has a secondary pathway that "originates in the pelvic cavity and penetrates inside the vertebral column all the way up to the upper back" (similar to the Penetrating vessel).

The primary pathway of the Governing vessel originates at CV-1 *(hui yin)* at the level of the perineum, then ascends along the spine up to the neck at GV-16 *(feng fu)*. There it penetrates the brain, ascends to the vertex, flows down the forehead and follows the nose along its midline.

From the pelvic cavity, the vessel descends toward the genital organs, meets CV-1 *(hui yin)*, traverses the coccyx and comes out at its tail end, goes around the buttocks, crosses the leg lesser yin channel which ascends along the medial aspect of the thigh, goes back to the interior along with the leg greater yang channel to penetrate inside the vertebral column, and ends in the Kidney Organ.

A third branch follows the leg greater yang channel starting at the inner canthus of the eye, ascends to the forehead and crosses the leg greater yang at the vertex, where it penetrates into the brain. Following the pathway of the leg greater yang channel, it goes down the neck then splits on either side of the spine and descends to the lumbar area, where it goes inside and reaches the Kidneys.

This last branch of the Governing vessel has no direct relationship with the spine.

The collateral of the Governing vessel originates at GV-1 *(chang qiang)*, ascends bilaterally on either side of the midline along the spinal processes up to the neck, and branches out at the vertex (FIG. 15-6).

The leg lesser yin (Kidney) channel originates in the sole of the foot, ascends along the medial aspect of the foot, leg and thigh, reaches the tip of the coccyx at GV-1 (chang qiang), and follows the spine up to the level of the Kidneys.

The collateral of the Kidney channel (FIG. 15-5) originates at KI-4 (da zhong) posterior to the medial malleolus and goes around the heel to meet the leg greater yang (Bladder) channel. Another branch ascends with the primary channel to an area located below the Pericardium, and then goes down to penetrate inside the lumbar area of the spine.

We should also note that the foot greater yang (Bladder) channel divergence (FIG. 15-7), which originates in the popliteal fossa, has a branch that follows the spine and diffuses into the Heart, then resumes its upward journey alongside the spine up to the neck, where it meets the leg greater yang primary channel. The leg lesser yin (Kidney) channel divergence has a deep branch that emerges at the level of the second lumbar vertebra to meet the Girdle vessel.

Musculoligamental Complex

The musculoligamental complex is frequently involved in lower back pain pathologies. It is essentially governed by the primary channels and the channel sinews.

Primary Channels

Leg Greater Yáng (Bladder) Channel

This channel splits into two branches at the level of the neck at BL-10 (tian zhu).

The medial branch traverses the spinal processes of C7 and T1, then follows a downward pathway lateral to the spinal processes to the pelvis at BL-30 (bai huan shu), goes back up to the first sacral foramen, then over the second, third and fourth sacral foramina, goes down to the medial third of the gluteal fold, and descends along the posterior aspect of the thigh to the lateral end of the popliteal fossa. The lateral branch proceeds downward parallel to the medial branch, spreads into the Spleen, reaches the buttock, meets GB-30 (huan tiao) at the trochanter, and goes down to the middle of the popliteal fossa and along the posterior aspect of the leg to end at the lateral corner of the fifth toe. Another deep branch penetrates into the lumbar area, follows the paravertebral

muscles to link with the Kidney Organ and then the Bladder Organ (FIG. 15-8).

Leg Lesser Yang (Gallbladder) Channel

The superficial branch of this channel, originating in the supraclavicular fossa at ST-12 (que pen), descends obliquely to the nipple line, follows the inferior costal border and then the iliac crest, goes around the buttock at GB-29 (ju liao), reaches the sacral foramina (BL-31~33), proceeds downward to the tip of the coccyx at GV-1 (chang qiang), reaches the trochanter at GB-30 (huan tiao), and descends along the medial aspect of the lower limb to the fourth toe (FIG. 15-9).

Channel Sinews and Collaterals

Leg Greater Yang (Bladder) Channel Sinew

This channel sinew governs all the paravertebral muscles (FIG. 15-10).

Leg lesser Yin (Kidney) Channel Sinew

This channel sinew follows the lateral aspect of the spine up to the neck, where it penetrates at the level of the occipital bone (FIG. 15-11).

Leg Greater Yin (Spleen) Channel Sinew

This channel sinew originates at the pubis, ascends to the navel, penetrates deeply along the sides of the abdominal wall where it meets the ribs and spreads inside the thorax, and links with the anterior aspect of the thoracic vertebrae (FIG. 15-12).

Leg Yang Brightness (Stomach) Channel Sinew

One branch of this channel sinew starts at the instep, ascends along the fibula, reaches the hip, meets the lower ribs which it follows up to the thoracic portion of the spine, and inserts at the posterior aspect of the thoracic vertebrae (FIG. 15-13).

Leg Lesser Yang (Gallbladder) Channel Sinew

A branch of this channel sinew originates at the lateral aspect of the hip and ends at the sacrum (FIG. 15-14).

Bladder Longitudinal Collateral

This vessel originates at BL-58 (fei yang), ascends along the leg greater yang (Bladder) primary channel up to the trunk, neck and head, then proceeds to the medial canthus of the eye and enters the mouth.

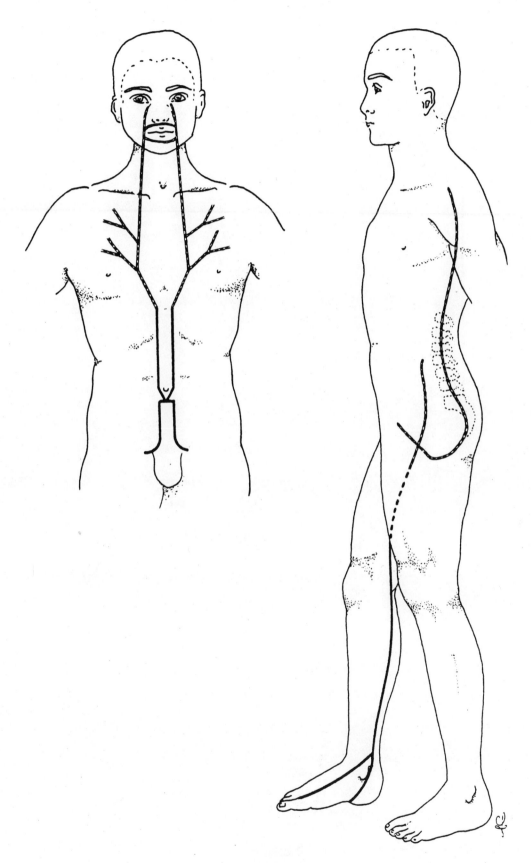

Fig. 15-1
Penetrating Vessel

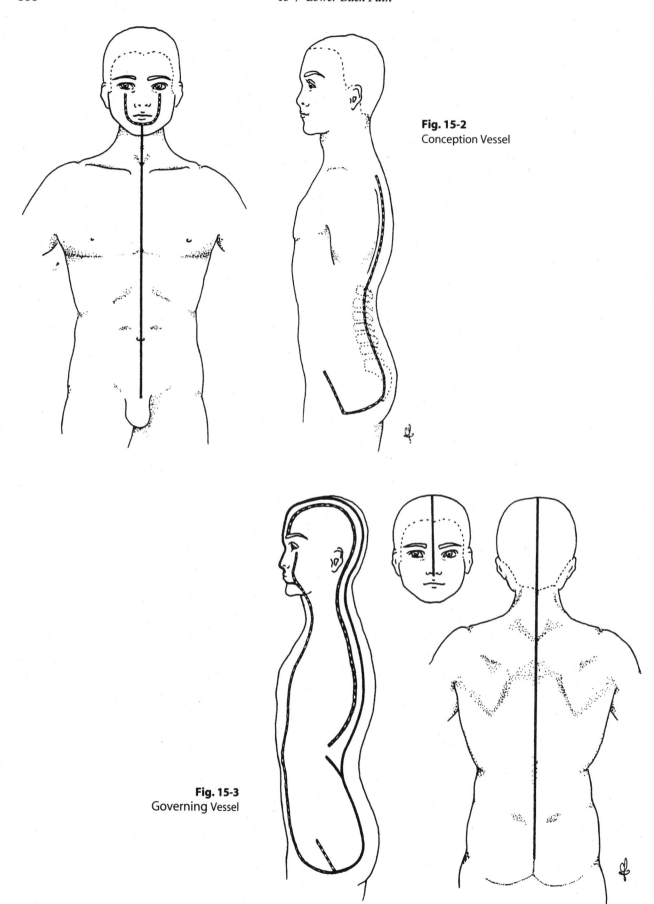

Fig. 15-2
Conception Vessel

Fig. 15-3
Governing Vessel

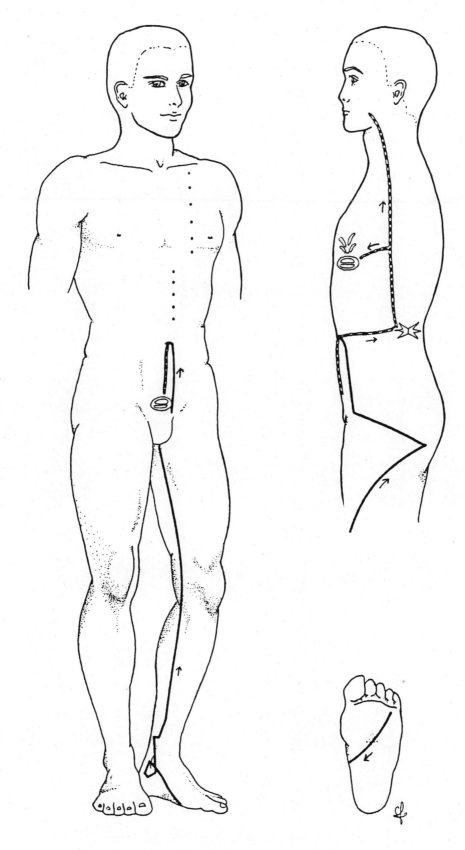

Fig. 15-4
Leg Lesser Yin (Kidney) Primary Channel

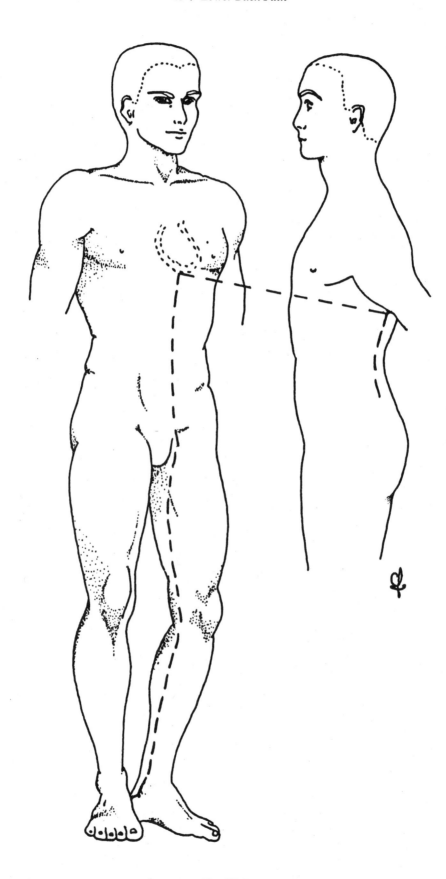

Fig. 15-5
Leg Lesser Yin Collateral

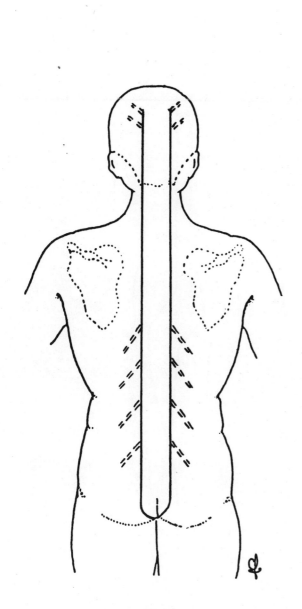

Fig. 15-6
Governing Vessel Collateral

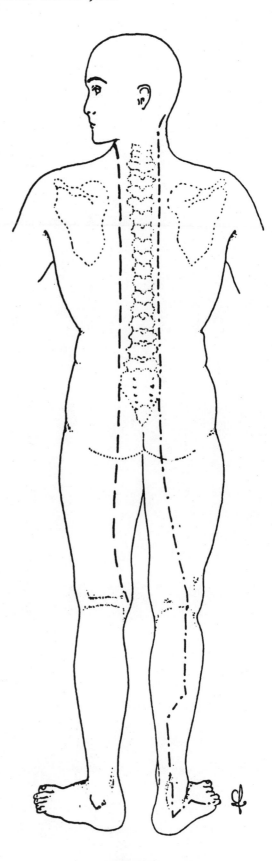

Fig. 15-7
Leg Greater Yang and Leg Lesser
Yang Channel Divergences

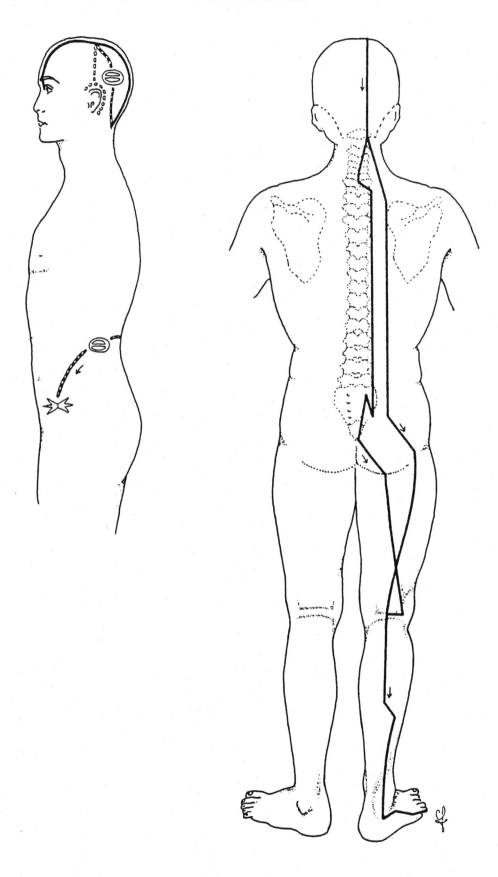

Fig. 15-8
Leg Greater Yang (Bladder) Primary Channel

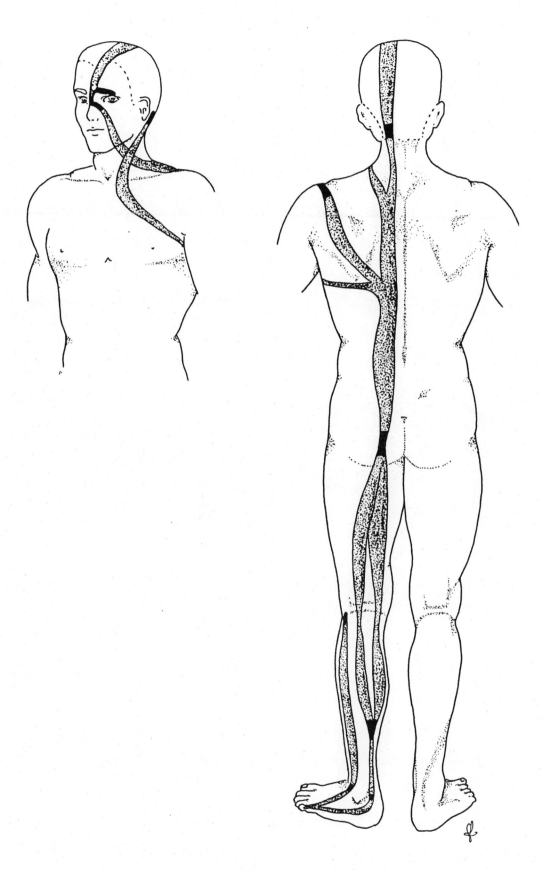

Fig. 15-9
Leg Lesser Yang (Gallbladder) Primary Channel

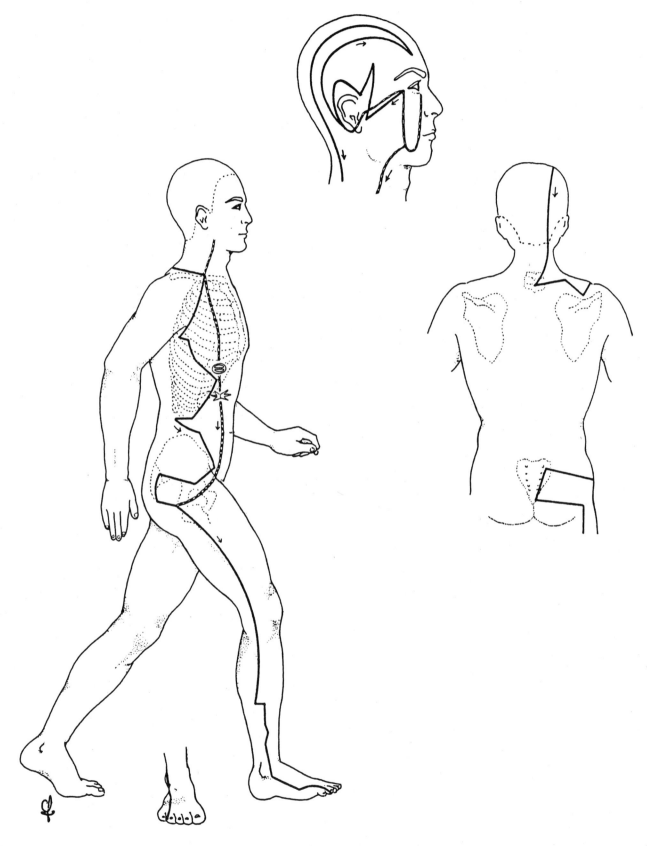

Fig. 15-10
Leg Greater Yang (Bladder) Channel Sinew

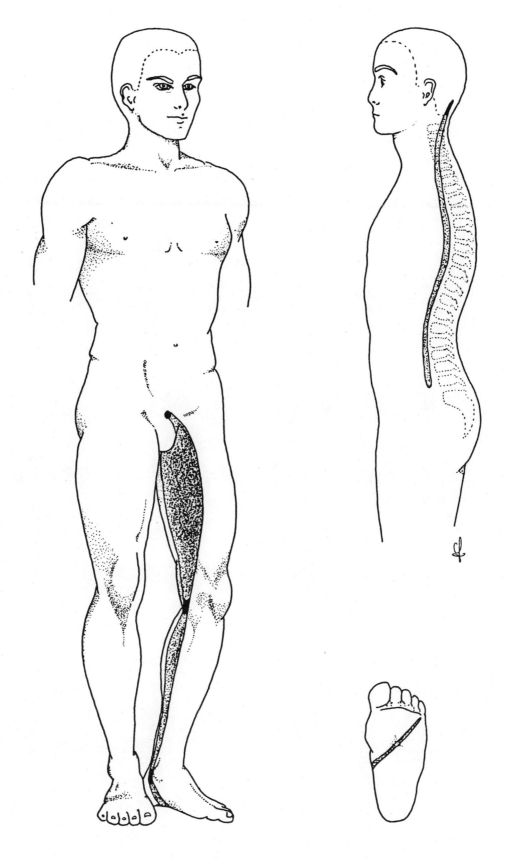

Fig. 15-11
Leg Lesser Yin (Kidney) Channel Sinew

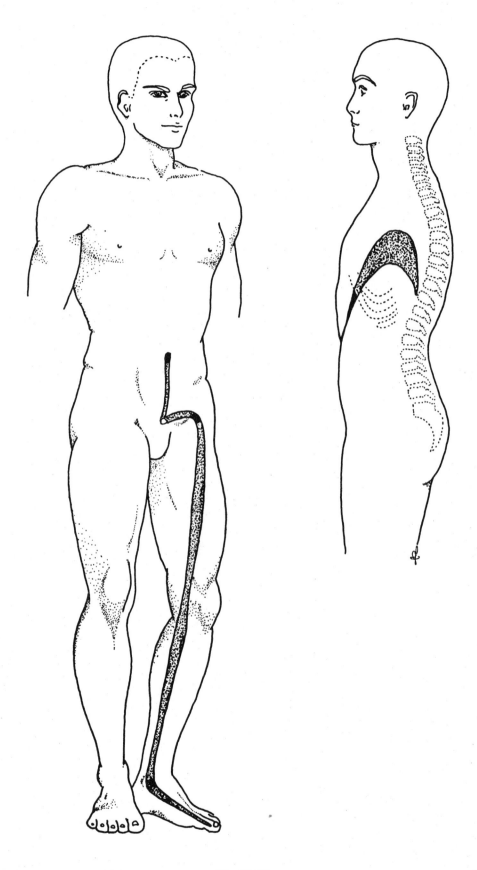

Fig. 15-12
Leg Greater Yin (Spleen) Channel Sinew

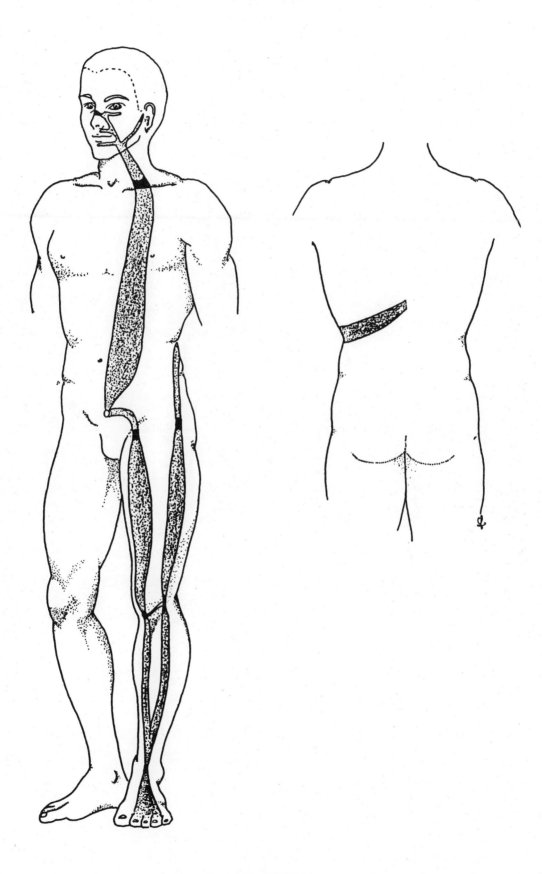

Fig. 15-13
Leg Yang Brightness (Stomach) Channel Sinew

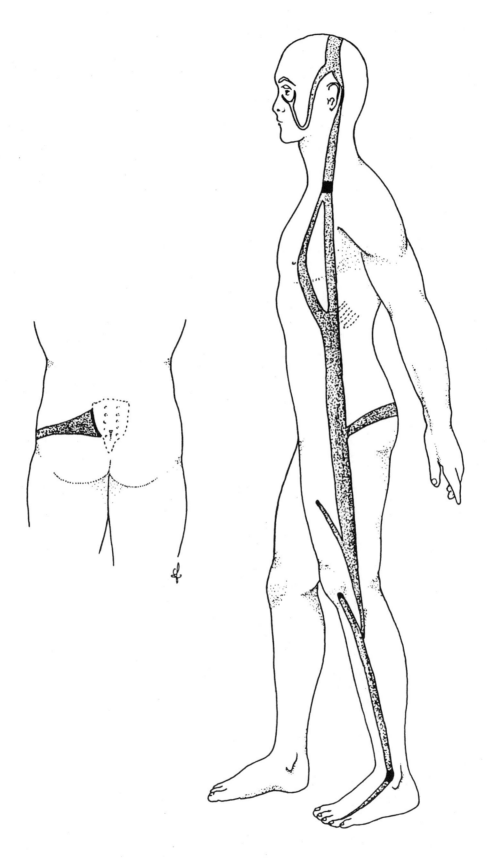

Fig. 15-14
Leg Lesser Yang (Gallbladder) Channel Sinew

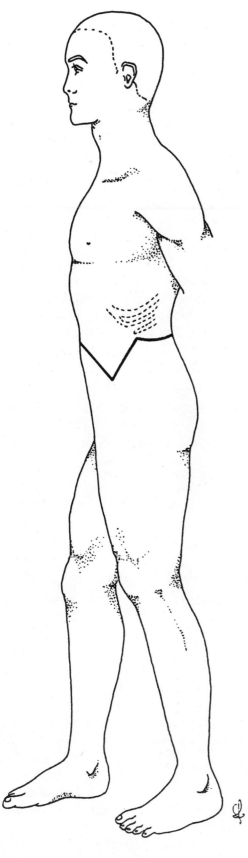

Fig. 15-15
Girdle Channel

Curious Vessels

Girdle Vessel

As indicated by its name, this vessel encircles the body in the lumbar area at the level of the second lumbar vertebra and below the floating ribs in the abdomen (FIG. 15-15). It crosses at GB-26 *(dai mai)*, GB-27 *(wu shu)* and GB-28 *(wei dao)*.

The other Curious vessels may also affect the spine due to their global actions.

STATIONARY SPINE

The spine exhibits four curvatures. The two yang are convex anteriorly or lordoses in the lumbar and cervical areas. The two yin are convex posteriorly or kyphoses in the thoracic and sacral areas. Thus an accumulation of yang in a yang area aggravates lordoses, and an accumulation of yin in a yin zone aggravates kyphoses. Scolioses indicate a poor left-right distribution of the yin and yang Qi.

Generally speaking, the spine has a relationship with the leg greater yang (Bladder) channel, which governs all muscle tonicity.

The three sections of the spine (lumbar, thoracic and cervical) are governed by:

- the lesser yin channel for the lower back, through the connecting point KI-4 *(da zhong)*
- the greater yin channel sinew for the middle and upper back, through the well point SP-1 *(yin bai)*
- the terminal yin channel for the neck, through the connecting point PC-6 *(nei guan)*
- generally speaking, GV-1 *(chang qiang)*, the connecting point of the Governing vessel.

Diagnosis: Acute Lower Back Pain

Diagnosis of lower back pain is arrived at through analysis of the pain topography, limitation of movement, antalgic attitudes, painful spots, duration of the pathology, and associated signs. These must, of course, utilize all the modern techniques provided by medical imaging and biomedicine.

For the sake of clarity, we have opted for a classification scheme that is based on the age of the problem. This scheme does have its limitations due to its arbitrary nature. For example, the topography of lower back pain is not always easy to pinpoint, the distinction between recent and old lower back pain mechanisms is far from being definite, and the greatest frequency of clinical observations are only a guideline. A disorder of the channel sinews should not be dismissed straightaway in the case of old lower back pain, and neither should disruption of the Conception vessel be overlooked in the case of a recent pattern. On the other hand, an acute pattern can always be the recurring result of a chronic condition, which therefore warrants a systematic investigation of intricate pathogenic mechanisms.

Transverse or Layered Lower Back Pain

Qi Movements

Obstruction of the Outward Movement of Yang Qi toward the Lower Limbs

This very common mechanism must be evoked in the case of strain-induced lower back pain. Straining one's back while in a static position blocks the exit of trunk yang Qi toward the lower limbs, causing an excess of yang in the pelvis. This manifests as lower back pain aggravated by coughing and straining, and referred pain on the posterior aspect of the lower limbs along the leg greater yang (Bladder) channel, often affecting one leg only. This imitates an L5 type sciatica. Needling BL-29 (zhong lu shu), which governs the pelvic yang movement toward the lower limbs, brings an immediate reduction in pain, and can be usefully combined with BL-36 (cheng fu) and BL-60 (kun lun).

Internally generated or externally contracted local Cold may obstruct the circulation of yang Qi; apply moxa at BL-31~34 (ba liao) or even at KI-13 (qi xue), which improves Cold-induced abdominal fullness.

For traumatic acute lower back pain, it is also worth noting the efficacy of needling GV-26 (ren zhong) while asking the patient to simultaneously perform pelvic movements of an ever-increasing magnitude.

Obstruction of the Movement of Yin Qi from the Lower Limbs toward the Trunk

The yin of the lower limbs, unable to return to the trunk, creates a local yin deficiency which manifests as a yang-type acute lower back which is ameliorated by cold and pressure. It is accompanied by a heavy sensation in the legs, cramps, often peripheral venous disorders, or even pain in the medial aspect of the thigh resembling an obturator neuralgia. Needling the barrier point LR-11 (yin lian), which promotes the movement of lower limb yin toward the trunk, immediately alleviates the pain.

If such a pattern lingers on, we must then look for a more global mechanism that is preventing the inner withdrawl of the Qi. This retreat is regulated by CV-3 (zhong ji), and when it is disrupted, pelvic, genital, urinary and intestinal disorders are predominant, due to yin deficiency.

Channel Pathology

Penetrating Vessel

The Penetrating vessel may be involved in cases of transverse lower back pain, one of its characteristic features being strain-induced lower back pain when a person attempts to lift a weight that is too heavy. This blocks the person in a semi-flexed posture. This pattern is an illustration of a Qi and Blood imbalance in the pelvis, which can be corrected by needling BL-38 (fu xi) and BL-39 (wei yang), and by bleeding the superficial blood vessels or nidi of the lower back. Note that BL-38 (fu xi) and BL-39 (wei yang) are used for this local disturbance in the Penetrating vessel, while the confluent and paired confluent points SP-4 (gong sun) and PC-6 (nei guan) are better used for more generalized or systemic perturbations of this vessel.

Yang Linking Vessel

This type of lower back pain often belongs in a context of diffuse joint pain, and is sensitive to changes in the weather, snow and storms. It is sometimes accompanied by a swelling sensation in the lower back. There is frequently a sensation of fever, chills and headaches, often indicating that the pathogenic influences attacking the leg greater yang and leg lesser yang channels have begun to spread into the yang Linking vessel. The pulse is floating.

The treatment principle is to open the yang Linking vessel by needling its confluent point TB-5 (wai guan) combined with its paired confluent point GB-41 (zu lin qi), and to promote circulation by needling the cleft point GB-35 (yang jiao).

Leg Lesser Yin Collateral

In cases of deficiency there is lower back pain. When the pathogenic influence residing in the collateral reaches the primary channel, it leaves the collateral in a state of deficiency. We should needle the primary channel's source point KI-3 (tai xi), and tonify its paired connecting point BL-58 (fei yang).

GV-26 *(ren zhong)*

In cases of acute recent lower back pain indicating a disruption in the circulation of the Governing and Conception vessels, needling GV-26 *(ren zhong)* may bring instant relief from the pain.

LONGITUDINAL LOWER BACK PAIN

Leg Greater Yang Channel Sinew

Symptomatology

There is sharp pain with a breaking sensation in the spine. The vertebral column is stiff and bent backward. Sometimes other signs along the channel pathway occur, such as pain in the posterior aspect of the lower limb, contractures of the neck sinews and muscles, difficulty in lifting the arm, stabbing pain in the armpit and the supraclavicular fossa, migraine and facial pain.

Treatment

The immediate improvement of symptoms while needling the well point BL-67 *(zhi yin)* constitutes a good diagnostic test; this rule can be extended to all channel sinews.

If the pain is of traumatic origin, add the river point BL-60 *(kun lun)*, insertion points surrounding the affected area, and possibly the main *ashi* point. BL-57 *(cheng shan)*, which governs muscle motricity, is also a very useful point for this indication.

If pathogenic influences (Wind-Damp-Cold) are the cause of the pathology, add the leg greater yang tonification point, which is also BL-67 *(zhi yin)* in this case, as well as the crossing point of the leg yang channels, SI-18 *(quan liao)*, in order to prevent the pathogenic influences from invading the other channel sinews.

Leg Lesser Yin Channel Sinew

Symptomatology

This is marked by paramedial pain, which is deep but not reproduced by palpation, and may be accompanied by contractures of the whole body or restricted to the soles of the feet, or even the medial aspect of the lower limbs.

If the condition affects the posterior and superficial aspects of the body, there will be a sensation of heaviness in the lower back and difficulty in bending forward. If it affects the anterior and deep aspects of the body, there is difficulty in bending backward.

Treatment

If the origin is traumatic, needle the well point KI-1 *(yong quan)*, the river point KI-7 *(fu liu)*, and possibly the main *ashi* point and insertion points which surround the painful area. If the origin is linked to the invasion of pathogenic Cold or Damp-Cold, needle KI-7 *(fu liu)* to tonify the Kidney channel, and the crossing points CV-2 *(qu gu)* and CV-3 *(zhong ji)* to prevent the pathogenic influences from spreading to the other channel sinews.

Leg Greater Yang Bladder Channel

Symptomatology

Sharp wrenching-type pain in the lower back and spine, with a breaking sensation in the lumbar area that is deeper than a channel sinew-related pain. Other painful areas are usually found along the channel pathway in the lower limbs, neck and head.

Treatment

If the condition is caused by invasion of pathogenic Cold, needle the well point BL-67 *(zhi yin)*, which is also the tonification point, and the river point BL-60 *(kun lun)*, and possibly the spring point BL-66 *(zu tong gu)*.

If Wind is predominant, eliminate Wind by needling the point where Wind penetrates, BL-12 *(feng men)*, and the stream point BL-65 *(shu gu)*.

If the channel condition is a repercussion of an internal disorder of the Bladder Organ, needle the lower sea point BL-40 *(wei zhong)*, and reinforce the effect with an etiological treatment. Regulating the condition can also be achieved by needling the source point BL-64 *(jing gu)* and its paired connecting point KI-4 *(da zhong)*.

If the Bladder channel condition stems from a greater yang-stage pathology, regulation is achieved by needling the stream and connecting points, BL-65 *(shu gu)* and BL-58 *(fei yang)*.

Leg Lesser Yin Kidney Channel

Symptomatology

The pain is deep, median, it affects the thoracic and lumbar vertebrae, and is sometimes accompanied by signs such as cold feet and painful soles of the feet, pain in the posteromedial aspect of the lower limb, sore throat and dry mouth.

Treatment

The channel dysfunction is usually the expression of

an internal Kidney Organ disorder, which can be addressed by needling the spring and stream points, KI-2 *(ran gu)* and KI-3 *(tai xi)*, combined with an etiological treatment of the Kidneys. A similar action is achieved by needling the source point KI-3 *(tai xi)*, combined with its paired connecting point BL-58 *(fei yang)*.

In cases of pathogenic Cold invasion, needle the well point KI-1 *(yong quan)* and the river point KI-7 *(fu liu)*, which is also the tonification point. If the Kidney channel dysfunction stems from a lesser yin-stage pathology, use the stream-connecting points needling technique: KI-3 *(tai xi)* and KI-4 *(da zhong)*.

Yang Heel Vessel

When this vessel is involved, the entire back is painful and the whole body is stiff. The lower back often feels as if it has been "pounded by a hammer," with a swelling sensation in the affected area. The patient will also experience difficulty in getting up and may develop an antalgic posture, bending toward the affected side. Other yang Heel signs may also exist, such as pain along the vessel pathway in the shoulder, insomnia, eye pain and lower limb contractures.

Treatment involves combining the confluent point BL-62 *(shen mai)* and the cleft point BL-59 *(fu yang)*, to which the paired confluent point SI-3 *(hou xi)* may be added.

Governing Vessel

In cases of excess in this vessel, the spine is stiff, the entire back is painful, and lying on one's back is difficult. If the pathogenic influence has invaded through GV-16 *(feng fu)*, the original clinical picture is a pseudo-flu syndrome with vertebral pain progressing down the spine. In this case, treat the entry barrier by needling GV-16 *(feng fu)*, draw the Governing vessel Qi upward by applying moxa at GV-20 *(bai hui)*, and promote circulation within the vessel by needling the confluent point SI-3 *(hou xi)*.

If the condition results from a leg greater yang invasion spreading to the Governing vessel, symptoms common to both locations will be found, particularly headaches and pain in the nape of the neck. In this case, also treat the leg greater yang primary channel.

It is useful to tonify the Kidney Qi in both cases.

Collateral of the Governing Vessel

In our experience this vessel controls a person's means of contact with the external world. It is often involved in lower back pain in people who feel poorly situated within themselves, or in the world. In cases of excess, there is stiffness and heaviness in the upper and lower back and the vertebral column, the body is bent, the head feels full and there is sensitivity at the vertex. Sometimes patients may experience seizures. This can be treated by needling GV-1 *(chang qiang)*.

SACROILIAC PAIN

Leg Lesser Yang Channel Sinew

Symptomatology

The pain is mostly located in the sacroiliac and sacral regions, radiating toward the buttocks and the lateral aspect of the thigh and leg, and can reach the fourth toe, with difficulty in bending the knee, and flank pain.

Treatment

If the condition is of traumatic origin, needle the well point GB-44 *(zu qiao yin)* in combination with the river point GB-40 *(qiu xu)*, the main *ashi* point and the insertion points surrounding the painful area.

If it is caused by the invasion of pathogenic influences, also tonify the leg lesser yang channel by needling GB-43 *(xia xi)* and the crossing point SI-18 *(quan liao)* to prevent the pathogenic influences from spreading to other lower limb yang channel sinews.

Leg Lesser Yang Gallbladder Channel

Symptomatology

The pain in the sacroiliac region radiates toward the lateral aspect of the lower limb, and may be accompanied by right hypochondriac pain, headaches, chills and vomiting.

Treatment

If Wind-Cold is responsible for the disorder, needle the well point GB-44 *(zu qiao yin)*, the river point GB-38 *(yang fu)*, the tonification point GB-43 *(xia xi)*, and GB-30 *(huan tiao)*.

If the condition is associated with an internal Gallbladder disorder, needle the sea point GB-34 *(yang ling quan)* in combination with an etiological treatment of the Gallbladder Organ. Regulation can also be achieved by needling the source point GB-40 *(qiu xu)* together with its paired connecting point LR-5 *(li gou)*.

If the entire lesser yang stage is involved, use the stream-connecting points harmonization technique: GB-41 *(zu lin qi)* and GB-37 *(guang ming)*.

THORACOLUMBAR PAIN

Leg Greater Yin Channel Sinew

Symptomatology

There is deep posterior thoracic pain, which may radiate toward the lower back and anterior thorax. In addition, there may be contracture of the big toe, twisting-type pain in the medial malleolus, pain in the medial aspect of the thigh, and a wrenching sensation in the genital organs that radiates toward the umbilicus and flanks.

Treatment

For trauma-induced pain, needle the well point SP-1 *(yin bai)*, the river point SP-5 *(shang qiu)*, the main *ashi* point and the insertion points surrounding the painful area.

If the pain is caused by pathogenic Dampness, add the leg greater yin tonification point SP-2 *(da du)* and the crossing points of the foot yin channels, CV-2 *(qu gu)* and CV-3 *(zhong ji)*, in order to prevent the Dampness from spreading to other lower limb channel sinews.

Leg Yang Brightness Channel Sinew

Symptomatology

The transverse pain is located in the lower middle back and gathers around the flanks, sometimes with pain on the anterior aspect of the lower limb and abdominal tension.

Treatment

If the condition is of traumatic origin, needle the well point ST-45 *(li dui)*, the river point ST-41 *(jie xi)* (which is also the leg yang brightness tonification point, and which needs to be tonified if the Cold or Hot pathogenic influences are involved), the main *ashi* point and the insertion points surrounding the painful area.

Leg Greater Yang Collateral

In cases of excess, there is middle and upper lumbar pain, with a stuffy nose and headaches.

The collateral is in a state of excess because of the pathogenic Qi, so we should drain the corresponding connecting point BL-58 *(fei yang)*.

Diagnosis: Recurrent or Chronic Lower Back Pain

REGIONAL PATHOLOGY

Pain from Nonentry of Lower Limb Yang

There are constant energy exchanges between the trunk and the lower limbs, corresponding to the entry and exit of the yin and yang. When the yang of the lower limbs cannot enter the trunk, there is a local deficiency of yang. This manifests as a yin-type dull lower back pain which improves with pressure, warmth and rest, and is aggravated by cold and strain. The presence of pain on the anterior aspect of the thigh along the yang brightness pathway (invoking a vastus intermedius myalgia) is not required for this diagnosis.

The treatment principle is to promote the entry of the yang into the trunk by needling the barrier point ST-31 *(bi guan)*. If treatment is unsuccessful, or if there is persistent lower back pain, we must seek a pelvic obstacle to the yang entry, which would explain its chronic nature by an excess or stagnation of yin and/or Blood (such as fibroma, ovarian cyst or prostatic adenoma).

Pain from Local Qi Stagnation

The chief feature of this type of lower back pain is its occurrence during rest, when sitting for long periods of time, while standing about, on arising in the morning with difficulty in getting started, along with a decrease in pain after a warm-up period of some duration. It also improves with walking, massage and warmth, and is aggravated by cold.

Activation or mobilization of the Qi is generally dependent on the lesser yang channels. The point that mobilizes yang stagnation at the lumbar and lower extremity level is GB-30 *(huan tiao)*. This point should be needled deeply. Whatever the case, it is recommended that you check whether this stagnation is part of a more general Qi stagnation pattern involving the Girdle vessel, the lesser yang stage, or whether it corresponds to the systemic obstruction of the yang Qi, which is governed by GB-25 *(jing men)*. This is the alarm point of the Kidneys, which correspond to winter. As such, this change or activation of the yang of the body corresponds to the movement that occurs each day at midnight, or each year at the winter solstice. In a similar fashion, needling CV-4 *(guan yuan)*, the alarm point of the Small Intestine, has an effect on the yin corresponding to that which occurs at noon or at the summer solstice.

One prominent feature of local Qi stagnation is pain in the sacroiliac joint, indicated by the presence of local fibrous nodules which are inflamed, painful to the touch, and which diminish after cupping. Manipulation of the sacroiliac joint is often required for satisfactory results.

Pain from Blood Stasis

This type of lower back pain is characterized by stabbing pain, which can evoke "dagger stabs" when very severe. It worsens at night, movement is difficult, in women relapses may occur during their ovulation or premenstrual period, and hemorrhoids are frequent. The tongue is deep purple or with purple spots, and the pulse is choppy.

The treatment principle is to circulate the Blood by needling BL-40 *(wei zhong)*, BL-17 *(ge shu)*, BL-53 *(bao huang)* and BL-32 *(ci liao)*. Bleeding the congested blood vessels in the lumbar area with a triangular needle may be beneficial.

If this pattern occurs within the context of a disruption of the Girdle vessel, needle GB-28 *(wei dao)*.

CHANNEL PATHOLOGY

Primary Channels

The primary channels discussed above in the section on recent lower back pain may be involved in this context, sometimes with involvement of several mechanisms, which explains the progression toward a chronic stage.

The leg greater yang may be involved, as it governs muscle tonicity and relates to vertebral posture. It is regulated by BL-11 *(da zhu)* and BL-57 *(cheng shan)*. We should always investigate possible involvement of the Governing vessel, in which case needling GV-3 *(yao yang guan)* and GV-14 *(da zhui)* is helpful.

Disruption of the greater yin-greater yang balance can be felt at the leg greater yang level as middle and lower back pain. To restore the balance, needle BL-57 *(cheng shan)* combined with SP-8 *(di ji)* or SP-5 *(shang qiu)*.

Qi constraint in a patient under constant pressure may manifest as contractures of the middle and lower back muscles at the level of the greater yang, and of the trapezius muscle. In such cases needle GB-23 *(zhe jin)*, which disperses yang excess in the chest, as well as SI-11 *(tian zong)* and BL-29 *(zhong lu shu)*, which open the upward and downward yang movements of the trunk respectively.

When the leg terminal yin channel is involved, the lower back pain prevents flexion or extension of the trunk. In men, this is accompanied by a scrotal condition and pruritus of the external genital organs. Women have a variety of pelvic pathologies. The main point to needle is the river point LR-4 *(zhong feng)*. This disorder is usually internally generated and, according to our reading of the classics, due to rebellious channel Qi. LR-2 *(xing jian)* is indicated in this case. Externally generated excess Liver channel lower back pain is rarer. It is characterized as being acute and of relatively recent origin.

Governing Vessel

According to J.–M. Kespi, the Governing vessel is the "sea of the yang channels" and sums up all the yang processes of the body. It is the governor that supports life and allows it to grow and develop. It represents the physical and mental framework of the human being, his structure, allowing him to rest physically and mentally against a strong, solid back, a spine that fulfills its mission as the tree of life.

When the Governing vessel is deficient, the patient suffers from chronic pain affecting the entire back. Such patients often have a history of scoliosis or problems such as Scheuerman's disease, and feel inadequately equipped to meet life's challenges. In such cases, the Governing vessel deficiency is often the consequence of a poor relationship with a father who was physically or spiritually absent during childhood, or who did not fulfill his role as a guide.

GV-1 *(chang qiang)* rules the Governing vessel as a place where life's yang finds the support to structure itself; needling or applying moxa at this point strengthens the human framework and reinforces the spine in its physical and mental supporting role. This point is often used in combination with BL-11 *(da zhu)*, the influential point for the bones, which shares similar functions.

Yin Heel Vessel

This type of lower back pain can be accompanied by pain in the lower abdomen and hip which radiates toward the genitals. In our experience, this symptomatology may be triggered by the different phases of the menstrual cycle, and may be reactivated during the ovulation or premenstrual period.

The recommended treatment is to needle the vessel's confluent point KI-6 *(zhao hai)*, the cleft point KI-8 *(jiao xin)* and possibly the paired confluent point LU-7 *(lie que)*.

Girdle Vessel

Lower back pain associated with the Girdle vessel typically encircles the waist and radiates toward the medial aspect of the thigh, with abdominal and periumbilical pain, and a sensation of sitting in cool water. Other characteristic signs include dysmenorrhea, leukorrhea and looseness of the ankles.

The recommended treatment is to needle GB-26 *(dai mai)*, the confluent point GB-41 *(zu lin qi)* and the paired confluent point TB-5 *(wai guan)*.

When the Girdle vessel is deficient, disability of the lower limbs is the predominant symptom, which calls for additional action at the yang brightness level (controlled by the Girdle vessel) by needling ST-30 *(qi chong)*, ST-36 *(zu san li)* and ST-37 *(shang ju xu)*.

Conception Vessel

According to chapter 41 of *Basic Questions*, lower back pain associated with the Conception vessel starts at the bottom of the back and is accompanied by profuse sweating; there is thirst when the sweat has dried, and the patient feels like walking after drinking. We have never observed these types of manifestations. The typical pathology associated with a disruption of the Conception vessel (various hernias, abdominal masses, gynecological and sexual disorders) indicates Qi deficiency, accumulation of Cold, and Blood stasis in the pelvis. This can manifest in deep lower back pain, usually on the midline, which is affected by the patient's sexual activity.

The treatment principle is to open the Conception vessel by needling LU-7 *(lie que)* combined with the paired confluent point KI-6 *(zhao hai)*, and to apply moxa at CV-4 *(guan yuan)* and CV-6 *(qi hai)*. When the lower back pain is associated with difficulty or inability to take charge of one's own responsibilities, needling CV-2 *(qu gu)* by itself is sometimes sufficient.

Yin Linking Vessel

Lower back pain associated with this vessel is accompanied by pain and swelling of the flanks, and pain in the chest and genital organs. The chief features to look for are a stabbing, piercing pain in the heart area (sometimes similar to being stabbed by a dagger) and headaches in patients who are tense and have trouble relaxing.

Needle the confluent point PC-6 *(nei guan)* in combination with the paired confluent point SP-4 *(gong sun)* and the cleft point KI-9 *(zhu bin)*.

ORGAN PATHOLOGY

Kidneys

As we have seen, the Chinese view the lower back as the "Kidneys' residence," and it is the Kidneys that govern the bones and marrow. When the Kidney Essence is deficient, the muscles, channels, bones and marrow are deprived of nourishment, which causes pain in the lumbar area. Depletion of Essence can occur in patients who have a characteristic prenatal or acquired weakness, who engage in excessively strenuous work, after a prolonged illness, or who are elderly. The lower back pain manifests mostly as stiffness and weakness in the lumbar area, which is ameliorated by light massage. The legs and knees are without strength. This pattern is aggravated by physical activity and improved by rest. There are frequent relapses.

If yang deficiency predominates, there are spasms in the lower abdomen, the face is pale, the extremities are cold, the tongue is pale, and the pulse is submerged and thin. The treatment principle is to warm and tonify the Kidneys by gentle application of moxa for fifteen to twenty minutes at BL-23 *(shen shu)*, GV-4 *(ming men)* and GV-20 *(bai hui)*.

If yin deficiency predominates, the lower back pain manifests within a context of worry, restlessness, insomnia, dry throat, dark urine, hot flashes, and heat in the palms and soles. The tongue is red, and the pulse is wiry, thin and rapid. The treatment principle is to nourish the Kidneys and the yin by needling BL-23 *(shen shu)*, BL-52 *(zhi shi)*, KI-15 *(zhong zhu)* and KI-3 *(tai xi)*.

The features of another type of lower back pain suggest a Kidney disorder, but the Kidney pulse is normal or, paradoxically, excessive. This is blockage of the Kidney Qi, which cannot ascend due to an obstruction in the pelvis related to fear, usually from an old fright. The presence of diarrhea associated with emotional stress is an excellent diagnostic sign. The recommended point is GV-5 *(xuan shu)*, which promotes the ascension of Kidney Qi.

Liver

Liver Qi stagnation can cause lower back pain radiating toward the flanks and abdomen, accompanied by abdominal distention and difficulty in standing up for long periods of time. Other characteristics include personality traits such as excessive prudence, worry about the future, being thin-skinned, and irritability or anger. Physical signs such as vertex headaches, visual disorders and cramps may also be present. The tongue is typically red with a thin coating, and the pulse is wiry or thin, or submerged and wiry.

The treatment principle is to promote the movement of Liver Qi by needling BL-18 (gan shu), LR-6 (zhong du) and LR-3 (tai chong).

Small Intestine

Heat excess in the Small Intestine causes abdominal pain radiating toward the back and spine, accompanied by abdominal distention, dark urine that is almost red, and pain in the external genitals. The tongue is yellow with a red tip and edges. The pulse is slippery and rapid. This Heat excess is usually endogenous, secondary to Heart Fire. In addition to the etiological treatment of Heart Fire, we must clear the Heat by needling the associated point BL-27 (xiao chang shu), the lower sea point ST-39 (xia ju xu) and the spring point SI-2 (qian gu).

Large Intestine

This is yang deficiency-type lower back pain, accompanied by digestive and intestinal transit disorders. The recommended point is GV-3 (yao yang guan). As the median point at the level of BL-25 (da chang shu), it reinforces the lower back and lower extremities while expelling Cold and Dampness, among other functions.

Spleen

Lower back pain associated with Spleen disorders is accompanied by a heavy sensation, stiffness in the limbs, facial pallor, poor appetite, and occasionally abdominal distention and diarrhea. The tongue coating is white and greasy, and the pulse is slippery and soggy.

The treatment principle is to tonify the Spleen, eliminate the Dampness and dissolve the Phlegm. Warm needles or moxa is recommended at BL-20 (pi shu), CV-12 (zhong wan), ST-40 (feng long) and SP-3 (tai bai).

If the Spleen pathology is secondary to Kidney yang deficiency, the Kidneys must be tonified first.

Exogenous Lower Back Pain, Painful Obstruction

The pathogenic influences Wind, Dampness, Cold and Heat can generate lower back pain after such events as exposure to bad weather, working or staying in a damp or cold environment, and profuse sweating. Onset is usually sudden. If the pathogenic influences are not eliminated,

the pattern may progress toward painful obstruction disorder. Stagnant Cold and Dampness can transform into Heat. Dampness is the most frequently encountered cause of lower back blockage, due to its sticky and stagnant nature. Damp-Cold and Damp-Heat are the most frequent patterns, while underlying Kidney deficiency is the norm.

Damp-Cold Lower Back Pain

This occurs when catching a cold or after exposure to dampness. The pain is accompanied by a cold and heavy sensation in the lower back, and progressively worsens. Rotation of the trunk is difficult. Resting in a recumbent position only partially alleviates the pain, and may even aggravate it. The pain increases in damp and cold weather. As the disorder progresses to the chronic stage, periods of crises and lulls alternate. The tongue coating is white and greasy, and the pulse is submerged and slow.

The treatment principle is to expel the Cold, eliminate the Dampness, warm the channels and open the collaterals. Among the points used in treating this pattern are BL-23 (shen shu), which, when warmed with moxa, regulates and strengthens the Kidney Qi and expels Damp-Cold; BL-40 (wei zhong), which expels Cold from the collaterals; BL-60 (kun lun), the Fire point on the leg greater yang channel; GV-3 (yao yang guan), which circulates the yang in the Governing vessel; GV-16 (feng fu), which disperses Wind and Cold and connects with the Governing vessel; SP-3 (tai bai), which eliminates Dampness; and possibly local ashi points.

Damp-Heat Lower Back Pain

The pain associated with this pattern is accompanied by a sensation of local heat, and a heavy feeling while walking. The pain is aggravated by hot and rainy weather. The joints may be red and swollen, and there are general signs of Heat such as thirst, restlessness, dark urine and constipation. The tongue coating is yellow and greasy, and the pulse is soggy and rapid.

The treatment principle is to clear Heat and eliminate Dampness. Needling is recommended at BL-23 (shen shu), BL-52 (zhi shi) and KI-3 (tai xi) to tonify the Kidney yin; BL-32 (ci liao) to eliminate Damp-Heat from the pelvis; BL-39 (wei yang) and BL-55 (he yang) to cool Heat and eliminate Dampness; KI-10 (yin gu) to cool Heat and tonify the Kidneys; and at the M-BW-35 (hua tuo jia ji) points in the affected area.

Damp-Phlegm Lower Back Pain

This type of lower back pain radiates toward the sacrum with a dull, heavy sensation that generally occurs when getting started or while standing about. Palpation reveals the presence of subcutaneous nodules in the painful area. The treatment principle is to tonify the Spleen to eliminate Phlegm. Needling is prescribed at SP-3 *(tai bai)*, the stream point of the Spleen, which eliminates Dampness; and at ST-40 *(feng long)*, the connecting point of the Stomach, which eliminates Phlegm. The nodules should be dissolved by using cupping or the triangular needle technique.

Lower Back Pain and Painful Obstruction

When the pathogenic influences penetrate inward and cause painful obstruction disorder, the lower back pain is but one of the symptoms, and the treatment protocol is similar to that for painful obstruction discussed in chapter 8.

Trigger Points

SERRATUS POSTERIOR INFERIOR MUSCLE

Referred Pain

Mildly stabbing pain in the posterior and inferior aspect of the rib cage, improved by twisting and stretching. The pain follows the pathway of the lateral branch of the leg greater yang channel and the leg yang brightness channel sinew (FIG. 15-16).

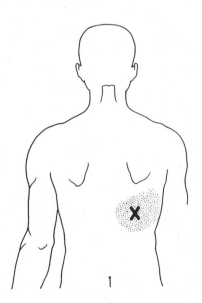

Fig. 15-16
Trigger Point Area for Serratus Posterior Inferior Muscle

Trigger Point

Located in the area of BL-48 *(yang gang)*.

ILIOCOSTALIS THORACIS MUSCLE

Referred Pain

Pain in the posterior and inferior aspect of the rib cage radiating along the spine. The pain follows the pathway of the leg greater yang channel, in the scapula and iliac fossa (FIG. 15-17).

Trigger Point

Located in the area of BL-49 *(yi she)*.

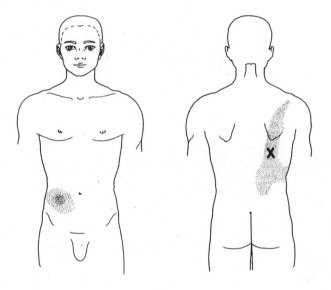

Fig. 15-17
Trigger Point Area for Iliocostalis Thoracis Muscle

ILIOCOSTALIS LUMBORUM MUSCLE

Referred Pain

Pain in the lower back and buttocks, following the pathway of the leg greater yang channel (FIG. 15-18).

Trigger Point

Located in the area of BL-51 *(huang men)*.

LONGISSIMUS THORACIS MUSCLE

Referred Pain

Pain in the lower back and buttocks, following the pathway of the leg greater yang channel. Pain in the lower back and the posterosuperior aspect of the iliac crest (FIG. 15-19).

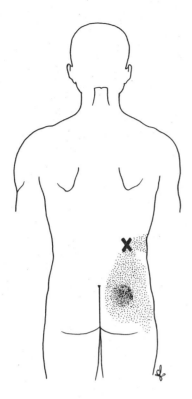

Fig. 15-18
Trigger Point Area for Iliocostalis Lumborum Muscle

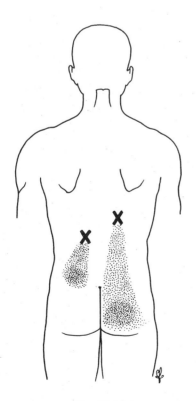

Fig. 15-19
Trigger Point Area for Longissimus Thoracis Muscle

Trigger Point

Located in the area of BL-49 *(yi she)* in the first case, and in the area of BL-22 *(san jiao shu)* in the second case.

MULTIFIDI AND ROTATORES MUSCLES

Referred Pain

Pain in the sacrococcygeal and buttocks area (FIG. 15-20).

Trigger Point

Located in the area of BL-30 *(bai huan shu)*.

Referred Pain

Lower back and abdominal pain, which may be confused with visceral pain (FIG. 15-20).

Trigger Point

Located in the area of BL-23 *(shen shu)*.

Referred Pain

Pain in the sacrococcygeal area, sensitive to pressure, which evokes a coccygodynia; on the posterior aspect of the thigh along the leg greater yang pathway; and in the hypogastrium (FIG. 15-20).

Trigger Point

Located in the area of BL-27 *(xiao chang shu)*.

RECTUS ABDOMINIS MUSCLE

Referred Pain

Bilateral pain in the lower posterior thoracic area encircling the body, sometimes with a sensation of abdominal fullness, epigastric pain, nausea and vomiting. According to Travell, the latter symptoms are more frequent when the trigger point is located on the left, in which case there may be precordial pain (FIG. 15-21).

Trigger Point

Located in the area of KI-21 *(you men)*.

Referred Pain

Lower back encircling pain.

Trigger Point

Located in the area of KI-11 *(heng gu)*.

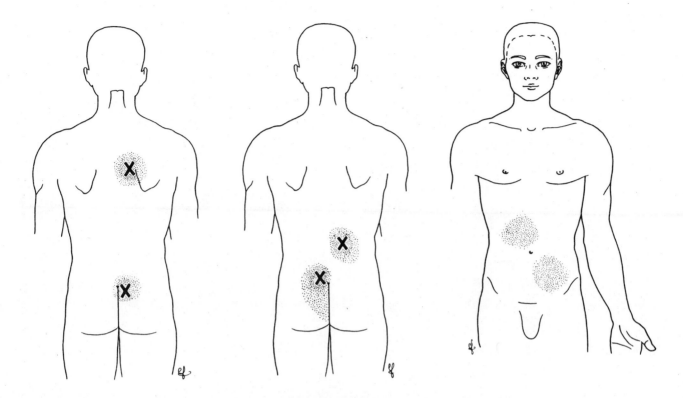

Fig. 15-20
Trigger Point Area for Multifidi and Rotatores Muscles

Chapter Notes

1. All of the quoted material in this chapter is drawn from Soulié de Morant (1972), unless otherwise noted.

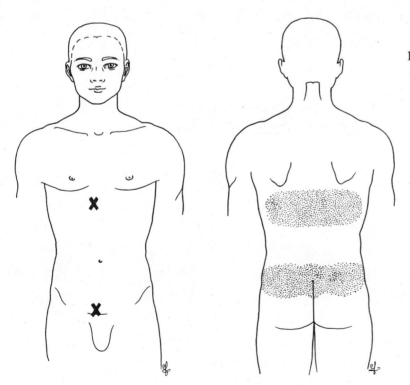

Fig. 15-21
Trigger Point Area for Rectus Abdominis Muscle

CHAPTER SIXTEEN

Sciatica

WE HAVE CHOSEN to present sciatica as it occurs in the daily practice of an acupuncturist. In this respect, we are presenting it in its energetic aspect with an L5 and S1 radicular pathway. In essence, this excludes other types of lower limb radicular pain.

It is important to bear in mind that although over 80 percent of sciatica cases are related to a discoradicular conflict, it would be a serious mistake to ignore the other serious etiologies such as neoplastic sciatica, neurinoma, ankylosing spondylitis of the sacroiliac joints, posterior interapophyseal degenerative joint disease, spondylolisthesis, lumbar spinal stenosis, nerve trunk sciatica, posterior spinal and nerve cord sciatica. Finally, we should note that the majority of sciatica cases that cannot be categorized clearly in biomedicine have a purely energetic etiology. This brief review underscores the necessity of performing a complete conventional medical, radiological and biochemical examination prior to any therapeutic intervention.

An osteopathic or similar structural exam is an important phase of the examination process. It allows us to diagnose and treat minor intervertebral disruption or other localized connective tissue problems. We must also bear in mind here that recurrences must lead us to look for an underlying energetic disorder. These are addressed in this chapter.

The above represents the preliminary stages of an energetic diagnosis, which involves an analysis of:

• the location of the pain
• the nature of the pain
• the regional and generalized eight parameters
• the clinical context and associated signs
• the patient's personal pathological history.

In this chapter, sciatica is divided temporally into acute and chronic types. This distinction should not be taken too rigidly. It is important to understand clearly and fully the specifics of each case.

Acute Sciatica

CHANNEL SINEW PATHOLOGY

This diagnosis is considered when the pain is superficial, usually recent, sharp and severe, presenting an acute blockage symptomatology. It is accompanied by muscle contractures. The onset is usually sudden, resulting from exposure to cold or subsequent to trauma, and is located along the muscles related to their channel, pointing to an L5 or S1 sciatica.

L5 Topography

Leg Lesser Yang Channel Sinew

There is painful contracture with stiffness of the fourth toe radiating toward the lateral aspect of the knee, difficulty in flexing or extending the knee, and pain in the lateral aspect of the thigh, hip and buttock up to the sacrum.

Treatment consists of needling the *ashi* points found below the iliac crest, in the areas around GB-29 *(ju liao)* or GB-30 *(huan tiao)*, or near GB-31 *(feng shi)* or GB-34 *(yang ling quan)*. It is possible to drain the local painful points, and it is recommended to combine treatment at these points with the well point GB-44 *(zu qiao yin)* and the river point GB-38 *(yang fu)*, and possibly to tonify the primary channel at GB-43 *(xia xi)*.

Leg Yang Brightness Channel Sinew

This condition affects the branch that separates at the instep, ascends along the lateral aspect of the leg, branches out at the fibula, climbs up the lateral aspect of the thigh and hip, travels along the flank and inserts at the spine. It manifests as painful stiffness with contracture of the three medial toes, and pain with a twisting sensation all along the pathway.

Treatment in this case is to look for the *ashi* points in the area of ST-36 *(zu san li)*, possibly to needle the local painful points, the well point ST-45 *(li dui)*, and to tonify the primary channel at ST-41 *(jie xi)*.

S1 Topography

Leg Greater Yang Channel Sinew

There is painful contracture of the small toe with a swelling sensation of the heel, pain along the channel pathway on the posterior aspect of the lower limb, and stiffness when hyperextending the spine. Additional signs may include pain in the cervical portion of the spine with difficulty in turning the head, and contractures in the axilla or supraclavicular fossa.

We should look for *ashi* points in the area around the M-BW-35 *(hua tuo jia ji)* paravertebral points, below the iliac crest, in the proximity of BL-38 *(fu xi)*, above the popliteal fossa, in the area of BL-57 *(cheng shan)*, or on the lateral border of the foot. In addition, we should tonify the primary channel at BL-67 *(zhi yin)* and needle the river point BL-60 *(kun lun)*.

Leg Lesser Yin Channel Sinew

The condition associated with this channel sinew affects the deep branch that travels along the lateral aspect of the spine up to the neck, or its distal plantar portion. It manifests as painful contractures in the sole of the foot and along the entire pathway of the channel, with diffi-

culty in bending the lumbar area. The problem is with forward bending for a superficial condition, and backward bending for a deeper one. The lateral aspects of the involved spinous processes are painful to the touch.

Treatment is to needle the well point KI-1 *(yong quan)*, the river point KI-7 *(fu liu)*, which is also the primary channel tonification point, and the *ashi* points in the areas around KI-1 *(yong quan)* and KI-2 *(ran gu)*.

PRIMARY CHANNEL PATHOLOGY

Leg Greater Yang (Bladder) Channel

The pain is sharp, severe, deep, like a fracture in the lumbar area, with a breaking, wrenching and exploding sensation along the pathway of the channel, suggesting an S1 topography. Other painful greater yang signs are sometimes associated, such as chills, headaches, stiff neck, stuffy nose and ocular pain.

If this symptomatology is the consequence of a direct invasion of Cold at the stream point, the pulse is tight and superficial, and the tongue is white. The symptoms can also result from Cold penetrating deeply into the muscles of the channels. Treatment is to needle the river point BL-60 *(kun lun)* and the sea point BL-40 *(wei zhong)*. In these cases one should bear in mind the need to tonify an underlying Kidney deficiency, which is probably present.

Regulation of the channel can also be achieved by utilizing the rule of midday-midnight. In this case, use the connecting point on the contralateral channel related by this rule, LU-7 *(lie que)*, along with the source point on the affected channel, BL-64 *(jing gu)*. This approach is especially helpful when no triggering factor has been identified. The host-guest rule can also be utilized by needling the host channel's source point, BL-64 *(jing gu)*, in combination with the guest channel's connecting point, KI-4 *(da zhong)*.

Leg Lesser Yang (Gallbladder) Channel

The pain is located along the lateral aspect of the lower limb in an L5 type topography, and in the sacroiliac joint. In this situation, we should also look for other symptoms pointing to a lesser yang disorder: vertigo, headaches, bitter taste in the mouth, poor hearing, chills and difficulty turning over in bed.

This pathology is often linked to pathogenic Wind-Dampness, which should be eliminated by needling points on this channel that eliminate Wind-Dampness, namely GB-38 *(yang fu)*, GB-34 *(yang ling quan)* and GB-30 *(huan tiao)*.

A possible Gallbladder Organ disorder affecting its associated channel should always be investigated. In cases of lesser yang stage disorder, it is preferable to use the stream-connecting points pairing technique, namely GB-41 *(zu lin qi)* and GB-37 *(guang ming)*.

Leg Yang Brightness (Stomach) Channel

The pain is located on the lateral aspect of the leg and on top of the foot, with difficulty in moving the second and third toes, and accompanied by a cold sensation in the leg, evoking a lateral popliteal sciatica. For this type of case, ST-38 *(tiao kou)* is particularly recommended to eliminate Damp-Cold.

CURIOUS VESSEL PATHOLOGY

It is perfectly legitimate to consider involvement of a Curious vessel in the case of a recent sciatica, but such involvement is limited to the yang Heel and Penetrating vessels. The other vessels are more involved in recurring or chronic sciatica. Moreover, pathology in any of the Curious vessels may indicate a deep disorder which often involves the patient's psyche.

Yang Heel Vessel

There is lower back pain with a sensation of being hit by a hammer, accompanied by stiffness of the entire body, difficulty in warming up in the morning, an ipsilateral flexion antalgic posture, contracture of the lateral aspect of the leg, and pain along the vessel's pathway. Accompanying sleep disorders are characteristic of this etiology.

Regulation is obtained by needling the confluent point BL-62 *(shen mai)*, the cleft point BL-59 *(fu yang)*, GB-29 *(ju liao)* along the trajectory of the pain, and possibly the paired confluent point SI-3 *(hou xi)*.

Penetrating Vessel

Straining while lifting a heavy object can disrupt the Penetrating vessel, causing a rod-type lower back pain with possible sciatica due to an anteroposterior imbalance. This situation can be resolved by needling BL-38 *(fu xi)* and BL-39 *(wei yang)*. If the imbalance lingers on, it could lead to a regional dysfunction.

ENERGETIC REGIONAL DYSFUNCTIONS

This category covers sciatica related to the obstruction of Qi circulation in the lumbar and pelvic areas, manifesting as local Qi stagnation or excess, which can be of a yang or a yin nature.

Yang Type

Qi trapped in the pelvis because of strain or an untimely movement is prevented from moving toward the lower limbs, which causes a yang excess-type pain in the lower back and abdomen, aggravated by pressure, coughing or local application of warmth, and spreading along the greater yang pathway to the lower limbs in an S1 type topography.

The treatment principle is to promote the outward movement of this energy by needling BL-29 *(zhong lu shu)*, BL-36 *(cheng fu)* and BL-60 *(kun lun)*.

Yin Type

Pathogenic Cold Obstruction

The "solidification" of circulation in the pelvis prevents the lower limb Qi from entering the trunk, which affects the greater yang level and causes an S1 type sciatica. There is a combination of yin excess signs in the pelvis and yang excess signs in the lower limbs.

The treatment principle in such cases is to expel the pathogenic Cold from the pelvis by applying moxa at CV-4 *(guan yuan)*, promote the circulation of Qi by needling KI-13 *(qi xue)* and BL-31 *(shang liao)*, and induce the lower limb yang to enter the trunk by needling ST-31 *(bi guan)*.

Blood Stasis

This type of Blood stasis is often the consequence of a dysfunction of the Penetrating vessel which disrupts the balance of Qi and Blood. The stabbing pain is often synchronized with the menstrual cycle in women, and indicates possible prostate pathology in men. In both sexes, hemorrhoids are a common feature. At any rate, this condition will progress toward a chronic stage if not treated in a timely manner.

The treatment principle is to open the Penetrating vessel by needling SP-4 *(gong sun)*, ST-30 *(qi chong)* and ST-36 *(zu san li)*, and to circulate the Blood by needling BL-53 *(bao huang)* and BL-37 *(yin men)*. Depending on the accompanying symptomatology, it may be advisable to add general command points for Blood circulation.

Chronic or Recurrent Sciatica

The chronic or recurring character of a sciatica implies

the involvement of any number of the following factors, in addition to the precipitant cause discussed above:

• an Organ pathology, especially of the Kidneys
• a painful obstruction-type rheumatic pathology
• a deep internal disorder which affects a Curious vessel.

KIDNEY DEFICIENCY

The usual symptoms are lower back pain and stiffness, which are aggravated by exhaustion and improve with rest, accompanied by weakness of the thighs and knees. All of these signs tend to recur frequently.

Kidney Yang Deficiency

The patient complains of spasms in the lower abdomen, the face is pale, the limbs are cold, and there may be spermatorrhea. The tongue is pale, and the pulse is submerged and thin.

Kidney Yin Deficiency

The patient presents signs of anxiety with restlessness and insomnia, dryness of the mouth, redness of the cheeks, heat in the palms and soles, a red tongue, and a wiry, thin and rapid pulse.

For Kidney yang deficiency, needle BL-23 (shen shu), GV-4 (ming men) and CV-4 (guan yuan). For Kidney yin deficiency, needle BL-23 (shen shu), KI-3 (tai xi), BL-52 (zhi shi) and BL-60 (kun lun). In both cases, it may be useful to needle and bleed BL-40 (wei zhong), as this point fortifies the lower back and is useful in the treatment of lower back pain associated with Kidney deficiency.

PAINFUL OBSTRUCTION DISORDERS

The presence of Wind-Damp-Cold painful obstruction should alert the practitioner to look for degenerative joint or even inflammatory manifestations in the lumbar area, which may be part of a larger problem.

Cold-predominant

The crises are severely painful, aggravated by exposure to cold, accompanied by a cold sensation in the lumbar area, and are not relieved by rest or standing up. The tongue coating is white, and the pulse is submerged and slow.

The treatment principle in such cases is to eliminate the Cold and tonify the protective Qi by applying moxa at BL-23 (shen shu) and GV-3 (yao yang guan), and needling BL-40 (wei zhong) and GB-39 (xuan zhong).

Damp-predominant

The pain is stabbing, with a swelling and heavy sensation through the entire body, and difficulty in moving. The painful crises are sensitive to changes in the weather, and occur mostly at night. The tongue has a thick, white, greasy coating, and the pulse is choppy. The elimination of pathogenic Dampness is always difficult and requires several sessions. Drying up Dampness can be achieved by using the method prescribed in Basic Questions: needle the yin river and stream points and the yang sea points, tonify the Spleen by applying moxa at BL-20 (pi shu), and tonify the essential Qi with moxa at CV-10 (xia wan), CV-12 (zhong wan) and CV-13 (shang wan).

CURIOUS VESSELS

Implication of a Curious vessel in chronic or recurring sciatica should always be a signal to look for a deep internal disorder involving the patient's psyche. The entire symbolic interpretation of the lumbar manifestation should be investigated. Thus a yang Heel vessel pathology occurs more frequently in patients who complain of having no "roots," who never feel at home anywhere; a Penetrating vessel pathology implies fundamental disorganization, a lack of structure in life among patients who can neither organize nor build it. The other involved Curious vessels are the Governing, yang Linking and Girdle vessels.

Governing Vessel

The vertebral pain is located in the midline, and is often accompanied by scoliosis- or kyphosis-type asymmetry disorders, marked spinal stiffness, and the possible addition of urinary disorders. The Governing vessel becomes the support that is lacking in individuals who feel that they are ill-equipped to meet life's challenges.

The important point to needle is GV-1 (chang qiang), to which BL-11 (da zhu) must be added.

Yang Linking Vessel

When disrupted, there is pain along the pathway of this vessel on the lateral aspect of the lower limb in accordance with an L5 topography. There is also a painful swelling sensation in the lumbar area, a local sensation of heat or generalized feverishness, and sensitivity to changes in the weather, such as snow and storms. This type of symptomatology occurs mostly in patients who are confused and who engage in frantic activity due to a lack of relationship with a superior order, or to an inability to put some distance between themselves and the external world.

To regulate this disorder, needle GB-35 *(yang jiao)* and TB-5 *(wai guan)*.

Girdle Vessel

Girdle vessel disorders usually lead to rod-type lower back pain that radiates around the beltline and is aggravated by movement. It is accompanied by weakness of the ankles, pelvic problems and a cold sensation in the buttocks and extremities. This belt vessel links the top and the bottom of the body, and becomes disrupted in individuals who feel isolated from the exterior world or who cannot find their place in society.

The classic prescription for regulating this disorder is to needle GB-26 *(dai mai)* and GB-41 *(zu lin qi)*.

SEQUELAE OF SCIATICA

The presence of a residual pain in the lateral aspect of the leg may indicate collateral deficiency of the leg yang brightness; one of its branches emerges at ST-40 *(feng long)*, travels along the lateral aspect of the lower limb, up the trunk, and ends in the head. The symptoms include emaciated and weak legs, and difficulty in flexing the knees. In this case, tonify ST-40 *(feng long)*.

Residual pain in the lateral aspect of the leg may also indicate collateral deficiency of the leg lesser yang, causing weakness in the lower limbs with muscular atrophy of the leg. In such cases, tonify GB-37 *(guang ming)*.

Post-operative Sciatica

Presence of post-operative sciatica should alert the practitioner to look for an underlying energetic disorder prior to the surgery, as discussed previously, especially a disorder of a Curious vessel, or Kidney deficiency. One particular aspect is represented by a pre-operative invasion of pathogenic Cold, generating local Blood stasis with all the associated risks of fibrosis. The treatment principle in such cases is to eliminate the local pathogenic Cold through the repeated application of moxa at CV-6 *(qi hai)*, BL-31 *(shang liao)* and BL-23 *(shen shu)*, or the use of the warm needle technique, or even suction cups.

Trigger Points

ILIOCOSTALIS LUMBORUM MUSCLE

Referred Pain

Pain in the lower back and buttocks (FIG. 16-1).

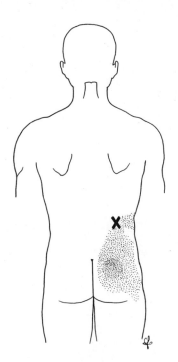

Fig. 16-1
Trigger Point Area for Iliocostalis Lumborum Muscle

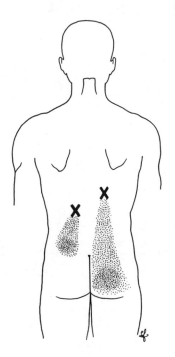

Fig. 16-2
Trigger Point Area for Longissimus Muscle

Trigger Point

In the area of BL-51 *(huang men)*.

LONGISSIMUS MUSCLE

Referred Pain

Pain in the lower back and buttocks (FIG. 16-2).

Trigger Point

In the area of BL-49 *(yi she)*.

GLUTEUS MAXIMUS MUSCLE

Referred Pain

Pain in the buttocks (FIG. 16-3).

Trigger Point

In the area of N-BW-34 *(bi kong)*.[1]

GLUTEUS MEDIUS MUSCLE

Referred Pain (according to Travell)

Pain in the buttocks (FIG. 16-4).

Trigger Point

In the area of M-BW-26 *(zhong kong)*.[2]

GLUTEUS MINIMUS MUSCLE

Referred Pain

Pain in the buttocks and lateral aspect of the lower limb along the pathway of the leg lesser yang (FIG. 16-5).

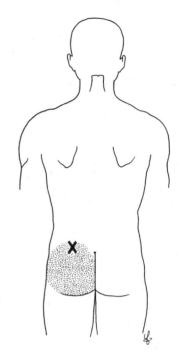

Fig. 16-4
Trigger Point Area for Gluteus Medius Muscle

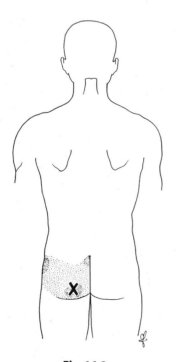

Fig. 16-3
Trigger Point Area for Gluteus Maximus Muscle

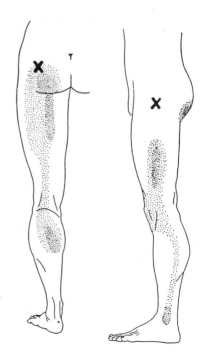

Fig. 16-5
Trigger Point Area for Gluteus Minimus Muscle

Trigger Point

In the area of N-LE-56 *(kuan jiu),*[3] or even around GB-29 *(ju liao).*

Referred Pain

Pain in the buttocks and posterior aspect of the thigh and calf along the pathway of the leg greater yang (FIG. 16-5).

Trigger Point

In the area of M-BW-33 *(tun zhong).*[4]

PIRIFORMIS MUSCLE

Referred Pain

Sacroiliac and buttock pain, which may radiate toward the posterior aspect of the thigh along the pathway of the leg greater yang, frequently encountered during pregnancy or postpartum (FIG. 16-6).

Trigger Point

In the area of GB-30 *(huan tiao).*

TIBIALIS ANTERIOR MUSCLE

Referred Pain

Pain along the tibial crest and big toe (FIG. 16-7).

Trigger Point

In the area of ST-36 *(zu san li).*

EXTENSOR DIGITORUM LONGUS MUSCLE

Referred Pain

Pain along the anterolateral aspect of the leg and three smaller toes (FIG. 16-8).

Trigger Point

In the area of N-LE-7 *(li wai).*[5]

PERONEUS LONGUS MUSCLE

Referred Pain

Pain along the lateral aspect of the leg along the pathway of the leg lesser yang (FIG. 16-9).

Trigger Point

In the area of GB-34 *(yang ling quan).*

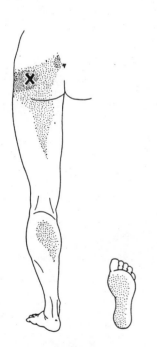

Fig. 16-6
Trigger Point Area
for Piriformis Muscle

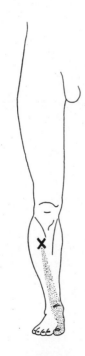

Fig. 16-7
Trigger Point Area for
Tibialis Anterior Muscle

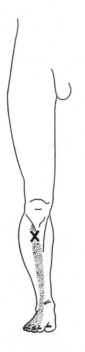

Fig. 16-8
Trigger Point Area for Extensor
Digitorum Longus Muscle

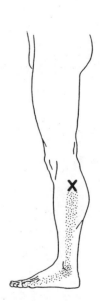

Fig. 16-9
Trigger Point Area for
Peroneus Longus Muscle

POSTERIOR SACROILIAC LIGAMENT

Referred Pain

Pain in the posterolateral aspect of the thigh, lateral aspect of the leg, and lateral border of the foot (FIG. 16-10).

Trigger Point

In the area of BL-26 (guan yuan shu), BL-27 (xiao chang shu), BL-28 (pang guang shu) and BL-53 (bao huang).

BICEPS FEMORIS MUSCLE

Referred Pain

Pain in the popliteal fossa and posterior aspect of the leg along the pathway of the leg greater yang. This pain is of a musculoligamental type, and should not be confused with radicular pain (FIG. 16-11).

Trigger Point

In the lower third of a line joining BL-37(yin men) to BL-40 (wei zhong).

SACROSPINOUS AND SACROTUBEROUS LIGAMENTS

Referred Pain

Pain in the posterior aspect of the thigh, calf and heel (FIG. 16-12).

Trigger Point

In the area of BL-30 (bai huan shu).

ILIOLUMBAR LIGAMENT AND SUPERIOR PORTION OF POSTERIOR SACROILIAC LIGAMENT

Referred Pain

Pain appears in the posterolateral aspect of the thigh, radiating toward the front down to the patella and the lateral aspect of the leg, but stopping before the malleolus. There may also be pain in the groin, genital organs, below the iliac crest, and in the trochanter area (FIG. 16-13).

Trigger Point

In the area of BL-26 (guan yuan shu) and BL-27 (xiao chang shu).

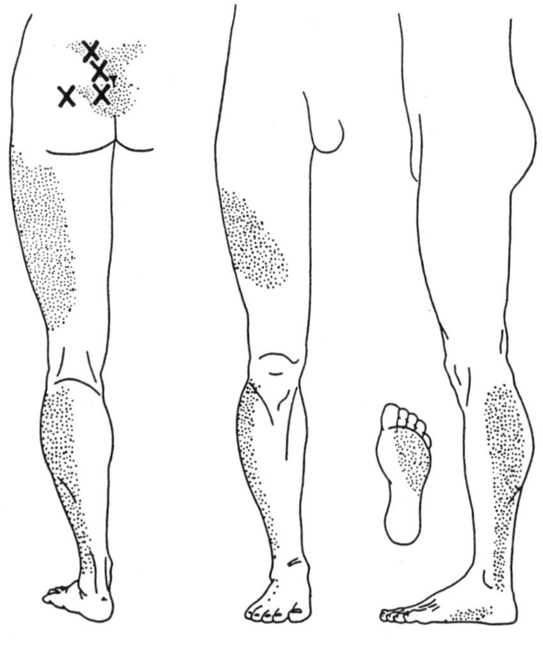

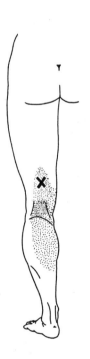

Fig. 16-10
Trigger Point Area for
Posterior Sacroiliac Ligament

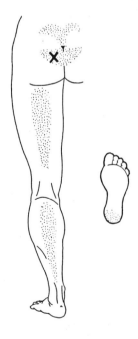

Fig. 16-11
Trigger Point Area for
Biceps Femoris Muscle

Fig. 16-12
Trigger Point Area
for Sacrospinous and
Sacrotuberous Ligaments

SACROSPINOUS AND SACROTUBEROUS LIGAMENTS, AND INFERIOR PORTION OF SACROILIAC LIGAMENT

Referred Pain

Pain in the posterior aspect of the thigh and calf, the posterolateral border of the calf down to the malleolus, the lateral border of the foot down to the fifth toe, and sometimes under the foot and toes, except for the big toe (FIG. 16-14).

Trigger Point

In the area of BL-28 *(pang guang shu)*, between that point and BL-53 *(bao huang)*; in the area of BL-30 *(bai huan shu)*, and one unit below that point. According to Hackett (1958), the point corresponding to BL-29 *(zhong lu shu)* is an important one for sciatica.

ARTICULAR LIGAMENT OF THE HIP

Referred Pain

Pain in the trochanter area, the posterolateral aspect of the thigh, the anterolateral aspect of the leg, the big toe and the medial half of the fourth toe (FIG. 16-15).

Trigger Point

In the area of GB-30 *(huan tiao)* and ST-31 *(bi guan)*.

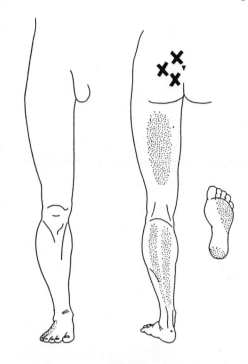

Fig. 16-14
Trigger Point Area for Sacrospinous and Sacrotuberous Ligaments and Inferior Portion of Sacroiliac Ligament

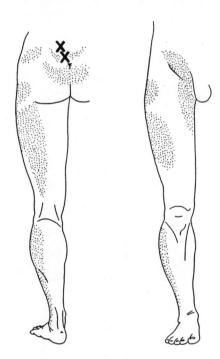

Fig. 16-13
Trigger Point Area for Iliolumbar Ligament and Superior Portion of Posterior Sacroiliac Ligament

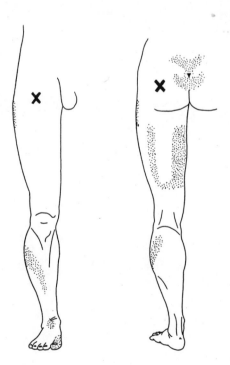

Fig. 16-15
Trigger Point Area for Articular Ligament of the Hip

Conclusion

In the presence of sciatica, modern biomedicine primarily looks for a radiculopathy related to disc disease. On an energetic level, however, the etiologies are far from being so uniform. We must learn not to fixate on the most obvious diagnosis, and remember that a deep internal disorder affecting the patient's very personality can cause recurring or chronic disorders. Failing to do so will unavoidably lead to many therapeutic failures. Because of the wealth of its diagnostic tools and therapeutic efficacy, acupuncture should today be a part of the medical treatment of sciatica.

Chapter Notes

1. This point is located 2 units lateral to the tip of the coccyx.
2. This point is located 3.5 units lateral to the spinous process of L5.
3. This point is located 0.5 units directly above the greater trochanter.
4. This point is located at the apex of an imaginary equilateral triangle whose base is a line drawn between the posterosuperior greater trochanter and the ischial tuberosity.
5. This point is located 1 unit lateral to ST-36 *(zu san li)*.

Neck Pain

Energetic Aspects of Neck and Cervical Spine

The neck is a crucial area of the body. Not only does it connect the head with the trunk, but it is the place where, both in biomedical anatomy and acupuncture energetics, important crossings are made. To understand how to treat neck pain, we must understand the salient energetic aspects of this region of the body.

RELATIONSHIP WITH CHANNEL SYSTEM

Primary Channels

Arm Yang Brightness (Large Intestine) Channel

After going around the shoulder, this channel connects with SI-12 *(bing feng)* in the suprascapular fossa, then with GV-14 *(da zhui)* below the seventh cervical spinal process. It then returns to the front toward ST-12 *(que pen)* in the supraclavicular fossa, from where it goes deep inside the body. From ST-12 *(que pen)*, a superficial branch ascends along the sternocleidomastoid muscle toward the mandible, and continues up to LI-20 *(ying xiang)* on the opposite side.

Leg Yang Brightness (Stomach) Channel

The descending branch starts from ST-5 *(dai ying)*,

goes through ST-9 *(ren ying)*, and then descends toward the supraclavicular fossa. From ST-11 *(qi she)* it goes back toward GV-14 *(da zhui)* below the seventh cervical spinal process, then returns toward the front to the supraclavicular fossa at ST-12 *(que pen)*, from which a deep branch and a descending superficial branch originate.

Leg Greater Yin (Spleen) Channel

The deep branch follows the esophagus and ascends to the root of the tongue.

Arm Lesser Yin (Heart) Channel

In its deep pathway a branch emerges from the Heart, ascends along the esophagus, passes through the larynx and goes toward the eye.

Arm Greater Yang (Small Intestine) Channel

From behind the shoulder joint this channel reaches the sub- and suprascapular fossae, then GV-14 *(da zhui)* below the seventh cervical spinal process, then it goes toward the front to the supraclavicular fossa, and from ST-12 *(que pen)* moves internally. Here emerges a superficial branch which ascends along the lateral aspect of the neck and continues up the face.

Leg Greater Yang (Bladder) Channel

The pathway of this channel on the head ends in the

nape of the neck at BL-10 *(tian zhu)*, where it separates into two branches. The medial branch goes through the seventh cervical and first thoracic spinal processes, and continues its downward pathway lateral to the spine. The lateral branch descends parallel and laterally to the medial branch.

Leg Lesser Yin (Kidney) Channel

A deep branch of this channel emerging from the Kidneys travels along the trachea and the throat, penetrates the base of the tongue, and connects with the greater yang channel at BL-10 *(tian zhu)*.

Arm Lesser Yang (Triple Burner) Channel

This channel arrives at the posterior aspect of the shoulder, travels along the trapezius muscle, and reaches GV-14 *(da zhui)* below the seventh cervical spinal process. It returns toward the front, crosses the leg lesser yang channel at GB-21 *(jian jing)*, and penetrates the supraclavicular fossa, where it travels internally.

A branch goes up from the chest to the supraclavicular fossa where it emerges, continues up the neck, reaches the anterior border of the mastoid process, and then separates into two branches.

Leg Lesser Yang (Gallbladder) Channel

The first portion of this channel on the head ends at the occiput at GB-20 *(feng chi)*, where it reaches SI-17 *(tian rong)* behind the angle of the jaw. It then travels backward, crosses the arm lesser yang channel at the superior border of the trapezius at GB-21 *(jian jing)*, and connects with GV-14 *(da zhui)* below the seventh cervical spinal process. From there it returns to the front toward the supraclavicular fossa, where both a superficial and deep branch originate. In another portion of its trajectory from the head, the channel descends from the mandibular angle to end at the supraclavicular fossa.

Leg Terminal Yin (Liver) Channel

The deep branch reaches the throat and pharynx, then ascends to the eye, forehead, and ends at the vertex at GV-20 *(bai hui)*.

Channel Sinews

Leg Greater Yang Channel Sinew

This channel sinew travels along the spine and ends at the nape of the neck, where one branch penetrates to connect with the base of the tongue. The main branch

inserts at the occipital bone, ascends to the top of the head, and descends to the ala nasi.

The branch that penetrates inside the axilla emerges at the supraclavicular fossa and goes upward to insert at GB-12 *(wan gu)*, posterior and inferior to the mastoid process. Another branch travels upward from the supraclavicular fossa and ascends obliquely to end by the side of the nose.

Leg Lesser Yang Channel Sinew

The main branch of this channel sinew ascends vertically in front of the axilla, goes through the supraclavicular fossa, emerges in front of the leg greater yang channel and ascends behind the ear to end at the temple.

Leg Yang Brightness Channel Sinew

A branch ascends from the supraclavicular fossa along the anterolateral aspect of the neck, goes around the mouth and inserts at the nose.

Leg Lesser Yin Channel Sinew

A branch travels deeply along the lateral aspect of the spine up to the neck to insert at the occipital bone, where it meets the leg greater yang channel.

Arm Greater Yang Channel Sinew

A branch goes behind the axilla and ascends around the scapula, along the neck, emerges in front of the leg greater yang channel sinew and inserts at GB-12 *(wan gu)*, posterior and inferior to the mastoid process.

Arm Lesser Yang Channel Sinew

This channel sinew travels along the lateral aspect of the neck to meet the arm greater yang channel.

Arm Yang Brightness Channel Sinew

The main branch ascends from LI-15 *(jian yu)* in front and below the lateral extremity of the acromion to the neck, and continues on the head to the angle of the jaw on the opposite side.

Curious Vessels

Governing Vessel

In its main pathway this channel ascends through the spinal processes of the vertebral column up to the neck at GV-16 *(feng fu)*. It enters the brain, ascends to the vertex, follows the forehead and descends along the midline of the nose.

A branch starts with the leg greater yang channel at

the inner canthus of the eye, ascends to the forehead, crosses the leg greater yang channel at the vertex, and enters the brain. It follows the same pathway as the leg greater yang channel down to the neck, and continues its downward trajectory on either side of the spine.

Conception Vessel

Following the midline of the body, this channel travels to the anterior aspect of the neck.

Penetrating Vessel

In the second portion of its trajectory, branching out at the thorax, this channel ascends through the neck to spread into the nasal cavities.

Yang Heel Vessel

This channel travels along the anterolateral aspect of the neck, then reaches the lips and the inner canthus of the eye. Together with the greater yang channel and the yin Heel vessel, it then goes up the head, through the hair, and down the nape of the neck to reach GB-20 *(feng chi)* below the occipital bone. From GV-16 *(feng fu)* located between the two tendons of the nape of the neck, it enters the brain.

Yin Heel Vessel

From the supraclavicular fossa, this channel goes up the throat in front of ST-9 *(ren ying)*, passes in front of the medial border of the cheek bone to reach the inner canthus of the eye where it meets the greater yang channel and the yang Heel vessel, which all together ascend to the brain.

Yang Linking Vessel

This channel goes up the lateral aspect of the neck through the two cervical barriers TB-15 *(tian liao)* and GB-21 *(jian jing)*, reaches the occipital gate at GV-15 *(ya men)* and GV-16 *(feng fu)*, and travels on the skull through the yang (lesser yang) level, from GB-20 *(feng chi)* to GB-13 *(ben shen)*.

There is a variant pathway that goes up behind the ear, reaches the forehead, then goes all the way back to GV-16 *(feng fu)*.

Yin Linking Vessel

In its last portion, the yin Linking vessel trajectory meets the Conception vessel pathway on the midline of the throat at CV-22 *(tian tu)* and CV-23 *(lian quan)*.

Collaterals

The arm yang brightness, arm lesser yin and leg yang brightness collaterals that ascend to the head all go through the neck. However, none has any particularly well-defined trajectory.

When deficient, the arm terminal yin collateral exhibits a typical symptom of "nape and neck stiffness." According to J.-M. Kespi, PC-6 *(nei guan)* governs the cervical portion of the spine.

The leg greater yang collateral, which starts from BL-58 *(fei yang)*, accompanies the primary channel through the nape of the neck. This pathway is not confirmed by the modern text prepared by the Shanghai College of Traditional Medicine (Roustan, 1979).

The collateral of the Governing vessel starts from GV-1 *(chang qiang)* at the tip of the coccyx, ascends alongside the spine to reach the nape of the neck, and branches out at the vertex.

Channel Divergences

The channel divergences are internally linked to the yin and yang Organs.

The channel divergences connected to the yang primary channels start in the four limbs and enter the chest and abdomen to communicate with the internal Organs. Most of them emerge at the level of the neck and connect with their own yang primary channels. The channel divergences connected to the yin primary channels rise out of their own primary channels, and travel parallel to their paired yang channel. This function of linking the primary yin channels with their paired yang channels is represented in their name as the six confluences *(liù hé)*.

The three leg yang channel divergences all pass through the Heart to ascend to the head. The three hand yin channel divergences all pass through the throat to ascend to the face and head.

All of the channel divergences go through the "window of the sky" points and promote the exchange of energy between the trunk and the head:

- ST-9 *(ren ying)* for the leg greater yin-leg yang brightness pair
- SI-16 *(tian chuang)* for the arm lesser yin-arm greater yang pair
- SI-17 *(tian rong)* for the leg terminal yin-leg lesser yang pair
- LI-17 *(tian ding)* for the arm yang brightness-arm greater yin pair

- TB-16 *(tian you)* for the arm lesser yang-arm terminal yin pair
- BL-10 *(tian zhu)* for the leg greater yang-leg lesser yin pair.

WINDOW OF THE SKY POINTS

The "window of the sky" points were first grouped together in chapter 2 of *Divine Pivot*, where they were simply listed as the major points in the area around the supraclavicular fossae. With the exception of LU-3 *(tian fu)* and PC-1 *(tian chi)*, they are all located at the junction of the head and neck. Their role is to promote the movement of Qi between the head and trunk, to connect humans with heaven.

BL-10 *(tian zhu)*: This point brings down the head and neck Qi toward the trunk and the lower part of the body. Its symptomatology is therefore related to a yang excess above (headache, vertigo) and a yin deficiency below (a sensation of losing one's legs, weakness of the legs).

ST-9 *(ren ying)*: This point promotes the passage of the trunk yang toward the head. Its symptomatology is therefore related to yang excess of the thorax (dyspnea, thoracic distention, blockage at the level of the neck with swelling and difficulty swallowing) with yin deficiency above.

SI-16 *(tian chuang)*: This point governs the influence of heaven on humans. This is particularly true at the level of the orifices of the head. Its symptomatology includes deafness, tinnitus, insanity, incoherent speech and warm facial skin.

SI-17 *(tian rong)*: This point governs the outward movement of the trunk yin toward the head. Its symptomatology is therefore related to yin excess of the trunk and neck with deficiency above. Among the possible symptoms are cough, surging of Qi toward the top, vomiting of sputum, a sensation of obstruction in the throat, dyspnea, goiter, painful obstruction of the throat and trismus.

TB-16 *(tian you)*: This point governs the yang external to humans (heavenly yang), which circulates the Qi in humans at the level of the head and neck. It is therefore indicated in all cases of stagnation of yin and/or yang in the face. This includes such problems as facial deviation, trismus, difficulty in opening the mouth, swelling of the cheeks, toothache and jaw pain.

LI-17 *(tian ding)*: This point promotes the passage of the termination of the yang in humans toward heaven and the external world. This function is illustrated by the symptomatology: sudden loss of voice, obstruction of Qi in the throat, gurgling in the throat and a suffocating sensation. The last symptom means to us that there has been an extremely sudden halt in the movement of a person toward the exterior.

CV-22 *(tian tu)*: This point governs the outward movement of all the Qi (yin or yang) from the trunk to the top. It is marked by such problems as sudden loss of voice, cough with surging of Qi toward the top, painful obstruction of the throat, throat spasms, excess in the thorax, heart pain and a flushed, warm face.

GV-16 *(feng fu)*: This is also a Wind point which is located at the occipital barrier level. It mobilizes the yin and yang Qi of the skull. On the one hand, it is used for externally contracted problems such as direct attack by pathogenic Wind, Wind-attack *(zhòng fēng)* with chills, sweating, and stiffness of the nape with difficulty in turning the head. On the other hand, it is used for stagnation of yin or yang in the skull marked by such symptoms as headache, vertigo, hemiplegia, agitation or hallucinations.

LOCAL QI MOVEMENTS

The nape and neck connect and separate the trunk and head, providing a place of constant Qi exchange between these two areas, which we shall study in greater detail in our discussion of cervical pathology below.

NAPE AND NECK SYMBOLISM

The importance of the neck area has been clearly and succinctly described by B. Cygler (1987):

> The neck is made of two elements, the nape and throat. The nape carries and supports the head; it is both its hinge and pillar. It is the nape that promotes the motility of the neck through the cervical vertebrae; it is the nape that rules and regulates man's sixth sense (balance), constantly adjusting the position of the head in space, and the position of the head above the nape. While the nape is the "hinge" area, the throat on the other hand is the "passage" area. More than an anatomical region, the throat is first and foremost an energetic crossroad through which travels the Qi moving from the trunk to the head and from the head to the trunk.

The head is separated from the neck by the "occipital gate," as noted by H. Maspero in the chapter on breathing in his book *Le Taoïsme et religions chinoises*. Maspero describes three types of gates: *dì guān*, or "earth's gate," which means the feet; *rén guān*, or "man's gate," which means the hands; and *tiān guān*, "heaven's gate," or the occiput.

From the perspective of its relationship with the external world, the occipital gate plays the same role as the hands and feet. According to Kespi (1982), the occipital gate includes three Governing vessel points:

- GV-15 (*ya men*), the "door of mutism," governs speech and silence
- GV-16 (*feng fu*), the "wind's palace," moves the intracranial Qi and Blood
- GV-17 (*nao hu*), the "brain's door" and "sea of marrow," governs the brain and coordinates our exchanges with the external world.

One of the fundamental aspects of the neck is its ability to rotate. Related to the yin and yang inversion law, the action of rotating or turning around accompanies any change of plane or state. The passage from anterior heaven (the prenatal state) to posterior heaven (post birth), from the unmanifested to the manifested, is precisely accompanied by this yin and yang inversion.

On the physical plane, the action of turning around manifests as a decussation of the medullary nerve fibers. On the energetic plane, it manifests as the crossing over of the yang Heel Curious vessel, the arm yang brightness primary channel, and the leg lesser yang channel sinew.

As noted by Kespi (1982), the spine has many levels of meaning. It is not only the vertical axis linking man to heaven, but also a transcendental path incarnating the return toward Oneness. It is the tree of life which allows the ascension of the self along its vertebral column and therefore its spiritual rebirth. In this ascension, the "7" cervical vertebrae are the means to achieve this realization. The "7" cervical vertebrae lead indeed to the skull and head, a place where one is "recapitulated." These "7" vertebrae lead to the superior cinnabar field (*dān tiān*), an important seat of consciousness in Daoist yoga, where one can merge with the universe.

Cervical Spine Pathology

LOCAL PATHOLOGY

Obstruction of the Qi's Downward Movement from the Head to the Trunk

The Qi descending from the head is originally greater yang and emerges at BL-10 (*tian zhu*); in its intermediate

lesser yang stage it is ruled by GB-21 (*jian jing*); and in its terminal yang brightness phase it enters the trunk at ST-11 (*qi she*). This downward movement can be disrupted by mechanical factors or external pathogenic influences such as Wind-Cold or Wind-Dampness (FIG. 17-1).

Obstruction of BL-10 (*tian zhu*) creates a yang excess at the occiput radiating down the leg greater yang channel with "horrendous pain in the shoulders and back," and a resultant deficiency of yang below with "stiff neck, spasms, torticollis." Obstruction at GB-21 (*jian jing*) frequently generates a contracture of the trapezius muscle, often due to nervous tension. This can radiate down the leg lesser yang channel, as in the case of torticollis. Obstruction of ST-11 (*qi she*) is responsible for sore throat with difficulty in tolerating anything tight around the neck.

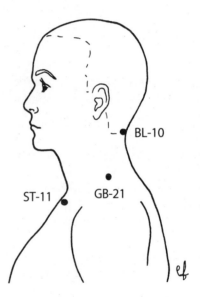

Fig. 17-1
Downward Movement of Qi from Head to Trunk

Obstruction of the Qi's Upward Movement from the Trunk to the Head

The Qi ascending from the trunk is originally greater yang and emerges at SI-14 (*jian wai shu*) on the arm greater yang; in its intermediate lesser yang phase it is ruled by TB-15 (*tian liao*); and in its terminal yang brightness stage it is governed by ST-3 (*ju liao*) (FIG. 17-2). Disruption of the Qi's upward movement can be caused by the same factors that disrupt its downward movement (see above); only a detailed eight parameter analysis can determine in which direction the obstruction occurs.

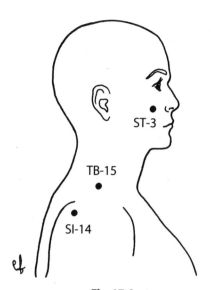

Fig. 17-2
Upward Movement of Qi from Trunk to Head

Obstruction of SI-14 (*jian wai shu*) causes yang excess upstream in the suprascapular fossa, radiating down the arm greater yang and/or arm lesser yang channel(s), and deficiency downstream in the nape of the neck with cervical stiffness, torticollis and a cold sensation in the nape. This can be a pattern suggesting a C7 type cervicobrachial neuralgia.

Obstruction of TB-15 (*tian liao*) prevents the intermediate yang from rising to the face. There is yang excess upstream with pain in the hand and leg greater yang channels in the nape, back and shoulders, and deficiency downstream which may be marked by numbness or coolness around the ear.

Obstruction of ST-3 (*ju liao*) generates more facial or maxillary symptoms than cervical ones.

Diffuse Yang Deficiency in the Nape of the Neck

Yang deficiency at the nape of the neck is frequently observed when cervical trauma cuts off the Qi circulation in the channels, requiring the patient to wear an orthopedic collar. The underlying cervical weakness manifests as pain under strain or exhaustion, which is improved by pressure and local application of warmth. The indicated treatment is to tonify the meeting point of the entire body's yang, GV-14 (*da zhui*). This is done through repeated applications of moxa, which quickly restores the nape's normal tonicity.

External Pathogenic Influences

A sudden onset of torticollis is often due to an invasion of pathogenic Wind-Cold at the nape of the neck. An example might be by exposure to wind or a draft, as when driving a car with the window rolled down. The principal point of penetration of the pathogenic influences is GV-16 (*feng fu*). In this case, the pain is in the nape of the neck, traveling downward symmetrically from GV-16 (*feng fu*) to the shoulders. Draining this point and then tonifying GV-14 (*da zhui*) is sufficient to quickly resolve the pathology. This process is described in a passage from chapter 60 of *Basic Questions*:

> When Wind enters from the outside, it causes people to shiver, sweat comes out, the head hurts, the body feels heavy and there is aversion to cold. The treatment for this is at *feng fu* to regulate the yin and yang by tonifying the insufficiency and draining the overabundance. When there is great Wind with a painful nape, needle *feng fu*, located above the superior vertebra.

Two other points are common sites in the upper part of the body for invasion by pathogenic influences: BL-12 (*feng men*) and SI-12 (*bing feng*). Disruption of the functions of these points is frequently responsible for pain in the cervical region of the spine. When the pathogenic Qi is not eliminated, it spreads through the leg greater yang and arm greater yang and causes severe cervicobrachial pain.

Channel Pathology

Primary Channels

The primary channels involved in cervical pathology are the leg greater yang, leg lesser yang and arm greater yang.

Leg Greater Yang (Bladder) Channel

Pathogenic Cold is usually the chief culprit; the pain in the nape is severe with a sensation of tearing apart, and often accompanied by headaches, pain in the spine, or even a breaking sensation in the lumbar portion of the spine. As described in chapter 49 of *Basic Questions*:

> For those with a unilateral deficiency, with winter cold they have extreme insufficiency. For this reason a unilateral insufficiency causes limping. For those with unyielding above [in the head and neck—meaning toriticollis] radiating toward the back, the yang ascends in one block and its struggle causes the unyielding above.

Regulating the leg greater yang is achieved by needling the transport points in accordance with the techniques presented in chapter 15.

One particular feature is discussed in chapter 63 of *Basic Questions*. When the pathogenic influence has settled inside the collateral of the Bladder channel, there is pain in the nape and shoulders; needle BL-67 *(zhi yin)* immediately, and if instant relief is not forthcoming, needle BL-63 *(jin men)* three times. For a unilateral condition, needle the opposite side.

Arm Greater Yang (Small Intestine) Channel

The cervical pain is more lateral. It is accompanied by a restriction in the rotation of the head, and pain in the shoulder and arm along the pathway of the channel, which may look like a cervicobrachial neuralgia.

Treatment generally consists of needling the well point SI-1 *(shao ze)*; the stream point SI-3 *(hou xi)*, which fights off the pathogenic invasion and is also the confluent point for the Governing vessel; and draining SI-12 *(bing feng)* through which the pathogenic influences tend to invade the body.

Among the different pathogenic modalities which may confirm the role played by the primary channel, remember to consider a midday-midnight imbalance, and, in this case, to needle on the opposite leg terminal yin Liver channel. One possibility is LR-10 *(zu wu li)*, which Soulié de Morant considered to have a relationship with the lateral muscles of the neck. Another is the cleft point LR-6 *(zhong du)*.

Leg Lesser Yang (Gallbladder) Channel

This type of lateral cervical pain occurs in a context of vertigo, headaches with polyarthralgia, flank and intercostal pain, pain along the pathway of the channel on the lower limb, difficulty in turning around, or even chills and fever. Painful swelling in the supraclavicular fossa is a typical feature. In addition to the regulation techniques of the primary channels discussed previously, we need to emphasize the importance of local points such as GB-20 *(feng chi)* and GB-21 *(jian jing)*. The former promotes the mobilization of the Qi; it is therefore especially indicated for stagnation-type pain which is typically improved with topical heat and massage.

Arm Yang Brightness (Large Intestine) and Arm Lesser Yang (Triple Burner) Channels

These primary channels are rarely involved in cervical pain. Instead, they tend to exhibit signs of swelling or painful obstruction of the throat *(hóu bì)*.

Channel Sinews

When manipulation of the cervical spine becomes a necessary therapeutic intervention, it is greatly enhanced if preceded by needling the channel sinews. This is because this type of treatment helps relax local muscle spasms. The major point used for treating channel sinew problems is the well point. Other points, especially the river points and those in the zone of the pain, are often added.

Leg Greater Yang Channel Sinew

These cervical spasms can be difficult to overcome and may extend to the supraclavicular fossa and the thoracic spine. The cervical column is bent backward, and it is difficult to turn the head left or right, or to lift the shoulders. If this condition is of mechanical or post-traumatic origin, needle the *ashi* or trigger points in accordance with the pain topography described at the end of this chapter, in addition to the well point BL-67 *(zhi yin)*.

If external Wind-Cold is involved, add BL-60 *(kun lun)* and also SI-18 *(quan liao)*, meeting point of the lower limb channel sinews. This will prevent the pathogenic Qi from spreading to other channel sinews.

Leg Lesser Yin Channel Sinew

When this channel is involved, the cervical pain is deep and flexion and extension of the neck is difficult or impossible. Use the well point SP-1 *(yin bai)*, the river point SP-5 *(shang qiu)*, the main *ashi* point and the insertion points surrounding the painful area. If there is an aspect of pathogenic Dampness, add the leg greater yin tonification point SP-2 *(da du)* and the crossing points of the foot yin channels, CV-2 *(qu gu)* and CV-3 *(zhong ji)*. This will prevent the problem from spreading to the other lower limb channel sinews.

Leg Lesser Yang Channel Sinew

Stiffness and contracture of the cervical spine and supraclavicular fossa are characteristic signs of an invasion of the leg lesser yang channel sinew. Needle the well point GB-44 *(zu qiao yin)* in combination with the river point GB-40 *(qiu xu)*, the main *ashi* point and the insertion points surrounding the painful area. If it is caused by the invasion of pathogenic influences, also tonify the leg lesser yang channel by needling GB-43 *(xia xi)* and the crossing point SI-18 *(quan liao)* to prevent these influences from spreading to other lower limb yang channel sinews.

Collaterals

The only collateral involved is the one pertaining to the Governing vessel, which, when in a state of excess, causes stiffness of the vertebral column, including the cervical spine. In such cases, needle GV-1 *(chang qiang)*.

Curious Vessels

Governing Vessel

In cases of obstruction, there is cervical and spinal stiffness; with deficiency, there are mostly headaches and vertigo. Needling the confluent point SI-3 *(hou xi)* promotes the free circulation of Qi in the Governing vessel.

Sometimes the Governing vessel is involved in problems in which the very frame of the body is deficient, as this vessel is the space where the yang finds the support to structure itself. In such cases the cervical pain is often the consequence of an underlying scoliosis. Here it might be useful to combine, often with moxa, BL-11 *(da zhu)* and GV-1 *(chang qiang)*.

Yin and Yang Heel Vessels

An imbalance in these vessels causes contractures of the muscles and tendons. This may manifest at the level of the cervical spine as pain with a sidebent antalgic posture. Sleep disorders, ocular problems and whole body stiffness are typical signs, but not always present.

Regulation is achieved by needling the cleft and confluent points, KI-6 *(zhao hai)* and KI-8 *(jiao xin)* for the yin Heel vessel, and BL-62 *(shen mai)* and BL-59 *(fu yang)* for the yang Heel vessel. Also needle local points along the pathway of these vessels, such as GB-20 *(feng chi)* or GV-16 *(feng fu)*.

Yang Linking Vessel

Cervical pain is typically sensitive to changes in the weather, snow and storms. It is frequently accompanied by occipitofrontal headaches and a febrile sensation.

Regulation of the yang Linking vessel is achieved by needling the confluent point TB-5 *(wai guan)* and the cleft point GB-35 *(yang jiao)*. Depending on the circumstances, it might be useful to needle one of the local pathway points: TB-15 *(tian liao)*, SI-10 *(nao shu)*, GB-21 *(jian jing)*, GB-20 *(feng chi)*, GV-15 *(ya men)*, GV-16 *(feng fu)*, GB-19 *(nao kong)* or GB-18 *(cheng ling)*.

Girdle Vessel

The Girdle vessel may be involved when the balance between the upper and lower parts of the body is disrupted. The pattern is one of yang excess above and yin excess below. The yin excess may be the most notable aspect, as the body type includes a very heavy lower half of the body, with a "riding breeches" look. In such cases, needle GB-41 *(zu lin qi)* in combination with GB-26 *(dai mai)*.

ORGANS

Pathogenic influences attacking the Kidneys can cause, along with abdominal distention and difficulty in defecation, pain in the neck, shoulders and back with occasional vertigo or dizziness. According to chapter 20 of *Divine Pivot*, the indicated treatment is to needle KI-1 *(yong quan)* and BL-60 *(kun lun)*.

PAINFUL OBSTRUCTION

If they are not eliminated from the body, external pathogenic influences will naturally evolve into painful obstruction. Localization in the cervical spine can be observed either in a degenerative or inflammatory context. The treatment is the same as for painful obstruction.

EXAMPLE: TORTICOLLIS

Torticollis *(luò zhěn* or *shī zhěn)* is described in chapter 60 of *Basic Questions*. In the Shanghai College of Traditional Chinese Medicine text (Roustan, 1979),[1] torticollis is characterized by muscle pain in the neck with impaired movement due to an invasion of the channels and vessels by Cold and Wind, which often occurs while sleeping. It can also result from bad posture disrupting the balance of Blood and Qi. The obstruction of the energetic circulation in turn causes muscle spasms. There is no redness or localized swelling, but mostly pain while moving or when firmly pressed. This condition manifests as soon as the patient wakes up, and is accompanied by neck rigidity and considerable functional disability.

The acupuncture treatment principle is to select local points on the arm and leg greater yang and lesser yang channels. According to a passage in chapter 26 of *Divine Pivot*, "When there is pain in the nape and the patient can neither flex nor turn the head, needle the leg greater yang channel. If rotation of the head becomes impossible, needle the arm greater yang channel."

The main points are M-UE-24 *(luo zhen)*, located between the second and third metacarpal bones, and local painful points. Secondary points are SI-3 *(hou xi)* and

GB-39 *(xuan zhong)*. Needle M-UE-24 *(luo zhen)* first with a strong to medium stimulation while asking the patient to move his neck. If pain persists, add points sensitive to the touch. Stimulation of M-UE-24 *(luo zhen)*, SI-3 *(hou xi)* and GB-39 *(xuan zhong)* can be performed alternately by rotating the needles. The warm needle technique can also be used on painful points, immediately followed by cupping.

Thousand Ducat Prescriptions (Qian jin yao fang) prescribes the following points: SI-1 *(shao ze)*, SI-2 *(qian gu)*, SI-3 *(hou xi)*, SI-5 *(yang gu)*, SI-4 *(wan gu)*, BL-60 *(kun lun)*, HT-3 *(shao hai)*, BL-2 *(zan zhu)*.

Classic of Nourishing Life with Acupuncture and Moxibustion (Zhen jiu zi sheng jing) prescribes BL-64 *(jing gu)*, BL-42 *(po hu)*, BL-11 *(da zhu)*, GB-21 *(jian jing)*, TB-16 *(tian you)*, SI-3 *(hou xi)*, BL-10 *(tian zhu)*, and, for pain radiating toward the back and shoulders, TB-10 *(tian jing)*.

Outline of Medicine (Yi xue gang mu) prescribes CV-24 *(cheng jiang)*, GV-16 *(feng fu)* and SI-3 *(hou xi)* for neck stiffness.

Spasmodic Torticollis

This particular case corresponds to a constant or intermittent contracture of the neck muscles, causing a rotation or inclination of the head. Besides the congenital type, the etiology varies and is often unidentified. Underlying psychological problems can occasionally be responsible for this syndrome. If this is the case, it indicates serious energetic disorders which can only be analyzed individually, taking into account the neck symbolism and issues relating to turning around. From a symptomatic point of view, SI-10 *(nao shu)*, which rules the "shoulders' door," can be a useful addition.

Trigger Points

TRAPEZIUS MUSCLE (SUPERIOR PORTION)

Referred Pain

Pain occurs on the posterolateral border of the nape and mastoid processs. This is the origin of most nape tensions. When the pain is severe, it radiates to the lateral aspect of the skull, the temple, and the bottom of the orbit in accordance with a leg lesser yang pathway, and sometimes to the mandibular angle (FIG. 17-3).

Trigger Point

In the area of TB-15 *(tian liao)* or GB-21 *(jian jing)*. For suboccipital pain radiating to the shoulder, the trigger point is below TB-15 *(tian liao)*.

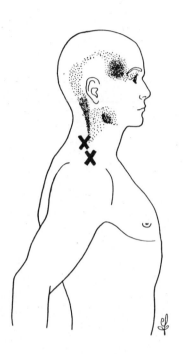

Fig. 17-3
Trigger Point Area for Superior Portion of Trapezius Muscle

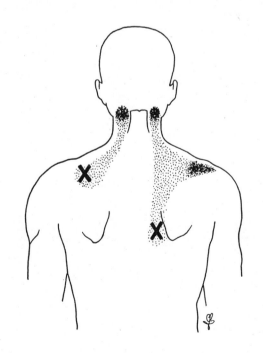

Fig. 17-4
Trigger Point Area for Inferior Portion of Trapezius Muscle

Trapezius Muscle (Inferior Portion)

Referred Pain

Suboccipital, retromastoidal pain, from the nape to the acromion (FIG. 17-4).

Trigger Point

In the area of BL-45 (yi xi).

Splenius Capitis Muscle

Referred Pain

Pain in the nape of the neck, particularly in the cervicoscapular angle (FIG. 17-5).

Trigger Point

At the level of the spinous process of C7, on the medial branch of the leg greater yang channel.

Multifidus Muscle

Referred Pain

Suboccipital pain descending to the cervicothoracic junction and the posterosuperior border of the shoulder (FIG. 17-6).

Trigger Point

In the area of N-BW-48 (xia xin shi).[2]

Levator Scapulae Muscle

Referred Pain

Pain at the cervicoscapular angle radiating along the vertebral border of the scapula and the posterior aspect of the shoulder (FIG. 17-7).

Trigger Point

In the area of SI-15 (jian zhong shu) and BL-41 (fu fen).

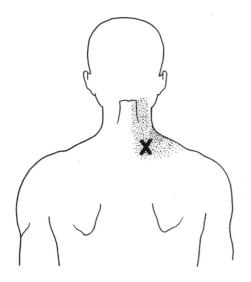

Fig. 17-5
Trigger Point Area for Inferior Portion
of Splenius Capitis Muscle

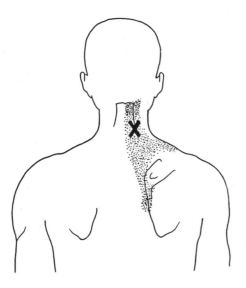

Fig. 17-6
Trigger Point Area for Inferior Portion
of Multifidus Muscle

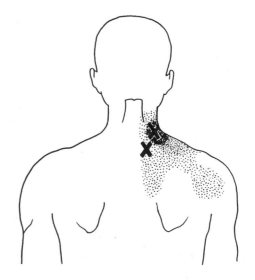

Fig. 17-7
Trigger Point Area for Inferior Portion
of Levator Scapulae Muscle

Chapter Notes

1. *Editors' note:* This refers to a book by the Shanghai College of Traditional Chinese Medicine published in 1974. The English language edition was translated and edited by John O'Connor and Dan Bensky under the title *Acupuncture: A Comprehensive Text* (Chicago: Eastland Press, 1981). This particular section is entitled "Stiff Neck" and can be found on pp. 661-62 of the English language edition.

2. This point is located 1.5 units lateral to the lower end of the spinous process of the fourth cervical vertebra.

CHAPTER EIGHTEEN

Shoulder Pain

Energetic Aspects of Shoulder

RELATIONSHIP WITH CHANNEL SYSTEM

Primary Channels

Arm Greater Yin (Lung) Channel

The superficial pathway of this channel ascends to the inferior border of the clavicle and descends along the anterior aspect of the upper limb.

Arm Yang Brightness (Large Intestine) Channel

The superficial pathway of this channel travels up the lateral aspect of the arm and deltoid muscle, crosses the acromioclavicular angle, and reaches the spinous process of T7 at GV-14 *(da zhui)*. From there, it descends to the supraclavicular fossa and goes internally at ST-12 *(que pen)*.

Arm Lesser Yin (Lung) Channel

The superficial pathway of this channel emerges in the pit of the axilla, and then travels along the ulnar border of the upper limb.

Arm Greater Yang (Small Intestine) Channel

The superficial pathway of this channel travels along the posterior aspect of the arm, emerges behind the shoulder joint and goes medially toward the middle of the subscapular fossa. It then goes upward, crosses the spine of the scapula at the junction of the middle third and the medial third, goes down to the subscapular fossa, crosses the leg greater yang channel at BL-41 *(fu fen)* and BL-11 *(da zhu)*, and reaches the seventh cervical vertebra at GV-14 *(da zhui)*. It then goes down the front to the supraclavicular fossa at ST-12 *(que pen)*, where it penetrates deep inside the body.

Leg Greater Yang (Bladder) Channel

The lateral branch of this channel travels along the medial border of the scapula.

Leg Lesser Yin (Kidney) Channel

The superficial branch of this channel reaches the inferior border of the clavicle.

Arm Terminal Yin (Pericardium) Channel

The superficial branch of this channel emerges one unit lateral to the nipple, reaches the axilla, and travels down the medial aspect of the upper limb.

Arm Lesser Yang (Triple Burner) Channel

The superficial branch travels along the lateral border of the upper limb, reaches the posterior aspect of the shoulder, follows the trapezius, and crosses the arm greater yang channel at SI-12 *(bing feng)*. The channel meets the seventh cervical vertebra at GV-14 *(da zhui)* and then goes down the front toward the supraclavicular fossa while crossing the leg lesser yang channel. The channel goes deep inside the body at ST-12 *(que pen)*.

Leg Lesser Yang (Gallbladder) Channel

At the end of its cephalic pathway, this channel reaches the occiput, goes down to the neck at SI-17 *(tian rong)*, travels back toward the superior border of the trapezius, reaches the seventh cervical vertebra at GV-14 *(da zhui)*, goes back to the shoulder through BL-11 *(da zhu)* and SI-12 *(bing feng)*, and returns to the front toward the supraclavicular fossa at ST-12 *(bing feng)*. A superficial branch emerges from the supraclavicular fossa and travels down the front of the axilla.

Channel Sinews

Arm Greater Yin Channel Sinew

A branch of the channel sinew ascends the anterior aspect of the arm, penetrates under the axilla, emerges at the supraclavicular fossa, spreads over the clavicle, inserts at LI-15 *(jian yu)*, and goes back to ST-12 *(que pen)*.

Arm Yang Brightness Channel Sinew

A branch ascends the lateral aspect of the arm and inserts at LI-15 *(jian yu)*. From this point, a secondary branch goes around the scapula and attaches to the side of the spine. The main branch goes from LI-15 *(jian yu)* up the neck along the superior border of the trapezius.

Leg Yang Brightness Channel Sinew

The vertical thoracic branch inserts at the supraclavicular fossa.

Arm Lesser Yin Channel Sinew

A branch of this channel goes up the medial aspect of the arm, then penetrates the axilla and reaches the thoracic wall.

Arm Greater Yang Channel Sinew

A branch goes behind the axilla, up and around the scapula, and then travels along the neck.

Leg Greater Yang Channel Sinew

Two branches of this channel sinew emerge from the thoracic region. One reaches the axilla, the supraclavicular fossa, and then the occipital region at GB-12 *(wan gu)*. The other inserts in the acromial region at LI-15 *(jian yu)*. A branch emerges from the supraclavicular fossa and ascends obliquely along the thorax.

Leg Lesser Yang Channel Sinew

The main (vertical) branch ascends in front of the axilla, goes through the supraclavicular fossa, and then travels toward the back of the ear.

Collaterals

Arm Yang Brightness Collateral

The collateral originates at LI-6 *(pian li)*, and reaches the shoulder at LI-15 *(jian yu)*. At the maxillary bone, it branches out into the teeth and penetrates into the ear.

Arm Lesser Yin Collateral

The collateral emerges at HT-5 *(tong li)* at the wrist, goes to the arm greater yang, travels along the primary channel, meets the axilla, penetrates the Heart, reaches the base of the tongue, and enters the eye.

Arm Greater Yang Collateral

The collateral starts at SI-7 *(zhi zheng)* and ascends the shoulder to reach LI-15 *(jian yu)*.

Arm Terminal Yin Collateral

The collateral originates at PC-6 *(nei guan)* and follows the pathway of the primary channel to reach the axilla and connect with the cardiovascular system.

Arm Lesser Yang Collateral

The collateral starts at TB-5 *(wai guan)*, ascends the lateral aspect of the upper limb to the shoulder, and enters the chest.

Curious Vessels

Yang Heel Vessel

The vessel ascends along the lateral aspect of the shoulder and neck, passing through SI-10 *(nao shu)*, LI-15 *(jian yu)* and LI-16 *(ju gu)*.

Yang Linking Vessel

The vessel travels along the sides of the body, enters the shoulder from back to front, and continues upward. It passes through SI-10 *(nao shu)*, TB-15 *(tian liao)* and GB-21 *(jian jing)*.

SHOULDER AND TRUNK

The shoulder is a physiological barrier for the continual exchange of Qi between the trunk and the upper limb. The yin and yang Qi emerge from the trunk toward the upper limb, and, conversely, move from the upper limb to enter the trunk.

Qualification of this entry and exit of energy is made in relation to its point of origin, in a greater *(tài)*, lesser *(shào)*, terminal *(jué)* or brightness *(míng)* sequence (see chapter 8). Thus, the yang Qi emerging from the trunk toward the shoulder is qualified as greater yang, and is governed by SI-11 *(tian zong)*. The yin Qi emerging from the trunk is labeled greater yin, and is governed by LU-2 *(yun men)*. The yang Qi entering the trunk is identified as yang brightness, and is governed by LI-15 *(jian yu)*. The yin Qi entering the trunk is labeled terminal yin, and is governed by PC-2 *(tian quan)*.

Shoulder and Body Symbolism

In body symbolism, the shoulders indicate strength and power. They represent the power to do, to act, to perform. The Bambaras people, who live in Senegal and Mali, consider the shoulders to be the seat of physical strength and even of violence.

Diagnosis of Shoulder Pain

As always, it is necessary to make a detailed study of the pain according to the local application of the eight parameters. In shoulder pain this process leads to two main clinical pictures.

Pain Matching Local Application of Eight Parameters

Barrier Disorders

When a barrier prevents the exchange of the yin or yang Qi between the trunk and the upper limb, the shoulder pain is diffuse. This is usually the case with a recent pain, although we must not rule out the same pathogenic mechanisms when there is an older pain.

Sharp Pain

Obstruction to the entry of the yang into the trunk

The Qi of the yang channels of the upper limb cannot go through the shoulder barrier and therefore cannot enter the trunk. The Qi then accumulates upstream and causes a yang-type pain in the shoulder due to a yang excess. This is marked by sharp pain which is aggravated by pressure, the lateral recumbent position, or application of topical warmth. It is ameliorated by cold. Needling LI-15 *(jian yu)* on the yang brightness channel brings instant relief.

Obstruction to the exit of the yin from the trunk

Because the yin Qi cannot proceed from the trunk to the upper limb, there is yang-type pain due to yin deficiency. This is marked by sharp pain which is ameliorated by pressure and the topical application of cold. It is aggravated by warmth. Needling LU-2 *(yun men)* on the greater yin channel sedates the pain immediately, which confirms the diagnosis. Depending on the circumstances, relief from pain may be quite prolonged or may not return at all.

Dull Pain

Obstruction to the exit of the yang from the trunk

Because the yang Qi cannot proceed from the trunk to the shoulder, there is yin-type pain in the shoulder due to yang deficiency. This is marked by dull pain which is ameliorated by pressure and the topical application of warmth. It is aggravated by cold and movement. Needling SI-11 *(tian zong)* on the greater yang channel promotes the outward movement of the trunk Qi and instantly alleviates the pain.

Obstruction to the entry of the yin into the trunk

Because the yin Qi of the upper limb cannot enter the trunk, it accumulates at the level of the shoulder, causing pain due to yin excess. This is marked by dull pain which is aggravated by pressure, the lateral recumbent position, or by cold. It is ameliorated by the topical application of warmth. Needling PC-2 *(tian quan)* on the terminal yin channel promotes the movement of yin Qi toward the trunk, and brings very fast relief from the pain.

Obstruction to the exit of the trunk yang toward the head

We must consider the possibility, under certain circumstances, of an obstruction to the movement of the trunk yang toward the head. This occurs when there is pain in the posterior aspect of the shoulder which radiates toward the upper limb along the arm greater yang channel, mimicking a C7 cervicobrachial neuralgia. Besides its location, there are signs that this yin-type pain is due to yang deficiency. The pain is dull, improved by pressure and warmth, and aggravated by the topical application of cold. The yang Qi accumulates underneath the scapula and may manifest as a sharp, burning or stinging pain.

Improvement of this clinical picture is brought by needling the point that promotes the upward movement of the yang Qi from the trunk to the head, SI-14 *(jian wai shu)* on the greater yang channel. It is often useful to combine this point with those on the other channels that share this function, TB-15 *(tian liao)* and ST-3 *(ju liao)*. The exact localization of the pain will determine which point will bring the best results.

Local Qi Stagnation

This type of pattern must be considered in the presence of a shoulder pain that worsens with rest and improves with movement.

In the case of yang Qi stagnation, the pain is sharp and manifests in the morning when waking up or when resting. Getting started is always difficult, but the pain rapidly improves with activity. Cold aggravates the pain, while topical warmth alleviates it.

Mobilization of the yang Qi in the shoulder is induced by needling TB-14 *(jian liao)* on the lesser yang channel. This yang Qi stagnation may be the consequence of pathogenic Cold, which must be expelled by the use of moxa.

In the case of yin Qi stagnation, the pain is relatively dull; getting started in the morning takes more time, and the pain is aggravated by topical warmth and massage. Mobilization of the stagnant yin Qi in the shoulder is induced by needling HT-1 *(ji quan)*.

PAIN NOT MATCHING LOCAL APPLICATION OF EIGHT PARAMETERS

Pain of Mechanical Origin

We shall not consider this cause as it points to a structural problem of the cervical spine. This type of problem requires manipulation and is beyond the scope of our discussion.

Disruption of Local Movement

When this occurs the pain in the shoulder does not seem to fit the schema of the eight parameters. A more detailed analysis indicates that the problem may be comprised of several components, each of which corresponds to one or more of the eight parameters. For instance, dull pain in the shoulder which worsens at night or when getting started, improves temporarily, and reappears when a repetitive movement is performed, suggests local yin stagnation (pain when resting) that the yang deficiency cannot mobilize (pain on movement). HT-1 *(ji quan)* should be needled in combination with SI-11 *(tian zong)*, which promotes the outward movement of the yang from the trunk to the upper limb. If the yang Qi is blocked at the level of the trapezius, GB-21 *(jian jing)*

should be added, which promotes the downward movement of the yang from the head to the trunk.

A similar condition is a sharp pain that worsens with pressure and improves with local application of cold (yang excess). Yet it also occurs during the second half of the night, worsens in the morning and when movement is initiated, improves as movement continues, and is relieved by local application of warmth, such as provided by a hot shower (yin stagnation). This commonly occurs when yin stagnation in the shoulder follows an attack of Wind-Cold. In such cases, HT-1 *(ji quan)* is needled to mobilize the yin, and LI-15 *(jian yu)* is added to facilitate the entry of yang.

Channel Sinews

Channel sinews are usually involved in shoulder pain of relatively recent origin, due to trauma or external pathogenic influences. The diagnosis is based upon the location of the pain and the fact that movement aggravates the condition.

A diagnostic test consists in needling the well point to find out whether it brings a reduction in pain or instant and marked improvement. The channel sinews most often involved are the arm greater yin for anterior and clavicular pain, arm yang brightness for lateral pain, and arm greater yang for posterior pain.

If the pain is of post-traumatic origin, needle the well point in combination with the river point, the insertion points surrounding the painful area, and possibly drain the *ashi* points.

If the pain is caused by the invasion of external pathogenic influences (such as Wind-Damp-Cold), also needle the tonification point of the corresponding primary channel and the meeting area of the upper limb yang or yin channels. This will prevent the condition from spreading to the other channel sinews.

For example, pain, spasms and twinges of the lateral aspect of the shoulder, which cannot be abducted, and limited cervical mobilization are symptoms of an arm yang brightness channel sinew disorder. If the pain is traumatic, needle the well point LI-1 *(shang yang)* in combination with the river point LI-5 *(yang xi)*, the insertion points surrounding the painful area, and possibly the *ashi* points.

If the pain is due to an invasion of external pathogenic influences, add the tonification point of the primary channel LI-11 *(qu chi)*, and the meeting area of the upper limb yang at GB-13 *(ben shen)*.

Primary Channels

Primary channel involvement must be considered for pain of an older origin than that affecting the channel sinews. It is often accompanied by signs that the corresponding Organ has been slightly affected, as well as by general signs.

Several mechanisms may be involved:

- penetration of external pathogenic influences, which may be an evolution or an aggravation of the channel sinew stage
- manifestation of an internal dysfunction of the corresponding Organ
- symptoms indicating that a particular energetic level has been affected
- loss of harmony between man and the macrocosm.

Continuing with the arm yang brightness example, the primary channel symptomatology is as follows: pain in the arm and behind the shoulder; redness, swelling and heat (or sometimes a sensation of cold) behind the shoulder; and difficulty in moving the index finger. There may also be toothache, swollen and sore throat, thirst, dry mouth, epistaxis and fever.

If pathogenic Cold is involved, needle the well point LI-1 *(shang yang)*, the river point LI-5 *(yang xi)* and the spring point LI-2 *(er jian)*. If Wind predominates, it must be eliminated by needling the Wind point of the shoulder, SI-12 *(bing feng)*, and the stream point LI-3 *(san jian)*.

If the condition is a repercussion of a Large Intestine disorder, in addition to pain in the abdomen and in the umbilical area, there may be borborygmus, diarrhea or loose stools. The treatment calls for needling the sea point LI-11 *(qu chi)*. This is because, as noted in chapter 43 of *Basic Questions*, when a disorder is located in a yang Organ (which is yang within yin), the sea points should be needled. In addition, the etiology of the Organ disorder must be treated. Regulation can also be achieved by needling the source point LI-4 *(he gu)* in combination with the paired connecting point LU-7 *(lie que)*.

If the arm yang brightness disorder is the result of a pathological problem affecting the yang brightness energetic axis, restoration of the balance is achieved by needling the stream and connecting points, LI-3 *(san jian)* and LI-6 *(pian li)*.

When the arm yang brightness disorder is part of a larger loss of harmony between man and the macrocosm at the level of the Metal phase, the pathology is acute, with a sudden onset, and without any apparent cause. According to chapter 63 of *Basic Questions*, we should needle the well point and the opposite connecting point. The problem is to find out if "opposite" here means a point on the ipsilateral paired channel in accordance with an interior/exterior relationship, or a point on the contralateral affected channel. We must therefore needle LU-7 *(lie que)* on the same side and LI-6 *(pian li)* on the opposite side. In addition, we should needle the contralateral connecting point KI-4 *(da zhong)* in accordance with the midday-midnight law.

In addition to this symptomatic treatment, we must treat the root cause centering on rebalancing the Metal phase by needling the transport points, in accordance with the "open" points of the stem and branch system, or the mother-child tonification or drainage rule. If the Metal phase is deficient, tonify the mother. This means the Earth phase, which is the river point of the yin channels, LU-9 *(tai yuan)*, and the sea point of the yang channels, LI-11 *(qu chi)*. If it is excessive, drain the child. In this case it is the Water phase, which is the sea point of the yin channels, LU-5 *(chi ze)*, and the spring point of the yang channels, LI-2 *(er jian)*.

Collaterals

When the arm greater yang collateral is in a state of excess, the elbow and shoulder joints are obstructed and the elbow cannot be bent or stretched. Needle the corresponding connecting point, SI-7 *(zhi zheng)*.

Curious Vessels

Yang Heel Vessel

There is pain in the shoulder with contracture and the necessity of a warm-up stage in the morning before the shoulder feels at all comfortable. This is usually part of a larger context of pain with stiffness in the lower limbs and back, sleep disorders, and ocular pain.

Treatment consists of combining the confluent point BL-62 *(shen mai)*, the cleft point BL-59 *(fu yang)*, possibly the paired confluent point SI-3 *(hou xi)*, and one of the local pathway points, SI-10 *(nao shu)*, LI-15 *(jian yu)* or LI-16 *(ju gu)*.

Yang Linking Vessel

The shoulder pain fits within the context of a polyarticular condition which is more or less severe, sensitive to changes in the weather, especially snow and storms, and is accompanied by a sensation of fever, chills and headaches which progress from back to front. It can follow after a previous leg greater yang or leg lesser yang condition.

Treatment consists of opening the yang Linking vessel by needling its confluent point TB-5 *(wai guan)*, combined with its paired confluent point GB-41 *(zu lin qi)*, and promoting circulation by needling the cleft point GB-35 *(yang jiao)*. The local pathway points, SI-10 *(nao shu)*, TB-15 *(tian liao)* and GB-21 *(jian jing)*, may also prove useful.

Organ Pathology

Theoretically, the Organs corresponding to the primary channels traveling through the shoulder may all be involved. In reality, this pathology concerns mostly the Lungs and Large Intestine, which are the body's administrators.

Painful Obstruction

The invasion of pathogenic Wind, Cold and Dampness obstructs the circulation of Blood and Qi. If they are not quickly eliminated, a painful obstruction disorder may appear, the shoulder being only one of several possible locations within a polyarticular syndrome (see chapters 8 and 9).

Shoulder and Gestural Expression

When all the previously mentioned etiologies have been ruled out, we can look at a dysfunction of shoulder mobility as a disruption of a person's mode of expression in the external world. From this perspective, the shoulder is governed by LI-14 *(bi nao)*, associated with ST-38 *(tiao kou)*, which governs all the joints as the motor expression in humans (Kespi, 1982).

The presence of bilateral pain moving downward, scarf-like, from the neck to the shoulders, with spasms of the trapezius, suggests, during an acute phase, an invasion of Wind-Cold at GV-16 *(feng fu)* or BL-12 *(feng men)*. On the other hand, the presence of an older or continuing similar condition invites us to consider the possible manifestation in the body of a psychological behavior in which the ego cannot "let go," and tries to control and master everything. In this case, applying moxa at GV-14 *(da zhui)*, the meeting point of all the body's yang, brings a remarkable reduction in pain.

Trigger Points

TRAPEZIUS MUSCLE (UPPER TRACT)

Referred Pain

High cervical pain radiating toward the posterior aspect of the shoulder (FIG. 18-1).

Trigger Point

This point is located below TB-15 *(tian liao)*.

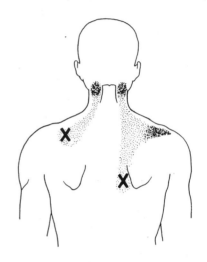

Fig. 18-1
Trigger Point Area for Trapezius Muscle: Upper Tract

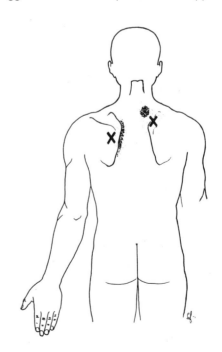

Fig. 18-2
Trigger Point Area for Trapezius Muscle: Middle Tract

TRAPEZIUS MUSCLE (MIDDLE TRACT)

Referred Pain

Superficial burning-type pain between the medial border of the scapula and the cervicothoracic hinge (FIG. 18-2).

Trigger Point

This point is located in the area of BL-42 *(po hu)*.

Referred Pain

Pain located in the acromion and superior aspect of the shoulder.

Trigger Point

This point is located in the area of LI-16 *(ju gu)*.

Referred Pain

Sensation of cold and piloerection on the lateral aspect of the arm (FIG. 18-2).

Trigger Point

This point is located in the area of SI-14 *(jian wai shu)*.

TRAPEZIUS MUSCLE (LOWER TRACT)

Referred Pain

Pain from the superior portion of the neck behind the mastoid process, radiating to the acromion and a place between the medial border of the scapula and the spine. The pain feels like numbness and makes the patient want to scratch (FIG. 18-3).

Trigger Point

This point is located below BL-45 *(yi xi)*.

Referred Pain

Burning-type pain at the medial border of the scapula.

Trigger Point

This point is located in the subscapular fossa, between SI-11 *(tian zong)*, BL-43 *(gao huang shu)* and BL-44 *(shen tang)*.

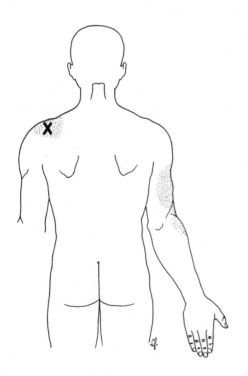

Fig. 18-3
Trigger Point Area for
Trapezius Muscle: Lower Tract

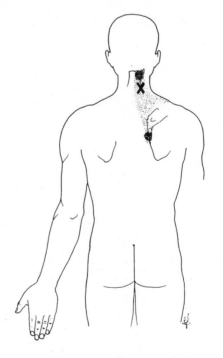

Fig. 18-4
Trigger Point Area for Semispinalis
Capitis and Multifidus Muscles

SEMISPINALIS CAPITIS AND MULTIFIDUS MUSCLES

Referred Pain

Suboccipital pain radiating toward the superior border of the shoulder and the medial border of the scapula (FIG. 18-4).

Trigger Point

This point is located in the area of N-BW-48 *(xia xin shi)*.[1]

LEVATOR SCAPULAE MUSCLE

Referred Pain

Posterolateral cervical pain radiating toward the posterior aspect of the shoulder and along the medial border of the scapula (FIG. 18-5).

Trigger Point

This point is located in the area of SI-15 *(jian zhong shu)*.

SCALENE MUSCLES (ANTERIOR, MIDDLE, POSTERIOR)

Referred Pain

Pain on the anterior portion of the pectoralis muscle going down toward the nipple, on the posterior aspect of the shoulder and arm, the radial aspect of the arm and forearm following the arm greater yang and arm yang brightness pathways, and on the posterior aspect of the first two fingers (FIG. 18-6).

Trigger Point

This point is located in the area of LI-17 *(tian ding)*.

SUPRASPINATUS MUSCLE

Referred Pain

Pain in the suprascapular fossa, deltoid muscle, lateral border of the arm and forearm, which may simulate a "tennis elbow" syndrome (FIG. 18-7A).

Trigger Point

This point is located in the area of SI-12 *(bing feng)* and SI-13 *(qu yuan)*.

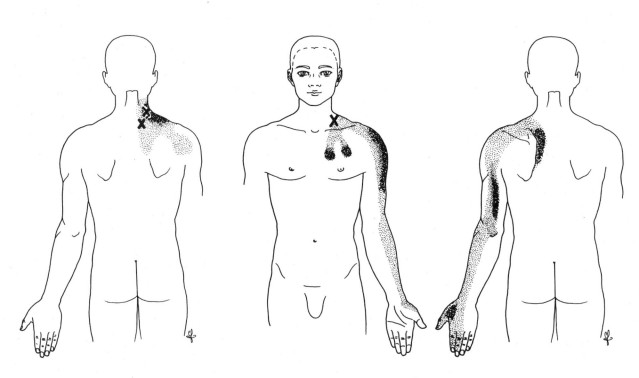

Fig. 18-5
Trigger Point Area for
Levator Scapulae Muscle

Fig. 18-6
Trigger Point Area for
Scalene Muscles

Referred Pain

Pain in the deltoid muscle area (FIG. 18-7B).

Trigger Point

This point is located in the area of TB-14 *(jian liao)*.

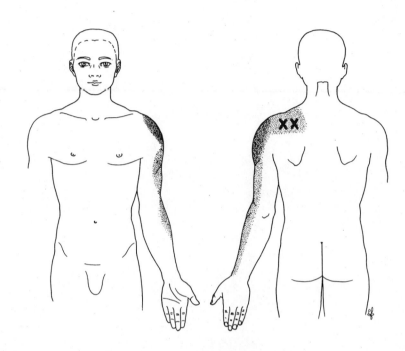

Fig. 18-7A
Trigger Point Area for Supraspinatus Muscle (A)

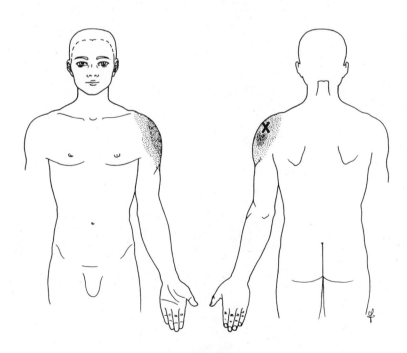

Fig. 18-7B
Trigger Point Area for Supraspinatus Muscle (B)

INFRASPINATUS MUSCLE

Referred Pain

Deep pain in the anterior aspect of the shoulder, the anterolateral aspect of the arm, the lateral border of the forearm, and sometimes in the fingers (FIG. 18-8).

Trigger Point

This point is located in the area of SI-11 *(tian zong)*.

Referred Pain

Pain in the medial border of the scapula.

Trigger Point

This point can be found lateral to BL-44 *(shen tang)*.

TERES MINOR MUSCLE

Referred Pain

Deep pain in the posterior aspect of the deltoid muscle. This point is extremely localized and is about the size of a quarter (FIG. 18-9).

Trigger Point

This point is located in the area of SI-9 *(jian zhen)*.

LATISSIMUS DORSI MUSCLE

Referred Pain

Pain in the tip of the scapula, the posterior and medial aspect of the upper limb, and in the two last fingers (FIG. 18-10A).

Trigger Point

This point is located in the area of GB-22 *(yuan ye)*.

Referred Pain

Pain in the anterior aspect of the shoulder and in the waist (FIG. 18-10B).

Trigger Point

This point is located in the area of GB-25 *(jing men)*.

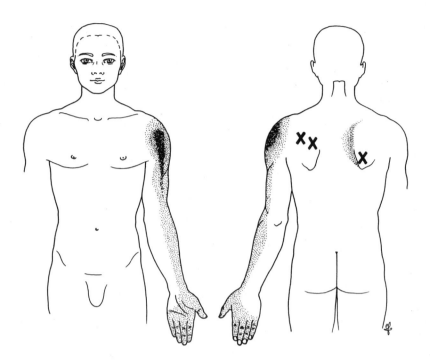
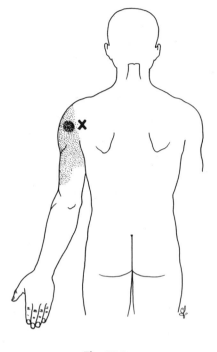

Fig. 18-8
Trigger Point Area for
Infraspinatus Muscle

Fig. 18-9
Trigger Point Area for
Teres Minor Muscle

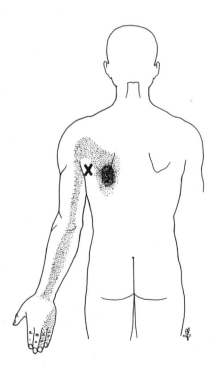
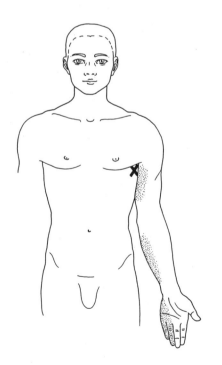
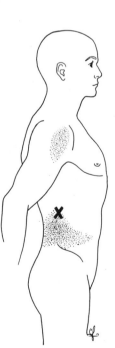

Fig. 18-10A
Trigger Point Area for
Latissimus Dorsi Muscle (A)

Fig. 18-10B
Trigger Point Area for
Latissimus Dorsi Muscle (B)

TERES MAJOR MUSCLE

Referred Pain

Pain in the posterior aspect of the shoulder and upper limb, following the arm lesser yang pathway (FIG. 18-11).

Trigger Point

This point is lateral to BL-46 *(ge guan)*.

Referred Pain

Pain in the stump of the shoulder (FIG. 18-11).

Trigger Point

This point is located in the posterior aspect of the axillary fossa.

SUBSCAPULARIS MUSCLE

Referred Pain

Pain in the posterior aspect of the shoulder, scapula, arm and wrist (FIG. 18-12).

Trigger Point

Three points can be found in the body of the subscapularis muscle, in the axilla.

MAJOR AND MINOR RHOMBOID MUSCLES

Referred Pain

Pain along the medial border of the scapula and in the suprascapular fossa (FIG. 18-13).

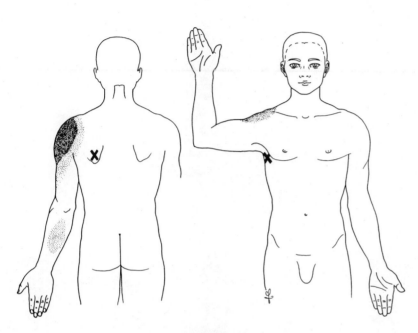

Fig. 18-11
Trigger Point Area for Teres Major Muscle

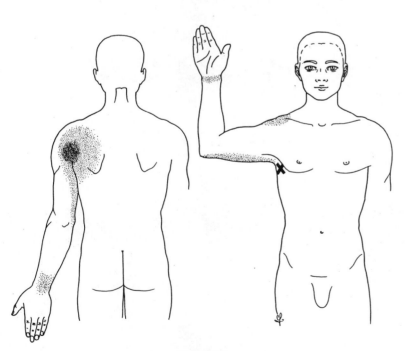

Fig. 18-12
Trigger Point Area for Subscapularis Muscle

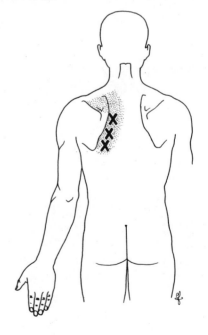

Fig. 18-13
Trigger Point Area for Major and Minor Rhomboid Muscles

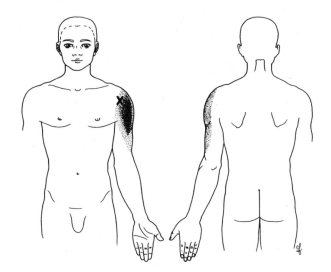

Fig. 18-14A
Trigger Point Area for Deltoid Muscle (A)

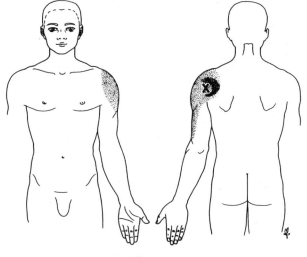

Fig. 18-14B
Trigger Point Area for Deltoid Muscle (B)

Trigger Point

This point can be found in the areas of BL-42 *(po hu)*, BL-44 *(shen tang)* and BL-45 *(yi xi)*.

DELTOID MUSCLE

Referred Pain

Pain in the anterior and medial aspect of the deltoid muscle and arm (FIG. 18-14A).

Trigger Point

This point can be found in the area of N-UE-11 *(tai jian)*.[2]

Referred Pain

Pain in the posterior aspect of the deltoid muscle and arm (FIG. 18-14B).

Trigger Point

This point can be found in the area of TB-14 *(jian liao)*.

CORACOBRACHIALIS MUSCLE

Referred Pain

Pain in the stump of the shoulder and on the posterior aspect of the upper limb following the arm lesser yang pathway (FIG. 18-15).

Trigger Point

This point can be found lateral to and below LU-2 *(yun men)*.

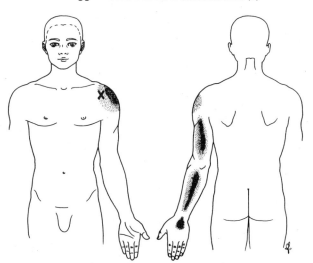

Fig. 18-15
Trigger Point Area for Coracobrachialis Muscle

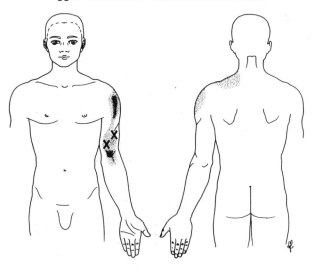

Fig. 18-16
Trigger Point Area for Biceps Brachii Muscle

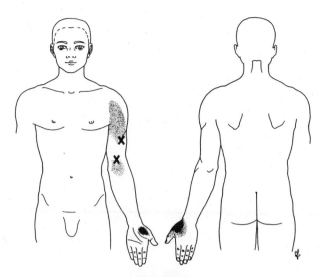

Fig. 18-17
Trigger Point Area for Brachialis Muscle

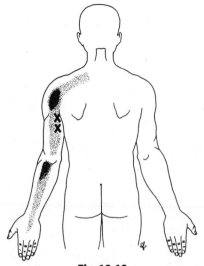

Fig. 18-18
Trigger Point Area for Triceps Brachii Muscle

Biceps Brachii Muscle

Referred Pain

Pain in the anterior aspect of the shoulder and arm, and in the suprascapular fossa (FIG. 18-16).

Trigger Point

This point can be found below LU-4 *(xia bai)* and lateral to HT-2 *(qing ling)*.

Brachialis Muscle

Referred Pain

Pain in the anterior aspect of the shoulder and deltoid muscle, in the elbow crease, and in the dorsal and palmar aspect of the base of the thumb (FIG. 18-17).

Trigger Point

This point can be found in the area of LU-4 *(xia bai)* and N-UE-25 *(xia xia bai)*.[3]

Triceps Brachii Muscle: Long Head

Referred Pain

Pain in the posterior aspect of the shoulder and upper limb (FIG. 18-18).

Trigger Point

This point can be found in the area of TB-13 *(nao hui)*.

Pectoralis Major Muscle: Clavicular Head

Referred Pain

Pain in the anterior aspect of the deltoid and subscapular muscles (FIG. 18-19).

Trigger Point

This point can be found in the area of LU-1 *(zhong fu)* and N-UE-10 *(ju bi)*.[4]

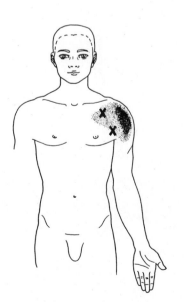

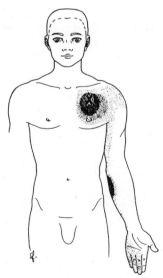

Fig. 18-19
Trigger Point Area for Pectoralis Major Muscle: Clavicular Head

Fig. 18-20
Trigger Point Area for Pectoralis Major Muscle: Sternal Head

PECTORALIS MAJOR MUSCLE: STERNAL HEAD

Referred Pain

Pain in the pectoralis muscle, in the anteromedial border of the upper limb, the palm of the hand, and the palmar aspect of the third, fourth and fifth fingers, following the arm terminal yin pathway (FIG. 18-20).

Trigger Point

This point can be found in the area of ST-15 *(wu yi)* and ST-16 *(ying chuang)*.

PECTORALIS MAJOR MUSCLE: COSTOABDOMINAL HEAD

Referred Pain

Pain in the mammary region with hypersensitivity of the nipple radiating toward the axilla (FIG. 18-21).

Trigger Point

This point can be found in the area of HT-1 *(ji quan)*.

SUBCLAVIUS MUSCLE

Referred Pain

Pain in the subclavicular area, the anterior aspect of the arm, the anterolateral border of the forearm and of the first three fingers, following the arm greater yin pathway (FIG. 18-22).

Trigger Point

This point can be found in the area of KI-27 *(shu fu)*.

PECTORALIS MINOR MUSCLE

Referred Pain

Pain in the anterior aspect of the deltoid muscle, the subclavicular fossa, the pectoral region, the anteromedial border of the upper limb, and the palmar aspect of the three last fingers (FIG. 18-23).

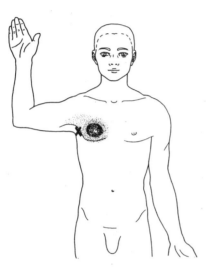

Fig. 18-21
Trigger Point Area for Pectoralis
Major Muscle: Costoabdominal Head

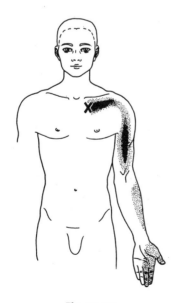

Fig. 18-22
Trigger Point Area for Subclavius Muscle

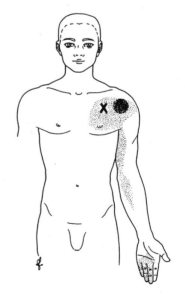

Fig. 18-23
Trigger Point Area for Pectoralis Minor Muscle

Trigger Point

This point can be found in the area of LU-1 *(zhong fu)*.

STERNALIS MUSCLE

Referred Pain

Pain in the manubrium radiating toward the anterior aspect of the shoulder and the anteromedial border of the arm (FIG. 18-24).

Trigger Point

This point can be found in the area of KI-24 *(ling xu)*.

SERRATUS POSTERIOR SUPERIOR MUSCLE

Referred Pain

Deep pain in the subscapular fossa, the posterior aspect of the shoulder, and the posterior aspect of the upper limb and little finger (FIG. 18-25).

Trigger Point

This point is located just below the scapular spine inferior to SI-12 *(bing feng)*.

SERRATUS ANTERIOR MUSCLE

Referred Pain

Pain in the subaxillary flank, radiating toward the medial border of the upper limb and the palmar aspect of the fourth and fifth fingers, and underneath the tip of the scapula (FIG. 18-26).

Trigger Point

This point is located in the area of SP-21 *(da bao)* or GB-22 *(yuan ye)*.

ILIOCOSTALIS THORACIS MUSCLE

Referred Pain

Pain in the tip of the scapula, along the medial border of the scapula, and in the thorax (FIG. 18-27).

Trigger Point

This point is located in the area of BL-45 *(yi xi)*.

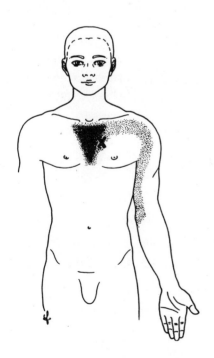

Fig. 18-24
Trigger Point Area for Sternalis Muscle

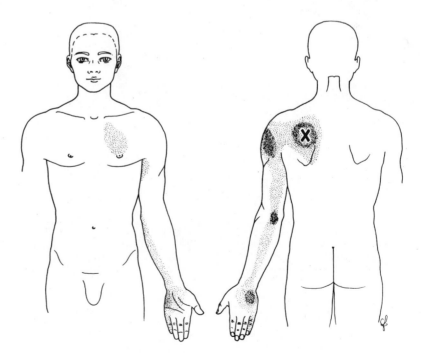

Fig. 18-25
Trigger Point Area for Serratus Posterior Superior Muscle

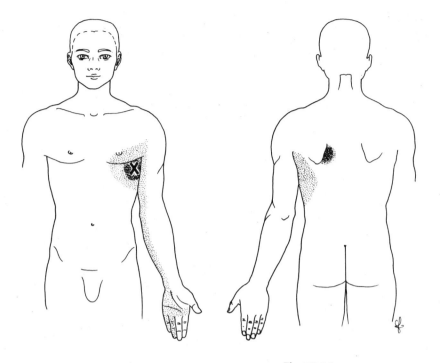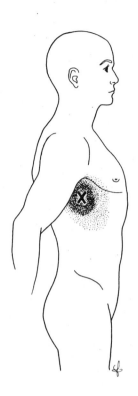

Fig. 18-26
Trigger Point Area for Serratus Anterior Muscle

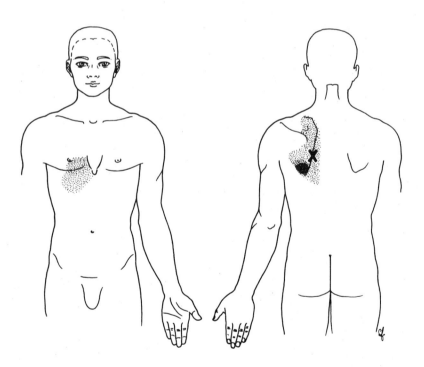

Fig. 18-27
Trigger Point Area for Iliocostalis Thoracis Muscle

Chapter Notes

1. This point is located 1.5 units lateral to the lower end of the spinous process of the fourth cervical vertebra.
2. This point is located 1.5 units below the acromion process.
3. This point is located on the upper arm, 3 units below LU-4 *(xia bai)*.
4. This point is located 3.5 units below the acromion process.

CHAPTER NINETEEN

Elbow Pain

Energetic Aspects of Elbow

RELATIONSHIP WITH CHANNEL SYSTEM

Primary Channels

The elbow is connected to the three yin and three yang channels of the upper limb in a very complete and straightforward manner. On the anterior aspect, there is the radial arm greater yin (Lung) channel, the ulnar arm lesser yin (Heart) channel, and the median arm terminal yin (Pericardium) channel. On the posterior aspect, there is the median arm lesser yang (Triple Burner) channel, the lateral arm yang brightness (Large Intestine) channel, and the medial arm greater yang (Small Intestine) channel.

Channel Sinews

Their pathways correspond to the trajectory of the primary channels.

Channel Divergences

The arm yang brightness is the only channel divergence to go through the elbow.

Collaterals

The arm lesser yin, arm terminal yin, arm yang brightness, arm greater yang and arm lesser yang collaterals go through the elbow.

Curious Vessels

No Curious vessel goes through the elbow.

ELBOW AND LOCAL CIRCULATION OF QI

Like the other joints, the elbow acts as a physiological barrier to the circulation of Qi in the upper limb. It is qualified as lesser yin or lesser yang in relation to the exchange of Qi between the arm and forearm.

Diagnosis of Painful Elbow

The most frequent elbow pathology is epicondylitis or "tennis elbow," for which acupuncture treatments are often sought. This chapter will focus on this topic, followed by a discussion of inflammation of the epitrochlea.

TENNIS ELBOW

The epicondyle is directly related to three channels: the arm yang brightness which overhangs the tip, the arm greater yin which passes in front of it, and, to a lesser degree, the arm lesser yang which goes behind it.

Channel Pathology

Channel Sinews

From a clinical standpoint, the channel sinew etiology is the most frequently encountered. Because of its pathway, the arm yang brightness is the channel sinew that is most often involved.

This diagnosis can be confirmed by a therapeutic test which consists of needling the well point LI-1 (shang yang). When the problem is due to a disturbance at the level of the channel sinew, this will almost immediately bring definite relief from pain. Treatment must then be completed by draining the river point LI-5 (yang xi), the muscle insertion points located above and below, as well as a central ashi point. If the pathology is recent, one to three sessions within a week should be enough to eliminate it.

In the presence of pathogenic Wind-Damp-Cold, one should also tonify the primary channel at LI-11 (qu chi) and needle the meeting point of the upper limb yang channels in the area of GB-13 (ben shen), to prevent the pathogenic influence from spreading to the other channels.

The arm greater yin channel sinew is less frequently involved in traumatic tennis elbow. However, it is more frequently involved when this pathology is due to exogenous pathogenic factors. The treatment principle remains the same.

Primary Channels

Primary channels are usually involved when the condition becomes chronic, and when no traumatic or microtraumatic factors have been identified. Here again, the arm yang brightness (Large Intestine) is the main channel involved, most often due to:

• aggravation of the previous etiology
• repercussion of a Large Intestine Organ pathology
• disruption of the yang brightness axis
• man and the macrocosm falling out of synchronization due to disruption of the Metal phase.

It is unnecessary to review the different descriptions and treatment principles here. They are the same as those discussed for shoulder pain in chapter 18.

Collaterals

Arm greater yang collateral

Problems of excess are marked by a dysfunction of the elbow or shoulder joint. The elbow can neither be flexed nor extended. Needle the corresponding connecting point SI-7 (zhi zheng).

Arm lesser yang collateral

Problems of excess are marked by contracture of the elbow joint. Needle the corresponding connecting point TB-5 (wai guan).

Problems of deficiency are marked by flaccidity of the elbow joint. Needle the source point on the corresponding channel, TB-4 (yang chi), and the connecting point on the paired yin channel, PC-6 (nei guan).

Disruption of Local Qi Circulation

Obstruction to the circulation of Qi between the arm and forearm is a frequent etiology in post-traumatic tennis elbow. An eight parameter diagnosis is not always easy to make for the elbow, although excess is commonly observed. The direction of any radiating pain is a valuable clue in determining whether the obstruction is between the arm and the forearm or the other way around.

If the yang Qi is obstructed between the arm and the forearm, the pain tends to radiate toward the forearm. Needle LI-9 (shang lian), the upper limb distal barrier point regulating the yang circulation between the trunk and the hand, along with TB-13 (nao hui).

If the movement of Qi is obstructed between the upper limb and the trunk, needle LI-15 (jian yu), the shoulder barrier point regulating this circulation, and add LI-8 (xia lian) or even the cleft point LI-7 (wen liu). TB-7 (hui zong) is also often useful.

Elbow and Gestural Expression

LI-12 (zhou liao) is the point which governs the elbow as a means of expression. This point should be used for tennis elbow with no precise triggering factor, when it suggests a disruption in the motor expression of the patient.

Cervical Spine

The cervical spine should be systematically examined in order to detect a possible minor intervertebral restriction. If any is found, it should be corrected by manipulation in conjunction with acupuncture treatment.

INFLAMMATION OF EPITROCHLEA

The pathogenic mechanisms of inflammation of the epitrochlea, or medial epicondyle of the humerus, overlap those of epicondyle pain, except that in this case it is the arm greater yang that is involved.

There is one particular etiology that should be highlighted. This relates to the upward movement of the Qi from the trunk to the head. The Qi coming out of the trunk is qualified as greater yang, and emerges from the arm greater yang channel at SI-14 *(jian wai shu)*. It then follows an intermediate, or lesser yang level, and emerges at TB-15 *(tian liao)*. Finally, it becomes terminal, or yang brightness, on the face, and is governed by ST-3 *(ju liao)*.

A closing of the SI-14 *(jian wai shu)* barrier creates yang excess upstream at the level of the scapula, deficiency downstream, and a spreading of the yang along the arm greater yang channel. This manifests as pain, which may be centered around the epithrochlea. Needling SI-14 *(jian wai shu)* releases the yang excess and makes the inflammation of the epithrochlea disappear.

Trigger Points

EPICONDYLE

Supraspinatus Muscle

Referred Pain

Epicondyle pain, pain in the deltoid muscle extending to the arm and suprascapular fossa (FIG. 19-1).

Trigger Point

This point is located in the area of SI-12 *(bing feng)* and SI-13 *(qu yuan)*.

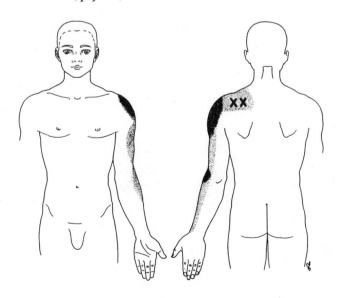

Fig. 19-1
Trigger Point Area for Suprapinatus Muscle

Infraspinatus Muscle

Referred Pain

The pain affects mostly the neck, the deltoid muscle, the lateral aspect of the upper limb, and may involve the epicondyle (FIG. 19-2).

Trigger Point

This point is located in the area of SI-11 *(tian zong)*.

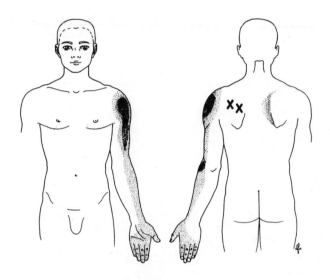

Fig. 19-2
Trigger Point Area for Infraspinatus Muscle

Coracobrachialis Muscle

Referred Pain

The pain affects the stump of the shoulder and the posterior aspect of the upper limb. It may also involve the epicondyle (FIG. 19-3).

Trigger Point

This point is lateral and inferior to LU-2 *(yun men)*.

Scalene Muscles (Anterior, Middle, Posterior)

Referred Pain

The pain affects the medial border of the scapula, the shoulder, the lateral aspect of the upper limb, and may involve the epicondyle (FIG. 19-4).

Trigger Point

This point is located in the area of LI-17 *(tian ding)*.

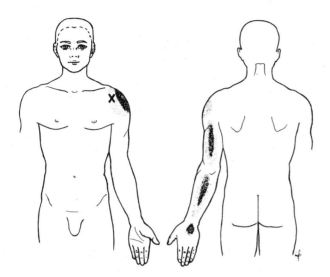

Fig. 19-3
Trigger Point Area for Coracobrachialis Muscle

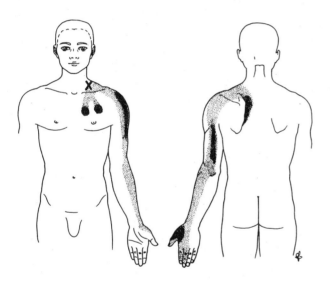

Fig. 19-4
Trigger Point Area for Scalene Muscles

Triceps Brachii Muscle: Long head

Referred Pain

Epicondyle pain, pain in the posterior aspect of the shoulder and upper limb, and possibly at the base of the neck (FIG. 19-5).

Trigger Point

This point is located in the area of TB-13 (nao hui).

Triceps Brachii Muscle: Medial head

Referred Pain

Epicondyle pain and pain on the radial aspect of the forearm (FIG. 19-6).

Trigger Point

This point is located in the area of TB-11 (qing leng yuan).

Triceps Brachii Muscle: Lateral Head

Referred Pain

Epicondyle pain (FIG. 19-7).

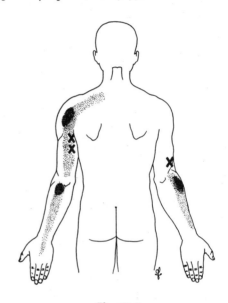

Fig. 19-5
Trigger Point Area for Triceps Brachii Muscle: Long Head

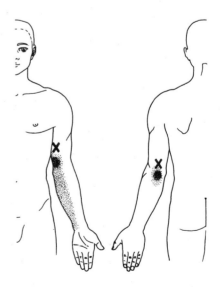

Fig. 19-6
Trigger Point Area for Triceps Brachii Muscle: Medial Head

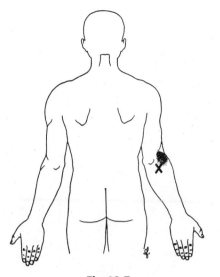

Fig. 19-7
Trigger Point Area for Triceps Brachii Muscle: Lateral Head

Brachioradialis Muscle

Referred Pain

Epicondyle pain and pain in the dorsal aspect of the first intermetacarpal space (FIG. 19-9).

Trigger Point

This point is located in the area of LI-10 *(shou san li)*.

Extensor Digiti Muscles

Referred Pain

Epicondyle pain and pain in the dorsal aspect of the fourth finger (FIG. 19-10).

Trigger Point

This point is located in the area of LI-9 *(shang lian)*.

Trigger Point

This point is located in the area of N-UE-7 *(ying xia)*.[1]

Extensor Carpi Radialis Longus Muscle

Referred Pain

Epicondyle pain and pain radiating toward the anatomical snuff box of the hand (FIG. 19-8).

Trigger Point

This point is located in the area of LI-11 *(qu chi)*.

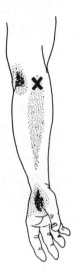

Fig. 19-9
Trigger Point Area for Brachioradialis Muscle

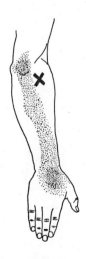

Fig. 19-8
Trigger Point Area for Extensor Carpi
Radialis Longus Muscle

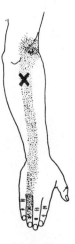

Fig. 19-10
Trigger Point Area for Extensor Digiti Muscles

Supinator Muscle

Referred Pain

Epicondyle pain and pain in the dorsal aspect of the first interosseous carpal space (FIG. 19-11).

Trigger Point

This point is located in the area of M-UE-31 *(ze xia)*.[2]

Subclavius Muscle

Referred Pain

Subclavicular pain and pain in the anterior aspect of the arm, the epicondyle, the anterolateral border of the forearm, and in the first three fingers (FIG. 19-12).

Trigger Point

This point is located in the area of KI-27 *(shu fu)*.

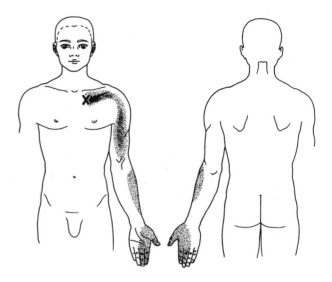

Fig. 19-12
Trigger Point Area for Subclavius Muscle

EPITROCHLEA

Pectoralis Major Muscle

Referred Pain

Pectoral pain in the sternal head, the anteromedial border of the upper limb and epitrochlea, and in the palmar aspect of the last three fingers (FIG. 19-13).

Trigger Point

This point is located in the area of ST-15 *(wu yi)*.

Pectoralis Minor Muscle

Referred Pain

Pectoral pain, and pain in the anterior aspect of the shoulder, the anteromedial border of the upper limb and epitrochlea, and in the palmar aspect of the last three fingers (FIG. 19-14).

Trigger Point

This point is located in the area of LU-1 *(zhong fu)*.

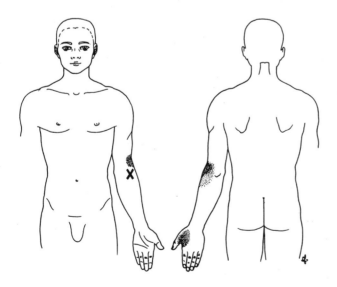

Fig. 19-11
Trigger Point Area for Supinator Muscle

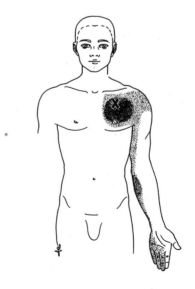

Fig. 19-13
Trigger Point Area for Pectoralis Major Muscle

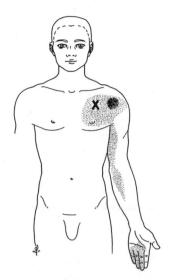

Fig. 19-14
Trigger Point Area for Pectoralis Minor Muscle

Serratus Anterior Muscle

Referred Pain

Pain in the medial border of the inferior angle of the scapula, the subaxillary flank, the medial border of the upper limb, the epitrochlea, and the palmar aspect of the fourth and fifth fingers (FIG. 19-16).

Trigger Point

This point is located in the area of SP-21 *(da bao)*.

Latissimus Dorsi Muscle

Referred Pain

Pain below the tip of the scapula, the medial border of the upper limb, and the epitrochlea (FIG. 19-17).

Trigger Point

This point is located in the area of GB-22 *(yuan ye)*.

Triceps Brachii Muscle: Medial Head

Referred Pain

Pain in the epitrochlea, the anteromedial border of the forearm, and the palmar aspect of the fourth and fifth fingers (FIG. 19-18).

Trigger Point

This point is located in the area of HT-2 *(qing ling)*.

Serratus Posterior Superior Muscle

Referred Pain

Pain in the subscapular fossa, the posterior aspect of the shoulder and arm, the epitrochlea, the posterior aspect and medial border of the forearm, and the fifth finger (FIG. 19-15).

Trigger Point

This point is located just below the scapular spine inferior to SI-12 *(bing feng)*.

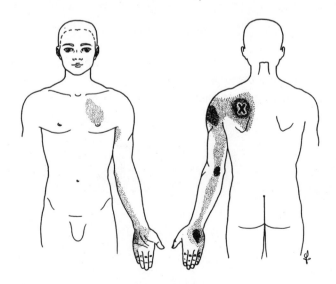

Fig. 19-15
Trigger Point Area for Serratus Posterior Superior Muscle

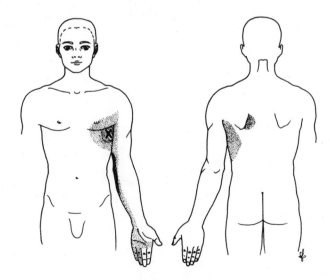

Fig. 19-16
Trigger Point Area for Serratus Anterior Muscle

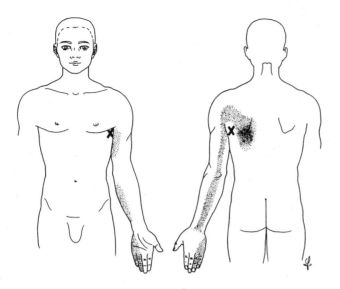

Fig. 19-17
Trigger Point Area for Latissimus Dorsi Muscle

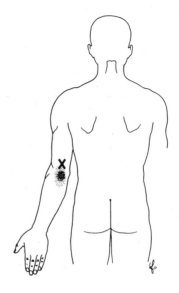

Fig. 19-19
Trigger Point Area for Triceps Brachii Muscle

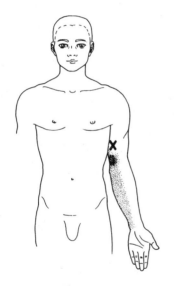

Fig. 19-18
Trigger Point Area for Triceps Brachii: Medial Head

OLECRANON

Triceps Brachii Muscle

Referred Pain

Pain in the olecranon (FIG. 19-19).

Trigger Point

This point is located in the area of TB-10 *(tian jing)*.

Chapter Notes

1. This point is located 3 units below the olecranon between the ulna and radius.
2. This point is located 2 units below LU-5 *(chi ze)*.

CHAPTER TWENTY

Wrist and Hand Pain

Energetic Aspects

RELATIONSHIP WITH CHANNEL SYSTEM

Primary Channels

Arm Greater Yin (Lung) Channel

From the anterior aspect of the upper limb, the channel reaches the radial groove, the thenar eminence, and ends at the lateral corner of the thumbnail. A secondary branch emerges from the inferior tuberosity of the radius and goes to the lateral corner of the thumbnail where it connects with the arm yang brightness, its paired yang channel.

Arm Lesser Yin (Heart) Channel

The channel travels along the ulnar side of the upper limb to the lateral corner of the fifth fingernail.

Arm Terminal Yin (Pericardium) Channel

The channel travels down the middle of the anterior aspect of the upper limb to the palm, follows the lateral side of the middle finger, and ends at the lateral corner of its nail. Another branch emerges from the palm, follows the medial side of the fifth finger, and connects at its tip with its paired yang channel, the arm lesser yang.

Arm Yang Brightness (Large Intestine) Channel

The channel starts at the tip of the two first fingers (thumb and index), follows the lateral side of the index finger and second metacarpal, and goes up the lateral side of the radius.

Arm Greater Yang (Small Intestine) Channel

The channel starts at the medial corner of the nail of the fifth finger, and follows its ulnar side up to the hand and wrist.

Arm Lesser Yang (Triple Burner) Channel

The channel starts at the medial tip of the fifth finger, emerges between the fourth and fifth metacarpals, follows the dorsal aspect of the hand, and arrives at TB-4 *(yang chi)*, lateral to the center of the crease of the wrist.

Channel Sinews

The pathways of the channel sinews correspond to those of their associated primary channels. They all follow a centripetal direction, beginning at the well points.

The three yang channel sinews meet in the frontoparietal area at GB-13 *(ben shen)*. The three yin channel sinews meet in the fourth intercostal space area, on a vertical line below the axillary at GB-22 *(yuan ye)*.

These hand channel sinews are involved in the movements of the wrist, hand and fingers as follows:

Wrist-hand:

- flexion: lesser yin, terminal yin
- extension: all three yang
- adduction: greater yang, lesser yang, lesser yin
- abduction: yang brightness, greater yin

Fingers:

- flexion of the thumb: greater yin
- flexion of the second and fifth fingers: terminal yin, lesser yin
- thumb opposition: greater yin
- fifth finger opposition: lesser yin
- extension of the fingers: all three yang

Collaterals

Arm Greater Yin Collateral

The channel emerges at LU-7 *(lie que)* at the level of the wrist, between the flesh and the skin, and connects with the arm yang brightness channel. It travels parallel to the arm greater yin to enter the palm of the hand, and spreads into the thenar eminence. Like the leg lesser yang collateral, it follows a centripetal pathway, and governs the hand in its relationship to the outside world. This collateral controls the hand as a gripping organ.

Channel Divergences

The arm yang brightness channel divergence is the only one to diverge from its primary channel to enter the hand.

Curious Vessels

The pathways of the Curious vessels do not involve either the hand or the wrist, yet it is at this level that the following confluent points are found:

- Conception vessel: LU-7 *(lie que)*
- Governing vessel: SI-3 *(hou xi)*
- Yin Linking vessel: PC-6 *(nei guan)*
- Yang Linking vessel: TB-5 *(wai guan)*

LOCAL CIRCULATION OF QI

Through its transport points, the hand is a place of exchange between the human Qi and that of the outside world, particularly through the Branch and Stem system, which monitors the synchronization of the human microcosm with that of the macrocosm.

The hand is classified as greater yin or greater yang with respect to the local movement of yin and yang Qi going from the hand toward the trunk. It is therefore governed by LU-6 *(kong zui)* or SI-6 *(yang lao),* both of which are cleft points.

Conversely, with respect to the circulation of yin and yang Qi from the hand to the upper limb, the hand is classified as either terminal yin and governed by PC-4 *(xi men),* or as yang brightness and governed by LI-9 *(shang lian).*

SYMBOLIC FUNCTIONS OF HAND

The hand is one of the most important mechanisms of human expression. In the hand-foot pair, the hand represents the yang aspect which enables us to act on the world, to transform it, to seize it, but also to protect us from it. The hand expresses ideas of action, as well as power and domination, strength and authority.

Square in shape, centered around HT-8 *(shao fu)* and PC-8 *(lao gong),* the hand symbolizes creation and potential. In every tradition, the hand is always linked to knowledge. Our discussion shall focus on the interpretation of the hand from a traditional Chinese perspective, and we shall refer our readers interested in general hand symbolism to investigate the ritual dances called "dance of the hands" of Southeast Asia, or the Hindu and Buddhist *mudras.*

Centered around HT-8 *(shao fu),* the hand demonstrates its relationship with knowledge. While the Heart-center is linked to intuitive knowledge, the hand itself has a connection with experimental knowledge. Along these lines, it is interesting to note that the word "manifestation" has the same Latin root as the word hand *(manus),* whereby what is manifested is that which can be seized by the hand, or *manipulated.* Yet experimental knowledge in itself is insufficient. As noted in Kespi (1982), "Everything that can become an object of our manifestation is there 'at hand,' but only if our hand is the extension of our Heart."

For all the above reasons, there seems to be a clear relationship between the hand and the Heart: the hand is the expression of the Heart. Similarly, there is a relationship between the eye and the Heart. Sight and touch lead to the knowledge that frees us.

It is important to remember that the hand represents an energetic microsystem, useful from a diagnostic and therapeutic point of view, and which corresponds to reflex zones in accordance with the holographic representation of anatomical structures. Several holographic patterns have been mapped out, but their description is beyond the scope of our discussion.

Specific Symptomatic Relationships of Hands

Traditional data relating the meaning of different types of hands are rare. The proper interpretation of the hands can only be arrived at in the context of a complete examination.

Eight Parameters and the Hands

Yin Hands

These are "silent" hands which remain closed. The patient keeps them in the pockets or close to the body. Gestures are slow and not demonstrative. To extend the hand obviously takes effort, and the handshake is limp. The hands are usually thick, short and small. They are often damp and cold, with little color to them, or they are almost cyanotic. These hands cannot tolerate cold. The fingers are short, stubby, knotted and stiff. Deformations are frequent.

Yang Hands

These are open hands, easily extended toward others; warm hands. Gestures and movements are quick. These hands "speak." The handshake is straightforward and strong. These hands are usually long and harmonious. They are warm and dry, with long, supple and nimble fingers.

Deficiency Hands

These are limp, hypotonic hands (yang deficiency) which become tired on exertion. To clench the fist or hold objects in the hand is difficult if not impossible. The hands are clammy and sweat easily (Blood deficiency). They have limited mobility, and gestures are slow and infrequent. There are few hairs (Blood deficiency). The skin exhibits atrophic disorders, is dry, and retains its creases (Blood deficiency); or, on the contrary, the skin is edematous (yang deficiency). Hyperextension of the fingers is weak, which indicates a problem of the corresponding channel.

Excess Hands

These are tonic hands, always in motion. The gestures are sharp and energetic (yang excess). The skin on the dorsal aspect of the hand is thin and supple, and the palm stays dry. A red hand indicates yang excess, while a deep red color points to Blood excess. A white, thick and painful hand indicates yin excess.

Cold Hands

These hands are icy-cold, white and numb. The fingers are stiff and painful. They often exhibit impaired sensitivity and a tendency toward cramping. The metacarpophalangeal joints are knotted and are often the location of arthritic nodules. Dupuytren's contracture is a good illustration of a local Cold accumulation which "coagulates" in the palmar fascia. The Blood collaterals (*xuè luò*) of the thenar eminence turn dark, indicating an accumulation of Cold at the Stomach level. Icy cold and slightly moist hands indicate Kidney deficiency. Cold hands are a manifestation of yin excess or stagnation, yang deficiency or Blood deficiency.

Hot Hands

These hands are warm, red and agitated. The fingers tremble or shake. This shows that there is a release of overabundant Heat from the Heart. These hands are often the site of such problems as eruptions, paronychia and abscesses, as they are predisposed to develop Damp-Heat. Warm, red and dry hands indicate a similar release of Heart yang. Hot and painful palms indicate an invasion of the arm lesser yin or arm terminal yin channels. When the Heat in the palms is combined with Heat in the soles of the feet and in the middle of the chest, a condition arises known as "five-center Heat." This is usually due to Kidney yin deficiency. Warm, red and damp hands indicate Lung excess. Hot palms indicate an excess of the arm greater yin collateral.

Interior-Exterior

Determining the internal or external location of a hand pathology is relatively easy, but specifying the internal or external origin of the condition requires a complete examination of the patient.

Five Phases and the Hands

Chinese chiromancy treatises provide the most comprehensive material on this subject. They identify five types of hands corresponding to the Five Phases and the Five Planets.

Metal-type Hands

The fingers and the palm have well-balanced proportions. The palmar aspect of the finger joints have a triple crease. The hand and fingers are rounded, without a lot of lines.

Wood-type Hands

These hands are hard and dry, with many apparent veins. The palms are furrowed by multiple parallel lines.

Fire-type Hands

The fingers are slender, thin and full of life.

Earth-type Hands

The fingers and palms are stubby, heavy, short, hard and lacking in elegance.

Water-type Hands

The fingers and palms are swollen, rounded and too full.

Diagnosis of Hand or Wrist Pain

The flow chart in Table 20-1 allows the practitioner to list the most frequent symptoms of hand or wrist pain which could benefit from acupuncture.

TABLE 20-1 DIFFERENTIAL DIAGNOSIS OF WRIST AND HAND PAIN

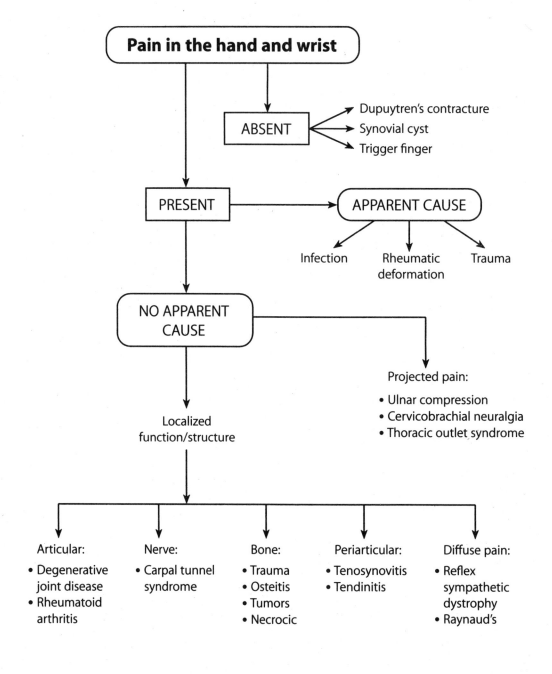

DUPUYTREN'S CONTRACTURE

Dupuytren's contracture is characterized by a thickening and retraction of the medial palmar fascia, leading to the irreducible flexion of one or several fingers. It is linked to a fibroplastic proliferation inside the fascia, occurring mostly in men over the age of fifty. It is often a bilateral condition. While common among northern Europeans, it is not seen in Asians or Africans.

Microtraumas are often involved in its etiology. Other times it is related to heredity and family history. It often affects diabetic and cirrhotic patients. It is sometimes associated with other fibromatous lesions such as those affecting the plantar aponeurosis (also known as Ledderhose's disease), fibrous pads of the phalanges, or fascia of the corpus cavernosum (Peyronie's disease). The association of Dupuytren's disease with these other localized fibroses has led to the concept of a "hereditary polyfibromatosis" or "Dupuytren's diathesis."

From an energetic point of view, Dupuytren's contracture corresponds to local Cold yin excess. The treatment principle is as follows:

* Draw the yang into the hand by needling the well points, or possibly LI-8 *(xia lian)*, or the connecting point of the upper limb yang, TB-8 *(san yang luo)*.
* Disperse local Cold by peripherally needling the local nodules as well as prolonged daily moxibustion on these nodules performed by the patient; this should be done until the nodules become soft.
* Treat the "flesh" layer by needling the leg greater yin spring and river points, SP-3 *(tai bai)* and SP-5 *(shang qiu)*.

This treatment deserves to be performed even when surgery has become necessary, as the softening of the fascial structures can only facilitate the surgeon's task. When Dupuytren's contracture affects the arch of the foot and the corpus cavernosum, the hand should be regarded as terminal yin.

In Peyronie's disease, the recommended principle is to treat the Penetrating vessel at ST-30 *(qi chong)* and SP-4 *(gong sun)*, the terminal yin channel at the connecting point LR-5 *(li gou)* or LR-12 *(ji mai)*, and to draw the yang into the pelvis by needling ST-29 *(gui lai)*.

TENDINITIS AND TENOSYNOVITIS

Overwork and trauma can cause lesions in the synovial sheath, thereby impairing the sliding motion of the tendons. The most frequent conditions are styloid tenosynovitis and tenosynovitis of the finger flexors. In traditional Chinese medicine, these are known by the term sinew painful obstruction. They are attributed to overwork affecting the collaterals and channel sinews, thereby disrupting the circulation of the Blood and Qi.

Painful Stenosing Tenosynovitis (Quervain's Disease)

This is an inflammation of the tendinous sheaths of the abductor pollicis longus and extensor pollicis brevis muscles, where they travel over the styloid process of the radius. This pathway follows the arm yang brightness channel sinew. The treatment principle is to needle the well and river points, LI-1 *(shang yang)* and LI-5 *(yang xi)*, as well as the *ashi* or trigger points.

The Shanghai College of Traditional Chinese Medicine text on acupuncture (1974) recommends activating the collaterals and relaxing the muscles by needling points which are sensitive to pressure in combination with LI-5 *(yang xi)*, LU-7 *(lie que)* and LI-4 *(he gu)*.

Tenosynovitis of the Finger Flexors

This condition affects the thumb, but also the middle and ring fingers. The corresponding channel sinew should be treated in accordance with the principles previously discussed.

CARPAL TUNNEL SYNDROME

This syndrome usually manifests as nocturnal acroparesthesia involving primarily the median aspect of the hand: palmar aspect of the hand, thumb, index, middle finger, and the lateral aspect of the ring finger. It corresponds to a compression of the median nerve in the osteofibrous band of the carpal tunnel, between PC-6 *(nei guan)* and PC-7 *(da ling)*.

The nocturnal aggravation of the symptoms indicates Qi stagnation, or a yin excess. Because both of these conditions are ameliorated by local application of warmth, differentiation is based on the effect of pressure and movement. Yin excess is aggravated by pressure and is not affected much by movement; Qi stagnation is improved by movement and not affected much by pressure.

For Qi stagnation, the treatment principle is to promote the circulation of Qi in the upper limb by needling SI-6 *(yang lao)* and LI-15 *(jian yu)*, and to harmonize the arm terminal yin and arm lesser yang channels by using the connecting point-source point combination technique, PC-6 *(nei guan)* with TB-4 *(yang chi)*.

For yin excess, the treatment principle is to promote its circulation by needling the group connecting point of the upper limb yang, TB-8 *(san yang luo)*, and the well point TB-1 *(guan chong)*. One can also needle the meeting point of the upper limb yin channels, PC-5 *(jian shi)*, the meeting point of the upper limb yang channels, TB-8 *(san yang luo)*, and the well point of the hand terminal yin channel, PC-9 *(zhong chong)*. Another method—less often used— is to promote circulation in the terminal yin by needling the cleft point PC-4 *(xi men)*, as well as HT-1 *(ji quan)*, which mobilizes the entire upper limb yin, and the arm lesser yin well point HT-9 *(shao chong)*.

REFLEX SYMPATHETIC DYSTROPHY OF HAND

The onset of this disorder is usually progressive, and its evolution may go through two stages: inflammatory and atrophic. In the hypertrophic inflammatory stage, we encounter painful dysfunction of the hand; diffuse edema pitting on pressure; cutaneous modifications (warm and ruddy skin, profuse sweating); an articular and muscular stiffness with difficulty in fully opening or closing the hands and fingers; and an absence of fever, adenopathy or neurological signs.

The atrophic stage begins after several weeks or months of progression. In this stage the pain decreases, the edema diminishes, and the atrophic disorders worsen. There is atrophy of the subcutaneous tissue, thinning, paling and smoothing of the skin, and loss of hair. At this point a neurotrophic condition settles in.

Upon analysis, the first stage corresponds to a disruption of the yin penetration, which stagnates; then, in a second stage, it contracts, causing local atrophic disorders.

Local treatment will focus on promoting the circulation of the yin by needling lesser yin points such as HT-1 *(ji quan)* and HT-9 *(shao chong)*; needling the group connecting point of the upper limb yang, TB-8 *(san yang luo)*; and promoting the penetration of yin Qi from the upper extremities into the trunk by needling PC-2 *(tian quan)*.

The etiological treatment is done on a case-by-case basis.

DEGENERATIVE JOINT DISEASE

Degenerative disease of the thumb is a painful obstruction disorder, and should be addressed as such. Prolonged moxibustion at LI-5 *(yang xi)* contributes to expulsion of the local Damp-Cold.

From a symptomatic point of view, needling M-UE-32 *(ze qian)*[1] brings instant cessation of the pain. This can be maintained with repeated treatment sessions.

If the arm lesser yin channel sinew is affected, needle the well point LU-11 *(shao shang)* and M-UE-13 *(ban men)*.[2]

If the greater yin axis is affected, regulate it by needling SP-3 *(tai bai)* and CV-12 *(zhong wan)*.

NODULAR DEGENERATIVE DISEASE

Swelling of the distal or proximal interphalangeal joints, more frequent in women, also corresponds to a painful obstruction disorder. The points M-UE-22 *(ba xie)*, located in the web of the fingers on the dorsal aspect of the hand, and M-UE-50 *(shang ba xie)*, located behind the metacarpophalangeal joints, in combination with LI-11 *(qu chi)*, LI-5 *(yang xi)* and TB-5 *(wai guan)*, are classically indicated for deforming rheumatism of the hands.

Trigger Points

SCALENE MUSCLES (ANTERIOR, MIDDLE, POSTERIOR)

Referred Pain

Pain in the thumb and index finger, or in the dorsal aspect of the wrist and five fingers (FIG. 20-1).

Trigger Point

This point is located in the area of LI-17 *(tian ding)*.

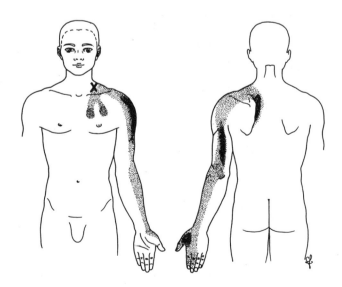

Fig. 20-1
Trigger Point Area for Scalene Muscles

Scalenus Minimus Muscle

Referred Pain

Pain in the lateral aspect of the arm, the posterior aspect of the forearm, and the dorsal aspect of the hand (FIG. 20-2).

Trigger Point

This point is located in the area of ST-10 *(shui tu)*.

Infraspinatus Muscle

Referred Pain

Pain in the radial aspect of the hand, occasionally of the fingers (FIG. 20-3).

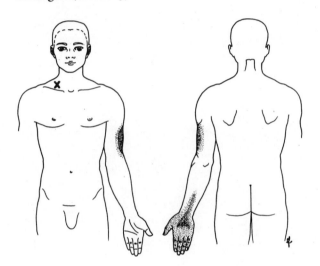

Fig. 20-2
Trigger Point Area for Scalenus Minimus Muscles

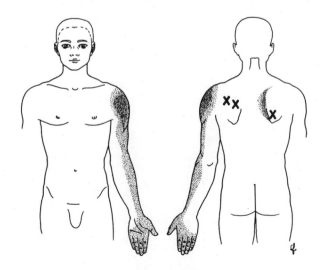

Fig. 20-3
Trigger Point Area for Infraspinatus Muscle

Trigger Point

This point is located in the area of SI-11 *(tian zong)*.

Latissimus Dorsi Muscle

Referred Pain

Pain in the medial border of the hand, and of the fourth and fifth fingers (FIG. 20-4).

Trigger Point

This point is located in the area of GB-22 *(yuan ye)*.

Subscapularis Muscle

Referred Pain

Pain in the wrist, mostly in the dorsal aspect (FIG. 20-5).

Trigger Point

This point is located in the body of the subscapularis muscle, in the posterior aspect of the axilla.

Coracobrachialis Muscle

Referred Pain

Pain in the dorsal aspect of the hand (FIG. 20-6).

Trigger Point

This point is lateral and inferior to LU-2 *(yun men)*.

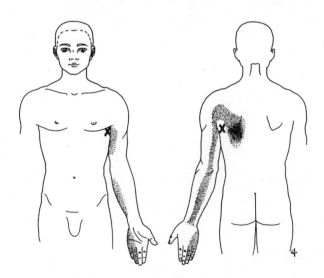

Fig. 20-4
Trigger Point Area for Latissimus Dorsi Muscle

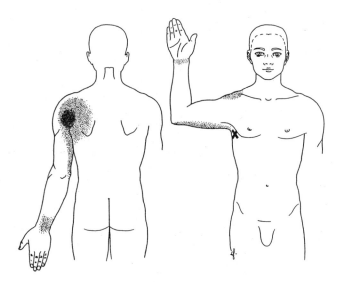

Fig. 20-5
Trigger Point Area for Subscapularis Muscle

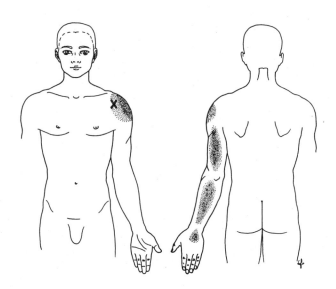

Fig. 20-6
Trigger Point Area for Coracobrachialis Muscle

BRACHIALIS MUSCLE

Referred Pain

Pain in the base and dorsal aspect of the thumb (FIG. 20-7).

Trigger Point

This point is located in the area of LU-4 (*xia bai*) and N-UE-25 (*xia xia bai*).[3]

TRICEPS BRACHII MUSCLE: LATERAL HEAD

Referred Pain

Pain in the dorsal aspect of the fourth and fifth fingers (FIG. 20-8).

Trigger Point

This point is located in the area of TB-12 (*xiao luo*).

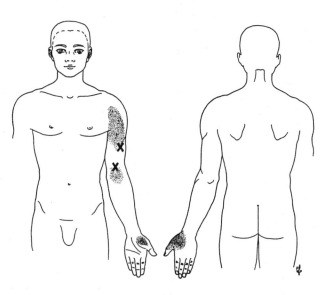

Fig. 20-7
Trigger Point Area for Brachialis Muscle

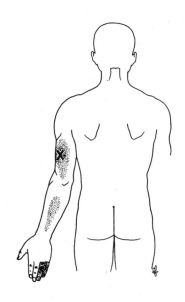

Fig. 20-8
Trigger Point Area for Triceps Brachii Muscle: Lateral Head

Triceps Brachii Muscle: Medial Head

Referred Pain

Pain in the palmar aspect of the fourth and fifth fingers (FIG. 20-9).

Trigger Point

This point is located in the area of HT-2 *(qing ling)*.

Extensor Carpi Ulnaris Muscle

Referred Pain

Pain in the ulnar border of the posterior aspect of the wrist (FIG. 20-10).

Trigger Point

This point is located between SI-7 *(zhi zheng)* and SI-8 *(xiao hai)*.

Extensor Carpi Radialis Brevis Muscle

Referred Pain

Pain in the dorsal aspect of the wrist (FIG. 20-11).

Trigger Point

This point is located in the area of N-UE-8 *(niu shang xue)*.[4]

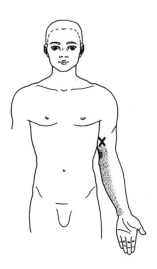

Fig. 20-9
Trigger Point Area for Triceps Brachii Muscle: Medial Head

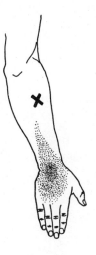

Fig. 20-11
Trigger Point Area for Extensor Carpi Radialis Brevis Muscle

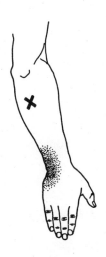

Fig. 20-10
Trigger Point Area for Extensor Carpi Ulnaris Muscle

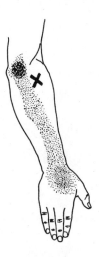

Fig. 20-12
Trigger Point Area for Extensor Carpi Radialis Longus Muscle

Extensor Carpi Radialis Longus Muscle

Referred Pain

Pain in the dorsal aspect of the hand and the anatomical snuff box (FIG. 20-12).

Trigger Point

This point is located in the area of LI-11 *(qu chi)*.

Brachioradialis Muscle

Referred Pain

Pain in the base of the thumb and first interdigital space (FIG. 20-13).

Trigger Point

This point is located in the area of LI-10 *(shou san li)*.

Extensor Digiti Muscles

Referred Pain

Pain in the dorsal aspect of the hand and fingers, except in the last phalanges (FIG. 20-14).

Trigger Point

This point is located in the area of N-UE-7 *(ying xia)*[5] and TB-5 *(wai guan)*.

Supinator Muscle

Referred Pain

Pain in the dorsal aspect of the thumb (FIG. 20-15).

Trigger Point

This point is located in the area of M-UE-31 *(ze xia)*.[6]

Palmaris Longus Muscle

Referred Pain

Pain in the palm of the hand (FIG. 20-16).

Trigger Point

This point is located on the arm lesser yin channel, 3 units below HT-3 *(shao hai)*.

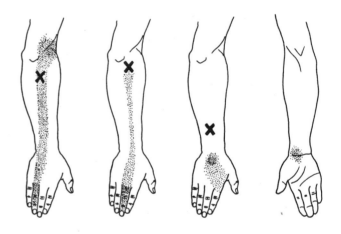

Fig. 20-14
Trigger Point Area for Extensor Digiti Muscles

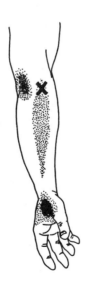

Fig. 20-13
Trigger Point Area for Brachioradialis Muscle

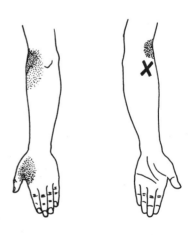

Fig. 20-15
Trigger Point Area for Supinator Muscle

FLEXOR CARPI RADIALIS MUSCLE

Referred Pain

Pain in the palmar aspect of the wrist (FIG. 20-17).

Trigger Point

This point is located in the area of N-UE-5 *(xi shang).*[7]

FLEXOR CARPI ULNARIS MUSCLE

Referred Pain

Pain in the hypothenar eminence (FIG. 20-18).

Trigger Point

This point is located on the arm lesser yin channel, 3 units below HT-3 *(shao hai).*

FLEXOR DIGITORUM MUSCLE

Referred Pain

Pain in the finger corresponding to the involved muscle head. There is no difference between the superficial and deep tract (FIG. 20-19).

Trigger Point

This point is located at the junction of the superior third and inferior two-thirds of the volar surface of the forearm.

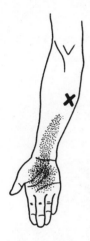

Fig. 20-16
Trigger Point Area for Palmaris Longus Muscle

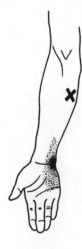

Fig. 20-18
Trigger Point Area for Flexor Carpi Ulnaris Muscle

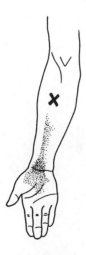

Fig. 20-17
Trigger Point Area for Flexor Carpi Radialis Muscle

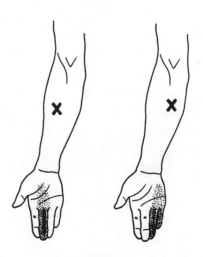

Fig. 20-19
Trigger Point Area for Flexor Digitorum Muscle

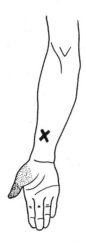

Fig. 20-20
Trigger Point Area for Flexor Pollicis Longus Muscle

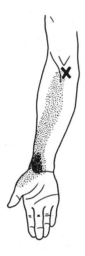

Fig. 20-21
Trigger Point Area for Pronator Teres Muscle

FLEXOR POLLICIS LONGUS MUSCLE

Referred Pain

Pain in the palmar aspect of the thumb and its extremity (FIG. 20-20).

Trigger Point

This point is located in the area of M-UE-29 *(er bai).*[8]

PRONATOR TERES MUSCLE

Referred Pain

Pain in the radial border of the palmar aspect of the wrist and thenar eminence (FIG. 20-21).

Trigger Point

This point is located in the area of M-UE-32 *(ze qian).*[9]

ADDUCTOR POLLICIS MUSCLE

Referred Pain

Pain in the lateral border of the thumb, its base, and thenar eminence (FIG. 20-22).

Trigger Point

This point is located in the palmar aspect of the first interosseous space.

OPPONENS POLLICIS MUSCLE

Referred Pain

Pain in the palmar aspect of the thumb, and the radial border of the palmar aspect of the wrist (FIG. 20-23).

Trigger Point

This point is located in the area of LU-10 *(yu ji).*

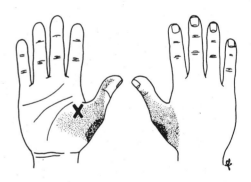

Fig. 20-22
Trigger Point Area for Adductor Pollicis Muscle

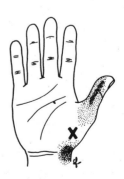

Fig. 20-23
Trigger Point Area for Opponens Pollicis Muscle

First Dorsal Interosseus Muscle

Referred Pain

Pain in the index finger, the dorsal and palmar aspect of the hand, and the dorsal aspect of the fifth finger (FIG. 20-24).

Trigger Point

This point is located in the area of N-UE-15 *(hu bian)*.[10]

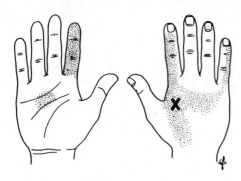

Fig. 20-24
Trigger Point Area for First Dorsal Interosseus Muscle

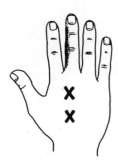

Fig. 20-25
Trigger Point Area for Second Dorsal Interosseus Muscle

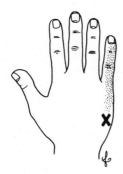

Fig. 20-26
Trigger Point Area for Abductor Digiti Minimi Muscle

Second Dorsal Interosseus Muscle

Referred Pain

Pain in the lateral border of the middle finger (FIG. 20-25).

Trigger Point

This point is located in the area of N-UE-19(a) *(yao tong #1)*[11] and M-UE-24 *(luo zhen)*.[12]

Abductor Digiti Minimi Muscle

Referred Pain

Pain in the posteriolateral aspect of the fifth finger (FIG. 20-26).

Trigger Point

This point is located in the area of N-UE-4 *(shang hou xi)*.[13]

Pectoralis Major Muscle

Referred Pain

The sternal head causes pain in the palm of the hand and in the palmar aspect of the third, fourth and fifth fingers (FIG. 20-27).

Trigger Point

This point is located in the area of ST-15 *(wu yi)*.

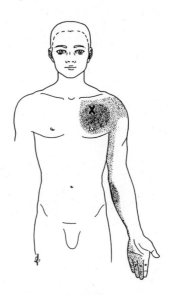

Fig. 20-27
Trigger Point Area for Pectoralis Major Muscle

Subclavius Muscle

Referred Pain

Pain in the first three fingers (FIG. 20-28).

Trigger Point

This point is located in the area of KI-27 *(shu fu)*.

Pectoralis Minor Muscle

Referred Pain

Pain in the palmar aspect of the last three fingers (FIG. 20-29).

Trigger Point

This point is located in the area of LU-1 *(zhong fu)*.

Serratus Posterior Superior Muscle

Referred Pain

Pain in the medial aspect of the hand and fifth finger (FIG. 20-30).

Trigger Point

This point is located inferior to the scapular spine, level with BL-41 *(fu fen)*.

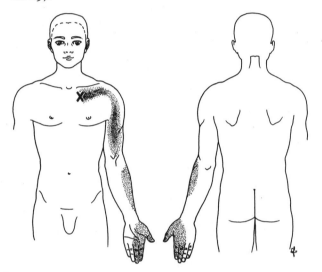

Fig. 20-28
Trigger Point Area for Subclavius Muscle

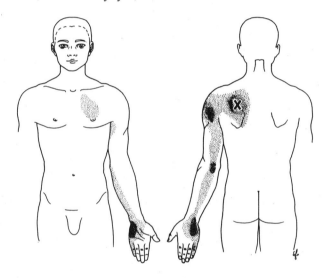

Fig. 20-30
Trigger Point Area for Serratus Posterior Superior Muscle

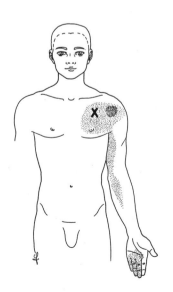

Fig. 20-29
Trigger Point Area for Pectoralis Minor Muscle

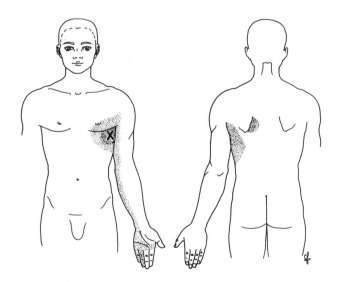

Fig. 20-31
Trigger Point Area for Serratus Anterior Muscle

Serratus Anterior Muscle

Referred Pain

Pain in the palmar aspect of the fourth and fifth fingers (FIG. 20-31).

Trigger Point

This point is located in the area of SP-21 *(da bao)*.

Chapter Notes

1. Located 1 unit distal and slightly medial to LU-5 *(chi ze)*, on a straight line from the middle finger.
2. Located on the palmar aspect of the hand in the first interosseous space.
3. Located on the upper arm, 3 units below LU-4 *(xia bai)*.
4. Located one-quarter the distance from LI-11 *(qu chi)* to TB-4 *(yang chi)*.
5. Located 3 units below the olecranon between the radius and ulna.
6. Located 2 units below LU-5 *(chi ze)*.
7. Located 3 units above PC-4 *(xi men)*.
8. Located 4 units proximal to the ulnar end of the transverse crease of the wrist. It is actually comprised of two points: the first between the two tendons and the second on the radial side of the tendons. It is the second one which is the trigger point here.
9. Located 1 unit distal and slightly medial to LU-5 *(chi ze)*, on a straight line from the middle finger.
10. Located between LI-3 *(san jian)* and LI-4 *(he gu)*.
11. Located on the dorsum of the hand between the proximal aspects of the second and third metacarpals.
12. Located on the dorsum of the hand approximately 0.5 unit proximal to and between the articulations of the second and third metacarpophalangeal joints.
13. Located on the lateral aspect of the dorsum of the hand between SI-3 *(hou xi)* and SI-4 *(wan gu)*.

CHAPTER TWENTY-ONE

Hip Pain

Energetic Aspects of Hip

RELATIONSHIP WITH CHANNEL SYSTEM

Primary Channels

The leg lesser yang (Gallbladder) channel follows the lateral aspect of the hip. The leg yang brightness (Stomach) channel proceeds down its anterior aspect, and the leg greater yang (Bladder) channel follows its posterior aspect. The three lower limb yin channels ascend the medial aspect of the thigh.

Channel Sinews

The pathways of the channel sinews roughly overlap the trajectory of the primary channels.

Channel Divergences

Leg Greater Yang Channel Divergence

The channel divergence originates at the popliteal fossa, ascends to a place 5 units below the coccyx, and then goes toward the anal area.

Leg Lesser Yin Channel Divergence

The channel divergence separates from the leg lesser yin channel behind the knee, ascends, and crosses the leg greater yang channel divergence.

Leg Yang Brightness Channel Divergence

The channel divergence emerges from the primary channel in the hip area and penetrates into the abdomen.

Leg Greater Yin Channel Divergence

The channel divergence separates from the leg greater yin primary channel at the hip, then crosses the leg yang brightness primary channel.

Leg Lesser Yang Channel Divergence

The channel divergence originates from its primary channel at the hip, goes around it in the front and penetrates the pubis, where it crosses the leg terminal yin primary channel.

Leg Terminal Yin Channel Divergence

The channel divergence emerges from its primary channel at the dorsum of the foot, and ascends to the pubis, where it crosses the leg lesser yang primary channel.

Curious Vessels

The yang Heel vessel and yang Linking vessel follow the lateral aspect of the hip. One branch of the Penetrating vessel emerges at the groin at ST-30 (*qi chong*) and descends along the medial aspect of the thigh. The yin Heel vessel and yin Linking vessel travel along the medial aspect of the thigh. From the level of the second lumbar vertebra, the belt-like pathway of the Girdle vessel proceeds downward in front of the iliac crest.

Collaterals

Leg Yang Brightness Collateral

The collateral emerges at ST-40 (*feng leng*), and travels down the lateral aspect of the leg.

Leg Greater Yang Collateral

The collateral diverges from BL-58 (*fei yang*), and one branch ascends alongside the pathway of the primary channel.

Leg Greater Yin, Leg Lesser Yin, And Leg Terminal Yin Collaterals

All three collaterals ascend the medial aspect of the thigh.

Hip and Local Circulation of Qi

The hip represents a physiological barrier to the entry and exit of Qi between the trunk and the lower limbs. The yin and yang Qi that come out of the trunk are described as greater (*tài*) at the hip, as it is the joint proximal to their origin. The yin and yang Qi of the lower limb that enter the trunk are described as terminal yin or yang brightness at the hip, as they are quite removed from their origin in the foot.

Hip pain that occurs during the course of walking, and that worsens as one tires, is often due to the failure of the yang Qi to exit from the trunk to the lower limb; this is especially the case when one cannot step backward without difficulty. The appropriate treatment is the barrier point BL-29 (*zhong lu shu*). Yin Qi not exiting from the trunk, on the other hand, is marked by inguinal pain with radiation toward the anterior aspect of the thigh. SP-12 (*chong men*) is indicated for this pattern. The two points are often used together. If the pain is most acute just as one starts walking, we use GB-30 (*huan tiao*) to mobilize the Qi in this area.

Hip Gate

All our structures, potential and paths are inscribed in our body, at all levels: life is One, and it is impossible to exclude or isolate a plane of manifestation.

One of these paths ascends, like sap in a tree, from our feet, our grounding roots, all the way to our hair, going through five different gates.

We follow this path through different ages and on different planes: on a somatic plane with our biological evolution from our birth to our death; a psychological plane with, for instance, the passage from childhood to adolescence to adulthood; and finally, a spiritual plane.... (J.-M. Kespi, 1982)

These gates are therefore stages which illustrate the temporal, physical, mental and spiritual evolution of the human being. It is manifested by ascending from the heels to the vertex, through the spinal pathway. The hip gate governs adolescence, the passage to adulthood, when one leaves the sheltered world of childhood to face the reality of the outside world.[1] This passage is governed by a point on the yang Heel vessel, GB-29 (*ju liao*).

Diagnosis of Hip Pain

We shall begin by using the modern biomedical approach to diagnosing a painful hip. From there we will deduce the probable energetic patterns of disharmony, and the appropriate principles of treatment.

With many possible causes for hip pain, it is particularly important to establish a precise diagnosis. The more precise the diagnosis, the more precise the prescription for correct treatment, and the better the therapeutic results. This diagnosis involves three stages:

• identifying the articular origin of the pain
• ruling out a regional pain which does not originate in the coxofemoral joint
• determining the etiology of the painful hip.

Pain of Coxofemoral Origin

In its typical form, the focal point of the pain is the groin, with radiation down the anterior aspect of the thigh, that is, the pathway of the leg yang brightness channel. The pain is accompanied by dysfunction with limited range of motion of the hip, and limping. This symptomatology strongly suggests a coxofemoral disorder.

When the problem is less typical, we need to specify the characteristics of the pain:

Location: Pain may be in the inguinal area, radiating to the anterior aspect of the thigh, and possibly to the knee. This pathway overlaps the trajectory of the leg yang brightness channel. Knee pain may predominate, hence the necessity of always examining the hip when the knee is painful. Gluteal pain, radiating to the posterior aspect of the thigh, follows the path of the leg greater yang channel. Trochanteric pain may be along the leg lesser yang channel, the yang Heel vessel or the yang Linking vessel.

Features: Most of the time, the pain follows a "mechanical" pattern. It occurs upon exertion or during extensive walking (suggesting a yang deficiency), or in getting started after prolonged immobilization. This "warming up" period is particularly pronounced in the morning in the case of Blood stasis. For other patients, the pain is more constant and worsens at night, due to yin stagnation and release of Heat during that time.

Pattern of progression: It is necessary to analyze the onset (progressive or sudden) as well as the presence of possible relapses. A simple dysfunctional impairment can cause a temporary limp, a missed step posteriorly, or a problem with the stance of the lower limb that can rekindle the patient's complaint.

Whatever the case, the pain must be analyzed according to the diagnostic rules of the eight parameters.

Often the pain in the groin or anterior aspect of the thigh is precipitated by movements involving the coxofemoral joint. It is always important to evaluate the range of motion of this joint by comparing it with that of the contralateral hip. The motions (with normal ranges in parentheses) are set forth below, followed by the name of the channel involved in dysfunctions:

• flexion (130°): leg yang brightness channel sinew
• adduction (over 30°): three leg yin channel sinews
• abduction (over 45°): leg lesser yang channel sinew
• internal rotation (over 30°): leg lesser yang channel sinew
• external rotation (over 30°): leg lesser yang channel sinew
• extension (10 to 15°): leg greater yang channel sinew.

REGIONAL PAIN OF NONCOXOFEMORAL ORIGIN

When the location of pain is different from that described above and the examination does not provoke coxofemoral pain, or if the joint moves freely, differential diagnosis then relies on:

• more thorough history of the patient's complaint
• looking for the precise point that recreates the pain
• complementary radiological and biochemical exams.

Pain in a Proximal Joint

Pubic symphysis dysfunction with spontaneous pain in the medial aspect of the thigh can involve one of three mechanisms. First, a problem with one of three yin primary channels or channel sinews. Second, sometimes the pain follows the trajectory of the Penetrating vessel, which means involvement of this vessel. Third, the pain may be attributable to a barrier to the exit of yin Qi from the trunk to the lower extremities. If this is the mechanism, the barrier point SP-12 *(chong men)* should be selected.

Pain in the sacroiliac joint usually involves the leg lesser yang channel sinew or primary channel. Another frequent mechanism is the development of sacroiliac fibrous nodules.

Tendinitis, Enthesitis and Bursitis

Tendinitis of the gluteus medius muscle involves the leg lesser yang channel sinew.

Tendinitis of the rectus femoris muscle involves the leg yang brightness channel sinew. Another possibility is the entry barrier point governing the movement of the yang Qi from the lower limb toward the trunk, ST-31 *(bi guan)*.

Tendinitis of the adductors involves one of the three leg yin channel sinews, or the entry barrier point governing the movement of the yin Qi of the lower limb toward the trunk, LR-11 *(yin lian)*.

Tendinitis of the psoas muscle involves the leg yang brightness channel sinew, or the exit barrier point governing the movement of the yin Qi of the trunk toward the lower limbs, SP-12 *(chong men)*.

Bony Lesions of the Pelvis

The bony structures of the pelvis can develop various problems. These structures include the ischiopubic and iliopubic rami, the iliac crest, the neck of the femur, the trochanter and the acetabulum. Any involvement of the bony structures points to a pathology of the bone in its various guises:

• as a Curious organ
• linked to the Kidneys
• related to the Water phase
• corresponding to winter.

Also note that with all osseus lesions there is demineralization and consequent loss of structure. As such, they involve a relatively intense loss of yin. This give them some relation to Heat and/or Fire.

Referred Pain

Femoral Pain

If there is femoral pain we should always check if it is the lower limb yang Qi being unable to move into the trunk. When this is the case there will be yang excess on the anterior aspect of the thigh corresponding to the yang brightness pathway, as well as yang deficiency lower back pain. Needling the barrier point ST-31 *(bi guan)* should provide quick improvement in such cases. This pathology should also direct us to look for pelvic yin excess or stagnation.

Meralgia Paraesthetica

This neuropathy (also known as Roth-Bernhardt's disease) is characterized by pain, paresthesia and various sensory disturbances in the area supplied by the lateral femoral cutaneous nerve. Its location on the lateral aspect of the thigh corresponds to the pathway of the leg lesser yang channel, yang Heel or yang Linking vessels.

Sciatica Radiating Toward the Gluteus Muscles

This problem may correspond to one of a few dysfunctions. It can be associated with either an endogenous or exogenous leg greater yang problem (direct or indirect), or the inability of the trunk yang to move out into the lower limbs. In either case, needling BL-29 *(zhong lu shu)* and BL-36 *(cheng fu)* should bring improvement.

Visceral and Pelvic Pain

The Kidneys, Bladder and Large Intestine, and the Conception, Penetrating, Girdle and Governing vessels should be examined. We should also look for possible Blood and Qi imbalance in the area of the pelvic cavity.

Inguinal or Femoral Hernia

In traditional Chinese medicine this pathology is related to the leg terminal yin channel or the Conception vessel.

Etiologic Diagnosis

PATIENTS WITH ABNORMAL RADIOLOGICAL FINDINGS

Narrowing of the Superior Joint Space

Senile Coxarthritis

Degenerative disease of the hip corresponds to a Wind-Damp-Cold painful obstruction disorder. In addition to analyzing the traditional signs differentiating Cold from Dampness, radiological images may supplement the diagnosis. Osteophytosis with well-defined outlines, pinching of a joint or osteosclerosis are all radiological findings suggesting the presence of Cold. More vague outlines, or the presence of cysts, suggest Dampness. Rapid destructive patterns are related to transformation of the disorder into Heat.

In the case of mild senile coxarthritis with no associated deformation, the therapeutic modality relies primarily on medical treatment, with an important role to be played by acupuncture. In more advanced cases, medical treatment, including acupuncture, should always be attempted as long as is practicable. If disability and pain become intolerable, or if there are associated deformations, surgery is then indicated.

The acupuncture treatment principle is to eliminate the Cold with repeated application of moxa at BL-23 *(shen shu)* and CV-4 *(guan yuan)*. If Dampness predominates, the treatment is longer and more complex, and requires the use of the warm needle technique at SP-5 *(shang qiu)*, ST-36 *(zu san li)* and BL-20 *(pi shu)*.

Specific action on the hip (in order to eliminate the pathogenic influences) is achieved through the leg lesser yang and leg greater yang channels. This is done by choosing GB-30 *(huan tiao)*, which should be needled deeply (up to 10cm) and stimulated until the *de qi* sensation is obtained; applying moxa at GB-31 *(feng shi)*; deeply needling GB-34 *(yang ling quan)* and GB-39 *(xuan zhong)*; and also needling BL-40 *(wei zhong)* and BL-60 *(kun lun)*. A passage in chapter 63 of *Basic Questions* advises that if the pathogenic influence "settles in the Gallbladder collateral, causing residing pain in [the area of] the center of the pivot[2] paralyzing the hip, use a filiform needle to needle that point."

Coxitis

Infectious coxitis requires the rapid implementation of antibiotic therapy.

Inflammatory coxitis, due to rheumatoid arthritis or ankylosing spondylitis, corresponds to a Hot painful obstruction disorder.

Paget's Disease of Bone

Although its treatment is similar to that of senile coxarthritis, this condition features certain distinct elements affecting the bone as the reservoir of marrow. This indicates a problem with the bone as a Curious Organ, and also the loss of Kidney Essence. The presence of cardiovascular and neurological complications further confirms this hypothesis.

Normal Joint Space but Abnormal Bone

Osteonecrosis of the Femoral Head

This diagnosis suggests local and systemic Blood stasis, as indicated by its sudden onset (as if "pierced by a dagger"), even more so if its origin is secondary to trauma or decompression disease.

Epiphysitis of the medulla of the femoral head, leading to osteochondritis deformans juvenilis (or Legg-Calvé-Phertes disease), is an aseptic osteonecrosis which manifests between the ages of 4 and 16, mostly in boys, and is of unknown origin. Its onset mechanism suggests a disruption of the yang Heel vessel. Besides the conventional medical treatment, it would make sense to further regulate this vessel by needling the confluent point BL-62 *(shen mai)*, the cleft point BL-59 *(fu yang)*, and first and foremost GB-29 *(ju liao)*, the point that governs the hip gate.

Reflex Sympathetic Dystrophy of the Hip

This hip pathology is rare and difficult to diagnose. Several factors are involved in its pathogenesis and it can be meaningfully discussed only on a case-by-case basis. In this condition we always find disruption of the local circulation of Qi, suggesting a barrier pathology with a two-stage progression. First there is yin stagnation followed by excess yang (Heat). This explains the pseudoinflammatory condition caused by swelling and vasomotor disturbances along with slight bone loss, followed later by retraction of the yin. This last symptom is marked by such signs as atrophy of the subcutaneous tissues, wasting of the musculature, thickening of the joint capsules and finally atrophic changes with severe demineralization of the bones.

Beginning Stage of Coxitis

This is another case of Hot painful obstruction.

PATIENTS WITH NORMAL RADIOLOGICAL FINDINGS

Hip pain with normal radiological findings can be seen in a variety of disorders. Some of the more common ones are osteoid osteoma, chondromatosis and pigmented villonodular synovitis. These conditions do not fall in the realm of acupuncture treatment, but can nonetheless benefit from an energetic interpretation.

Trigger Points

EXTERNAL ABDOMINAL OBLIQUE MUSCLE

Referred Pain

Pain in the iliac fossa, hypochondriac area, groin and testicle (FIG. 21-1).

Trigger Point

This point is located in the area of GB-26 *(dai mai)* and GB-27 *(wu shu)*.

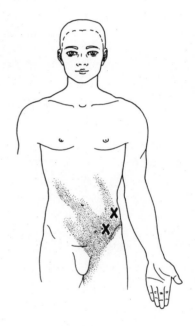

Fig. 21-1
Trigger Point for the External Abdominal Oblique Muscle

ILIOPSOAS MUSCLE

Referred Pain

Pain in the iliac fossa and groin (FIG. 21-2).

Trigger Point

This point is located in the area of SP-12 *(chong men)*.

ADDUCTOR MAGNUS MUSCLE

Referred Pain

Pain in the inguinal region and in the anteromedial aspect of the thigh (FIG. 21-3).

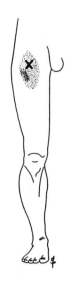

Fig. 21-2
Trigger Point for the Iliopsoas Muscle

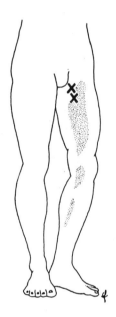

Fig. 21-3
Trigger Point for the Adductor Magnus Muscle

Trigger Point

This point is located in the area of LR-10 *(zu wu li)* and LR-11 *(yin lian)*.

GLUTEUS MINIMUS MUSCLE

Referred Pain

Pain below the trochanter and in the posterior aspect of the thigh (FIG. 21-4).

Trigger Point

This point is located in the area of GB-29 *(ju liao)*.

GLUTEUS MEDIUS MUSCLE

Referred Pain

Localized pain in the buttock.

Trigger Point

This point is located in the area of M-BW-26 *(zhong kong)* (FIG. 21-5).

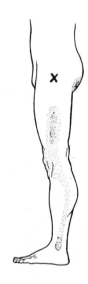

Fig. 21-4
Trigger Point for the Gluteus Minimus Muscle

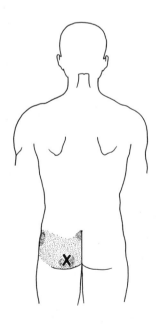

Fig. 21-5
Trigger Point for the Gluteus Medius Muscle

ILIOLUMBAR LIGAMENT

Referred Pain

Pain around the trochanter, the groin, the medial aspect of the thigh and the external genital organs (FIG. 21-6).

Trigger Point

This point is located in the area of BL-26 *(guan yuan shu)*.

Chapter Notes

1. For a fuller discussion of this topic, see Kespi (1982), pp. 227-31. The gates are BL-61 *(pu can)* for the feet; GB-29 *(ju liao)* for the hips (or Kidneys); SI -10 *(nao shu)* for the shoulders; CV-23 *(lian quan)* for the pharynx; and GV-15 *(ya men)* for the ears.

2. *Shū zhōng*, "center of the pivot," is an alternate name for GB-30 *(huan tiao)*.

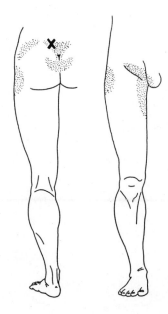

Fig. 21-6
Trigger Point for the Iliolumbar Ligament

CHAPTER TWENTY-TWO

Knee Pain

Energetic Aspects of Knee

RELATIONSHIP WITH CHANNEL SYSTEM

Primary Channels

Leg Yang Brightness (Stomach) Channel

The superficial branch of this channel goes down the anterior aspect of the thigh, enters the patella, and follows the lateral border of the tibia. A secondary branch emerges below the knee from ST-36 *(zu san li)*, follows a parallel course lateral to the main branch, and ends in the third toe.

Leg Greater Yin (Spleen) Channel

The superficial trajectory of this channel ascends along the medial aspect of the knee.

Leg Greater Yang (Bladder) Channel

The medial branch of this channel goes down from the trochanter at GB-30 *(huan tiao)* to the posterior aspect of the thigh, and ends at the lateral border of the popliteal fossa at BL-38 *(fu xi)* and BL-39 *(wei yang)*. Its lateral branch meets GB-30 *(huan tiao)* in the buttock, descends along the posterior aspect of the thigh, reaches the middle of the popliteal fossa at BL-40 *(wei zhong)* and then travels down the posterior aspect of the leg.

Leg Lesser Yin (Kidney) Channel

This channel ascends along the medial aspect of the knee behind the leg greater yin channel, enters the popliteal fossa and travels up the medial aspect of the thigh.

Leg Lesser Yang (Gallbladder) Channel

A superficial branch of this channel descends along the lateral aspect of the thigh and knee.

Leg Terminal Yin (Liver) Channel

This channel ascends to the medial aspect of the knee between the leg greater yin (anteriorly) and the leg lesser yin (posteriorly).

Channel Sinews

Leg Yang Brightness

One channel sinew branch ascends along the lateral aspect of the leg, spreads into the fibula, inserts at the lateral aspect of the knee, and then finally at the hip joint. A second branch emerges from the dorsum of the foot, and inserts in the anterior aspect of the knee. Another branch starts from there, meets the first branch, inserts at the head of the fibula, and connects with the leg lesser yang channel.

Leg Greater Yin

This channel sinew runs parallel to the primary channel in the medial aspect of the knee.

Leg Greater Yang

This channel sinew starts at the small toe, inserts at the lateral malleolus, travels obliquely up toward the head, inserts at the lateral aspect of the knee, then goes down again along the lateral aspect of the leg. One branch descends to and inserts in the middle of the calf, then goes up to the medial aspect of the popliteal fossa. The two branches ascend together to the posterior aspect of the thigh.

Leg Lesser Yin

This channel sinew runs parallel to the primary channel.

Leg Lesser Yang

This channel sinew starts at the fourth toe, inserts at the lateral malleolus, ascends along the lateral aspect of the leg, and inserts at the lateral border of the knee. Another branch emerges above the lateral condyle of the femur, travels up and anteriorly in an oblique fashion, and inserts anteriorly above ST-32 (fu tu).

Leg Terminal Yin

This channel sinew attaches at the knee, at the head of the tibia, and ascends along the medial aspect of the thigh.

Channel Divergences

Leg Greater Yang Channel Divergence

This channel divergence separates from the leg greater yang primary channel at the popliteal fossa, and proceeds up the thigh.

Leg Lesser Yin Channel Divergence

This channel divergence separates from the leg lesser yin primary channel behind the knee, ascends, and then crosses the leg greater yang channel divergence.

Collaterals

Leg Yang Brightness Collateral

This collateral diverges from ST-40 (feng long) and meets the leg greater yin channel. One branch travels along the lateral aspect of the leg and knee, and goes toward the head.

Leg Greater Yin, Leg Terminal Yin and Leg Lesser Yin Collaterals

These three collaterals follow their primary channels' pathways in the medial aspect of the knee.

Curious Vessels

Penetrating Vessel

The complex pathway of the Penetrating vessel includes a branch that emerges at ST-30 (qi chong), follows the medial aspect of the thigh, enters the popliteal fossa, and descends the medial aspect of the tibia toward the sole of the foot.

Yang Heel Vessel

This vessel starts below the lateral malleolus at BL-62 (shen mai) and travels along the lateral aspect of the lower limb and knee.

Yin Heel Vessel

This vessel starts below the medial malleolus at KI-6 (zhao hai) and travels up the medial aspect of the lower limb and knee.

Yang Linking Vessel

This vessel starts at BL-63 (jin men) and ascends the lateral aspect of the leg, knee and thigh.

Yin Linking Vessel

This vessel starts at KI-9 (zhu bin) and travels up along the medial aspect of the leg, knee and thigh.

KNEE AND LOCAL CIRCULATION OF QI

The knee joint represents communication between humans and the external world. It works as a barrier regulating the exchange of Qi between the leg and thigh. As we have seen before, there are both inward and outward movements of yin and yang Qi between the trunk and lower limbs.

Thus, for exchanges between the trunk and the lower limbs, the yang Qi that emerges from the trunk is:

• most characteristic of its origin (greater yang) at the hip
• intermediate (lesser yang) at the knee
• least characteristic of its origin (yang brightness) at the ankle

The yang Qi that enters the trunk is:

• most characteristic of its origin (greater yang) at the ankle

- intermediate (lesser yang) at the knee
- least characteristic of its origin (yang brightness) at the hip.

Similarly, the yin Qi that emerges from the trunk is:

- greater yin at the hip
- lesser yin at the knee
- terminal yin at the ankle.

The yin Qi that enters the trunk is:

- greater yin at the ankle
- lesser yin at the knee
- terminal yin at the hip.

The knee, as a place of exchange of Qi, is therefore qualified as lesser yang or lesser yin according to which point of reference is used.

Diagnosis of Knee Pain

LOCAL CAUSES

Local Disruption of Qi Circulation

Under certain circumstances the knee joint, the physiological barrier to the exchange of Qi between the thigh and leg, may pathologically obstruct such exchange. If it impairs the circulation of yang from the thigh to the leg, there is pain in the knee due to yang deficiency. This type of pain is aggravated by movement, and improved by the topical application of warmth and supporting bandages. Needling the barrier point on the lesser yang channel, GB-33 *(xi yang guan)*, which promotes the downward movement of the yang, brings instant relief from the pain. Its action can be reinforced by needling ST-37 *(shang ju xu)*.

If, on the other hand, yin circulation from the leg to the thigh is obstructed, there will be pain in the knee due to yin deficiency, which often predominates in the medial aspect. It may be accompanied by an underlying painful noninfectious cellulitis, which indicates local accumulation of yin. Needling the cleft point KI-5 *(shui quan)* on the lesser yin channel should be combined with LR-7 *(xi guan)*. Both of these points restore circulation of yin Qi through the knee and alleviate the pain.

When there is knee pain caused by local disruption in the circulation of Qi, it is often useful to combine GB-33 *(xi yang guan)* and LR-7 *(xi guan)* for their synergistic effects.

Local Qi Stagnation

In this case, the knee pain appears upon initiation of movement, and abates after getting started. It is also improved by the topical application of warmth, and by massage. The pain is alleviated by needling the Wind point GB-31 *(feng shi)*, which promotes the circulation of Qi in the lower limb.

Channel Sinews

The channel sinews in the lower limb all bear a close relationship with the knee. We must therefore suspect their involvement in any case of knee pain of rather recent origin along a linear pathway matching one of their channels. We must also consider them for pain that does not correspond to the local analysis of the eight parameters.

Tendinitis of the pes anserinus, for example, suggests involvement of the leg greater yin channel sinew. Its treatment consists of needling the well point SP-1 *(yin bai)*, the river point SP-5 *(shang qiu)*, the muscle insertion points above and below the painful area, and performing local sedation with the plum-blossom needle.

If the origin is not traumatic, but related to a local invasion of Damp-Cold, we should also tonify the primary channel at SP-2 *(da du)*, and prevent the pathogenic Qi from spreading to the other channel sinews by needling the crossing point CV-2 *(qu gu)*.

Tendinitis of the patella affects the leg yang brightness channel sinew, and is treated according to the same therapeutic principles.

Tendinitis of the biceps femoris is felt as spontaneous pain in the lateral aspect of the knee, primarily during rotation. It is treated by stimulating the leg lesser yang channel sinew.

A popliteal cyst that impairs the motion or causes pain in the posterior aspect of the knee, or impairs flexion of the knee, indicates a disruption of the leg greater yang channel sinew.

Painful Knee in Children

A traction apophysitis of the tibial tuberosity (Osgood-Schlatter disease) manifests in children between the ages of 10 and 15, usually after engaging in strenuous athletic activities. Treating the leg lesser yang or leg yang brightness channel sinews speeds up the healing process, but even better results are achieved when stimulating the yang Heel vessel. The most important point is BL-61 *(pu shen)*, which, according to J.-M. Kespi, governs the foot gate, that is, the first stage in a person's growth.

REGIONAL CAUSES

Obstruction of the Lesser Yang Level

Yang excess in the lower limb may be due to an obstruction at the lesser yang level in its "hinge of the yang" function. After prolonged physical effort, pain and contraction manifest in the knee. Needling GB-32 *(zhong du)* brings definite improvement. According to J.-M. Kespi, this point governs the free flowing of the yang in the lower limb.

Foot Problems

Pain in the knee should motivate the practitioner to look systematically for a postural imbalance due to a problem with the foot. The examination should include that for such problems as pes planus and pes cavus. This finding suggests a disruption of the yin and yang Heel vessels, which must be confirmed by associated signs and significant morning stiffness.

Hip Problems

Any unexplained knee pain should lead to a systematic examination of the coxofemoral joint. If the cause is Wind-Damp-Cold painful obstruction of the hip affecting the knee, the general treatment will be greatly enhanced by deeply needling GB-30 *(huan tiao)*, which promotes the movement of yang Qi in the lower limb. According to *Great Compendium of Acupuncture and Moxibustion (Zhen jiu da cheng)*, this point is indicated for Wind-Damp rheumatism, lower back pain with pain in the hip, and pain in the knee with difficulty in extending or flexing the knee.

Sometimes radicular pains are only experienced on one part of a nerve's trajectory. For this reason, hip problems affecting the femoral nerve may manifest only as an isolated pain in the knee. From an energetic point of view, many of these pains correspond to an obstruction preventing the lower limb yang from entering the trunk. Common signs may include yang excess-type pain in the hip, thigh and knee accompanied by yang deficiency-type dull pain in the lumbar region. This symptomatology disappears after needling the barrier point governing the movement of the yang from the lower limb to the trunk, ST-31 *(bi guan)*. This diagnosis demands that we look in all cases for a pelvic yin excess which obstructs the entry of the lower limb yang. When this excess is due to energetic phenomena, it recedes when CV-4 *(guan yuan)* is needled. The organic excess (uterine fibroma, prostatic hypertrophy) requires specific treatment.

Another type of problem is due to an obstruction that prevents the lower limb yin Qi from entering the trunk. This pattern causes pain in the medial aspect of the thigh, suggesting an obturator neuralgia. In addition, there is pain in the medial aspect of the knee due to yin excess with contracture of the thigh adductors. Only LR-11 *(yin lian)*, the barrier point governing the movement of the yin Qi from the lower limb to the trunk, can alleviate this pain.

Circulatory Factors

Although disruption of venous circulation does not lead to a diagnosis of painful knee, it is an aggravating factor that should systematically be identified. It should be treated by needling BL-56 *(cheng jin)*. This point governs the yang that circulates the Blood from the bottom to the top of the body, the venous blood circulation. In our opinion, this point is more useful for this indication than is ST-32 *(fu tu)*, the meeting point of the veins, particularly because, according to *Great Compendium of Acupuncture and Moxibustion*, BL-56 *(cheng jin)* is indicated for painful obstruction of the leg.

GENERAL CAUSES

Primary Channels or Axes

In order to diagnose the involvement of a primary channel in the genesis of knee pain, the following general signs must be present.

Leg Yang Brightness

According to chapter 10 of *Divine Pivot*, all conditions pertaining to the bones of the leg are related to this channel. Among the problems associated with this channel are swollen and painful knee, pain in the chest, groin, the anterior thigh, the lateral aspect of the leg and on the dorsum of the foot. The two middle toes may also be difficult to move.

Leg Greater Yin

There is a cold sensation in the medial aspect of the knee. According to chapter 10 of *Divine Pivot*, when this channel is affected the standing posture is difficult to maintain because it causes swelling and pain in the medial aspect of the thigh and knee. The big toe may also be difficult to move.

Leg Greater Yang

There is pain in the thigh, popliteal fossa, calf and foot. According to chapter 10 of *Divine Pivot*, the hips cannot flex, the popliteal fossa feels knotted up, and there is a shearing pain in the calf. All calf disorders are related to this channel.z

Leg Lesser Yin

The posterior aspect of the lower limb is painful. All bone disorders are related to this channel through its connection with the Kidneys.

Leg Lesser Yang

There is pain in the hip, knee and the lateral aspect of the lower limb. According to *Divine Pivot*, all bone diseases are related to this channel. In addition, there is pain in the side of the thorax, hip, lateral aspect of the knee, leg and lateral malleolus. The joints are painful, and the fourth toe is difficult to move.

Leg Terminal Yin

Classically, the symptoms related to pathogenic Qi entering the Liver are deep pain in both sides of the body, and a deep cold sensation. Movement of the joints is impaired when walking, and the lower limbs are sometimes swollen.

In all cases it is essential to differentiate between an invasion by pathogenic influences of the channels and a pathology of their corresponding Organs. We shall not review here all the different clinical signs used to establish the appropriate diagnosis, as they are abundantly described in the reference books listed in the bibliography. Treatment of the primary channels has already been discussed above.

On closer inspection, a disorder of the primary channels may reveal an imbalance in an axis. In this case, the symptomatology manifests both in the arm and leg channels. A passage in chapter 5 of *Divine Pivot* observes that the greater yang serves as an opening, the yang brightness serves as a closing, and the lesser yang serves as the hinge or pivot. If the opening fails, the flesh and joints waste away, and disease settles in abruptly.

The same passage goes on to say that failure of the hinge/pivot means a shaking of the bones (*gŭ yáo*), and the inability to maintain an upright position. That is why we needle the lesser yang axis for laxity of the joints, while monitoring excesses and deficiencies. Shaking of the bones means laxity of the joints and immobility. It results from a loosening. We must try to identify its origin. Treatment of the axis may be done by using the root and termination technique, or the stream point-connecting point combination.

If a primary channel affliction indicates a disruption in the synchronization between man and macrocosm, the pain in the knee is sharp, the onset is sudden, but the local clinical examination is negative. It may be part of a historical pattern that resolves itself as suddenly as it appears. The treatment principle is to needle the well point on the affected channel, and the connecting point on three channels—the same channel contralaterally, the exterior-interior related channel ipsilaterally, and the midday-midnight channel ipsilaterally.

Treatment of the root cause involves regulating the disrupted phase and ensuring prevention, by using the transport points in relation to their opening and closing, according to the Stem and Branch system.

Curious Vessels

Yin and Yang Heel Vessels

Among the symptomatology of the yin and yang Heel vessels are pain in the knee with morning stiffness and sleep disorders. A lack of grounding, of a feeling of belonging or integration in a community, or rejecting it, are all factors that further disrupt the function of these vessels. These can be summarized as problems relating to support.

Restoring the free circulation of Qi in these vessels is achieved by needling their confluent and cleft points, KI-6 (*zhao hai*) and KI-8 (*jiao xin*) for the yin Heel vessel, and BL-62 (*shen mai*) and BL-59 (*fu yang*) for the yang Heel vessel. The paired confluent points may also be added, LU-7 (*lie que*) and SI-3 (*hou xi*) respectively.

Yang Linking Vessel

Knee pain related to the yang Linking vessel usually fits within a polyarticular syndrome, which is characterized by sensitivity to changes in the weather. This is usually but one element in a general state of sensitivity which manifests on an emotional and psychological level. A feverish sensation during these painful crises is not rare.

Regulation of this vessel is achieved by needling the confluent point TB-5 (*wai guan*), the cleft point GB-35 (*yang jiao*) and the paired confluent point GB-41 (*zu lin qi*).

Girdle Vessel

This vessel, related to the lesser yang axis, facilitates the mobilization of yin which has stagnated in the lower portion of the body. Its involvement should be suspected where there is pain in the lower limbs which is aggravated upon getting started, and by cold, and is ameliorated by movement and warmth. It is accompanied by belt-like lower back pain radiating down to the medial aspect of the thigh, together with laxity and weakness of the ankles. In women, dysmenorrhea and leukorrhea are revealing symptoms.

The treatment principle is to needle GB-26 (dai mai), the confluent point GB-41 (zu lin qi) and the paired confluent point TB-5 (wai guan).

Penetrating Vessel

This vessel is likely to be involved when the pain is predominantly in the medial aspect of the knee. Other manifestations include cold feet and legs, Blood stasis-induced lower back pain, gastralgia and dyspepsia, and marked genital and gynecological pathology.

The treatment consists of needling the confluent point SP-4 (gong sun), ST-30 (qi chong) or CV-4 (guan yuan), and ST-36 (zu san li).

Yin Linking Vessel

Headaches, stabbing precordial pain and frequent bouts of anger suggest a possible involvement of the yin Linking vessel, which travels up the medial aspect of the knee. Regulation of this vessel is achieved by needling the confluent point PC-6 (nei guan), the cleft point KI-9 (zhu bin) and the paired confluent point SP-4 (gong sun).

Painful Obstruction

The knee is one of the preferred locations for painful obstruction, the most frequent cause of knee pain, since it partially covers degenerative joint disease and arthritis. Painful obstruction is often the diagnosis for chronic knee pain which cannot be diagnosed by local application of the eight parameters. This condition follows the invasion of pathogenic Wind, Cold and Dampness, promoted by a deficiency of protective Qi. An underlying disruption in one of the Five Phases explains the dominant location of the pathology in the bones, sinews or muscles. General analysis and treatment principles are similar to those described in chapter 8, with certain particular features in cases of localized pain in the knee.

One of the possible treatment approaches consists of:

- eliminating the pathogenic influences by needling the river and stream points on the foot yin channels, and the sea points on the leg yang channels
- using warm needle technique at M-LE-27 (he ding) in the middle of the superior border of the patella, and ST-35 (du bi) and M-LE-16 (xi yan), both "eyes" of the knee on either side of the lower border of the patella
- tonifying the protective Qi and Kidney Qi by stimulating CV-7 (yin jiao), CV-12 (zhong wan) and BL-23 (shen shu)
- regulating the disrupted phase by stimulating the corresponding channel that has more Blood than Qi. The pertinent characteristics of these phases are as follows:

Water phase: bone disorders, hair loss, hearing loss, urinary dysfunction, lower back pain. Treatment is by the transport points on the leg greater yang channel in accordance with their physiological functions, BL-60 (kun lun) and BL-64 (jing gu). For action on the bone structure, treat BL-11 (da zhu), CV-3 (zhong ji) or GB-39 (xuan zhong).

Wood phase: disorders affecting the sinews, cramps, vision disorders, brittle nails, hepatobiliary disorders, difficulty in getting started. Treatment is by the transport points on the leg terminal yin channel, LR-2 (xing jian) and LR-3 (tai chong). For action on the sinew structure, treat GB-34 (yang ling quan).

Earth phase: disorders affecting the muscles, distention, diarrhea, dry lips, obsessive tendencies. Treatment is by the transport points on the leg yang brightness channel, ST-41 (jie xi) and ST-45 (li dui). For action on the muscular structure, treat BL-57 (cheng shan).

Organ Pathology

Two Organs are especially involved in knee pathologies: the Liver, which governs the sinews, and the Kidneys, which govern the bone and marrow. The Spleen may also be involved.

Kidneys

Classically, it is said that when the Kidney Essence is deficient, the marrow and bone are no longer nourished. This leads to weakness in the legs and knees, stiffness, and a weak lower back. This disorder is aggravated by exertion and improves with rest, and there are frequent relapses. This occurs mostly in older patients and in cases of constitutional or acquired deficiencies, particularly after a prolonged illness.

If yang deficiency predominates, the extremities are cold, the face is pale, sexual drive diminishes, the tongue is pale, and the pulse is submerged and thin. If yin deficiency predominates, there is a feeling of worry, insomnia, tinnitus, vertigo, dizziness, poor memory, dry mouth and throat, hot flashes, heat sensations in the palms of the hands and soles of the feet, and night sweats. The tongue is red, and the pulse is wiry, thin and rapid. This yin deficiency leads to a depletion of Fluids, causing the yang to flare up, which explains the symptomatology.

In cases of Kidney yang deficiency, we should tonify by using moxibustion at BL-23 *(shen shu)*, GV-4 *(ming men)*, CV-6 *(qi hai)*, GB-39 *(xuan zhong)* and ST-36 *(zu san li)*. For Kidney yin deficiency, tonify BL-23 *(shen shu)*, BL-52 *(zhi shi)*, KI-3 *(tai xi)* and CV-4 *(guan yuan)*.

Liver

Involvement of the Liver is suspected when there are signs of pain in the ligamentous structures, hypermobility of the knee with a sensation of instability, and the sinews are fragile. The Liver governs the sinews, and their trophic state is governed by Liver Blood.

If there is Liver yin deficiency, the weakness in the legs and knees is accompanied by lower back stiffness, cramps, brittle nails, insomnia, vivid dreams, excessive irritability, headaches, vertigo, palpitations, or other symptoms related to a blazing up of Liver yang which a deficient yin can no longer contain.

If there is Liver Qi stagnation, the patient is tense and irritable, complains of pain in the flanks and lower back, standing up is difficult, the abdomen is distended, the tongue is red, the coating is thin, and the pulse is wiry.

For Liver yin deficiency, nourish the Liver Blood, and possibly sedate the Liver yang, by needling BL-18 *(gan shu)*, LR-2 *(xing jian)*, LR-3 *(tai chong)*, GB-34 *(yang ling quan)* and SP-10 *(xue hai)*. If there is Liver Qi stagnation, promote the circulation of Qi by needling BL-18 *(gan shu)*, LR-6 *(zhong du)* and GB-34 *(yang ling quan)*.

Spleen

The function of the Spleen is to transform and transport the food essence in order to create and nourish the muscles and flesh. Disruption of this process is described in the following passage from chapter 29 of *Basic Questions*:

> The limbs all receive Qi from the Stomach. However, it does not directly go to the channels, but must first go through the Spleen and only then can they get nourishment. Now, if the

Spleen is ill, it cannot circulate the Fluids from the Stomach, and the limbs are unable to get the Qi of liquids and grains. Their Qi becomes weaker every day and the pulse pathways close down. The sinews, bones, muscles and flesh are all without Qi to generate their vitality, and become useless.

In this case, the knee pathology belongs to a more complex pattern which, besides its bilateral aspect and its extension to the whole limb, must be accompanied by other Spleen-related symptoms such as asthenia, obsessive tendencies, heaviness in the body, diarrhea or loose stools, turban-type headaches, lack of appetite, a swollen and tooth-marked tongue, and a frail and moderate pulse.

Tonification of the Spleen can be achieved by needling BL-20 *(pi shu)*, KI-17 *(shang qu)*, SP-3 *(tai bai)*, ST-36 *(zu san li)* and SP-9 *(yin ling quan)*, which has a particular action on the Fluids.

Knee and Fluids

Knee pathology may be part of a broader pattern of disruption of Fluid metabolism, and more particularly the *yè* portion of the Fluids. When this is the case, the mechanisms of pathogenesis and the ensuing treatment principles are to be found in the Organs involved in Fluid metabolism: the Spleen, Kidneys and Lungs.

Bone Structure

The knee may be involved in a primary affliction of the bone structure, which is governed by BL-11 *(da zhu)*. This is the meeting point for the bones, the name of which means "great shuttle." This point governs the body's structure, its framework, as represented by the bones. The point is needled to strengthen our being, whether from a mental or physical perspective (J.-M. Kespi).

According to *Great Compendium of Acupuncture and Moxibustion*, the symptomatology is as follows: pain in the knee with difficulty in bending that joint, lower back and spinal pain, and a stiff neck with difficulty bending forward and backward.

Support Problems

Any joint pathology, as any somatic localization, may be the physical manifestation of an improper integration of our being with our environment. Thus an unaccountable pain in the knee suggests a support problem in an individual who does not feel supported in their life, accompanied by the typical procession of associated functional signs. In our experience, CV-5 *(shi men)* ("stone gate") is the point that promotes the resolution of the symptomatology associated with this condition. We first came upon this by looking for the symbolism in the name of the point. Stone and rock form the foundation and the base of any building. This point, located in the pelvis, which is the foundation of the trunk and the base of an individual, has a similar function. This interpretation has been borne out over and over again in practice.

Along the same lines, knee pain may indicate Kidney deficiency, the Kidneys being the Organ which represents our strength, power and sturdiness, and also expresses the whole creative potential of our being. KI-14 *(si man)* and BL-23 *(shen shu)* are treated to engage the Kidneys in their creative function.

Gestural Dysfunctions

The joints support gestural expression, which is controlled in its overall function by ST-38 *(tiao kou)*, whereas ST-35 *(du bi)* governs the knee in its specific function. The latter is to be needled in cases of joint motility pathology when it symbolizes a dysfunction in expression. This expression can take different forms. Many traditions regard the knee as the seat of the body's force, as well as the symbol of authority and social power. For example, to bend one's knee is an act of humility, while making another bend their knee is to impose your will upon them.

Overlapping Factors

Chronic knee pain should always cause the practitioner to suspect a number of overlapping and intertwining factors, all of which should be analyzed in order to arrive at an appropriate treatment plan. For example, in a given patient the following factors could all signal support problems: Kidney deficiency, Damp-Cold pathogenic influence, or local barrier obstruction.

Trigger Points

ADDUCTOR LONGUS MUSCLE

Referred Pain

Pain in the anteromedial aspect of the thigh and leg, and in the medial aspect of the knee. The pathway of the pain may suggest a more generalized leg problem (FIG. 22-1).

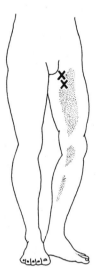

Fig. 22-1
Trigger Point for the Adductor Longus Muscle

Trigger Point

This point is located in the area of LR-11 *(yin lian)* and LR-10 *(zu wu li)*.

VASTUS MEDIALIS MUSCLE

Referred Pain

Pain in the anterior inferomedial aspect of the thigh, and in the medial aspect of the knee (FIG. 22-2).

Trigger Point

This point is located in the area of LR-9 *(yin bao)*.

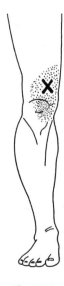

Fig. 22-2
Trigger Point for the Vastus Medialis Muscle

Biceps Femoris Muscle

Referred Pain

Pain in the popliteal fossa, radiating down the posterior aspect of the leg (FIG. 22-3).

Trigger Point

This point is located in the lower third of a line joining BL-37 *(yin men)* and BL-40 *(wei zhong)*.

Rectus Femoris Muscle

Referred Pain

Pain in the anterior aspect of the thigh and knee (FIG. 22-4).

Trigger Point

This point is located in the area of N-LE-23 *(mai bu)*.[1]

Chapter Notes

1. This point is located at the lateral margin of the rectus femoris muscle and the vastus lateralis muscle, about 3 units below ST-31 *(bi guan)*.

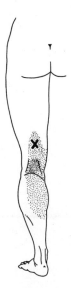

Fig. 22-3
Trigger Point for the Biceps Femoris Muscle

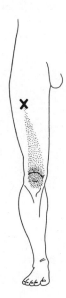

Fig. 22-4
Trigger Point for the Rectus Femoris Muscle

CHAPTER TWENTY-THREE

Foot Pain

Energetic Aspects of Foot

RELATIONSHIPS WITH CHANNEL SYSTEM

Primary Channels

Leg Yang Brightness (Stomach) Channel

The channel travels along the anterolateral border of the tibia down to the dorsum of the foot and in the second interdigital space, ending at the lateral corner of the second toenail at ST-45 *(li dui)*. A secondary branch emerges from ST-36 *(zu san li)* and descends to the tip of the third toe. Another branch separates from the dorsum of the foot and ends at the lateral corner of the big toenail.

Leg Greater Yin (Spleen) Channel

The channel starts at the medial corner of the big toenail at SP-1 *(yin bai)*, travels along the medial aspect of the foot, goes in front of the medial malleolus, and then ascends along the medial aspect of the tibia.

Leg Greater Yang (Bladder) Channel

In its descending pathway, the channel goes through the calf muscles, emerges behind the lateral malleolus, follows the fifth metatarsal and the fifth toe, and ends at the lateral corner of the fifth toenail at BL-67 *(zhi yin)*.

Leg Lesser Yin (Kidney) Channel

The channel starts under the fifth toe, goes to the middle of the sole of the foot at KI-1 *(yong quan)*, travels under the navicular tuberosity at KI-2 *(ran gu)*, goes behind the medial malleolus and spreads in the heel, and then ascends along the medial aspect of the lower limb.

Leg Lesser Yang (Gallbladder) Channel

The channel descends from the lateral aspect of the lower limb to the front of the lateral malleolus, and follows the dorsum of the foot to the lateral corner of the fourth toenail at GB-44 *(zu qiao yin)*. Another branch emerges from the dorsum of the foot at GB-41 *(zu lin qi)*, goes to the first intermetatarsal space, and ends at the medial corner of the big toenail at LR-1 *(da dun)*.

Leg Terminal Yin (Liver) Channel

The channel originates at LR-1 *(da dun)* at the medial corner of the big toenail, travels up the dorsum of the foot, passes one unit in front of the medial malleolus, and ascends along the medial aspect of the lower limb.

Channel Sinews

All the channel sinews follow a centripetal movement and start at the well points. The three yang lower limb channel sinews meet in the vicinity of GB-22 *(yuan ye)*, and the three yin lower limb channel sinews meet near CV-2 *(qu gu)*.

Leg Greater Yang

The leg greater yang channel sinew has a more complex pathway in the foot than that of the primary channel. It originates at the small toe, attaches at the lateral malleolus, travels obliquely toward the hip, and inserts at the lateral aspect of the knee. It then descends along the lateral aspect of the leg, attaches at the heel and at the lateral aspect of the foot, ascends from the heel, and attaches at the lateral aspect of the popliteal fossa.

Leg Yang Brightness

The channel sinew originates at the second, third and fourth toes, attaches at the instep, and then splits into two main branches.

The leg lesser yang channel sinew, as well as those of the yin channels, have pathways similar to their primary channels at the level of the foot.

Curious Vessels

The Curious vessels can be divided into two groups. One group originates in the area between, anterior and inferior to the Kidneys, and is governed by the gate of vitality (mìng mén). The other group originates at the foot. Both the Kidneys and the foot are shaped like seeds or embryos, and are related to procreative functions.

According to J.-M. Kespi, the group of Curious vessels originating at the foot (yin and yang Heel vessels, yin and yang Linking vessels) corresponds to the original creative influences of heaven (yang) and earth (yin).

The Linking vessels have a relationship with heaven, as indicated by their Chinese name which means "the main rope of a net" or the "linking cord" to which everything is connected. The Heel or "grounding" vessels correspond to earth, from whence life springs. Thus the celestial Linking vessels govern space, while the terrestrial Heel vessels govern time. In addition, the Linking vessels harmonize the yin and the yang, and the Heel vessels promote the return of the yang into the yin and the exit of the yin toward the yang.

Yang Heel Vessel

The vessel starts below the lateral malleolus at BL-62 (shen mai) on the leg greater yang channel, reaches BL-61 (pu shen), the foot gate, travels behind the malleolus, and then ascends along the lateral aspect of the lower limb.

Yin Heel Vessel

The vessel originates at KI-6 (zhao hai) on the leg lesser yin channel below the medial malleolus, and then ascends along the medial aspect of the lower limb.

Yang Linking Vessel

The vessel begins at the crossing point of the three yang channels. Its Qi emerges at BL-63 (jin men) on the leg greater yang channel, and then ascends along the lateral aspect of the lower limb.

Yin Linking Vessel

The vessel originates at the crossing point of the three yin channels.

Penetrating Vessel

This Curious vessel has five branches, one of which extends to the back of the medial malleolus and travels to the sole of the foot, while another reaches the dorsum of the foot and spreads into the big toe.

Collaterals

Leg Lesser Yang Collateral

The collateral starts at GB-37 (guang ming), five units above the lateral malleolus, connects with the leg terminal yin channel, and spreads into the dorsum of the foot. Along with the arm greater yin collateral, it is the only collateral to reach the distal extremity of a limb. It governs the foot in its function of contact and exchange with the outside world.

Leg Greater Yin Collateral

The collateral emerges at SP-4 (gong sun), one unit behind the big toe joint, and connects with the leg yang brightness channel. Another branch penetrates the abdomen to connect with the Intestines and Stomach.

Leg Lesser Yin Collateral

The collateral starts at KI-4 (da zhong) behind the medial malleolus and goes around the heel to connect with the leg greater yang channel. Another branch ascends with the primary channel to the Pericardium and penetrates in the lumbar aspect of the spine.

Channel Divergences

The leg terminal yin is the only channel divergence to have a pathway that connects with the foot. It diverges from the dorsum of the foot, ascends along the medial aspect of the lower limb, and continues upward to the face.

LOCAL CIRCULATION OF QI

Through its transport points, the foot is a place of exchange between human Qi and universal Qi. This is particularly true when viewed through the system of Stems and Branches which promotes the synchronization of the human microcosm with the universal macrocosm.

From the perspective of the local circulation of the yin or yang Qi from the foot toward the trunk, the foot is regarded as greater yin or greater yang respectively, and is governed by SP-8 *(di ji)* or BL-63 *(jin men)*, the cleft points of the leg greater yin and greater yang channels. Conversely, as far as the circulation of yin or yang Qi outward toward the foot is concerned, the foot is regarded as terminal yin and governed by LR-6 *(zhong du)*, or yang brightness and governed by ST-37 *(shang ju xu)*.

THE FOOT AND ITS SYMBOLIC FUNCTIONS

The foot is primarily associated with walking, movement toward the outside world, from yin to yang, and as such constitutes one of our modes of communication.

In supporting the principle of the body in the walking mode, the foot is not only the symbol of grounding, but also of our inner strength in the sense that it supports the upright position which characterizes humans, but also our vulnerability, as in the myth of Achilles' heel, or the lame Hephaistos.

The feet are shaped like seeds, as are the Kidneys. This further illustrates the relationship between the two groups of Curious vessels which originate in the feet and Kidneys, and which participate in all human procreative functions. The name of the only primary acupuncture point which is in direct contact with the earth, KI-1 *(yong quan)* or "gushing spring," is highly significant.

Our first stage of growth, whether physical, mental or spiritual, is defined as the feet, as they are the first gate to open during adolescence. This function is governed by BL-61 *(pu shen)*. The foot establishes contact with the earth through manifestation. From a more practical point of view, it represents a certain sense of reality, as when we say that someone has their feet firmly planted on the ground.

The footsteps that we leave on the ground bear witness to the path, good or bad, that we choose according to our own free will. This explains the ritual washing of the feet, a rite of purification. Finally, the sexual connotation associated with the feet by psychoanalysts can be traced back to the Chinese custom of binding the feet.

The foot is regarded as a microcosm within itself, mapping the entire human body, which is the basis for foot acupuncture or foot reflexology. Although this representation falls outside the scope of our discussion, it serves to illustrate the importance of this anatomical region.

Foot Pathology

The purpose of this presentation is not to list all possible foot pathologies. Such a list would necessarily be incomplete and artificial, especially since a major portion of them fall within the scope of orthopedic treatment, rehabilitation or even surgery. Some foot pathologies are of a rheumatic nature, and others have more generalized effect.

POSTURAL IMBALANCE

Metatarsalgia Due to Postural Imbalance

These modifications affect the anterior arch of the foot which may be collapsed, leading to a frontal flat foot or, inversely, to a frontal rounded foot. The metatarsophalangeal joint of the second toe is most often affected. Collapse of the anterior arch promotes the formation of painful plantar calluses and bursitis. This type of problem can be isolated, or it can be associated with another postural disorder, such as pes cavus. It can also be involved in a syndrome, frequently observed in postmenopausal women, of general musculoligamentous weakness of the foot.

This symptomatology is the result of local yang deficiency. The yang needs to be brought down to this area by needling ST-37 *(shang ju xu)* or ST-39 *(xia ju xu)*. In addition, we should nourish the Penetrating vessel by tonifying the yang brightness channels, and harmonize the yang brightness and lesser yin channels by selecting a few points among the following: ST-30 *(qi chong)*, SP-4 *(gong sun)*, ST-41 *(jie xi)*, ST-42 *(chong yang)*, KI-1 *(yong quan)*, KI-3 *(tai xi)*.

Flat Foot (Pes Planus)

Postural functional valgus flat foot is primarily the consequence of a weakness in the musculoligamentous structures in charge of maintaining foot stability. Hypotonia of the tibialis posterior and peroneus longus muscles promotes the collapse of the medial arch.

Similarly, distention of the long plantar ligament plays a significant role. Flat foot is rarely painful. When it does become painful, it indicates decompensation of the deformation or the emergence of a complication.

Painful flat foot during adolescence coincides with a growth spurt, increased athletic activity, or a change of life style. The patient complains of pain in the medial mediotarsal region in the evening. Treated incorrectly or left untreated, this form of functional flat foot can progress more or less rapidly toward insensitivity. This is by far the most frequent outcome. Sometimes the postural imbalance decompensates more severely. This is the case in contracted flat foot. Contracted flat foot is accompanied by acute medial tarsalgia, limping, and reluctance to rest on the deformed foot. Clinical examination reveals a painful spot on the talonavicular line in the area of KI-6 *(zhao hai)*. If the patient receives appropriate treatment, this acute phase is resolved within a few weeks, but the foot remains vulnerable for several months. Refractory flat foot is a permanent pathogenic attitude which can create severe pain.

In addition to conventional treatment, it is possible to use acupuncture in order to tonify the leg lesser yin channel sinew, and possibly to tonify the Kidney yang. Needling KI-2 *(ran gu)*, which corresponds to the insertion of the tibialis posterior muscle, BL-63 *(jin men)*, which relates to the peroneus muscles, and GB-37 *(guang ming)*, which governs the foot, are essential additions, as well as needling the trigger points presented at the end of this chapter.

A flattening of the foot may occur after menopause, as part of the general slackening of the body's tone. Should this occur, it is also necessary to regulate the Penetrating vessel.

Pes Cavus

Pes cavus is defined as an accentuation of the concavity of the medial anteroposterior arch. Most of the time it is asymptomatic and becomes painful for reasons similar to those that make a flat foot painful. In this case, we can observe signs of local contracture at the level of the anterior tarsals, often accompanied by signs of mediotarsal and metatarsophalangeal joint pain, hyperkeratosis by compression under the metatarsal heads, and claw-foot. Acupuncture treatment follows the same principles as those for flat foot.

Deformation of the Frontal Part of the Foot

Abnormal Toes

Toes can be abnormal by their number or their length. These variations are not necessarily pathological, but can simply be anatomical variants. Still, they can sometimes lead to the emergence of abnormalities or deformations at or distant to the toes, and promote the early onset of a degenerative disease of the metatarsophalangeal joint. Regulation of the corresponding channel sinews, as well as needling the trigger points described below, may bring a reduction in the pain associated with these deformations.

Hallux Valgus

Hallux valgus is by far the most frequent deformation of the big toe. It is the source of pain associated with mechanical factors, synovial articular or periarticular reactions, degenerative disease of the metatarsophalangeal joint (sometimes involving the sesamoid bone), or a combination of all of these factors. There is no real medical treatment for hallux valgus, nor any other toe deformation. Surgery is not always a viable option.

Analysis of the pain according to the eight parameters often reveals local yin excess, which can be mobilized by needling KI-5 *(shui quan)* or ST-37 *(shang ju xu)*, combined with regulation of the leg greater yin channel by needling the cleft point SP-8 *(di ji)*. If there is local Damp-Heat excess, SP-3 *(tai bai)* is the most appropriate point. When the leg greater yin channel sinew is involved, we should needle the well point, SP-1 *(yin bai)*, and a tender point in the area of SP-4 *(gong sun)*.

As is the case for any degenerative disease at the root of a digit, hallux valgus may indicate disruption of the greater yin axis. This can be rebalanced by needling the origin point SP-1 *(yin bai)* and the termination point CV-12 *(zhong wan)* of the greater yin.

PERIARTICULAR CONDITIONS

In these conditions, the pathology affects tissues around the joints. Clinical and imaging examination will demonstrate that the joints themselves are basically normal.

Tendinitis

This disorder can occur in isolation or be encountered as part of a rheumatic disease.

Tendinitis of the Achilles Tendon

This disorder is treated by stimulation of the leg greater yang channel sinew.

Tendinitis of the Tibialis Anterior Muscle

This disorder is treated by stimulation of the leg yang brightness channel sinew. This is the same treatment as that for bursitis of the Achilles tendon.

Tendinitis of the Tibialis Posterior Muscle

This disorder is treated by stimulation of the leg greater yin channel sinew.

Tendinitis of the Peroneus Muscles

This disorder is treated by stimulation of the leg lesser yang channel sinew. When the condition is chronic or relapses frequently, or when there is sensitivity to changes in the weather, a yang Linking vessel disorder is indicated.

Tenosynovitis

This disorder is usually encountered within the context of rheumatic disease, and therefore of painful obstruction. For more information, see chapter 8.

Posterior and Plantar Heel Pain

These disorders are diagnosed in accordance with the local circulation of Qi. Most often this indicates a yin excess, eliminated by needling KI-5 *(shui quan)*. Acute crises may correspond to a yang excess which can be drained by needling BL-63 *(jin men)*.

The Shanghai College of Traditional Chinese Medicine (Roustan, 1979) recommends using BL-57 *(cheng shan)*, KI-3 *(tai xi)* and BL-60 *(kun lun)*.[1] If the leg lesser yin channel sinew is involved, needle the well point KI-1 *(yong quan)* and M-LE-5 *(shi mian)*.[2] It is important to identify systematically the involvement of one of the two Heel vessels, which can be regulated by needling BL-61 *(pu shen)* for the yang Heel vessel, and KI-2 *(ran gu)* and KI-8 *(jiao xin)* for the yin Heel vessel.

Tarsal Tunnel Syndrome

This condition is related to pain in the posterior tibial nerve trunk, or in its emerging branches in the tarsal tunnel. It presents dysesthesia-type symptomatology, which is aggravated by pressure. This suggests local yin excess, which is resolved by needling KI-5 *(shui quan)* and ST-37 *(shang ju xu)*. The yin Heel vessel is sometimes involved.

Nodular Plantar Fibromatosis or Ledderhose's Disease

This is the foot equivalent of Dupuytren's contracture in the hand (see chapter 20). If both conditions occur simultaneously, they must be interpreted as a disruption of the terminal yin. Peyronie's disease, a similar condition affecting the penis, is more likely to involve the Penetrating vessel. Locally, this condition corresponds to a local Cold yin excess due to yang insufficiency.

The treatment principle is to:

- attract the yang by needling the well points
- bring the yang down to the foot by needling the barrier point ST-37 *(shang ju xu)*
- disperse the local Cold by using moxa on the plantar nodules
- treat the flesh level by needling the stream and river points on the leg greater yin, as well as SP-3 *(tai bai)* and SP-5 *(shang qiu)*
- act on the point that governs the foot, GB-37 *(guang ming)*.

Plantar Neuralgia or Morton's Neuroma

This condition is the consequence of a local irritation process, of a mechanical nature, occurring not only on the intermetatarsal plantar nerve, but also on the associated arteries. In any case, the pain of Morton's neuroma is neuralgia-like: acute stabbing-type pain, electrical sensation, knife stabbing-type pain in the heart. This symptomatology is characteristic of a local yang excess, which can be mobilized by needling BL-63 *(jin men)*. Regulation of the yin Linking vessel is sometimes required.

PLANTALGIA DUE TO CHRONIC VENOUS INSUFFICIENCY

This condition is often found among obese menopausal women. The patient complains of a heavy or burning plantar pain, frequently associated with cramps, and nocturnal paresthesia with "restless legs." Clinical examination reveals edema of the entire foot reaching up to the ankle, which is also the location of a perimalleolar lipomatous infiltration. Besides varicose veins, the usual atrophic signs are also frequently encountered: stasis dermatitis, scars from ulcerated varicosities, and thinning of the skin above the ankles. From an energetic perspective, this condition corresponds to Blood stasis in the foot which is not mobilized by the yang.

The treatment principle is to bring the yang down to the foot by needling GB-39 *(xuan zhong)*, promote venous return by needling BL-56 *(cheng jin)*, and harmonize the terminal yin and the lesser yang by using the stream point-connecting point technique, LR-3 *(tai chong)* and GB-37 *(guang ming)*.

SPRAINED ANKLE

Acupuncture is the preferred treatment modality for uncomplicated sprains. The most frequently encountered sprains involve the lateral collateral ligament with its anterior branch (anterior talofibular ligament) corresponding to the leg lesser yang channel sinew, and its middle and posterior branches (calcaneofibular and posterior talofibular ligaments) corresponding to the leg greater yang channel sinew. On the other hand, the deltoid ligament corresponds to the leg lesser yin channel sinew. In any case, simple sprains are treated by stimulating the channel sinews. The presence of hematoma indicates an involvement of the corresponding primary channel, which can be treated by needling the river and cleft points.

Quoting from *Traité général de l'acupuncture*, Chamfrault states that in the case of protracted pain and swelling of the ankles, we must needle the two confluent points GB-41 *(zu lin qi)* and TB-5 *(wai guan)*, and then LR-2 *(xing jian)* and BL-62 *(shen mai)*. For swelling of the lateral malleolus, needle the two confluent points and then BL-60 *(kun lun)*, GB-40 *(qiu xu)* and KI-6 *(zhao hai)*. For pain and swelling of the medial malleolus, needle the two confluent points and then KI-3 *(tai xi)*, GB-40 *(qiu xu)* and BL-60 *(kun lun)*.

OSSEOUS AND ARTICULAR PATHOLOGIES

Osteodystrophy

Developmental problems with the epiphyses of the foot primarily involve the navicular and the second metatarsal head. Other locations are rarer. This condition occurs in children between the ages of 3 and 15. It progresses in a cyclical fashion and seems to be linked to ossification disorders. It manifests primarily as moderate, spontaneous pain which is aggravated by walking, with inconstant and partial limitation in the range of motion of the joint.

The circumstances in which they occur suggest, in our opinion, the involvement of the yin or yang Heel vessels, which need to be harmonized through the foot gate, governed by BL-61 *(pu shen)*. In any case, it is also essential to tonify the Kidneys.

Rheumatic Foot

Degenerative Joint Disease

Degenerative joint disease is one of the frequent complications of postural or post-traumatic disorders of the foot. It should be analyzed within the framework of painful obstruction. Within this framework, the M-LE-8 *(ba feng)* points have an interesting symptomatic effect.

Inflammatory Rheumatisms

Such diseases as rheumatoid arthritis, psoriatic arthritis and Reiter's syndrome belong to the traditional category of painful obstruction. For ankylosing spondylitis, posterior heel pain is a common complaint at the onset. This, in our opinion, is highly indicative of yang Heel vessel involvement. Infectious arthritis shall only be mentioned in passing, as it is our opinion that this problem should be treated with conventional medicine.

Bone Tumors

Bone tumors are never treatable by acupuncture. Their occurrence suggests that the bone, as a Curious Organ related to the Kidneys, has been affected.

MISCELLANEOUS CONDITIONS LEADING TO CHRONIC FOOT PAIN

Reflex Sympathetic Dystrophy of the Foot

Decalcifying reflex sympathetic dystrophy of the foot is a vasomotor and trophic painful syndrome. In approximately half the cases it follows local trauma or prolonged immobilization. Cases for which no cause is known in conventional medicine are numerous. In this condition, we always find a disruption of the local circulation of Qi, suggesting a barrier pathology with a two-stage progression. There is first yin stagnation, followed by yang excess (Heat). This explains the pseudoinflammatory condition caused by swelling and vasomotor disturbances along with slight bone loss, followed later by a retraction of the yin. This last stage is marked by such signs as atrophy of the subcutaneous tissues, wasting of the musculature, thickening of the joint capsules, and finally atrophic changes with severe demineralization of the bones.

Gout

This pathology is discussed in chapter 14.

Diabetic Arthropathy or Osteopathy

Diabetes is a condition that was recognized long ago by the Chinese. *Inner Classic* mentions this pathology under the name *xiāo kě*, which can be translated as "wasting and thirsting." It always indicates a disruption of the Fluids. The joint or bone complications of diabetes belong to the "wasting away of the lower burner" category, with Kidney yin deficiency and excess Fire.

Trigger Points

SOLEUS MUSCLE

Referred Pain

Pain in the heel climbing up the Achilles tendon (FIG. 23-1).

Trigger Point

This point is located in the area of N-LE-10 *(jiu wai fan)*[3] and BL-58 *(fei yang)*.

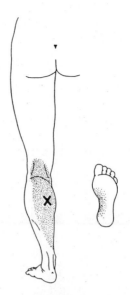

Fig. 23-2
Trigger Point for the Gastrocnemius Muscle

TIBIALIS ANTERIOR MUSCLE

Referred Pain

Pain in the big toe, instep, and the anterolateral aspect of the leg (FIG. 23-3).

Trigger Point

This point is located in the area of ST-36 *(zu san li)*.

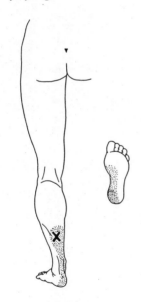

Fig. 23-1
Trigger Point for the Soleus Muscle

GASTROCNEMIUS MUSCLE

Referred Pain

Pain in the hollow of the arch of the foot radiating to the posteromedial aspect of the leg (FIG. 23-2).

Trigger Point

This point is located in the area of BL-56 *(cheng jin)*.

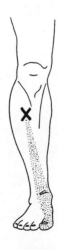

Fig. 23-3
Trigger Point for the Tibialis Anterior Muscle

EXTENSOR DIGITORUM LONGUS MUSCLE

Referred Pain

Pain in the toes, instep, and the anterolateral aspect of the leg (FIG. 23-4).

Trigger Point

This point is located in the area of N-LE-7 *(li wai).*[4]

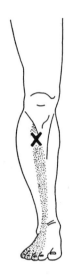

Fig. 23-4
Trigger Point for the Extensor Digitorum Longus Muscle

EXTENSOR DIGITORUM BREVIS MUSCLE

Referred Pain

Pain in the lateral border of the foot and in front of the lateral malleolus, following the leg lesser yang pathway (FIG. 23-5).

Trigger Point

This point is located in the area of GB-40 *(qiu xu).*

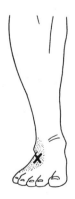

Fig. 23-5
Trigger Point for the Extensor Digitorum Brevis Muscle

PERONEUS LONGUS MUSCLE

Referred Pain

Pain in the lateral aspect of the leg and in the lateral malleolus, following the leg lesser yang pathway (FIG. 23-6).

Trigger Point

This point is located in the area of GB-34 *(yang ling quan).*

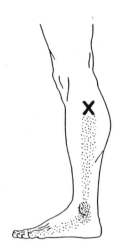

Fig. 23-6
Trigger Point for the Peroneus Longus Muscle

ABDUCTOR HALLUCIS LONGUS MUSCLE

Referred Pain

Pain in the big toe, and in the anterior and medial aspect of the sole of the foot (FIG. 23-7).

Trigger Point

This point is located in the area of KI-2 *(ran gu).*

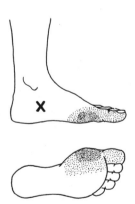

Fig. 23-7
Trigger Point for the Abductor Hallucis Longus Muscle

Chapter Notes

1. *Editors' note:* The English language edition of this book was translated by John O'Connor and Dan Bensky under the title *Acupuncture: A Comprehensive Text* (Chicago: Eastland Press, 1981). This information can be found on p. 663 of the English edition.

2. Located at the center of the plantar surface of the heel.

3. Located 1 unit medial to B-57 *(cheng shan)*.

4. Located 1 unit lateral to ST-36 *(zu san li)*.

PART FOUR

Classic Texts in
Traditional Chinese
Medicine

PART FOUR

Introduction

To our knowledge, there is no traditional Chinese medical treatise dedicated exclusively to rheumatology. This is so even though this branch of pathology is one of the few that was differentiated at the very beginning of Chinese medicine. Indeed, there is a description of rheumatism in *Basic Questions (Su wen)*, chapter 43 ("On Painful Obstruction"). This chapter has been referred to and commented on by other authors in other times. Chapter 41 of the same book is devoted to the use of acupuncture in the treatment of lower back pain. Among the different rheumatic conditions, this is the only disorder accorded the status of an individual clinical entity, probably because of the privileged relationship between the lower back and the Kidneys.

Our selection of chapters from the classics dealing with rheumatism is by no means exhaustive; rather, it represents what we feel is relevant. The Chinese have great respect for ancient authors, and because of this, the description of a problem in *Basic Questions* has remained the basic reference point for all later discussion. And while a great many authors have gone back and commented on how *Basic Questions* describes painful obstruction and lower back pain, few have shed new light on the subject or explored complementary developments. Those who did are the ones we have selected.

To begin our discussion, we will briefly place all of the texts in their historical perspective.

Note on Translation Style for Premodern Texts

Translation of premodern texts requires a slightly different style than that of contemporary works. In the main body of this book we have capitalized certain terms to distinguish traditional concepts from modern ones. For example, Heart refers to the traditional yin Organ; heart to the biomedical conception. However, in premodern texts there is only one idea of "heart," so capitalization is unnecessary. In addition, we have used as simple and literal a translation scheme as possible in order to convey the original flavor of these works.

Yellow Emperor's Inner Classic
(Huang di nei jing)

This is the oldest transmitted Chinese medical book. It was composed from medical manuscripts elaborated during the Warring States period (403-222 B.C.) and formalized under the Han dynasty (221 B.C.-220 A.D.) Its traditional attribution to the Yellow Emperor, Huang Di, the legendary founder of Chinese civilization, is actually without any historical validity. Presented as a dialogue between the emperor and his minister Qi Bo (among others), this exchange of questions and answers lays the foundation of Chinese medical thought.

This work, made up of 18 divisions (literally *juǎn* or rolls), is presented in two parts: *Basic Questions (Su wen)* and *Divine Pivot (Ling shu)*. *Basic Questions* establishes the foundation of medical theory, while *Divine Pivot* is devoted to the practice of acupuncture.

Today, the most widely used edition of *Basic Questions* is the one annotated by Wang Bing in 762, later amended by Lin Yi in the eleventh century.

For chapters 41 ("On Lower Back Pain") and 43 ("On Painful Obstruction") of *Basic Questions,* we have utilized the French translation by A. Husson (1973) as the basis of our work. This has been supplemented by modern Chinese editions. For chapter 27 ("Encompassing Painful Obstruction") of *Divine Pivot,* we translated from the original.

In *Basic Questions,* painful obstruction disorders are described in four chapters. They are presented in a particular order, which is generally followed in subsequent texts:

• Chapter 42, "On Wind," discusses conditions related to the invasion or generation of Wind in the body. This corresponds to such modern biomedical pathologies as cerebrovascular accident.
• Chapter 43, "On Painful Obstruction," corresponds to the modern biomedical concept of rheumatism.
• Chapter 44, "On Atrophy," describes pathologies dominated by paralysis and atrophy.
• Chapter 45, "On Inversion," is devoted to pathologies with syncope or sudden cold of the four limbs.

DISCUSSION OF COLD-INDUCED DISORDERS
(Shang han lun)

Discussion of Cold-induced Disorders and Miscellaneous Diseases (Shang han za bing lun) is a book composed of ten divisions written by Zhang Zhong-Jing (150–219), also known as the Chinese Hippocrates. It was partially destroyed during the period known as the Three Kingdoms (222–265). Reorganized by Wang Shu-He (210–285), author of *Pulse Classic (Mai jing)*, it was divided into two distinct treatises, *Discussion of Cold-induced Disorders (Shang han lun)* and *Essentials from the Golden Cabinet (Jin gui yao lue)*. The most widely used edition is that annotated by Cheng Wu-Ji in 1144.

Discussion of Cold-induced Disorders is an elaboration of chapter 31 of Basic Questions, "On Feverishness." It discusses febrile diseases due to invasion of pathogenic Cold, spreading inside in accordance with the *liù jīng* system, which is variously translated as Great Channel, Six Stages

or Six Warps. According to this system, the order of penetration is from greater yang to yang brightness, to lesser yang, to greater yin, to lesser yin, to terminal yin. Each of the six modalities of propagation of the pathogenic influence is presented with its corresponding pattern, diagnostic method, and herbal-based therapy.

Painful obstruction resulting from a febrile disease is described primarily as an aspect of a greater yang disorder. Our work is based on the translation by Catherine Despeux (1985).

ESSENTIALS FROM THE GOLDEN CABINET
(Jin gui yao lue)

This book, also reorganized by Wang Shu-He, is composed of six divisions and organized into three parts. The first part deals with febrile and epidemic diseases, the second with miscellaneous illnesses, and the third with gynecological disorders.

In this book, rheumatic pathology is linked to Wind diseases, and is not clearly distinguished from what we would consider neurological disorders. It is included in the generic term *lì jié bìng* (literally "diseases traversing the joints"), which is translated in English as panarthralgia.

SYSTEMATIC CLASSIC OF ACUPUNCTURE AND MOXIBUSTION
(Zhen jiu jia yi jing)

This book, written by Huang-Fu Mi (215–281), returns to *Basic Questions*, and more particularly *Divine Pivot*, which it enriches considerably. To this day, it is a major reference text for acupuncturists.

The author emphasizes the importance of Wind, Cold and Dampness in the genesis of rheumatism, and analyzes the symptomatology of each different clinical picture, its relation to the yin and yang Organs, and the therapeutic principles.

The information from this text that we use is related to chapter 27 of *Divine Pivot*, "Encompassing Painful Obstruction."

DISCUSSION OF THE ORIGINS OF SYMPTOMS OF DISEASE
(Zhu bing yuan hou lun)

This book by Chao Yuan-Fang, published in 610, is the first known Chinese medical treatise specializing in the study of disease etiology. It is composed of 50 divisions, further sudivided into 67 chapters and 1720 articles, in which are described the etiology, symptoms and mode of progression of each disease, as well as preventive therapeutic methods and physical and breathing exercises. Diseases are classified into four categories (external, internal, gynecological, pediatric) according to either their location or dominant symptom.

Rheumatic disorders are linked in this book to the pathogenic influences of Wind, Cold and Dampness.

CONFUCIANS' DUTIES TO THEIR PARENTS
(Ru men shi qin)

In this book written by Zhang Zi-He (also known as Zhang Cong-Zheng, 1156–1228), the author emphasizes the importance of the six external pernicious influences in the genesis of disease. These are to be eliminated by using diaphoretic, purgative and emetic therapeutic methods.

Zhang is highly critical of physicians who adopt a generalized attitude in their prescriptions, without paying enough attention to the specific pathogenic mechanisms of disease. Modeling his book after *Basic Questions*, painful obstruction is included in the same chapter with Wind, atrophy and inversion disorders.

INTRODUCTION TO MEDICINE
(Yi xue ru men)

The author Li Yan, also known as Li Zhai-Jian, was born in Nanfeng in Jiangxi province. A physician of the sixteenth century (the book was published in 1575), he summarized the prescriptions of his era in 18 categories. Writing about painful obstruction, Li emphasized the importance of Phlegm and Blood stasis in advanced cases, and analyzed the causative factors of paresthesia and numbness.

ESSENTIAL READINGS FOR THOSE IN THE MEDICAL LINEAGE
(Yi zong bi du)

Written by Li Zhong-Zi (also known as Li Shi-Cai), this book was published in 1637 and is composed of ten divisions. The first division is devoted to the sources and theory of traditional Chinese medicine, and presents several illustrations. The second division deals with the pulse and complexion. The third and fourth divisions discuss materia medica. Divisions five through ten focus on internal diseases and Cold-induced disorders, as well as the diagnosis and clinical presentation of 36 different types of illness. The subject of rheumatism is incorporated into an elaboration of chapter 43 of *Basic Questions*, which is devoted to painful obstruction.

PRECEPTS FOR PHYSICIANS
(Yi men fa lü)

In this book published in 1658, author Yu Chang explains the diagnostic and therapeutic principles of disease based on the totality of symptoms and clinical signs. He points out common mistakes, and suggests which practices are forbidden. For painful obstruction disorders, Yu emphasizes the fact that the pathogenic influences are located in the yin.

GREAT COMPENDIUM OF ACUPUNCTURE AND MOXIBUSTION
(Zhen jiu da cheng)

This book, composed of ten divisions, is the most complete work on acupuncture published to date. It is attributed to Yang Ji-Zhou (1522–1619) and was published in 1601. Joint pathology is mentioned frequently, accompanied by numerous therapeutic indications.

From this book we have elected to present portions which discuss the use of acupuncture in the treatment of painful obstruction disorders.

CHAPTER TWENTY-FOUR

Basic Questions (*Su wen*)

(C. 200 B.C.–100 A.D.)

"On Painful Obstruction"

(CHAPTER 43)

The Yellow Emperor stated, "How is painful obstruction generated?"

Qi Bo answered, "The three influences wind, cold and dampness arrive in various ways, intermingle and constitute painful obstruction. When the wind influence predominates it is moving painful obstruction; when the cold influence predominates it is severe painful obstruction; when the dampness influence predominates it is fixed painful obstruction."

The Yellow Emperor stated, "But are there not five of them?"

Qi Bo said, "The one that is encountered in winter is bone painful obstruction; that in spring, sinew painful obstruction; that in summer, vessel painful obstruction; that at the ultimate yin time,[1] flesh painful obstruction; and that in fall, skin painful obstruction."

The Yellow Emperor said, "When it settles inside the five yin and six yang organs, what qi causes it to be that way?"

Qi Bo stated, "The yin organs all have [some tissue] that they are associated with. When a disease stays for a long time and does not leave, it will settle in that with which it is associated. Thus, for bone painful obstruction that does not improve, if the person repeatedly contracts

pathogenic influences [the painful obstruction] will settle internally in the kidneys. For sinew painful obstruction that does not improve, if the person repeatedly contracts pathogenic influences [the painful obstruction] will settle internally in the liver. For vessel painful obstruction that does not improve, if the person repeatedly contracts pathogenic influences [the painful obstruction] will settle internally in the heart. For flesh painful obstruction that does not improve, if the person repeatedly contracts pathogenic influences [the painful obstruction] will settle internally in the spleen. For skin painful obstruction that does not improve, if the person repeatedly contracts pathogenic influences [the painful obstruction] will settle internally in the lungs. As for those things that are considered painful obstruction, each occurs when a person contracts wind, cold or dampness at its particular season.

"As for painful obstruction that resides in the five yin organs:

"Those with lung painful obstruction have irritability, fullness, panting and vomiting. In those with heart painful obstruction, the vessels fail to afford passage, there is irritability with epigastric throbbing, sudden, violent rising of qi causing panting, dryness of the throat with a tendency to sigh, and when inversion qi ascends there is fear. Those with liver painful obstruction are frightened when they go to bed at night, drink a lot, urinate frequently, and have an upward pulling sensation as if pregnant.

Those with kidney painful obstruction have a tendency toward bloating, and [the body is all huddled up] with the coccyx in the place of the heels and the back in the place of the head. Those with spleen painful obstruction have weak and tired limbs, expulsion of liquid during coughing fits, and chest congestion. Those with intestine painful obstruction have frequent craving for drinks which cannot be evacuated. The qi struggles inside, causing panting and sometimes urgent diarrhea. Those with gestation membrane[2] (bāo 胞) painful obstruction, in terms of their lower abdomen and bladder, when pressed there is pain inside like a spilling out of boiling water, roughness in regards to urination, and above have clear nasal discharge.

"When the yin qi is serene the [visceral] spirits are stored, when agitated they are lost. Overeating injures the intestines and the stomach. When the circulation of qi is improper and there is panting, painful obstruction will cluster in the lungs. When the circulation of qi is improper and there is sadness and preoccupation, painful obstruction will cluster in the heart. When the circulation of qi is improper and there is leakage of urine, painful obstruction will cluster in the kidneys. When the circulation of qi is improper and there is fatigue and exhaustion, painful obstruction will cluster in the liver. When the circulation of qi is improper and there is collapsed flesh, painful obstruction will cluster in the spleen. All painful obstruction that does not improve spreads internally. When wind predominates, the person will improve more easily."

The Yellow Emperor said, "Among cases of painful obstruction, there are fatal cases, cases of prolonged suffering, and cases in which a cure is easily obtained. Why is that?"

Qi Bo said, "Fatal cases are those in which it [the painful obstruction] enters the yin organs. Prolonged pain is due to cases in which it resides between the sinews and bones. When it resides in the skin, cure is easy to obtain."

The Emperor said, "And when it resides in the six yang organs?"

Qi Bo said, "Diet and the place of residence are the root cause of these diseases. Each of the six yang organs also has an associated point (shū 俞). If, while conditions of food and drink resonate with them, the wind, cold or damp qi penetrate into the associated point, [the pathogenic influences] will follow the associated point and enter, each settling into its respective yang organ."

The Yellow Emperor said, "How do you treat them with needles?"

Qi Bo said, "There are the stream points (shū 輸) for the yin organs, and the sea points (hé 合) for the yang organs. They are distributed along the course of the vessels. Each has the place where it manifests and each treats its [particular] transgression so that diseases can be healed."

The Emperor said, "Do the nutritive and protective qi also cause people to have painful obstruction?"

Qi Bo said, "The nutritive is the essential qi of food and drink. It harmonizes and is regulated by the yin organs, while permeating throughout the yang organs before it is able to enter into the vessels. Therefore it follows the course of the vessels above and below, passes through the five yin organs, and connects with the six yang organs. The protective is the qi of food and drink that has prowess; its qi is urgent, rapid, slippery and quick and cannot enter into the vessels, so it circulates between the skin and flesh divisions, fumes in the vitals membrane,[3] to spread through the thorax and abdomen. When the qi flows rebelliously there is disease; when the qi flows the way it should, there is recovery. As long as they are not mixed with wind, cold or dampness, there is no painful obstruction."

The Yellow Emperor said, "Good. Painful obstruction may be painful, may be not painful, may have numbness, or cold, or heat, or dryness, or dampness. What is the reason for this?"

Qi Bo said, "When it is painful, there is much cold qi. As there is cold so there is pain. When there is no pain but numbness, the disease is old and has entered deeply. The circulation of the nutritive and protective [qi] becomes rough, but as the channels and collaterals are sometimes open there is no pain, only the skin is not nourished, so there is numbness. When there is cold, there is little yang qi and abundant yin qi. This state reinforces that of the disease so there is cold. When there is heat, the yang qi is abundant and there is little yin qi, the disease qi dominates and yang overcomes yin, so the painful obstruction is hot. When there is profuse sweating so that the person is soaked, this is due to meeting intense dampness. There is little yang qi and the yin is overabundant. The two qi influence each other leading to profuse sweating so that the person is soaked."

The Emperor said, "As for painful obstruction without pain, what about that?"

Qi Bo said, "If the painful obstruction is in the bone, there is heaviness; if it is in the vessels, the blood congeals and does not flow; if it is in the sinews, there is bending but no extension; if it is in the flesh, then there is numbness; if it is in the skin, then there is cold. Therefore, those who have one of these five do not have pain. In all types of painful obstruction, when they meet cold there is a tightness and urgency; when they meet heat there is a laxity.

The emperor said, "Good."

"Needling Lower Back Pain"
(CHAPTER 41)

When the leg greater yang vessel leads to lower back pain, it radiates from the back of the neck to the buttocks, and the back feels heavy. Needle the middle of the cleft on the main greater yang channel [BL-40 *(wei zhong)*][4] so that blood emerges. Do not bleed in spring.

When the lesser yang leads to lower back pain, it feels like needles are stuck into the skin; it spreads and disrupts so that the person cannot bend down or straighten up, nor can they rotate. Needle at the tip of the lesser yang well-formed bone *(chéng gǔ* 成骨, proximal tibia) so that blood emerges. The well-formed bone is the isolated bony protuberance on the outer aspect of the knee [GB-34 *(yang ling quan)*]. Do not bleed in summer.

When the yang brightness leads to lower back pain, the person is unable to rotate; when they rotate it is like they see something and are saddened. Needle three times in front of the tibia [ST-36 *(zu san li)*]. To harmonize it above and below, bleed. Do not bleed in the fall.

When the leg lesser yin leads to lower back pain, it radiates along the internal aspect of the spine. Needle twice above the medial malleolus [KI-7 *(fu liu)*]. Do not bleed in spring. If you bleed too profusely, they will not recover.

When the vessel of the terminal yin leads to lower back pain, the lower back feels like the string of a fully stretched bow. Needle the vessel of the terminal yin outside the "fish belly" between the calf and the heel [LR-5 *(li gou)*], following along until it is like pearls strung together, and needle there. This disease leads people who are talkative to become mute. Needle three times.

When the dispersed *(jiě* 解)vessel[5] leads to lower back pain, the pain radiates to between the shoulders, there is blurry vision and occasional urinary incontinence. Needle the dispersed vessel at the transverse vessel of the lateral aspect of the cleft that separates the knee sinews [BL-39 *(wei yang)*]; bleed until the blood changes color. When the dispersed vessel leads to lower back pain and the pain circles around the body, often as if the back were broken, and the person has a tendency to be afraid, needle a vascular nodule the size of a grain of millet in the mid-

dle of the cleft [BL-40 *(wei zhong)*]. When you bleed it the blood will shoot out black. Stop bleeding when the blood turns red.

When the vessel that accompanies the yin[6] leads to lower back pain, the pain is like having a small awl inside with sudden, intense swelling. Needle the vessel that accompanies the yin at the tip where the bone ends *(jué gǔ,* an alternate name for GB-39 *[xuan zhong])*[7] above the lateral malleolus, three times.

When the yang linking vessel leads to lower back pain, the pain ascends with sudden, intense swellings. Needle the yang linking vessel where it meets the greater yang channel, below the calf, one foot above the ground [BL-57 *(cheng shan)*].

When the vessel of the transverse collateral[8] leads to lower back pain, the person cannot bend down or straighten up; when they attempt to straighten up they become afraid they might fall. The cause is an injury to the lower back while straining to lift a heavy weight: the transverse collateral is severed, and bad blood accumulates there. Needle in the interval between the sinews at the yang [lateral aspect of the] cleft [BL-39 *(wei yang)*] and above the cleft several inches[9] [BL-37 *(yin men)*]. Make the blood come out of the vessel twice.

When the vessel of the perineum leads to lower back pain, the pain ascends and there is continuous sweating. When the sweat dries, the person wants to drink; once he drinks, he feels like running.[10] Needle three times on the vessel of the direct yang.[11] If, in the transverse area above the ankle which is five inches below the cleft, one sees congestion, bleed.[12]

When the vessel of the flying yang[13] leads to lower back pain, the pain ascends so that the person is upset, and, in serious cases, there is deep sorrow and fear.[14] Needle the vessel of the flying yang five inches above the medial malleolus in front of the lesser yin at the meeting point with the yin linking vessel [KI-9 *(zhu bin)*].

When the flourishing *(chāng* 昌*)* yang vessel leads to lower back pain, the pain radiates to the chest, and the vision is blurry. In serious cases, there is curling back of the whole body and coiling of the tongue, so that the person cannot talk. Needle twice the medial sinew, in front of the big sinew which is above the medial malleolus and two inches from it, behind the greater yin [KI-7 *(fu liu)*].[15]

When the dispersed vessel leads to lower back pain, there is also feverishness. When the feverishness is intense it leads to irritability. The lower part of the lower back feels like there is a transverse wooden rod inside, and, in serious cases, there is leakage of urine. Needle three times the dispersed vessel between the muscle and bone in front of the knee, on the ligature channel that connects with the lateral aspect [SP-8 *(di ji)*].

When the vessel of the inner patterns of the flesh[16] leads to lower back pain, the pain prevents coughing, as that causes muscle spasms. Needle this vessel twice lateral to the greater yang and posterior to the lesser yang GB-39 *(xuan zhong)* [at GB-38 *(yang fu)*].

For lower back pain that goes along the spine, such that the pain goes to the head, which becomes heavy, accompanied by visual disturbances and a tendency to fall down, bleed the leg greater yang cleft [BL-40 *(wei zhong)*]. For lower back pain with cold in the upper part of the body, needle the leg greater yang and yang brightness. If accompanied by heat in the upper part of the body, needle the leg terminal yin. If they cannot bend down or straighten up, needle the leg lesser yang. With penetration of heat and panting, needle the leg lesser yin and bleed the cleft.

For lower back pain with cold in the upper part of the body and inability to look behind, needle the leg yang brightness. With heat in the upper part of the body, needle the leg greater yin. With penetration of heat and panting, needle the leg lesser yin. With difficulty in bowel movements, needle the leg lesser yin. With fullness in the lower abdomen, needle the leg terminal yin. If the pain feels as if there is a fracture and the person cannot bend down or straighten up or get up, needle the leg greater yang. With radiation to the internal aspect of the spine, needle the leg lesser yin.

For lower back pain that radiates to the lower abdomen and pulls on the flanks, thereby preventing one from bending backward, needle the intersection of the lower back and sacrum [either BL-34 *(xia liao)* or BL-31~34 *(ba liao)*] and above the buttocks [BL-30 *(bai huan shu)*]. Needle as many times as there have been days since the new moon, or until the next new moon. As soon as the needle is taken out, it will immediately be better. For problems on the left, use the right; for problems on the right, use the left.

Miscellaneous Excerpts from *Basic Questions*

FROM "ON THE HEAVENLY TRUTH OF HIGH ANTIQUITY" (CHAPTER 1)

The Yellow Emperor said, "Is it the exhaustion of their strength and vigor or the fate of numbers that makes old men unable to have children?"

Qi Bo stated, "For girls at age seven, the kidney energy is vigorous, the teeth change, the hair lengthens. At two times seven [14 years], heavenly dew *(tiān guǐ 天癸)* appears.[17] The conception vessel opens up, the penetrating vessel is vigorous, and the monthly periods regularly flow. At three times seven [21 years], the kidney energy is steady with the formation of the true [wisdom] teeth. At four times seven [28 years], the sinews and bones are firm, the hair reaches its longest length, and the body is vigorous and strong. At five times seven [35 years], the yang brightness channel declines, the complexion starts to dry out and the hair starts to fall out. At six times seven [42 years], the three yang channels fade away in the upper part of the body, the whole face becomes dry and the hair starts to turn white. At seven times seven [49 years], the conception vessel is deficient, the penetrating vessel becomes weak and meager, the heavenly dew is exhausted, the earth passageways [of the menstrual period] are blocked, so the form is wasted and there is infertility.

"For boys at age eight, the kidney qi is full, the hair lengthens, and the teeth change. At two times eight [16 years], the kidney energy is vigorous, the heavenly dew arrives, and the essence [sperm] overflows and leaks out. After sexual encounters there can be children. At three times eight [24 years], the kidney qi is steady, the sinews and bones are powerful and strong, and the true [wisdom] teeth are fully developed. At four times eight [32 years], the sinews and bones are well-defined and vigorous and the flesh is full and firm. At five times eight [40 years], the kidney qi declines, the hair falls out, and the teeth go bad. At six times eight [48 years], the yang qi is exhausted in the upper part of the body, the face dries out, and the temples get white. At seven times eight [56 years], the liver qi declines, the sinews are unable to move [properly], the heavenly dew is exhausted, the essence becomes meager, the kidney organ declines, and the physical form and structure are both near their end. At eight times eight [64 years], there is no more teeth or hair. The kidneys govern water, they receive and preserve the essences of the five yin organs and six yang organs. They cannot produce if the yin organs are not vigorous. Now they are all weakened, the sinews and bones are tired, and the heavenly dew is finished. Therefore, the temples become white, the body becomes heavy, the gait is uneven, and there are no more children."

FROM "ON THE QI OF LIFE PENETRATING TO HEAVEN" (CHAPTER 3)

That which generates the yin is rooted in the five flavors; the five palaces of the yin[18] are damaged by the five flavors. Therefore, with too much sour flavor the liver qi overflows and the spleen qi is therefore cut off. Too much salty flavor fatigues the big bones, draws in the muscles, and the heart yin is restrained. With too much sweetness the heart qi is full and choked, and creates an imbalance in the kidneys while darkening the complexion. With too much bitter flavor the spleen qi dries up and the stomach qi then thickens. Too much pungent flavor loosens the sinews and vessels while exhausting the essence and spirit. Therefore, with careful harmonization of the five flavors the bones grow straight and the sinews become flexible, the qi and blood flow, and the interstices become tight. When it is like this the qi of the bones will be subtle. Respecting the way ensures a long life.

FROM "ON THE BIRTH AND MATURATION OF THE FIVE YIN ORGANS" (CHAPTER 10)

All the various vessels are connected to the eyes, all the marrow to the brain, all the sinews to the liver,[19] all the blood to the heart, all the qi to the lungs. Morning and evening the blood and qi circulate in the eight hollows of the limbs.[20] Thus, during sleep, the blood goes back to the liver, which enables one to see. When they receive the blood, the legs can walk, the hands can seize, the fingers can grasp. If one is exposed to wind right after arising, when the blood congeals in the skin it constitutes painful obstruction; if it congeals in the vessels, it constitutes a bind *(qì* 泣*)*;[21] if in the legs, it constitutes inversion *(jué* 厥*)*. In all three cases, the circulating blood cannot go back to its cavities, and that is the cause of painful obstruction and inversion.

FROM "EXPLANATIONS ON THE FIVE QI" (CHAPTER 23)

These are the contraindications for the five flavors. Pungence rushes the qi; do not eat too much pungent food when there is a disease of the qi. Saltiness rushes the blood; do not eat too much salty food when there is a disease of the blood. Bitterness rushes the bones; do not eat too much bitter food when there is a disease of the bones. Sweetness rushes the flesh; do not eat too much sweet food when there is a disease of the flesh. Sourness rushes the sinews; do not eat too much sour food when there is a disease of the sinews. This is what is referred to as the five contraindications.

FROM "ON THE GREATER YIN AND YANG BRIGHTNESS" (CHAPTER 29)

The Yellow Emperor said, "Why are the limbs useless when the spleen is sick?"

Qi Bo said, "The limbs receive qi from the stomach that must go through the spleen before entering the channels. Now if the spleen is sick, it is unable to promote movement of the fluids on behalf of the stomach. If the limbs are deprived of the qi from food and drink, their qi becomes weaker day after day, and the pulse passageways close down. The sinews, bones and flesh are deprived of their vitality and become useless."

FROM "ON REBELLIONS AND REGULATIONS" (CHAPTER 34)

The Yellow Emperor said, "There are patients who are cold who cannot become hot near hot water or fires, nor warm with thick clothing. However, there are no chills. What disease is this?"

Qi Bo said, "People like this have an elemental predominance of kidney qi which takes water as its activity. The greater yang weakens, the renal fat withers and does not last. One water cannot surpass two fires. The kidneys are water, they generate the bones. If the kidneys are unproductive, the marrow cannot fill the bones and the cold reaches all the way to them. The absence of chills is due to the fact that the liver constitutes one yang [it is yin within yang] and the heart a second yang [it is yang within yang]. The kidneys [yin within yin] are left alone to store. One water cannot surpass two fires, hence the inability to have chills. This disease is called bone painful obstruction and it causes stiffness in the joints."

FROM "ON SKIN REGIONS" (CHAPTER 56)

In general the twelve channels and collaterals [define] the regions of the skin. For this reason the genesis of the myriad diseases must first be in the skin and hair. When a pathogenic influence attacks, the interstices and pores open; when they open, then it enters to reside in the collateral vessels. If it remains there and does not leave, it is transmitted to the channel. If it remains there and does not leave, it is transmitted to the yang organs and accumulates in the intestines and stomach. When the pathogenic influence starts to invade the skin, the shivering causes a piloerection that opens the cutaneous orifices. When the pathogenic influence enters the collaterals, it changes the color of the collateral vessel that it fills. When it resides in the channels, the person feels deficient and then drops. When it stays between the sinews and bones, if it is very cold, the sinews become stiff and the bones hurt; if it very hot, the sinews are lax and the bones melt, the flesh liquefies, the rolls of flesh disappear, and the hair falls out.

FROM "ON QI CAVITIES" (CHAPTER 58)

The Yellow Emperor said, "Good. I would like to hear about the connections of the hollows and valleys."

Qi Bo said, "The major confluences in the flesh are the valleys, the lesser ones are the hollows. They are located in the interstices of the flesh and circulate the nutritive qi and protective qi which connect with the great qi . If the pathogenic influences overflow, the qi is clogged, the vessels heat up, and the flesh deteriorates. When the nutritive and protective qi can no longer circulate, pus must form, the marrow melts inside, and the rolls of flesh disappear outside. If the pathogenic influences settle in the joint confluences, the joints become useless. The nutritive and protective qi have no more room, and where cold accumulates, the flesh gets twisted, the sinews retract, the limbs can no longer stretch out. Internally, there is bone painful obstruction, and externally, numbness. This is called insufficiency due to great cold settling in the hollows and valleys. The hollows and valleys connect the 365 cavities and have the same number as the days of the year. When a minor[22] painful obstruction runs wanton and circulates back and forth in the vessels, subtle needling will get at it, just as the methods prescribe."

FROM "ON BONY HOLLOWS" (CHAPTER 60)

The Yellow Emperor asked, "I have heard that wind is at the origin of the myriad diseases. How do we treat them with needles?"

Qi Bo replied, "When wind enters from the outside, it causes people to shiver, sweat comes out, the head hurts, the body feels heavy, and there is aversion to cold. The treatment for this is at GV-16 (feng fu) to regulate the yin

and yang. Tonify for insufficiency and drain for overabundance. When there is great wind with a painful nape, needle GV-16 (feng fu) located above the superior vertebra. If there is sweating with great wind, moxa BL-45 (yi xi) which is three inches to the side of the lower dorsals; when you press it with the finger, the patient will cry "eee shee,"[23] the vibration of which can be felt with the hand. For aversion to wind from encountering wind, needle the head of the eyebrow [BL-2 (zan zhu)]. Stiff neck is treated between the top of the shoulder and the transverse bone [ST-12 (que pen)] and at the median point which is located in the spine, level with a line drawn between the two bent elbows [GV-3 (yao yang guan)], where moxa is applied. If there is painful tension in the flanks which travels from the floating ribs to the lower abdomen, needle BL-45 (yi xi). For lower back pain preventing movement and rotation, with an acute sensation radiating down to the testicles, needle the eight sacral foramina and the painful areas. The eight holes are distributed between the lower back and the coccyx. . . .

"For difficulty in walking when the knee extends but does not bend, treat the bolt. For pain of the knee in the sitting position, treat the mechanism. When the joint feels hot and dislocated when standing, treat the skeletal gate. For pain in the knee extending to the big toe, treat the popliteal fossa [BL-40 (wei zhong)]. If, in the sitting position, there is pain as if there were a foreign object in a joint, treat the gate. Knee pain with inability to flex or extend the knee is treated in the back [BL-11 (da zhu)]. If the skeletal connection feels as if it were broken, treat the bony hollow which is the point in the middle of the yang brightness.[24] We can also treat the spring points of the grand [greater] yang [BL-66 (zu tong gu)] and of the lesser yin [KI-2 (ran gu)]. If prolonged standing causes numbness and pain in the legs, treat the lesser yang linking [GB-37 (guang ming)] which is five inches above the lateral malleolus.

"The bolt is above the condyles and below the pubis [ST-31 (bi guan)]. The mechanism frames the pelvic bones [GB-30 (huan tiao)]. The skeletal gate continues down a line drawn from the knee [GB-33 (xi yang guan)]. The skeletal connection is at the junction of the knee bones. . . ."

FROM "ON ECCENTRIC NEEDLING" (CHAPTER 63)

The Yellow Emperor asked, "I have heard about eccentric (miù 繆) needling but not yet understood its meaning. What is referred to as eccentric needling?"

Qi Bo replied, "When a pathogen comes to reside in the physical form, it must at first lodge in the skin and body hair. If it stays and does not leave it will enter to lodge in the minute vessels. If it stays and does not leave it will enter to lodge in the collaterals. If it stays and does not leave it will enter to lodge in the channels, internally connect with the five yin organs, disperse through the stomach and intestines. In this way when the yin and yang are all involved the five yin organs will then be injured. This is the order by which a pathogen entering through the skin and body hair and not leaving, finally ends up in the five yin organs. When things go like this we needle the channel appropriate to it.

"Now, if a pathogen resides in the skin and body hair and then lodges in the minute vessels and collaterals, staying and not leaving, it may lead to [vessels] being stuffed up and obstructed. In these cases it cannot enter the channels and overflows into the great collaterals, which leads to the generation of odd diseases.[25] When the pathogen resides in the big collaterals, it flows from the left to the right, from the right to the left, mutually connecting with the channels and spreading to the limbs. Its qi is not localized and does not flow through the command points of the channels. This is the case for eccentric needling."

The Yellow Emperor said, "I would like to hear all about eccentric needling when one chooses the right for the left and the left for the right. How is it different from grand needling?"[26]

Qi Bo said, "If the pathogen resides in a channel and is overabundant on the side opposite to the affected one, this is also a case of contralaterality where the disease on the left is not yet finished while the vessel on the right is already diseased. Here you must use grand needling on it as it is necessary to target the channels and not the collaterals. For those with a collateral disease, the pain is off the mark of the channels, hence the technique is called eccentric needling."

The Yellow Emperor said, "I would like to hear how eccentric needling is done. How does one go about performing it?"

Qi Bo said, "When the pathogen resides in the collateral of the leg lesser yin, it causes people to have sudden heart pain, violent distention, and a feeling of fullness in the flanks without accumulation. Bleed in front of KI-2 (*ran gu*). The problem should be better in the time it takes to eat a meal. For problems on the left choose the right, for those on the right choose the left. For relapses, do this for five days and it will be better.

"When the pathogen resides in the collateral of the arm lesser yang, there is throat painful obstruction, coiling of the tongue, dryness of the mouth, irritability, and pain in the lateral aspect of the arm making it impossible to raise the hand to the head. Needle the ring finger above the nail, at a distance of a leek leaf away from the extremity [TB-1 (*guan chong*)]. In robust [patients], relief is instantaneous, whereas it takes more time for the elderly. For problems on the left choose the right, for those on the right choose the left. For relapses, needle for several days and it will improve.

"When the pathogen resides in the collaterals of the leg greater yang, there will be pain in the head, nape and shoulders. Needle the little toe above the nail, where it meets the flesh [BL-67 (*zhi yin*)] . If there is no instant relief, needle three times below the lateral malleolus [BL-63 (*jin men*)]. For problems on the left choose the right, for those on the right choose the left. Relief will be felt in the time it takes to have a meal.

"When the pathogen resides between the arm and the palm, preventing the flexion of the wrist, needle behind the [styloid] process after first using your finger to find the painful point. Needle it a number of times corresponding to the number of the lunar day: once for the first day, twice for the second day, fifteen times for the fifteenth day, and fourteen times for the sixteenth day.

"In all cases of painful obstruction that moves around without a fixed place, needle the painful area, in the flesh intervals. Do this a number of times corresponding to the number of the lunar day, as this number corresponds to the abundance or weakness of qi. If we exceed it, there is a sloughing of qi, and if we do not reach it, the qi is not drained. For problems on the left choose the right, for those on the right choose the left. If the disease is not better, repeat with the same technique: needle once on the first day of the month, twice on the second day, increasing the number of needlings by one each day until fifteen times on the fifteenth, then fourteen times on the sixteenth day, and thereafter decreasing the number by one each day.

"When the pathogen resides in the collateral of the leg greater yin, causing lower back pain radiating to the abdomen, pulling on the flanks, and making it impossible to breathe with the trunk erect, needle M-BW-23 (*yao yi*) at the junction of the lower back and sacrum, above the buttocks, a number of times corresponding to the lunar phase. Relief is instantaneous; the disease ceases immediately. For problems on the left choose the right, for those on the right choose the left.

"When the pathogen resides in the collateral of the leg greater yang, there are spasms and tightness in the upper back with pain radiating to the flanks. When needling, start at the nape and [go down] the sides of several vertebrae. When you reach a tight area that is painful to the touch, needle three times to the side. Relief is instantaneous.

"When the pathogen resides in the collateral of the leg lesser yang, pain stays at the center of the pivot [GB-30 (huan tiao)] and the hip cannot be raised. Needle that point with a filiform needle. If there is cold, retain the needle for a long period. Needle it a number of times corresponding to the number of the lunar day. Relief is instantaneous.

"For treating the various channels, needle them [directly], and, if what extends past them is not diseased, then use eccentric needling on them.

"In general, the method of needling is to inspect first the channels and vessels by palpating and following along them. By regulating them, examine their deficiency and excess. Those that are not regulated, needle directly. For those with pain but no disease of the channels, use eccentric needling. If you notice a vascular network on the cutaneous region, you must use it. Such is the eccentric needling method."

Chapter Notes

1. *Editors' note:* This refers to the third month of summer, which is the sixth lunar month.
2. *Editors' note:* See discussion of this term in chapter 8.
3. *Editors' note:* The term here is *huāng mò*, which is believed to refer to the membrane above the diaphragm and below the heart.
4. *Editors' note:* Throughout this section of the book, point designations placed between brackets are inferred from the text. When the text designates a point by name, the normal format is followed.
5. *Editors' note:* The commentators interpret the dispersed vessel to be an alternate name for the channel divergence of the greater yang channel.
6. *Editors' note:* The commentators interpret this to mean a divergent connecting channel of the leg lesser yang vessel.
7. *Editors' note:* Even though the alternate name of GB-39 (xuan zhong) is used here, many commentators interpret this as referring to GB-38 (yang fu).

8. *Editors' note:* Some commentators interpret this to mean an external divergent connecting channel of the Bladder channel; others take it to mean the Girdle vessel.
9. *Editors' note:* Throughout this part of the book, we will use "inch" for the Chinese unit of measurement *cūn*, and "foot" for the Chinese unit of measurement *chí*.
10. *Editors' note:* According to some commentators, this is a mistake and should read "urinate."
11. *Editors' note:* According to some commentators, this is a mistake and should read "vessel of the perineum."
12. *Editors' note:* Some commentators believe that this last sentence refers to two points that should be needled, BL-62 (shen mai) and BL-56 (cheng jin).
13. *Editors' note:* "Flying yang" refers to the divergence from the Bladder channel at BL-58 (fei yang), which goes to the Kidney channel.
14. *Editors' note:* The yin Linking vessel connects the Heart (sadness) with the Kidneys (fear).
15. *Editors' note:* "Flourishing yang" (chāng yáng) is an alternate name for KI-7 (fu liu).
16. *Editors' note:* Some commentators suggest that this is related to the yang Linking vessel.
17. *Editors' note:* "Heavenly dew" refers to sexual energy.
18. *Editors' note:* Commentators interpret this as referring to the five yin Organs.
19. *Editors' note:* This is based on an alternate text. The original version of *Basic Questions* uses "joints" instead of liver.
20. *Editors' note:* This refers to the elbow, wrist, knee and ankle areas.
21. *Editors' note:* Commentators interpret this as a condition marked by poor Blood flow.
22. *Editors' note:* Commentators interpret this as a superficial painful obstruction affecting the minute collaterals.
23. *Editors' note:* The sound "eee shee" (yi xi) is how this point got its name.
24. *Editors' note:* Some take this to mean ST-36 (zu san li), while others consider it to be the middle of the transport point, ST-43 (xian gu).
25. *Editors' note:* This is interpreted by most commentators as "one-sided" disease.
26. *Editors' note:* Contralateral needling is understood to mean needling the connective vessels; grand needling (jù cì) is also done contralaterally, but works on the primary channels.

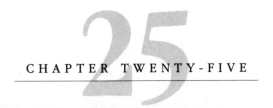

CHAPTER TWENTY-FIVE

Divine Pivot *(Ling shu)*

(C. 200 B.C.–100 A.D.)

From "Encompassing Painful Obstruction" (CHAPTER 27)

The Yellow Emperor asked Qi Bo, "When encompassing painful obstruction *(zhōu bì* 周痹*)* is located in the body, it moves from top to bottom, following the vessels. The painful symptoms are found from top to bottom, from left to right, so that no space is left alone. I wish to know if this pain is caused by pathogens located in the blood vessels or in the intramuscular spaces? What is its cause? The pain moves so rapidly that we do not have enough time to needle. If the pain is concentrated in one area, as soon as we determine the therapeutic method, the pain is already gone. What are the reasons that cause it to be like this? I wish to ask about its cause."

Qi Bo replied, "This is a multitudinous painful obstruction *(zhòng bì* 眾痹*)*, not an encompassing painful obstruction."

The Yellow Emperor said, "I wish to hear about the multitudinous painful obstruction."

Qi Bo replied, "One of the characteristics [of multitudinous painful obstruction] is that the pain has several fixed locations; the pain can manifest and recede; when it is on the right it may resonate on the left, and vice-versa. The pain cannot circulate [throughout the body—be encompassing], it manifests and then ceases."

The Yellow Emperor said, "Good. How does one needle [in such cases]?"

Qi Bo replied, "In such cases, although the pain has already stopped, we must needle the area [that was painful] to prevent a recurrence."

The Yellow Emperor said, "Good. I wish to hear what an encompassing painful obstruction is like."

Qi Bo replied, "Encompassing painful obstruction resides in the blood vessels;[1] it follows their course to ascend and descend; it cannot go left or right, neither can it have a fixed location."

The Yellow Emperor said, "How does one needle it?"

Qi Bo replied, "When the pain goes down from top to bottom, start by needling the bottom to overcome it, then needle the top to eradicate it. When the pain ascends from bottom to top, start by needling the top to overcome it, and then the bottom to eradicate it."

The Yellow Emperor said, "Good. What generates this pain? For what reason does it have this name?"

Qi Bo replied, "Wind, cold, and damp [pathogenic] qi settle externally in the intramuscular layers, press upon [the fluids] and produce a thick humor *(mò* 沫*)*. This condenses in the presence of cold, which distends the intramuscular spaces. This leads to cracks which cause pain. With the pain the spirit[2] returns there. When the spirit returns, there is heat. With this heat the pain is relieved. Although the pain has been relieved there is inversion (*jué* 厥) and the painful obstruction manifests in another location. When they develop, they have similar features."

The Yellow Emperor said, "Good. I have understood its meaning."

[Qi Bo said,] "This internal [pathological state] does not involve the organs, and does not manifest externally at the level of the skin. It is solely located within the muscular layers. The true qi cannot circulate around [encompass], hence the name encompassing painful obstruction.

"That is the reason why, when we treat painful obstruction with acupuncture, in order to regulate [the vessels] we must first palpate along the six channels below[3] to observe their deficiency and excess, including where the blood in the great collaterals is knotted and blocked, or where they are deficient with the pulses fallen and empty, and regulate them. Use heat to unblock them. In cases of muscle contracture, you can use acupuncture or massage to mobilize it [the qi]."

The Yellow Emperor said, "Good. I have understood its meaning and also learned how to deal with it."

Chapter Notes

1. *Editors' note:* Chinese commentators interpret "blood vessels" here to mean the channels.
2. *Editors' note:* Some commentators interpret this to mean the protective qi.
3. *Editors' note:* Some commentators interpret this to mean the six channels of the leg, others the six great channels.

CHAPTER TWENTY-SIX

Discussion of Cold-induced Disorders
(Shang han lun)
C. 200 by ZHANG ZHONG-JING

From "Greater Yang Disorders"

§ 116

When a patient exhibits a faint and rapid pulse, be careful and do not apply moxa, because the fire stirs up pathogenic influences and causes agitation and inversion [of the qi]. As this fire chases away the deficiency and pursues the excess, the blood disperses in the vessels, and the qi of the fire, although weak, forcefully attacks the interior of the body, withering the bones and damaging the sinews. The blood will recover its original state with difficulty.

If the pulse is floating, it is appropriate to release with sweating; if moxibustion is used to cauterize it, the pathogenic influences have no opportunity to come out, and the fire becomes more vigorous. The illness then becomes worse below the waist and transforms into painful obstruction. This is called fire rebellion. When the patient is on the way to recovery, he becomes agitated at first, starts sweating, and then releases it. How does one know this? Because the pulse is floating, therefore one knows that sweating will release it.

§ 174

At the eighth or ninth day of cold damage, when wind and dampness contend with each other, there is pain and irritability throughout the body, it is difficult to turn oneself over, there is no vomiting, a lack of thirst, and the pulse is floating, deficient and choppy, use Cinnamon Twig and Prepared Aconite Decoction *(gui zhi fu zi tang)*. If the stools are hard and urination is without difficulty, use Remove Cinnamon Twig plus Atractylodes Decoction *(qu gui jia zhu tang)*.

§ 175

When wind and dampness contend with each other, the bones and joints are painful to the point that flexion-extension is impossible, pain is aggravated by pressure, there is sweating, shortness of breath, difficult urination, and aversion to wind with reluctance to get undressed. The body may become slightly swollen. Use Licorice and Prepared Aconite Decoction *(gan cao fu zi tang)*.

Cinnamon Twig and Prepared Aconite Decoction
(guì zhī fù zǐ tāng)

桂枝附子湯

Ramulus Cinnamomi Cassiae *(gui zhi)* . . . . 4 *liang*[1]
Radix Lateralis Aconiti Carmichaeli
   Praeparata *(fu zi)* . . . . 3 roots
Rhizoma Zingiberis Officinalis Recens
   (sheng jiang). . . . . 3 *liang*
Fructus Zizyphi Jujubae *(da zao)* . . . . 12 pieces
Honey-toasted Radix Glycyrrhizae
   Uralensis *(zhi gan cao)*. . . . . 2 *liang*

Remove Cinnamon Twig plus Atractylodes Decoction
(*qù guì jiā zhú tǎng*)

去桂加朮湯

Radix Lateralis Aconiti Carmichaeli
 Praeparata (*fu zi*) . . . . 3 roots
Rhizoma Atractylodis Macrocephalae
 (*bai zhu*) . . . . 4 *liang*
Rhizoma Zingiberis Officinalis Recens
 (*sheng jiang*) . . . . 3 *liang*
Honey-toasted Radix Glycyrrhizae
 Uralensis (*zhi gan cao*). . . . . 2 *liang*
Fructus Zizyphi Jujubae (*da zao*) . . . . 12 pieces

Licorice and Prepared Aconite Decoction
(*gān cǎo fù zǐ tǎng*)

甘草附子湯

Honey-toasted Radix Glycyrrhizae
 Uralensis (*zhi gan cao*). . . . . 2 *liang*

Radix Lateralis Aconiti Carmichaeli
 Praeparata (*fu zi*) . . . . 2 roots
Rhizoma Atractylodis Macrocephalae
 (*bai zhu*) . . . . 2 *liang*
Ramulus Cinnamomi Cassiae (*gui zhi*) . . . . 2 *liang*

Chapter Notes

1. There is some controversy as to the meaning of these terms of measurement. The prevailing view is that during the late Han when this book was written, one *liang* was equivalent to three grams. However, another view is that one *liang* was equivalent to 37.5 grams. There are four *fen* in one *liang*.

CHAPTER TWENTY-SEVEN

Essentials from the Golden Cabinet
(Jin gui yao lue)
C. 200 by ZHANG ZHONG-JING

"Direct Wind Attack and Panarthralgia" (CHAPTER 5)

When wind is involved in the illness, there is hemiplegia. If only the arms are paralyzed, it is painful obstruction. If the pulse is faint and rapid, a direct wind attack caused it to be this way.[1]

When the pulse is floating and tight, tight means cold and floating means deficiency. When the cold and deficiency struggle together, the pathogenic influence resides in the skin. When [the pulse] is floating, there is blood deficiency and the pirate pathogenic influence is not drained out. It is located either on the right or on the left side. [The side with the] pathogenic qi is conversely lax, while it is the side where the normal qi [is present] that is urgent and tight. The normal qi brings along the pathogenic, resulting in the mouth and face being awry and paralyzed.

When the pathogenic influence is located at the collateral level, there is numbness of the skin and muscles. When it is at the level of the channels, there is an unshakable sensation of heaviness. When it is at the level of the yang organs, the patient does not recognize people. When it enters the yin organs, speech is difficult and there is drooling.

Hou's Black Powder *(hou shi hei san)* is suggested to treat wind attack with heaviness and restlessness in the four limbs and aversion to cold at the level of the heart in cases with deficiency.

Hou's Black Powder *(hóu shì hēi sǎn)*

侯氏黑散

Flos Chrysanthemi Morifolii *(ju hua)* . . . . 40 *fen*[2]
Rhizoma Atractylodis Macrocephalae *(bai zhu)* . . . . . 10 *fen*
Herba cum Radice Asari *(xi xin)* .3 *fen*
Sclerotium Poriae Cocos *(fu ling)* . . . . .3 *fen*
Concha Ostreae *(mu li)* . . . . .3 *fen*
Radix Platycodi Grandiflori *(jie geng)* . . . . 8 *fen*
Radix Ledebouriellae Divaricatae *(fang feng)* . . . . 10 *fen*
Radix Ginseng *(ren shen)* . . . . .3 *fen*
Alumen *(ming fan)* . . . . .3 *fen*
Radix Scutellariae Baicalensis *(huang qin)* . . . . 5 *fen*
Radix Angelicae Sinensis *(dang gui)* . . . . .3 *fen*
Rhizoma Zingiberis Officinalis *(gan jiang)* . . . . .3 *fen*
Radix Ligustici Chuanxiong *(chuan xiong)* . . . . .3 *fen*
Ramulus Cinnamomi Cassiae *(gui zhi)* . . . . .3 *fen*

When the pulse is slow and lax, slow means cold and lax means deficiency. When the nutritive is lax,[3] it is from loss of blood. When the protective is lax,[4] it is a direct wind attack. When the pathogenic qi directly attacks the channels, pruritus and urticaria appear, and the heart qi is insufficient. When the pathogenic qi enters the middle, the chest feels full and there is shortness of breath.

319

Wind-Leading Decoction (*feng yin tang*) eliminates heat, paralysis and convulsions.

Wind-Leading Decoction (*fēng yǐn tāng*)
風引湯

Radix et Rhizoma Rhei (*da huang*) . . . . 4 *liang*
Rhizoma Zingiberis Officinalis (*gan jiang*) . . . . 4 *liang*
Os Draconis (*long gu*) . . . . 4 *liang*
Ramulus Cinnamomi Cassiae (*gui zhi*) . . . . 3 *liang*
Radix Glycyrrhizae Uralensis (*gan cao*) . . . . 2 *liang*
Concha Ostreae (*mu li*) . . . . 2 *liang*
Calcitum (*han shui shi*) . . . . 2 *liang*
Talcum (*hua shi*) . . . . 2 *liang*
Halloysitum Rubrum (*chi shi zhi*) . . . . 2 *liang*
Kaolin (*bai shi zhi*) . . . . 2 *liang*
Fluoritum (*zi shi ying*) . . . . 2 *liang*
Gypsum (*shi gao*) . . . . 2 *liang*

Stephania and Rehmannia Decoction (*fang ji di huang tang*) treats diseases like mania, wildly walking around, speaking to oneself nonstop, without cold or heat, but with a floating pulse.

Stephania and Rehmannia Decoction (*fáng jǐ dì huáng tāng*)
防己地黃湯

Radix Stephaniae Tetrandrae (*han fang ji*) . . . . 1 *qian*
Ramulus Cinnamomi Cassiae (*gui zhi*) . . . . 3 *qian*
Radix Ledebouriellae Divaricatae (*fang feng*) . . . . . . 3 *qian*
Radix Glycyrrhizae Uralensis (*gan cao*) . . . . 2 *qian*

Head-Wind Rubbing Powder (*tou feng mo san*) treats headache and attacks of vertigo.

Head-Wind Rubbing Powder (*tóu fēng mō sǎn*)
頭風摸散

Radix Lateralis Aconiti Carmichaeli
  Praeparata (*fu zi*) . . . . 1 root
Salt . . . . amount equal to weight of *fu zi* root

These ingredients are ground into a powder and rubbed onto the affected area of the head.

When the pulse is submerged and frail, submerged means that it is connected to the bone, and frail that it is connected to the sinews. Submerged means kidneys, while frail means liver. If there is contact with water after sweating, the water may injure the heart, and a yellowish sweat [liquid] appears throughout the joints, so it is called panarthralgia.[5]

When the dorsal leg yang [dorsal pedis] pulse is floating and slippery, slippery means that the grain qi is in excess, floating that there is spontaneous sweating.

When the lesser yin [posterior tibialis] pulse is floating and frail, frail means that the blood is insufficient, floating means wind. When the wind and blood struggle together, there is then flashing pain.

There are abundant [obese] people with a choppy and small pulse, shortness of breath, spontaneous sweating, and pain in the various joints with difficulty in bending or extending. All these symptoms are the consequence of exposure to wind after excessive consumption of alcohol and sweating.

When the various joints of the limbs are sore and painful, the body is crooked and gaunt, the legs are swollen as if they are about to fall off, and there is vertigo, shortness of breath, and a constant feeling of nausea with a frequent desire to vomit, use Cinnamon Twig, Peony, and Anemarrhena Decoction (*gui zhi shao yao zhi mu tang*).

Cinnamon Twig, Peony, and Anemarrhena Decoction (*guì zhī shào yào zhī mǔ tāng*)
桂枝芍藥知母湯

Ramulus Cinnamomi Cassiae (*gui zhi*) . . . . 4 *liang*
Radix Paeoniae (*shao yao*) . . . . 3 *liang*
Radix Glycyrrhizae Uralensis (*gan cao*) . . . . 2 *liang*
Herba Ephedrae (*ma huang*) . . . . 2 *liang*
Rhizoma Zingiberis Officinalis Recens
  (*sheng jiang*) . . . . 5 *liang*
Rhizoma Atractylodis Macrocephalae
  (*bai zhu*) . . . . 5 *liang*
Rhizoma Anemarrhenae Asphodeloidis
  (*zhi mu*) . . . . 4 *liang*
Radix Ledebouriellae Divaricatae
  (*fang feng*) . . . . 4 *liang*
Radix Lateralis Aconiti Carmichaeli
  Praeparata (*fu zi*) . . . . 2 *liang*

The sour taste damages the sinews and the damaged sinews become lax; this is called flux (*xiè* 泄). The salty taste damages the bone and the damaged bone dries up; this is called withering (*kū* 枯). When flux and withering combine, this is severing flux (*duàn xiè* 斷泄).

When the nutritive qi is blocked and the protective qi does not move alone, both the nutritive and protective qi are weak. The three burners lack a place of safeguarding,[6] the four limbs are deprived of their support, the body is crooked and gaunt, only the feet are swollen and enlarged, yellow sweat emerges, and the legs are cold. If there is fever, this is panarthralgia.

For panarthralgia, when the joints cannot bend or extend and there is pain, the recommended prescription is Aconite Decoction *(wu tou tang)*.

Aconite Decoction *(wū tóu tāng)*

烏頭湯

Herba Ephedrae *(ma huang)*......................3 *liang*
Radix Paeoniae *(shao yao)*........................3 *liang*
Radix Astragali Membranacei *(huang qi)* ....3 *liang*
Honey-toasted Radix Glycyrrhizae
 Uralensis *(zhi gan cao)*........................3 *liang*
Radix Aconiti Carmichaeli Praeparata
 (zhi chuan wu) ....5 pieces

Chapter Notes

1. *Editors' note:* The wind described in this paragraph is generally considered to be internal Wind generated by a transformation of Liver yang.
2. There is some controversy as to the meaning of these terms of measurement. The prevailing view is that during the late Han when this book was written, one *liang* was equivalent to three grams. However, another view is that one *liang* was equivalent to 37.5 grams. There are four *fen* in one *liang*.
3. *Editors' note:* This refers to a submerged, lax pulse.
4. *Editors' note:* This refers to a floating, lax pulse.
5. *Editors' note:* Modern Chinese commentators interpret this to be a description of how dampness (water) can reach the Heart Qi through the pores and vessels when there is Liver and Kidney deficiency. Obstruction of the sweating process causes the production of Damp-Heat, which spreads to the joints and creates joint pain with swelling.
6. *Editors' note:* Most commentators interpret this to mean that they are not nourished.

CHAPTER TWENTY-EIGHT

Systematic Classic of Acupuncture and Moxibustion
(Zhen jiu jia yi jing)

C. 250 by HUANG-FU MI

"Development of Painful Obstruction When the Yin is Affected by Disease"
(DIVISION 10, CHAPTER 1, PART 1)[1]

The Yellow Emperor asked Qi Bo, "When encompassing painful obstruction (zhōu bì 周痹) is located in the body, it moves from top to bottom, following the vessels. The painful symptoms are found from top to bottom, from left to right, so that no space is left alone. I wish to know if this pain is caused by pathogens located in the blood vessels or in the intramuscular spaces? What is its cause? The pain moves so rapidly that we do not have enough time to needle. If the pain is concentrated in one area, as soon as we determine the therapeutic method, the pain is already gone. What are the reasons that cause it to be like this? I wish to ask about its cause."

Qi Bo replied, "This is a multitudinous painful obstruction (zhòng bì 眾痹), not an encompassing painful obstruction. One of the characteristics of [mulitudinous painful obstruction] is that the pain has several fixed locations; the pain can manifest and recede; when it is on the right it may resonate on the left, and vice-versa. The pain cannot circulate [throughout the body—be encompassing], it manifests and then ceases. In such cases, although the pain has already stopped, we must needle the area

[that was painful] to prevent a recurrence."

The Yellow Emperor said, "And encompassing painful obstruction?"

Qi Bo said, "Encompassing painful obstruction resides in the blood vessels;[2] it follows their course to ascend and descend; it cannot go left or right, neither can it have a fixed location. When the pain goes down from top to bottom, start by needling the bottom to stop it, then needle the top to eradicate it. When the pain ascends from bottom to top, start by needling the top to stop it, and then the bottom to eradicate it."

The Yellow Emperor said, "How does this illness [encompassing painful obstruction] occur, and why is it called that name?"

Qi Bo said, "Wind, cold, and damp [pathogenic] qi settle in the intramuscular spaces, press upon [the fluids] and produce a thick humor. This condenses in the presence of cold, which distends the intramuscular spaces. This leads to cracks which cause pain. When pain appears, the spirit returns there.[3] When the spirit returns, there is heat. With this heat the pain is relieved. Although the pain has been relieved there is inversion (jué 厥) and the painful obstruction manifests in another location. When they develop, they have similar features. This internal [pathological state] does not involve the organs, and does not manifest externally at the level of the skin. It is solely located within the muscular layers. The true qi cannot circulate around [encompass], hence the name encompassing painful obstruction.

"So when needling a painful obstruction, it is necessary to first palpate up and down along the great channels and observe deficiency or excess to where the blood in the great collaterals is knotted and blocked, or where they are deficient with the pulses fallen and empty, and regulate them. Use heat to unblock them. In cases of muscle contracture, you can use acupuncture or massage to mobilize it [the qi]."

The Yellow Emperor said, "How do you examine in order to determine whether a person can easily fall ill with painful obstruction?"

Qi Bo said, "People with coarse pores and interstices and flesh that is not firm can easily contract painful obstruction. That is the reason why in order to determine the location of the painful obstruction at the top or at the bottom, we must examine the three parts."[4]

The Yellow Emperor said, "For needling, there are three different methods; what are they?"

Qi Bo said, "You can needle the nutritive qi, the protective qi, and the cold painful obstruction which lodges in the channels. To needle the nutritive qi, let out blood. To needle the protective qi, let out qi. To needle the cold painful obstruction, you must warm up internally."

The Yellow Emperor said, "What are the characteristics of the nutritive qi, protective qi, and cold painful obstruction?"

Qi Bo said, "As for nutritive qi generating disease, there are chills, feverishness, little qi, and the blood goes up and down. As for protective qi generating disease, there is qi-type pain which comes and goes, along with tension and intestinal borborygmus. Wind-cold resides in the intestines and stomach. As for cold painful obstruction as the disease, it lodges and will not leave. Sometimes there is pain and the skin is numb."

The Yellow Emperor said, "How do we proceed to induce internal heat when needling cold painful obstruction?"

Qi Bo said, "To needle the cotton cloth-clothed,[5] use fire to warm them directly; to needle the great ones, warm with herbs.

"The prescription uses twenty *sheng*[6] of full-bodied wine, one *sheng* of Fructus Zanthoxyli Bungeani *(shu jiao)*, one *sheng* of Rhizoma Zingiberis Officinalis *(gan jiang)*, and one *sheng* of Ramulus Cinnamomi Cassiae *(gui zhi)*. Finely grind up these four and soak them in clear wine. Add to this mixture one *jin*[7] of silk fiber and four *chi* and two *zhang*[8] of fine white cloth. Keep it in a tightly closed container and do not let the qi drain off. Simmer on a low flame using horse droppings as fuel; after five days and five nights, remove the silk and cloth and dry them in the sun. Once dry, soak them again in the alcohol for one day and one night. Repeat the process being sure that the silk and cloth are dry before soaking them again. Then cut the cloth up into six pieces and make six small bags out of it, in which are placed the fiber and the dregs of the herbs. Warm these bags with mulberry tree coal, then apply them topically over the area affected by the cold painful obstruction so that the heat reaches the sick area. Once cooled down, heat them up again and repeat this operation thirty times. At that time, the patient will be sweating. After the sweating, warm up the bags to wipe the body dry thirty times. Then the patient must walk in a closed room, sheltered from drafts. At each needling session, proceed in the same manner until the cure is obtained. That is how the 'inner warming' process is performed."

The Yellow Emperor stated, "How is painful obstruction generated?"

Qi Bo answered, "The three influences wind, cold and dampness arrive in various ways, intermingle and constitute painful obstruction. When the wind influence predominates it is moving painful obstruction; when the cold influence predominates it is severe painful obstruction; when the dampness influence predominates it is fixed painful obstruction."

The Yellow Emperor stated, "But are there not five of them?"

Qi Bo said, "The one that is encountered in winter is bone painful obstruction; that in spring, sinew painful obstruction; that in summer, vessel painful obstruction; that at the ultimate yin time,[9] flesh painful obstruction; and that in fall, skin painful obstruction."

The Yellow Emperor said, "When it settles inside the five yin and six yang organs, what qi causes it to be that way?"

Qi Bo stated, "The yin organs all have [some tissue] with which each is associated. When a disease stays for a long time and does not leave, it will settle in that [tissue] with which it is associated. Thus for bone painful obstruction that does not improve, if the person repeatedly contracts pathogenic influences [the painful obstruction] will settle internally in the kidneys. For sinew painful obstruction that does not improve, if the person repeatedly contracts pathogenic influences [the painful obstruction] will settle internally in the liver. For vessel painful obstruction that does not improve, if the person repeatedly contracts pathogenic influences [the painful obstruction] will settle internally in the heart. For flesh painful obstruction that does not improve, if the person repeatedly contracts pathogenic influences [the painful obstruction] will settle internally in the spleen. For skin painful obstruction that does not improve, if the person repeatedly contracts pathogenic influences [the painful obstruction] will settle internally in the lungs. As for those things that are considered painful obstruction, each occurs when a person contracts wind, cold or dampness at its particular season. All painful obstruction that does not improve spreads internally. When wind predominates, the person will improve more easily."

The Yellow Emperor said, "Among [the cases of] painful obstruction, there are lethal cases, cases of prolonged pain, and cases in which a cure is easily obtained. Why is that?"

Qi Bo said, "Lethal cases are those in which it [the painful obstruction] enters the yin organs. Prolonged pain is found in those cases in which it resides between the sinews and bones. When it resides in the skin, cure is easy to obtain."

The Yellow Emperor said, "And when it resides in the six yang organs?"

Qi Bo said, "Diet and the place of residence are the root causes of these diseases. Each of the six yang organs also has an associated point (*shū* 俞). If, while conditions of food and drink resonate with them, the wind, cold or damp qi penetrate into the associated point, [the pathogenic influences] will follow the associated point and enter, each settling into its respective yang organ."

The Yellow Emperor said, "How do you treat them with needles?"

Qi Bo said, "There are the stream (*shū* 輸) points for the yin organs, and the sea (*hé* 合) points for the yang organs. They are distributed along the course of the vessels. Each has a place where it manifests, and each treats its [particular] transgression so that diseases can be healed."

The Yellow Emperor said, "Do the nutritive and protective qi also cause people to have painful obstruction?"

Qi Bo said, "The nutritive is the essential qi of food and drink. It harmonizes and is regulated by the yin organs, while permeating throughout the yang organs before it is able to enter into the vessels. Therefore it follows the course of the vessels above and below, passes through the five yin organs, and connects with the six yang organs. The protective is the qi of food and drink that has prowess; its qi is urgent, rapid, slippery and quick and cannot enter into the vessels, so it circulates between the skin and flesh divisions, fumes in the vitals membrane,[10] collects in[11] the thorax and abdomen. When their qi flows rebelliously there is disease; when their qi flows the way it should, there is recovery. As long as they are not mixed with wind, cold or dampness, there is no painful obstruction."

"Development of Painful Obstruction When the Yin is Affected by Disease"
(DIVISION 10, CHAPTER 1, PART 2)[12]

The Yellow Emperor asked, "Painful obstruction may be painful, may be not painful, may have numbness, or cold, or heat, or dryness, or dampness. What is the reason for this?"

Qi Bo replied, "When it is painful there is much cold qi. As there is cold so there is pain. When there is no pain but numbness, the disease is old and has entered deeply. The circulation of the nutritive and protective [qi] becomes rough, but as the channels and collaterals are sometimes open there is no pain, only the skin is not nourished, so there is numbness. When there is cold, there is little yang qi and abundant yin qi. This state reinforces that of the disease so there is cold. When there is heat, the yang qi is abundant and there is little yin qi, the pathogenic qi dominates and yang overcomes yin, so the painful obstruction is hot. When there is profuse sweating so that the person is soaked, this is due to meeting intense dampness. There is little yang qi and the yin is overabundant. The two qi influence each other so there is profuse sweating such that the person is soaked.

"If the painful obstruction is in the bone, there is heaviness; if it is in the vessels, the blood congeals and does not flow; if it is in the sinews, there is bending but no extension; if it is in the flesh, then there is numbness; if it is in the skin, then there is cold. Therefore, those who have one of these five do not have pain. In all types of painful obstruction, when they meet cold there is tightness and urgency; when they meet heat there is laxity."[13]

The Yellow Emperor said, "Sometimes the disruption of a single channel or a single vessel can be the source of scores of diseases: sometimes pain, sometimes an abscess, sometimes heat, sometimes cold, sometimes itching, sometimes painful obstruction, and sometimes numbness. There is an unlimited number of transformations. What is the reason for this?"

Qi Bo said, "All of these are generated by pathogenic qi."

The Yellow Emperor said, "Man has true qi, normal qi and pathogenic qi. What do they refer to?"

Qi Bo said, "True qi is what is received from heaven. When matched with the qi of water and grains, it is what fills the body. The normal qi is the normal wind that comes from a certain direction. It is not the deficient wind.[14] The pathogenic qi is the deficient wind. As for the deficient wind plundering and harming people, when it penetrates it does so deeply and cannot go away by itself. As for the normal wind striking into people, it does so superficially and goes away by itself. Its qi is soft and weak and cannot harm the true qi, so it goes away by itself.

"As for a deficient pathogenic [qi] penetrating into people, there is at first shivering that shakes the frame, raises the body hair, and opens up the pores and interstices; later, it enters deeply. If it gets to the bone, then there is bone painful obstruction. If it gets to the sinews, then there are contractures of the sinews. If it gets into the vessels so that the blood is blocked and does not flow, then there are abscesses. If it gets to the flesh, it struggles against the protective qi: if the yang qi predominates, there is fever; if the yin qi predominates, there is cold. If there is cold the true qi goes; when it goes there is deficiency; when there is deficiency there is cold. When it gets to the skin, its qi is released toward the exterior, the pores and interstices open, the hairs become agitated. When the pathogenic qi moves back and forth, it causes itching. When it stays and does not go away, there is painful obstruction. When the protective qi does not circulate, there is numbness.

"When the disease resides in the bones, the bones are heavy and cannot be lifted, the marrow is painful, and cold qi arrives there. It is called bone painful obstruction. Needling must be deep [to the bone], while being careful not to injure the vessels and flesh. The way [to the right place] is following the intramuscular spaces.[15] When the bone feels hot, the disease is gone.

"When the disease resides in the sinews, the sinews contract and the joints are painful so that the person cannot walk. This is called sinew painful obstruction. The needle must reach the superficial part of the sinews; needle the intramuscular groove without touching the bone; as soon as there is a sensation of heat felt in the sinews, the disease is gone [and needling] can be stopped.

"When the disease resides in the muscles and skin, all the muscles and skin hurt. This is called muscle painful obstruction. The injury comes from cold and dampness,

and the intramuscular spaces must be needled several times and deeply, until there is a sensation of heat in the affected area; be careful not to harm the sinews and bones. If the sinews and bones are harmed [to the point that] there are pathological changes, abscesses will develop. The emergence of a hot sensation in the various intramuscular grooves means that the disease is healed [and that needling] can be stopped."

The Yellow Emperor said, "Some people [are cold] even though they do not wear thin clothes and do not have cold qi inside them. How is cold generated from inside?"

Qi Bo said, "These people have suffered frequent painful obstruction, the yang qi is meager and the yin qi profuse. Therefore the body is cold as if it came out of the water."

The Yellow Emperor said, "Some people are cold such that [neither] soups nor fire can heat them nor thick clothes warm them. Given this, they do not shiver with cold. What kind of disease is this?"

Qi Bo said, "As for these people, it is simply that their kidney qi dominates and that they use water in their work. The greater yang qi weakens and the kidney fat becomes desiccated so that it does not grow. The kidneys are water and focus [their effects] on the bones. When the kidneys do not generate, the bone marrow is no longer filled and the cold sensation can spread all the way to the bone. As to why they are not shivering from cold, the liver is one yang, the heart is another yang, and the kidneys are a single organ. One water cannot overcome two fires, so the person cannot shiver. This disease is called bone painful obstruction and the patients should have contracture of the joints.

"When fixed painful obstruction does not go away and long-term cold is not resolved, it constitutes stagnation; if the cold becomes chronic and is not eliminated, it turns into tibial painful obstruction.[16]

"In bone painful obstruction the different joints are disabled and painful, there is profuse sweating and irritability of the heart, choose the three yin channels and tonify them.

"In inversion painful obstruction (jué bì 厥痹) the inversion qi ascends to the abdomen. Choose the yin and yang collaterals, determine which channel is primarily involved, sedate the yang channels, and tonify the yin channels.

"When wind painful obstruction worsens, it gradually progresses toward an incurable stage. The patient feels as if his legs are either icy or soaked in hot water, the leg bones are painful, and the legs have no strength. There is irritability of the heart, headache, occasional vomiting, and an occasional stifling sensation. If prolonged there will be vertigo. When the vertigo stops there is sweating. There is a combination of sadness, elation and anger, along with shortness of breath and inability to feel pleasure. Death will occur in less than three years.

"For legs and hips that cannot be raised, treat in the lateral recumbent position at the door-leaf of the pivot [GB-30 *(huan tiao)*] with round and sharp needles, not with big needles.

"For knee pain, select ST-35 *(du bi)* using round and sharp needles. Needle every other day. As the needle is as thick as an ox's hair, the knees can be needled without any hesitation.

"For numb legs, needle GV-16 *(feng fu)*.

"If there is coolness and numbness from the lower back all the way down to the feet, such that [the person] cannot sit or get up nor raise the buttocks, the main point is GV-2 *(yao shu)*.

"For painful obstruction, the main points are CV-1 *(hui yin)*, LU-9 *(tai yuan)*, TB-12 *(xiao luo)*, KI-6 *(zhao hai)*.

"For a constant desire to lie down when the body cannot move around due to great dampness, the main point is TB-8 *(san yang luo)*.

"For bone painful obstruction with restlessness and fullness, the main point is SP-5 *(shang qiu)*.

"For a hot sensation in the sole of the foot, inability to stand for a long period of time with pain in the tibia, due to damp painful obstruction with inability to walk, the main point is SP-6 *(san yin jiao)*.

"For pain in the medial aspect of the knee that radiates to the patella, with inability to flex and extend, and that links to the abdomen and radiates to the entire throat, the main point is LR-7 *(xi guan)*.

"If painful obstruction is accompanied by edema of the leg, flaccidity of the dorsum of the foot, and heel pain, the main point is ST-39 *(xia ju xu)*.

"For pain in the tibia and lax feet that lose their shoes, damp painful obstruction, a hot sensation in the sole of the foot, inability to stand for a long period of time, the main point is ST-38 *(tiao kou)*.

"For a troubling, tortuous painful obstruction of the tibia such that the knee cannot flex or extend nor be used in walking, the main point is ST-34 *(liang qiu)*.

"For a knee which has cold painful obstruction and numbness such that it cannot flex or extend, the main point is ST-31 *(bi guan)*.

"For pain, atrophy and painful obstruction of the skin, the main point is GB-36 *(wai qiu)*.

"For pain in the lateral aspect of the knee with inability to flex or extend, painful obstruction of the tibia with numbness, the main point is GB-33 *(xi yang guan)*.

"For hip painful obstruction that radiates pain down the lateral aspect of the thigh and knee, numbness, and very tense sinews, the main point is GB-34 *(yang ling quan)*.

"For cold qi located between the intramuscular grooves, causing pain to attack up and down, sinew painful obstruction, and numbness, the main point is GB-32 *(zhong du)*.

"For pain inside the hip joint and inability to lift the leg, use fine needles. If cold lodges there, needle as many times as there have been days since the new moon, or until the next new moon. The disease ceases immediately.

"For pain and tightness that pulls between the lower back and the ribs, contracture of the hip sinews, a painful lower leg that cannot be flexed or extended, painful obstruction, and numbness, the main point is GB-30 *(huan tiao)*.

"For wind-cold that starts from the small toe, vessel painful obstruction that goes up and down, and nonfixed chest and rib pain, the main point is BL-67 *(zhi yin)*.

"When there is traumatic injury to the big toe due to getting down from a cart with harm to the entire dorsum down to the extremities, it becomes sinew painful obstruction. The main point is ST-41 *(jie xi)*."

Chapter Notes

1. The first portion of this chapter is drawn from a source similar to chapter 27 of *Divine Pivot* (translated here in chapter 25), the final portion from a source similar to chapter 43 of *Basic Questions* (translated in chapter 24), and the middle portion is related to chapter 46 of *Divine Pivot* (not translated in our book).

2. *Editors' note:* Chinese commentators interpret "blood vessels" here to mean the channels.

3. *Editors' note:* Many commentators interpret "spirit" here to refer to the protective Qi, the most yang of the various bodily types of Qi.

4. *Editors' note:* Commentators interpret this to mean the upper, middle and lower parts of the human body. The purpose of the examination is to look for areas of weakness.

5. *Editors' note:* This refers to the common people, as opposed to those who wear silk, the "great ones" mentioned later in the passage.

6. *Editors' note:* One ancient *sheng* is thought to correspond to 200ml.

7. *Editors' note:* One ancient *jin* is thought to correspond to 250g.

8. *Editors' note:* One ancient *zhang* is thought to correspond to 33cm, and 10 *zhang* make up one *chi*.

9. *Editors' note:* This refers to the third month of summer, which is the sixth lunar month.

10. *Editors' note:* The term here is *huāng mò*, which is believed to refer to the membrane above the diaphragm and below the heart.

11. *Editors' note:* The parallel passage from *Basic Questions* has *sǎn,* "to spread through."

12. Note that some of the material in this chapter is drawn from sources similar to chapter 34 of *Basic Questions* (translated here in chapter 24), chapter 75 of *Divine Pivot,* and also chapters 34 and 55 of *Basic Questions.*

13. *Editors' note:* The Chinese commentary notes that in general, pain is the master symptom of painful obstruction, because pain appears when Wind, Cold and Dampness obstruct the Blood and Qi. The presence of pain indicates that normal Qi still has the ability to oppose pathogenic Qi. When the pain disappears, it is because the Qi and Blood are in a state of deficiency. Clinical observation has shown that painful obstruction without pain is more difficult to treat than acutely painful obstruction.

14. *Editors' note:* Normal winds are those that blow from the direction appropriate to the season, e.g., from the east in springtime. Deficient winds are those that blow from an inappropriate direction, e.g., from the west in springtime.

15. *Editors' note:* Literally, the large and small divisions. Chinese commentators interpret this to mean the places where the large and small muscles come together.

16. *Editors' note:* In the original text this reads "liver painful obstruction" *(gān bì),* which is thought to be a mistake. The intended words are understood to be "tibial painful obstruction" *(gàn bì).*

CHAPTER TWENTY-NINE

Discussion of the Origins of Symptoms of Disease
(Zhu bing yuan hou lun)

C. 610 by CHAO YUAN-FANG

From "Wind" (DIVISION 1)

"WIND-DAMP PAINFUL OBSTRUCTION WITH MOVEMENT IMPAIRMENT OF THE BODY AND LIMBS" (ARTICLE 16)

Wind, cold and dampness combine to form painful obstruction. These three pathogenic factors may attack simultaneously, or one of them may predominate. When wind and dampness predominate, it is wind-damp painful obstruction. If wind and dampness attack a patient whose pores and interstices are in a state of deficiency, there is a struggle at the level of the blood and qi. The blood and qi can no longer circulate or spread. The true qi and the pathogenic qi fight each other at the level of the muscles; that is the reason why the skin and muscles are sore.

Moreover, the role of the different yang channels is to circulate and spread the yang qi throughout the whole body. When wind and dampness settle in the skin, this at first creates painful obstruction. If they injure the various yang channels, the circulation of yang qi is slowed down, its mechanism slackens, the sinews and muscles are no longer governed. This is why in wind-damp painful obstruction the movements of the body and limbs are impaired.

"WIND PAINFUL OBSTRUCTION WITH MOVEMENT IMPAIRMENT OF THE LIMBS" (ARTICLE 17)

The combination of wind, cold and dampness forms painful obstruction. The predominance of wind generates wind painful obstruction. Wind painful obstruction symptomatology is characterized by pain of the skin and muscles. The various yang channels begin and end at the hands and feet, and travel throughout the entire body.

Wind and cold settle in the muscles and skin; at first, they create painful obstruction, later they injure the yang channels and follow them to stagnate in the deficient areas. When they struggle against the blood and qi, the circulation of the qi and blood is slowed down and their mechanisms become slack. This is why with wind painful obstruction the movements of the hands and feet are impaired.

"WIND WITH MOVEMENT IMPAIRMENT IN HALF OF THE BODY" (ARTICLE 18)

In cases of hemiplegia, the spleen and stomach qi are weak, the blood and qi tend to be deficient, and pathogenic wind takes advantage of the situation. The spleen and stomach are the sea of water and grain; the essence of the water and grain is transformed into blood and qi which moisten and nourish the entire body. Because of the weakness of the spleen and stomach, the essence of water and grain cannot fulfill its nutritive function, thus leading to blood and qi deficiency. Then, with the invasion of wind, there is hemiplegia.

When feeling their radial pulse, if it is submerged and thin, it is called yin within yang. The patient suffers from hurtful sadness and lack of pleasure, he cannot tolerate the sounds of other people, his breathing is shallow, he occasionally sweats, and he cannot lift his upper limbs. If the radial pulse is collapsed, the limb is completely disabled. If both distal pulses are collapsed, he cannot be treated.

"One-Sided Wind" (article 19)

In case of one-sided wind, the pathogenic wind resides in half of the body. Certain people exhibit a deficiency in half of the body; the pathogenic wind takes advantage of the situation to injure it, thus creating one-sided wind. The symptomatology is characterized by insensitivity to pain or itching, flaccidity, or the pain of painful obstruction.

"Wind Numbness" (article 21)

Wind numbness is due to deficiency of the nutritive qi and excess of the protective qi. Wind and cold enter the muscles and prevent the blood and qi from disseminating and flowing. Its symptomatology is that scratching the skin feels like being rubbed through cloth. If the radial pulse is lax, then the skin is numb. If with numbness the pulse is deficient and rapid, survival is possible; those with a confined and racing pulse will die.

"Wind-Damp Painful Obstruction" (article 22)

The symptomatology of wind-damp painful obstruction may be either a thickening of the skin or muscle aches and pain. Wind, cold and dampness combine to form painful obstruction. If wind and dampness predominate over cold, it is wind-damp painful obstruction. It is because the blood and qi are deficient that the person is susceptible to wind-dampness and this disease develops. If it persists for a long time and is not healed, it enters into the channels and collaterals, fights in the yang channels, and may lead to a functional disability of the body, hands and feet.

"Wind-Dampness" (article 23)

Wind-dampness is the consequence of the simultaneous invasion of the body by wind and dampness. This wind is the deficient wind of the eight cardinal points. The dampness is the vapor of water dampness; it comes from the dampness of the ground that is covered by a little frost, so that the mountain water vaporizes with the addition of warmth, causing people to retire and the pores and interstices to be open, so that they are susceptible to wind-dampness. Its symptomatology includes fatigue and disorientation. If it becomes chronic in the channels, there may be flaccidity of the four limbs which become disabled. If it enters the organs there may be voice loss with loss of control of the mouth and tongue. There may also be painful obstruction and weakness of the feet, which can progress to leg qi.

"Wind Painful Obstruction" (article 24)

Painful obstruction is the simultaneous attack of the three influences wind, cold and dampness. The symptomatology is characterized by a sensation of thickening of the muscles and flesh. There may be pain. The pores are open due to a deficiency of the body, so there is susceptibility to pathogenic wind. When the illness resides in the yang, it is called wind, when it is in the yin,[1] it is called painful obstruction. When both yin and yang are affected at the same time, it is called wind painful obstruction.

Painful obstruction encountered in spring is sinew painful obstruction; the sinews retract. If it does not heal and there is renewed exposure to pathogenic influences, the disease spreads into the liver. The symptomatology is fright at night after going to bed, excessive drinking, and frequent urination.

Painful obstruction encountered in summer is vessel painful obstruction; the blood congeals and does not flow leading to a wan, yellowish complexion. If it does not heal and there is renewed exposure to pathogenic influences, the disease spreads into the heart. The symptomatology is the drumlike qi under the heart, exploding upward against the flow with wheezing [and] without [normal] passage, a dry throat, and belching.

Painful obstruction encountered in midsummer[2] is muscle painful obstruction. If it does not heal and there is renewed exposure to pathogenic influences, muscle painful obstruction spreads into the spleen. The symptomatology is fatigue of the four limbs, coughing, and vomiting of sputum.

Painful obstruction encountered in autumn is skin painful obstruction; the skin is unaware of anything. If it does not heal and later there is renewed exposure to pathogenic influences, the disease spreads into the lungs. The symptomatology is that the qi scurries and there is pain.

Painful obstruction encountered in winter is bone painful obstruction; the bones are heavy and can no longer be lifted, there is pain and disability. If it does not heal and there is renewed exposure to the pathogenic influences, it spreads into the kidneys. The symptomatology is a tendency toward distention.

When taking the pulse, if it is large and choppy, it is painful obstruction. If it comes racing, it is also painful obstruction.

Chapter Notes

1. *Editors' note:* Here, yang refers to the skin, while yin refers to the sinews and bones.
2. *Editors' note:* This is probably an error and should instead be "Indian summer," the season corresponding to the Spleen.

CHAPTER THIRTY

Confucians' Duties to their Parents
(Ru men shi qin)

C. 1200 by ZHANG ZI-HE

From "Contemporary Mistaken Impenetrable Theories on Wind, Painful Obstruction, Atrophy Disorder, and Inversion Disorder"
(DIVISION 1, CHAPTER 2)[1]

As for wind, painful obstruction, atrophy disorder and inversion disorder, they have already been described in detail in the *Inner Classic*, and it may seem redundant to discuss them at this point. This is not true, however, as many practitioners today have not read the *Inner Classic*, assuming it to contain mistaken and impenetrable concepts. These four disorders are fundamentally different, yet many contemporary [physicians] cannot distinguish among them, treating all as patterns of wind-cold, and tonifying what is deficient below. This is why there are those who are not cured for interminable days and endless years.

When the four limbs are affected, if there is movement and agitation, it is wind; if there is numbness or pain, it is painful obstruction; if there is weakness and atrophy, it is atrophy disorder; if there is rebellion[2] with heat and cold, it is inversion disorder.

This demonstrates that the clinical manifestations are not identical and that the sources are also very different. In wind, there must be a combination of wind and heat; in painful obstruction, there must be a combination of wind, cold and dampness; in atrophy disorder, the fire must dominate the metal; and in an inversion disorder, whether it is cold or hot, all start below and ascend.

Practitioners today do not analyze these origins. When they observe that the limbs are limp, they assume it is a wind disorder. However, was it not already stated in [the Warring States period book] *Zuo Commentary (Zuo zhuan)* that "with wind pernicious influence the extremities become ill"? How can anyone not know that any of the six types of qi—wind, summerheat, dryness, dampness, fire, cold—can cause the diseases of the four extremities? Let us review these elements in detail below.

WIND

Wind is characterized by its mobility and its changing nature. According to *Inner Classic*, when wind causes instability and vertigo, this is directly related to the liver-wood.[3] Are not the movements related to the sense of balance and resulting from vertigo manifestations of wind and wood? Are not bending and rigidity manifestations of wind and wood? When there are spasms and tremors of the hands and feet, eyes and mouth awry, extremely tense and contracted sinews, convulsions, frightful seizures, [things that come without] pattern, opisthotonos; when severe spitting up froth, or crying or singing, bouts of uncontrollable elation or anger, with sudden stiffness, falling and loss of consciousness—are not all of these manifestations of wind and wood?

That is why that which is mobile and changing is related to the terminal yin liver. However, when the liver-wood is in excess at this point, it is not entirely due to wind. The lung-metal is controlled by the heart-fire and therefore cannot overcome the wood.

These diseases usually appear every year during the twelfth month after the great cold period, between the third and fourth months, and between the ninth and tenth months. Why do I say this?

After the great cold period, the terminal yin is the main qi, the fourth and tenth months also correspond to the terminal yin. They are all times when the wind is in command. Between the third and fourth months, there are many violent winds and showers. Hail storms follow these damages. Between the ninth and tenth months, it is the time of changing when the leaves fall. For these reasons, when the wind is constrained to its utmost limits, it waits for these three times to manifest. In general, those with wind disease have a pulse that is similar to a tight bowstring and forceful. Who would dare to still use herbs of a hot nature that may increase its [wind's] strength?

Today, when some practitioners obtain by chance an improvement two or three times in a row with a formula, they then assume that they have mastered the treatment principle. But even when you use moxa or utilize acupuncture, how can it be sufficient to just follow a disease! These doctors strive to convince the patient to follow their methods without analyzing the hard or soft nature of the ingredients, the relative dosage of the chief and assistant herbs, and without knowing which organs, channels, areas or qi they involve. Each time they observe a wind pattern with hemiplegia, deviation of the mouth and eyes, drooling, and dimming of consciousness they automatically prescribe medicines such as Divine Treasure *(ling bao)*,[4] Greatest Treasure *(zhi bao)*,[5] Clear the Heart *(qing xin)*,[6] and Prolong Life *(xu ming)*.[7] Do they not realize that there are ginger and cinnamon in Clear the Heart formula, actinolitum and sulfur in Greatest Treasure, and that aconite is hidden in Minor Prolong Life Decoction? Only the nature of the Greatest Treasure is not quite warm. The *Inner Classic* states that to treat internal pathogenic wind, we must use acrid and cool herbs.[8] Why use mineral and intensely hot herbs to treat wind? Some practitioners add heat to treat heat. Doing it once is already excessive; how can they repeat it yet again?

That is why the contemporary physician Liu He-Jian[9] made Ledebouriella Powder that Sagely Unblocks *(fang feng tong sheng san)* and Apprehend Wind Pill *(sou feng wan)*, while Cheng Can-Zheng[10] recommends Dispel Wind Pill *(qu feng wan)* and Change Bone Special Pill *(huan gu dan)*. These have been used successfully by those who prescribed them. However, in an attempt to confuse the facts, numerous attacks have been leveled against them.

I have also read in chapter 69[11] of *Inner Classic* that, when the five constraints arrive at their extreme expression, they cause disease. Furthermore, wind illnesses are characterized by sudden onset and rapid transformation. This is why the three therapeutic methods of sweating, purging and vomiting are effective to cure wind-fright and convulsive disorders. These methods are clearly discussed in *Inner Classic*.

In terms of the five constraints, when the wood is constrained it should be spread out. Vomiting is used to narrowly spread its stagnation out. Through sweating, wind follows the sweat out. Purging expels the old to regenerate the new. These are the three methods of sweating, purging and vomiting. Wind diseases cured by these three methods are countless, so why abandon them and not use them? I am afraid that physicians to come will denigrate these methods, so I have laid them out here.

In the past, a Mr. Yen had a wind illness that manifested as spasms and convulsions starting in the right arm and then in the right leg. These occurred between sixty and seventy times during each attack. After a certain period of time, the left side became affected with the same frequency. The disease did not heal and the patient started to stare straight ahead, with bouts of loss of consciousness. He consulted me after a few months. First, I expelled the cold-phlegm (3 to 4 *sheng* of it). Then I used Lead Out Water Pill or Powder with the Effectiveness of Yu[12] *(dao shui yu gong wan san)* to induce twenty purgings. After that I used the acrid, cool formula Ledebouriella Powder that Sagely Unblocks. After a few days, he was cured. Therefore I wrote this to demonstrate it.

PAINFUL OBSTRUCTION

The manifestations of painful obstruction are paresthesia and numbness. It is produced by the combination of pathogenic wind, dampness and cold.

Inner Classic states that when the wind pernicious influence predominates, it is moving painful obstruction.[13] The wind is received by the yang, so this painful obstruction moves. It is worse during the day and calmer at night. The common-run do not recognize it and instead call it rushing and pouring (*zǒu zhù* 走注) or the disease with pain like a tiger bite.

When pathogenic cold predominates, it is severe painful obstruction. The cold is received by the yin, so the painful obstruction is intensely painful. The pain is calmer during the day and worse at night. The common-run do not recognize it and instead call it ghost's defiance (*guǐ wǔ* 鬼忤).

When pathogenic dampness predominates, it is fixed painful obstruction. The dampness is received by the sinews, vessels, skin and muscles, so this painful obstruction is fixed and does not go away. It penetrates the muscles and settles in the bones. The common-run do not recognize it and instead call it hemilateral withering (*piān kū* 偏枯).

The onset of this disease usually occurs during the rainy period of the four seasons, in the third and ninth months, the months when the greater yang, water and cold are activated. This is why the disease predominates when the grasses are withered and the water is cold, when people work in damp areas, when there is overexertion, when they are exposed to the wind and rain, or when they lay down in damp places and dampness penetrates from the outside. In addition, over the entire territory, there are differences in environmental qi such as cold and heat, hard and supple endowments, diets, and living circumstances. None of these does not play adversely off the others. Thus, each received pathogen has its own depth. Sometimes there may be pain; sometimes not. Sometimes there may be feeling; sometimes numbness. Sometimes the sinews are contracted and cannot relax, or they are loose and cannot contract. When they meet with cold there is tightness and urgency; when they meet with heat there is laxity. Do not confuse them.

If skin painful obstruction does not heal, it transforms into muscle painful obstruction. If muscle painful obstruction does not heal, it becomes vessel painful obstruction. If vessel painful obstruction does not heal, it becomes sinew painful obstruction. If sinew painful obstruction does not heal, it transforms into bone painful obstruction. When the disease becomes chronic, it lodges in its corresponding organ. If the different yin and yang organs are both affected, even a competent physician will not be able to provide an effective remedy. In general, patients with painful obstruction have a submerged and choppy pulse.

Nowadays, people who discuss formulas, when they come upon the various painful obstruction disorders, treat them as leg qi. Do they not know that *Inner Classic* never talks about leg qi? Some people claim that many texts mention leg qi, and prescribe corresponding formulas. If we only take *Basic Questions* into account, does this mean that all the other texts are wrong?

They say that the source of painful obstruction is damp-heat, and that wind and cold are additional. When the three pathogenic influences join, they create painful obstruction. How can it be that those who treat it do not investigate the channels and collaterals, do not distinguish the yin from the yang organs, do not differentiate between exterior and interior, and just go along treating it as damp-cold leg qi? They aconite it, frankincense it, myrrh it, using every type of drying hot substance to attack it, moxa it at CV-12 (*zhong wan*), cauterize it under the umbilicus, and use fire at ST-36 (*zu san li*) on it, steam it, iron it, put hot water on it, put hot bricks on it until they have led to roughness and stagnation such that both the front and back [urine and stool] are closed, deficiency and dryness have turned more severe, and the flesh daily wastes away. When there is a pronounced lack of appetite, the pathogenic qi invades from the exterior and, even if a Bian Que or Hua Tuo[14] were to treat the patient, they would be of no help.

How does this come about? It is the stagnation of cold-phlegm between the chest and diaphragm. Painful obstruction itself is not terminal; death is due to the mistakes of physicians. Although the steam treatment is also used, you must first get rid of the cold-phlegm. Thereafter all the various therapies become effective.

Inner Classic says that the five yin organs have their stream (*shū* 輸) points and the six yang organs have their sea (*hé* 合) points.[15] By following the root division of the channel, we find that each thing has its starting point; if we use stone probes to tonify, the painful obstruction disease is cured. This has been clearly described in *Inner Classic*; why not mention it?

When the civil servant Wei De-Xin went to take an exam in winter, he caught a major cold on the way. His true qi was fundamentally weak, and added to this he stayed in damp places, and his diet was unbalanced. As all these factors occurred in winter, he developed bone painful obstruction. The bones are governed by the kidneys. The high bone of the lumbars was bad and useless. The hips were as if they were broken. His face was as black as ashes, and he had pain in the front and the back. He had atrophy, inversion and a strong desire to sleep. The physicians he saw had all treated his condition as kidney deficiency. I first used the "ling-long"[16] ironing and steaming method for several days. Next, I prescribed bitter herbs; once the upper drainage was completed, he had eliminated two to three *sheng* of cold phlegm. When the bottom is deficient and the top is excessive, it is clear to see. Next, I prescribed blander herbs: Rhizoma Atractylodis Macrocephalae *(bai zhu)* to eliminate the spleen dampness, Sclerotium Poriae Cocos *(fu ling)* to nourish the kidney water, Ramulus Cinnamomi Cassiae *(gui zhi)* to attack the wood wind. When pathogenic cold predominates, add Rhizoma Zingiberis Officinalis Recens *(sheng jiang)* and Radix Lateralis Aconiti Carmichaeli Praeparata *(fu zi)*; if there is no excess, do not add them. In addition, I needled BL-23 *(shen shu)* and KI-3 *(tai xi)* every other day. Within a month, everything was back to normal.

I often use the three methods of treating cold damage—sweating, vomiting and purging—to treat wind, painful obstruction, atrophy disorder and inversion disorder. A cure is frequently obtained.

FORMULAS

Ledebouriella Powder that Sagely Unblocks

(*fáng fēng tōng shèng sǎn*)

防風通聖散

Radix Ledebouriellae Divaricatae *(fang feng)*	1 *liang*[17]
Fructus Forsythiae Suspensae *(lian qiao)*	1 *liang*
Herba Ephedrae *(ma huang)*	1 *liang*
Herba Menthae Haplocalycis *(bo he)*	1 *liang*
Herba seu Flos Schizonepetae Tenuifoliae (*jing jie*)	1 *liang*
Rhizoma Atractylodis Macrocephalae *(bai zhu)*	1 *liang*
Fructus Gardeniae Jasminoidis *(zhi zi)*	1 *liang*
Radix Ligustici Chuanxiong *(chuan xiong)*	1 *liang*
Radix Angelicae Sinensis *(dang gui)*	1 *liang*
Radix Paeoniae Lactiflorae *(bai shao)*	1 *liang*
Radix et Rhizoma Rhei *(da huang)*	1 *liang*
Mirabilitum *(mang xiao)*	1 *liang*
Gypsum *(shi gao)*	1 *liang*
Radix Scutellariae Baicalensis *(huang qin)*	1 *liang*
Radix Platycodi Grandiflori *(jie geng)*	1 *liang*
Radix Glycyrrhizae Uralensis *(gan cao)*	2 *liang*
Talcum *(hua shi)*	3 *liang*

Grind to a fine powder, measure two qian, add three slices of fresh ginger and boil.

Apprehend Wind Pill (*sōu fēng wán*)

搜風丸

Radix Ginseng *(ren shen)*
Sclerotium Poriae Cocos *(fu ling)*
Rhizoma Arisaematis *(tian nan xing)*
Rhizoma Pinelliae Ternatae *(ban xia)*
Rhizoma Zingiberis Officinalis *(gan jiang)*
Alumen *(ming fan)*
Calcitum *(han shui shi)*
Concha Cyclinae Sinensis *(hai ge ke)*
Herba Menthae Haplocalycis *(bo he)*
Herba Agastaches seu Pogostemi *(huo xiang)*

Dispel Wind Pill (*qū fēng wán*)

祛風丸

Radix Astragali Membranacei *(huang qi)*
Fructus Citri Aurantii *(zhi ke)*
Radix Ledebouriellae Divaricatae *(fang feng)*
Radix Paeoniae Lactiflorae *(bai shao)*
Fructus Lycii *(gou qi zi)*
Radix Glycyrrhizae Uralensis *(gan cao)*
Cortex Lycii Radicis *(di gu pi)*
Radix Rehmanniae Glutinosae *(sheng di huang)*
Radix Rehmanniae Glutinosae Conquitae *(shu di huang)*

Change Bone Special Pill (*huàn gǔ dān*)

換骨丹

Os Tigris *(hu gu)*	1 *liang*
Radix Ledebouriellae Divaricatae *(fang feng)*	1 *liang*
Radix Achyranthis Bidentatae *(niu xi)*	1 *liang*
Radix Angelicae Sinensis *(dang gui)*	1 *liang*
Radix et Rhizoma Notopterygii *(qiang huo)*	1 *liang*
Radix Angelicae Pubescentis *(du huo)*	1 *liang*
Plastrum Testudinis *(gui ban)*	1 *liang*
Radix Gentianae Qinjiao *(qin jiao)*	1 *liang*
Rhizoma Dioscoreae Hypoglaucae *(bei xie)*	1 *liang*
Excrementum Bombycis Mori *(can sha)*	1 *liang*
Lignum Pini Nodi *(song jie)*	1 *liang*
Fructus Lycii *(gou qi zi)*	2.5 *liang*
Radix Solani Melongenae *(qie gen)*	2 *liang*

Lead Out Water Pill or Powder with the Effectiveness of Yu (*daǒ shuǐ yǔ gōng wán [sǎn]*)

導水禹功丸[散]

Talcum *(hua shi)*	4 *liang*
Semen Pharbitidis *(qian niu zi)*	4 *liang*

Radix et Rhizoma Rhei *(da huang)* . . . . 2 *liang*
Radix Scutellariae Baicalensis *(huang qin)* . . . . 2 *liang*

Grind to a fine powder, add water drop by drop to make pills the size of Semen Sterculiae Scaphigerae *(pang da hai)*. Take 50 pills each time with warm water before going to bed. The dosage may be doubled.

Chapter Notes

1. *Editors' note:* Only the first two sections of this chapter, regarding wind and painful obstruction, are translated here.
2. *Editors' note:* "Rebellion" here means that the extremities are drawn toward the trunk instead of extending.
3. *Editors' note:* This is a paraphrase of a statement found in chapter 74 of *Basic Questions*.
4. *Editors' note:* It is unclear which formula this refers to.
5. *Editors' note:* It is unclear which formula this refers to. While there is a common formula known as Greatest Treasure Special Pill *(zhi bao dan)* used for Windstroke, it does not contain Actinolitum *(yang qi shi)*.
6. *Editors' note:* It is unclear which formula this refers to. None of the formulas in our sources with the words "clear the heart" *(qīng xīn)* in their names contain any form of cinnamon.
7. *Editors' note:* This probably refers to Minor Prolong Life Decoction *(xiao xu ming tang)*.
8. *Editors' note:* This quotation is drawn from chapter 74 of *Basic Questions*.
9. *Editors' note:* Better known as Liu Yuan-Su (c. 1120–1200), he is one of the four great masters of the Jin-Yuan period.
10. *Editors' note:* It is unclear who this physician is.
11. *Editors' note:* Modern Chinese commentators have noted that this discussion is actually found in chapter 71 of *Basic Questions*, not in chapter 69, as stated here.
12. *Editors' note:* Yu is one of the great cultural heroes of China. Among his many achievements was the taming of the great flood.
13. *Editors' note:* This quotation is drawn from chapter 43 of *Basic Questions*, which is translated in chapter 24 of this book.
14. *Editors' note:* These are two famous physicians. The former is a legendary figure of the Warring States period, and the latter lived at the end of the Han dynasty.
15. *Editors' note:* This quotation is drawn from chapter 43 of *Basic Questions*, which is translated in chapter 24 of this book.
16. *Editors' note:* "Ling-long" is the sound of tinkling jade. We are unfamiliar with the specifics of this method.
17. Note on measurements: one *liang* (37.5g) equals 10 *qian*; one *qian* equals 10 *fen*.

CHAPTER THIRTY-ONE

Introduction to Medicine
(Yi xue ru men)

C. 1575 by LI YAN

"PAINFUL WIND"[1]

In those who are timid and thin, painful wind is primarily related to the internal cause of blood deficiency with fire. In those intrepid ones with well filled-out bodies, it is usually related to the external cause of wind-dampness generating phlegm. Since it can circulate throughout the entire body, it is called panarthralgia. When the pain is very intense and feels like a tiger bite, it is called white tiger wind. The pain will be more intense at night, as the blood circulates in the yin.

If there is more pain, it means that there is a lot of phlegm-fire; if there is swelling, there is more wind-dampness. As for phlegm-fire, while the internal factors of the seven emotions and the six desires may be present, or exhaustion of the fluids after an illness, with heat in the blood becoming agitated, its manifestation depends nonetheless on the action of externally contracted pathogens. When the bones and joints are extremely painful, after a long period the hands and feet will then become contracted and twisted.

Although wind-dampness is secondary to external causes such as walking in the cold, sitting in damp places, cooling off in drafts, only after the blood is hot is there congealing, stagnation and turbidity. This is what makes the pain. When it is severe there are blocks of nodules in the body.

In the presence of both phlegm-fire and wind-dampness, use the old Dragon and Tiger Special Pill (long hu dan).

If there is cold damage with pain throughout all of the body's joints, wind-cold has invaded the muscles and bones.

If there are miscellaneous diseases with generalized body pain, it is stagnation of wind-phlegm; prescribe the Two-Cured Decoction (er chen tang), adding Rhizoma Arisaematis (tian nan xing), Radix et Rhizoma Notopterygii (qiang huo), Rhizoma Atractylodis (cang zhu), Radix Angelicae Dahuricae (bai zhi), wine-fried Radix Scutellariae Baicalensis (jiu huang qin), Succus Bambusae (zhu li) and ginger juice. If there is also blood stasis, add Semen Persicae (tao ren) and Flos Carthami Tinctorii (hong hua).

If the damp-phlegm and blood stasis are everywhere in the body with pain running through both flanks, prescribe Control Mucus Special Pill (kong xian dan), adding Semen Persicae (tao ren) paste to prepare the pills, or use Minor Stomach Special Pill (xiao wei dan) to purge them.

[The text continues by specifying herbal prescriptions appropriate for each location at the level of the trunk and limbs.]

"Painful Obstruction"

Painful obstruction means that the qi is blocked and obstructed and cannot flow smoothly. There may be pain and itching, numbness and paresthesia, or weakness of the hands and feet similar to atrophy. However, atrophy is related to internal causes associated with blood deficiency and blazing fire with scorched lungs. Painful obstruction is due to invasion of pathogenic wind, cold and dampness. However, the external pernicious influences can only invade the body if there is an underlying weakness of the qi and blood; that is the reason why chronic painful obstruction may progress toward atrophy disorder.

Painful obstruction is also one type of wind attack. However, in a pure wind attack, it is the yang that is affected, whereas in the case of painful obstruction which combines pathogenic wind, cold and dampness, it is the yin that is affected. That is why this condition is more serious, as exemplified in the case of the great Song dynasty physician Qian Zhong-Yang,[2] who was himself affected by encompassing painful obstruction with hemiplegia and could not completely cure himself.

The *Classic*[3] specifies that in the spring, it is sinew painful obstruction; in summer, vessel painful obstruction; during late summer, muscle painful obstruction; in autumn, skin painful obstruction; in winter, bone painful obstruction. This shows that the skin, vessels, muscles, sinews and bones are affected by pathogenic wind, cold and dampness at different times. In general, wind-dampness affects mostly the upper part of the body with numbness and paresthesia of the shoulders and back, along with painful stiffness of the hands and wrists. Damp-cold affects mostly the lower part, with legs and feet feeling heavy and wooden. When there is simultaneous invasion of the upper and lower parts, the body [feels] as if trapped in a vise and the legs feel as if they are weighed down by stones. We must treat according to whether wind, cold or dampness predominates. With wind the pain moves around. With cold there is severe pain with whole body stiffness, along with cold and painfully obstructed hands and feet. It is like painful wind. With dampness there is usually edema with heaviness that is fixed and does not move.

When wind predominates, use Lindera Powder to Smooth the Flow of Qi *(wu yao shun qi san)*, Three Painful Obstruction Decoction *(san bi tang)*, Maidservant from Yue Decoction *(yue bi tang)*, Solo Siegesbeckia Pill *(dan xi xian wan)*. When cold predominates, use Five-Accumulation Powder *(wu ji san)* plus Rhizoma Gastro-diae Elatae *(tian ma)* and Radix Lateralis Aconiti Carmichaeli Praeparata *(fu zi)* or Remove Painful Obstuction Decoction *(juan bi tang)*. For damp-cold, use Five-Accumulation Interchange and Additions Powder *(wu ji jiao jia san)*.[4] When dampness predominates, use Ligusticum and Poria Decoction *(chuan xiong fu ling tang)*, Tangkuei Decoction to Draw Out Pain (dang gui nian tong tang), Stephania and Astragalus Decoction *(fang ji huang qi tang)*, Notopterygium Decoction to Overcome Dampness *(qiang huo sheng shi tang)*, or Dipsacus Pill *(xu duan wan)*.

Painful obstruction with cold such that the body is cold and cannot get warm, along with heaviness and cold in the lower back and lower limbs, is severely cold painful obstruction. Use Three Painful Obstruction Decoction *(san bi tang)* combined with Three-Five-Seven Powder *(san wu qi san)*; or use Comfort the Channels Decoction *(shu jing tang)*[5] or Prepared Aconite Pill to Regulate the Middle *(fu zi li zhong tang)*.

For hot painful obstruction, or heat produced from dampness, or wind-cold constraint generating heat with a sensation like a mouse crawling through the entire body, slackening of the lips, and changes in the color of the muscles and flesh, prescribe Decoction that Disseminates and Brightens with Cimicifuaga *(xuan ming sheng ma tang)*.[6]

For wind-cold-damp-hot painful obstruction, we prescribe Two-Marvel Powder *(er miao san)* taking equal amounts of Rhizoma Atractylodis *(cang zhu)* and Cortex Phellodendri *(huang bai)*, adding Os Tigris *(hu gu)* and half the dosage of Radix Ledebouriellae Divaricatae *(fang feng)*.

When pathogenic wind-cold-dampness attack simultaneously and settle in the skin, they are tenacious yet imperceptible. With exposure to cold there is a tightness and urgency; with heat, a laxity. It resonates with the lungs and manifests as dyspnea and fullness in the chest.

When it is located in the vessels, there is blood stasis, the six pulses are tight and choppy, and the complexion lacks color. It resonates with the heart and manifests as irritability of the heart, ascending qi, dry throat and belching.

When it is located in the muscles, there is numbness of the four limbs. It resonates with the spleen and manifests as a weary sensation and vomiting. When it is located in the sinews, there is flexion with inability to extend. It resonates with the liver and manifests as nocturnal fright, dysuria and hypogastric pain.

When it is located in the bones, there is a heavy sensation with difficulty in lifting the limbs, and the coccyx [feels as if it] is where the heel should be and the spine where the head belongs. It resonates with the kidneys and manifests as epigastric and abdominal bloating and fullness.

When the pernicious influences first penetrate the skin and blood vessels, they are mild and the disease is easy to treat. When they stagnate in the sinews and bones, in a chronic phase without causing pain but with numbness, the disease is difficult to treat. If it goes on for a very long time without a cure and the five painful obstructions are again subjected to the three pathogens, the condition will spread to the five yin organs. When the patient becomes bedridden, has profuse diarrhea and a poor appetite, and is like an organ-stroke, he will die.

At the onset of the disease, if there is stiffness and pain, disperse the wind and dislodge the phlegm. If there is a heavy sensation, eliminate the dampness and promote the circulation of qi. If the illness is chronic, distinguish between deficiency and excess of the qi or blood, and between the relative amounts of phlegm and blood stasis.

For those with qi deficiency and painful obstruction, the joints are not irrigated and the body feels like it has emerged out of water. This is yang deficiency with yin excess. Use Four-Gentlemen Decoction *(si jun zi tang)* plus Cortex Cinnamomi Cassiae *(rou gui)* and Radix Lateralis Aconiti Carmichaeli Praeparata *(fu zi)*; or use Aconite and Lateral Aconite Pill *(chuan fu wan)*.

For those with blood deficiency and painful obstruction, there is paresthesia of the skin. Prescribe Ledebouriella Decoction from *Formulas to Aid the Living* *(ji sheng fang feng tang)*[7] or Astagalus Decoction to Construct the Middle *(huang qi jian zhong tang)*, replacing Maltose *(yi tang)* with Ramulus Cinnamomi Cassiae *(gui zhi)*.

If there is concurrent blood stasis, prescribe Four-Substance Decoction *(si wu tang)*, adding Semen Persicae *(tao ren)*, Flos Carthami Tinctorii *(hong hua)*, Succus Bambusae *(zhu li)* and ginger juice.

If there is concurrent phlegm, the hands and feet have numb painful obstruction, hypersomnia and vertigo. Use Poria Decoction from *Formulas to Aid the Living* *(ji sheng fu ling tang)*[8] or Two-Cured Decoction *(er chen tang)* with the addition of Succus Bambusae *(zhu li)* and ginger juice.

If the kidney fat[9] dries up and does not move and the marrow is sparse and the sinews weak with chills, spasms and tension, use All-Inclusive Great Tonifying Decoction *(shi quan da bu tang)* or Earth Immortal Special Pill *(di*

xian dan),[10] in combination with the five painful obstructions massage method.

If, at the onset of the illness, Radix Ginseng *(ren shen)*, Radix Astragali Membranacei *(huang qi)*, Radix Angelicae Sinensis *(dang gui)* and Radix Rehmanniae Glutinosae Conquitae *(shu di huang)* are prescribed too quickly, they may cause stagnation of the qi and blood with the pathogen being confined in the channels and collaterals, instead of being dispersed. In cases of deficiency, use Aconite Porridge *(wu tou zhou)*[11] and Powder to Promote Movement of Dampness and Flow of Qi *(xing shi liu qi san)*.

Paresthesia corresponds to qi deficiency, whereas numbness corresponds to a coagulation of phlegm; these are general concepts. Sometimes when pathogenic wind, cold and dampness invade the organism by taking advantage of deficiency, there is both paresthesia and numbness. Sometimes with both qi deficiency and blood deficiency, there is numbness without insensibility. When the numbness is like painful obstruction, although the patient does not feel pain or itchiness, they still feel a slight flowing of qi. For the arms, wind and dampness often combine; for the legs, it is usually cold and dampness. When one has numbness, not only is there no pain or itchiness, but also no sensation of qi flowing.

Constant numbness corresponds to an obstruction of the qi by the blood, whereas intermittent insensibility corresponds to damp-phlegm. In all cases there is coagulation and stagnation in the channels and collaterals, and loss of flow through the blood vessels. This is called insensibility *(bù rén* 不仁*)*. When there is additional fire from deficiency, the muscles will twitch. Do not erroneously treat it as wind.

When the pain and paresthesia circulate throughout the body, it is called encompassing painful obstruction *(zhōu bì* 周痹*)*. The liver qi does not circulate properly, so we must first cause sweating and then tonify. Use Astragalus Decoction *(huang qi tang)*. If, when the eyes are open, the paresthesia and numbness disappear gradually, but when the eyes are closed they become more intense, use Raise the Yang and Harmonize the Middle Decoction *(sheng yang he zhong tang)*.

For paresthesia of the skin, use Tonify the Qi Decoction *(bu qi tang)*. For paresthesia of the limbs with qi deficiency, use Tonify the Middle and Augment the Qi Decoction *(bu zhong yi qi tang)*, removing Radix Angelicae Sinensis *(dang gui)* and Pericarpium Citri Reticulatae *(chen pi)*, and adding Fructus Schisandrae Chinensis *(wu wei zi)*, Radix Paeoniae Lactiflorae *(bai* shao) and Radix Glycyrrhizae Uralensis (gan cao). For serious deficiency with the addition of wind, use Tonify the Middle and Augment the Qi Decoction (bu zhong yi qi tang), adding Radix Lateralis Aconiti Carmichaeli Praeparata (fu zi), Radix Linderae Strychnifoliae (wu yao), Radix et Rhizoma Notopterygii (qiang huo), Radix Ledebouriellae Divaricatae (fang feng) and Rhizoma Gastrodiae Elatae (tian ma).

If all ten fingers have paresthesia and numbness, it indicates that there is damp-phlegm and dead blood stasis at the level of the stomach. Use Two-Cured Decoction (er chen tang), adding Rhizoma Atractylodis Macrocephalae (bai zhu), Rhizoma Atractylodis (cang zhu), Semen Persicae (tao ren), Flos Carthami Tinctorii (hong hua) and a little Radix Lateralis Aconiti Carmichaeli Praeparata (fu zi) to promote movement in the channels.

If there is hemiplegia and pain of the limbs on the left side, associated with deviation of the mouth and eyes to the right, it indicates the presence of wind in the exterior. Use Gastrodia and Astragalus Deoction (tian ma huang qi tang).

For paresthesia in both legs, use Conduct the Qi Decoction (dao qi tang). For paresthesia of both feet with a burning sensation, use Three-Marvel Powder (san miao san).

When the sour taste injures the sinews, there is loosening; when the salty taste injures the bones, there is atrophy. This can cause the person to become feverish and transform into such problems as severe painful obstruction, paresthesia and numbness. Those who are cautious about the disease must avoid fish, seafood, noodles, sauces and alcohol. Meat is yang and aids fire, but can be eaten in moderation. If there is an excess of strong tastes, there will be an excess of elimination at the bottom, and an accumulation and sensation of fullness at the top. First use Two-Cured Decoction (er chen tang) with the addition of Radix Paeoniae (shao yao) and Rhizoma Coptidis (huang lian) to direct the fire downward. Then use herbs according to the symptoms.

PRESCRIPTIONS

Dragon and Tiger Special Pill (lóng hǔ dān)
龍虎丹

Radix Aconiti Kusnezoffii (cao wu) .... 1 liang[12]
Rhizoma Atractylodis (cang zhu) .... 1 liang
Radix Angelicae Dahuricae (bai zhi) .... 1 liang
Gummi Olibanum (ru xiang) .... 2 qian

Myrrha (mo yao) .... 2 qian
Radix Angelicae Sinensis (dang gui) .... 5 qian
Radix Achyranthis Bidentatae (niu xi) .... 5 qian

Grind all the ingredients into a powder, add water and mix well, then add wine to make marble-sized pills. Ingest with warm wine.

Two-Cured Decoction (èr chén tāng)
二陳湯

Pericarpium Citri Reticulatae (chen pi) .... 2 qian
Rhizoma Pinelliae Ternatae (ban xia) .... 1 qian
Sclerotium Poriae Cocos (fu ling) .... 8 fen
Radix Glycyrrhizae Uralensis (gan cao) .... 4 fen

Add three slices of ginger, boil in water and drink warm.

Control Mucus Special Pill (kòng xián dān)
控涎丹

Radix Euphorbiae Kansui (gan sui)
Radix Euphorbiae seu Knoxiae (da ji)
Semen Sinapis Albae (bai jie zi)

Grind equal amounts of the above to make small pills. Take in one qian doses at bedtime.

Minor Stomach Special Pill (xiǎo wèi dān)
小胃丹

Flos Daphnes Genkwa (yuan hua) .... 5 qian
Radix Euphorbiae Kansui (gan sui) .... 5 qian
Radix Euphorbiae seu Knoxiae (da ji) .... 5 qian
Radix et Rhizoma Rhei (da huang) .... 5 qian
Cortex Phellodendri (huang bai) .... 3 liang

Prepare pills the size of castor oil seeds. Take 20 to 30 pills each time.

Lindera Powder to Smooth the Flow of Qi
(wū yào shùn qì sǎn)
烏藥順氣散

Herba Ephedrae (ma huang) .... 2 liang
Pericarpium Citri Reticulatae (chen pi) .... 2 liang
Radix Linderae Strychnifoliae (wu yao) .... 2 liang
Bombyx Batryticatus (jiang can) .... 1 liang
Radix Ligustici Chuanxiong (chuan xiong) .... 1 liang
Fructus Citri Aurantii (zhi ke) .... 1 liang
Radix Glycyrrhizae Uralensis (gan cao) .... 1 liang
Radix Angelicae Dahuricae (bai zhi) .... 1 liang
Radix Platycodi Grandiflori (jie geng) .... 1 liang

Quick-fried Rhizoma Zingiberis
Officinalis (*pao jiang*). . . . . .5 *qian*

Grind into a fine powder, measure and boil three *qian* with three slices of ginger and one jujube fruit, and drink.

Three Painful Obstruction Decoction (*sān bì tāng*)
三痹湯
Cortex Eucommiae Ulmoidis (*du zhong*) . . . . .8 *fen*
Radix Ledebouriellae Divaricatae (*fang feng*) . . . . . . .8 *fen*
Cortex Cinnamomi Cassiae (*rou gui*). . . . . .8 *fen*
Radix Dipsaci Asperi (*xu duan*) . . . . .8 *fen*
Radix Ginseng (*ren shen*). . . . . .8 *fen*
Radix Angelicae Sinensis (*dang gui*) . . . . .8 *fen*
Radix Gentianae Qinjiao (*qin jiao*) . . . . .8 *fen*
Radix Ligustici Chuanxiong (*chuan xiong*) . . . . .8 *fen*
Sclerotium Poriae Cocos (*fu ling*). . . . . .8 *fen*
Dry-fried Radix Paeoniae Lactiflorae
(*chao bai shao*) . . . . .8 *fen*
Dry-fried Radix Astragali Membranacei
(*chao huang qi*). . . . . .8 *fen*
Herba cum Radice Asari (*xi xin*). . . . . .8 *fen*
Radix Angelicae Pubescentis (*du huo*) . . . . .8 *fen*
Wine-fried Radix Achyranthis Bidentatae
(*jiu chao niu xi*) . . . . .8 *fen*
Radix Rehmanniae Glutinosae (*sheng di huang*) . . . . .8 *fen*
Honey-toasted Radix Glycyrrhizae Uralensis
(*zhi gan cao*) . . . . .8 *fen*

Mix with two bowls of water, two to three slices of ginger, and one jujube fruit. Boil down to half the quantity, drain and drink.

Maidservant from Yue Decoction (*yuè bì tāng*)
越婢湯
Herba Ephedrae (*ma huang*). . . . . .6 *liang*[13]
Gypsum (*shi gao*). . . . . .0.5 *jin*
Rhizoma Zingiberis Officinalis Recens
(*sheng jiang*). . . . . .3 *liang*
Radix Glycyrrhizae Uralensis (*gan cao*) . . . . .2 *liang*
Fructus Zizyphi Jujubae (*da zao*) 15

Solo Siegesbeckia Pill (*dān xī xiān wán*)
單豨薟丸
Grind Herba Siegesbeckiae (*xi xian cao*) into a powder, heat up and concentrate the honey, and make small pills. Take 40 pills each time on an empty stomach with wine.

Five-Accumulation Powder (*wǔ jī sǎn*)
五積散
[See formulas at end of chapter 5.]

Remove Painful Obstuction Decoction (*juǎn bì tāng*)
蠲痺湯
[See formulas at end of chapter 5.]

Ligusticum and Poria Decoction
(*chuān xiōng fú líng tāng*)
川芎茯苓湯
Sclerotium Poriae Cocos (*fu ling*). . . . . .2 *liang*
Cortex Mori Albae Radicis (*sang bai pi*). . . . . .2 *liang*
Radix Ledebouriellae Divaricatae
(*fang feng*) . . . . .1 *liang* 5 *qian*
Ramulus Cinnamomi Cassiae (*gui zhi*). . . . . .1 *liang* 5 *qian*
Radix Ligustici Chuanxiong (*chuan xiong*). .1 *liang* 5 *qian*
Radix Paeoniae Lactiflorae (*bai shao*) . . . . . .1 *liang* 5 *qian*
Herba Ephedrae (*ma huang*). . . . . .1 *liang* 5 *qian*

Grind into a powder, mix five *qian* with a bowl of water and one Fructus Zizyphi Jujubae (*da zao*), boil down to three-quarters of the volume, drain, and drink warm with ginger. The effect is obtained as soon as there is sweating.

Tangkuei Decoction to Draw Out Pain
(*dāng guī niān tòng tāng*)
當歸拈痛湯
[See formulas at end of chapter 7.]

Stephania and Astragalus Decoction
(*fáng jǐ huáng qí tāng*)
防己黃蓍湯
Radix Aristolochiae Fangchi (*fang ji*) . . . . .1 *liang*[14]
Radix Astragali Membranacei (*huang qi*) . . . . .1 *liang* 1 *fen*
Honey-toasted Radix Glycyrrhizae
Uralensis (*zhi gan cao*) . . . . .5 *qian*
Rhizoma Atractylodis Macrocephalae
(*bai zhu*) . . . . .7 *qian* 5 *fen*

Grind into a powder, add four slices of Rhizoma Zingiberis Officinalis Recens (*sheng jiang*) and one Fructus Zizyphi Jujubae (*da zao*). Boil in water. Drink in two portions.

Notopterygium Decoction to Overcome Dampness
(*qiāng huó shèng shī tāng*)
羌活勝濕湯
Rhizhoma et Radix Notopterygii (*qiang huo*) . . . . . .1 *qian*

Radix Angelicae Pubescentis (*du huo*)............. 1 *qian*
Radix Glycyrrhizae Uralensis (*gan cao*)............. 5 *fen*
Rhizoma et Radix Ligustici (*gao ben*)............. 5 *fen*
Radix Ligustici Chuanxiong (*chuan xiong*).......... 5 *fen*
Radix Ledebouriallae Divaricatae (*fang feng*)....... 5 *fen*
Fructus Viticis (*man jing zi*)..................... 3 *fen*

Dipsacus Pill (*xù duàn wán*)

續斷丸

Radix Dipsaci Asperi (*xu duan*).................. 2 *liang*
Rhizoma Dioscoreae Hypoglaucae (*bei xie*)........ 2 *liang*
Radix Achyranthis Bidentatae (*niu xi*)............. 2 *liang*
Fructus Chaenomelis Lagenariae (*mu gua*)........ 2 *liang*
Cortex Eucommiae Ulmoidis (*du zhong*).......... 2 *liang*

Grind into a powder, heat up and concentrate in honey, and make into pills (four pills per *liang*). Chew one pill with warm wine each time.

Three-Five-Seven Powder (*sān wǔ qī sǎn*)

三五七散

Radix Ginseng (*ren shen*)..................... 3 *liang*
Radix Lateralis Aconiti Carmichaeli
    Praeparata (*fu zi*)....................... 3 *liang*
Herba cum Radice Asari (*xi xin*)................ 3 *liang*
Radix Glycyrrhizae Uralensis (*gan cao*).......... 5 *qian*
Rhizoma Zingiberis Officinalis (*gan jiang*)........ 5 *qian*
Fructus Corni Officinalis (*shan zhu yu*).......... 5 *qian*
Radix Ledebouriellae Divaricatae (*fang feng*)...... 5 *qian*
Radix Dioscoreae Oppositae (*shan yao*)........... 5 *qian*

Grind into a powder. Take two *qian* in warm wine before meals.

Prepared Aconite Pill to Regulate the Middle
(*fù zǐ lǐ zhōng tāng*)

附子理中湯

Radix Lateralis Aconiti Carmichaeli
    Praeparata (*fu zi*)....................... 3 *liang*
Rhizoma Zingiberis Officinalis (*gan jiang*)........ 3 *liang*
Radix Ginseng (*ren shen*)..................... 3 *liang*
Rhizoma Atractylodis Macrocephalae
    (*bai zhu*)............................. 3 *liang*
Honey-toasted Radix Glycyrrhizae
    Uralensis (*zhi gan cao*)................... 3 *liang*

Grind into a powder and make into one *qian* pill with honey. Take one pill as a draft on an empty stomach.

Two-Marvel Powder (*èr miào sǎn*)

二妙散

[See formulas at end of chapter 6.]

Four-Gentlemen Decoction (*sì jūn zǐ tāng*)

四君子湯

Radix Ginseng (*ren shen*)..................... 1 *qian*
Rhizoma Atractylodis Macrocephalae (*bai zhu*).... 2 *qian*
Sclerotium Poriae Cocos (*fu ling*)............... 2 *qian*
Radix Glycyrrhizae Uralensis (*gan cao*)........... 6 *fen*

Add three slices of ginger and two Fructus Zizyphi Jujubae (*da zao*). Prepare as a decoction and drink warm.

Aconite and Lateral Aconite Pill (*chuān fù wán*)

川附丸

Radix Aconiti Carmichaeli Praeparata
    (*zhi chuan wu*)......................... 1 *liang*
Radix Lateralis Aconiti Carmichaeli
    Praeparata (*fu zi*)....................... 1 *liang*
Cortex Cinnamomi Cassiae (*rou gui*)............ 1 *liang*
Fructus Zanthoxyli Bungeani (*chuan jiao*)........ 1 *liang*
Rhizoma Acori Graminei (*shi chang pu*).......... 1 *liang*
Radix Glycyrrhizae Uralensis (*gan cao*)........... 1 *liang*
Rhizoma Drynariae (*gu sui bu*)................. 5 *qian*
Rhizoma Gastrodiae Elatae (*tian ma*)............ 5 *qian*
Rhizoma Atractylodis Macrocephalae (*bai zhu*).... 5 *qian*

Astagalus Decoction to Construct the Middle
(*huáng qí jiàn zhōng tāng*)[15]

黃蓍建中湯

Ramulus Cinnamomi Cassiae (*gui zhi*)........... 3 *liang*
Honey-toasted Radix Glycyrrhizae
    Uralensis (*zhi gan cao*)................... 3 *liang*
Radix Paeoniae Lactiflorae (*bai shao*)............ 6 *liang*
Maltose (*yi tang*)........................... 1 *sheng*
Radix Astragali Membranacei
    (*huang qi*)......................... 1 *liang* 5 *qian*
Fructus Zizyphi Jujubae (*da zao*)............... 12 pieces
Rhizoma Zingiberis Officinalis
    Recens (*sheng jiang*).................... 3 *liang*

Prepare as a decoction and drink in three doses.

Four-Substance Decoction (*sì wù tāng*)

四物湯

[See formulas at end of chapter 5.]

All-Inclusive Great Tonifying Decoction
(*shí quán dà bǔ tāng*)

十全大補湯

Radix Ginseng (*ren shen*)

Cortex Cinnamomi Cassiae (*rou gui*)

Radix Ligustici Chuanxiong (*chuan xiong*)

Radix Rehmanniae Glutinosae Conquitae (*shu di huang*)

Sclerotium Poriae Cocos (*fu ling*)

Rhizoma Atractylodis Macrocephalae (*bai zhu*)

Honey-toasted Radix Glycyrrhizae Uralensis (*zhi gan cao*)

Radix Astragali Membranacei (*huang qi*)

Radix Angelicae Sinensis (*dang gui*)

Radix Paeoniae Lactiflorae (*bai shao*)

Take equal amounts of the above ingredients, coarsely grind, and take two *qian* as a decoction with three slices of Rhizoma Zingiberis Officinalis Recens (*sheng jiang*) and two Fructus Zizyphi Jujubae (*da zao*).

Powder to Promote Movement of Dampness and Flow of Qi (*xíng shī liú qì sǎn*)

行濕流氣散

Rhizoma Atractylodis (*cang zhu*) . . . . 1 *liang*

Radix et Rhizoma Notopterygii (*qiang huo*) . . . . 1 *liang*

Radix Ledebouriellae Divaricatae (*fang feng*) . . . . 1 *liang*

Radix Aconiti Carmichaeli Praeparata
(*zhi chuan wu*) . . . . 1 *liang*

Semen Coicis Lachryma-jobi (*yi yi ren*) . . . . 2 *liang*

Sclerotium Poriae Cocos (*fu ling*) . . . . 1 *liang* 5 *qian*

Grind into a powder, and take two *qian* with warm wine or a soup of Bulbus Allii Fistulosi (*cong bai*).

Astragalus Decoction (*huáng qí tāng*)

黃蓍湯

Radix Astragali Membranacei
(*huang qi*) . . . . small quantity

Radix Ginseng (*ren shen*) . . . . small quantity

Radix Paeoniae Lactiflorae (*bai shao*) . . . . 2 *liang*

Cortex Cinnamomi Cassiae (*rou gui*) . . . . 2 *liang*

Rhizoma Zingiberis Officinalis Recens
(*sheng jiang*) . . . . 6 *liang*

Fructus Zizyphi Jujubae (*da zao*) . . . . 12 pieces

Raise the Yang and Harmonize the Middle Decoction
(*shēng yáng hé zhōng tāng*)

昇陽和中湯

Radix Astragali Membranacei (*huang qi*) . . . . 5 *qian*

Radix Ginseng (*ren shen*) . . . . 3 *qian*

Radix Glycyrrhizae Uralensis (*gan cao*) . . . . 4 *qian*

Herba Gnaphalii Affinis (*shu qu cao*) . . . . 4 *qian*

Pericarpium Citri Reticulatae (*chen pi*) . . . . 2 *qian*

Rhizoma Atractylodis Macrocephalae (*bai zhu*) . . . . 2 *qian*

Radix Angelicae Sinensis (*dang gui*) . . . . 2 *qian*

Rhizoma Atractylodis (*cang zhu*) . . . . 5 *fen*

Semen Alpiniae Katsumadai (*cao dou kou*) . . . . 5 *fen*

Cortex Phellodendri (*huang bai*) . . . . 1 *qian*

Rhizoma Cimicifugae (*sheng ma*) . . . . 1 *qian*

Sclerotium Poriae Cocos (*fu ling*) . . . . 1 *qian*

Radix Bupleuri (*chai hu*) . . . . 1 *qian*

Rhizoma Alismatis Orientalis (*ze xie*) . . . . 1 *qian*

Tonify the Qi Decoction (*bǔ qì tāng*)

補氣湯

Radix Paeoniae Lactiflorae (*bai shao*) . . . . 1 *liang* 5 *qian*

Pericarpium Citri Reticulatae (*chen pi*) . . . . . . 1 *liang* 5 *qian*

Honey-toasted Radix Glycyrrhizae
Uralensis (*zhi gan cao*) . . . . 1 *liang*

Radix Astragali Membranacei (*huang qi*) . . . . 1 *liang*

Rhizome Alismatis Orientalis (*ze xie*) . . . . 5 *qian*

Tonify the Middle and Augment the Qi Decoction
(*bǔ zhōng yì qì tāng*)

補中益氣湯

[See formulas at end of chapter 5.]

Gastrodia and Astragalus Deoction
(*tiān má huáng qí tāng*)

天麻黃蓍湯

Rhizoma Gastrodiae Elatae (*tian ma*) . . . . 3 *fen*

Radix Paeoniae Lactiflorae (*bai shao*) . . . . 3 *fen*

Massa Fermentata (*shen qu*) . . . . 3 *fen*

Radix et Rhizoma Notopterygii (*qiang huo*) . . . . 3 *fen*

Sclerotium Poriae Cocos (*fu ling*) . . . . 3 *fen*

Radix Ginseng (*ren shen*) . . . . 4 *fen*

Rhizoma Coptidis (*huang lian*) . . . . 4 *fen*

Radix Angelicae Sinensis (*dang gui*) . . . . 5 *fen*

Radix Astragali Membranacei (*huang qi*) . . . . 6 *fen*

Radix Glycyrrhizae Uralensis (*gan cao*) . . . . 6 *fen*

Rhizoma Cimicifugae (*sheng ma*) . . . . 6 *fen*

Radix Puerariae (*ge gen*) . . . . 6 *fen*

Cortex Phellodendri (*huang bai*) . . . . 6 *fen*

Rhizoma Atractylodis (*cang zhu*) . . . . 6 *fen*

Rhizome Alismatis Orientalis (*ze xie*) . . . . 7 *fen*

Radix Bupleuri (*chai hu*) . . . . 7 *fen*

Conduct the Qi Decoction *(dǎo qì tāng)*

導氣湯

Radix Paeoniae *(shao yao)* . . . . .1 *liang*
Radix Angelicae Sinensis *(dang gui)* . . . . .5 *qian*
Radix et Rhizoma Rhei *(da huang)* . . . . .1.5 *qian*
Radix Scutellariae Baicalensis *(huang qin)* . . . . .1.5 *qian*
Rhizoma Coptidis *(huang lian)* . . . . .1 *qian*
Radix Aucklandiae Lappae *(mu xiang)* . . . . .1 *qian*
Semen Arecae Catechu *(bing lang)* . . . . .1 *qian*

Three-Marvel Powder *(sān miào sǎn)*

三妙散

[See formulas at end of chapter 5.]

Chapter Notes

1. *Editors' note:* We have taken this from division 226 of *Medical Section of the Grand Compilation of Ancient and Contemporary Works (Gu jin tu shu ji cheng yi bu)*, which can be found at p. 191 in volume 6 of the modern edition.

2. *Editors' note:* This physician is better known as Qian Yi. He lived during the northern Song dynasty (c. 1032-1113) and is especially remembered for his work in pediatrics. He is the author of *Craft of Medicinal Treatment for Childhood Disease Patterns (Xiao er yao zheng zhen jue)*.

3. *Editors' note:* "Classic" here refers to chapter 43 of *Basic Questions*, which is translated in chapter 24 of this book.

4. *Editors' note:* We have no information about this formula.

5. Ibid.

6. Ibid.

7. Ibid.

8. Ibid.

9. *Editors' note:* The concept of Kidney fat goes back to chapter 34 of *Basic Questions*. It is thought to refer to the Essence stored by the Kidneys.

10. *Editors' note:* We have no information about this formula. It is quite possible that the words *dì xiān* in the name, which we have translated as "Earth Immortal," refer instead to two particular herbs.

11. *Editors' note:* We have no information about this formula. It is probably rice porridge made with Radix Aconiti *(wu tou)*.

12. Note on measurements: one *liang* (37.5g) equals ten *qian*; one *qian* equals ten *fen*. For the formulas drawn from *Essentials from the Golden Cabinet* and *Discussion of Cold-induced Disorders*, there is some controversy regarding the meanings of the terms of measurement. The majority view is that, at the time they were written, one *liang* was equivalent to three grams. Another view, however, holds that one *liang* was equivalent to 37.5 grams, as in later periods. We do know that, at the time these books were written, there were 16 *liang* in one *jin* and four *fen* in one *liang*. One *sheng* was approximately 200ml.

13. This formula is drawn from *Essentials of the Golden Cabinet* .

14. Ibid.

15. This formula is drawn from *Discussion of Cold-induced Disorders*.

32

Essential Readings for Those in the Medical Lineage *(Yi zong bi du)*

C. 1637 by LI ZHONG-ZI

"Painful Obstruction"

(DIVISION 10)

Editors' note: This division begins with a review of chapter 43 of *Basic Questions,* "On Painful Obstruction" (see chapter 24 for translation). It then proceeds as follows:

When *Inner Classic (Nei jing)* discusses painful obstruction, it says that the cardinal influences of the four seasons can all become pathogenic influences, and that the qi of any of the five yin organs can be affected. Among the six external pathogenic factors, wind, cold and dampness represent half of them. When it says "arrive in various ways" and "intermingle," then one knows that it is not that one can just receive one qi and get painful obstruction. It also says that when wind predominates, it is moving painful obstruction, when cold predominates, it is severe painful obstruction, and when dampness predominates, it is fixed painful obstruction. By this we know that it is merely relating the relative strengths [of the pathogenic influences] and not denying that the three pathogenic influences arrive in various ways, intermingle, and constitute the disease.

The skin, flesh, sinews, bones and vessels correspond to different organs. At the onset of the disease, it resides on the outside. When it lasts a long time and does not leave, it settles inside in the corresponding organ. When the disease is on the outside, it is still easy to dispel; when it enters into the organs, attacking it is truly difficult. When treating a disease that is on the outside, it is urgent to disperse the pathogenic influences. When treating the organs, first nourish the normal [qi].

When treating moving painful obstruction, the main point is to disperse the wind; do not neglect, however, to ensure protection from the cold and to promote the elimination of dampness. Generally speaking, use formulas that tonify the blood. In addition, to treat the wind we must first treat the blood; when the blood moves properly, the wind disappears.

To treat severe painful obstruction, the main point is to scatter the cold, but eliminating wind and drying dampness cannot be ignored. Generally speaking, use formulas that tonify the fire. Without these very spicy and hot ingredients, it is not possible to shake off the harmful influence of the congealing cold.

To treat fixed painful obstruction, the main point is to promote the elimination of dampness, but dispelling wind and relieving cold cannot be ignored. Generally speaking, use formulas that tonify the spleen and tonify the qi. The strengthened earth can conquer dampness, and when the qi is sufficient it can overcome the numbness itself.

Such are the general principles mentioned in the book. The different treatments are listed separately below.

Sinew painful obstruction is a [type of] wind painful obstruction: it roams and moves without being fixed from top to bottom and from left to right, following the deficiency and pathogenic influence. Struggling with the blood and qi, it clusters at the level of the joints. They may be red or swollen, while the sinews and vessels become loose and lax. Of old this was called rushing and pouring (*zǒu zhù* 走注); it is now referred to as flowing fire (*liú hǔo* 流火). The main formula for this is Ledebouriella Decoction (*fang feng tang*). [Others are] Powder that Sagely Unblocks as Desired (*ru yi tong sheng san*), Cinnamon Core Powder (*gui xin san*), Myrrh Powder (*mo yao san*), Tiger Bone Pill (*hu gu wan*), Ten-Fresh Special Pill (*shi sheng dan*), One-Tael Gold Special Pill (*yi li jin dan*) and Frankincense Powder to Respond to Pain (*ru xiang ying tong san*).

Vessel painful obstruction is a [type of] hot painful obstruction: the heat moves to the yin and yang organs and meets external pathogenic influences. The struggle takes place at the level of the channels and collaterals where the pernicious influence lingers, hence painful obstruction. The muscles and flesh are extremely hot, the lips chapped, and the skin changes color. The main formula for this is Cimicifuga Decoction (*sheng ma tang*).

Muscle painful obstruction is a fixed painful obstruction, a [type of] damp painful obstruction: it lingers and does not migrate. There is profuse sweating, the four limbs are loose and weak, the skin is numb, the essential spirit is blurry and blocked. Currently this is called paresthesia and numbness. The main formula for this is Magically Effective Astragalus Decoction (*shen xiao huang qi tang*).

With skin painful obstruction the pathogenic influence settles in the skin and hairs, with hidden rashes or wind sores. It itches but is not painful. It is appropriate to disperse the wind and nourish the blood.

Bone painful obstruction is a [type of] cold painful obstruction, severe painful obstruction: the suffering and pain cut to the heart. The four limbs are contracted and there is floating edema around the joints. The main formula is Five-Accumulation Powder (*wu ji san*).

For intestine painful obstruction, use Five-Ingredient Powder with Poria (*wu ling san*) with the addition of Cortex Mori Albae Radicis (*sang bai pi*), Caulis Mutong (*mu tong*) and Tuber Ophiopogonis Japonici (*mai men dong*).

For painful obstruction of the gestation membranes or bladder, use Fixed Kidney Decoction (*shen zhuo tang*) or Kidney Trickle Decoction (*shen li tang*).

For painful obstruction of the five yin organs, use Five-Painful Obstruction Decoction from *Essential Readings* (*wu bi tang*).

For liver painful obstruction, add Semen Zizyphi Spinosae (*suan zao ren*) and Radix Bupleuri (*chai hu*).

For heart painful obstruction, add Radix Polygalae Tenuifoliae (*yuan zhi*), Sclerotium Poriae Cocos (*fu ling*), Tuber Ophiopogonis Japonici (*mai men dong*) and Cornu Rhinoceri (*xi jiao*).

For spleen painful obstruction, add Cortex Magnoliae Officinalis (*hou po*), Fructus Citri seu Ponciri Immaturus (*zhi shi*), Fructus Amomi (*sha ren*) and Massa Fermentata (*shen qu*).

For lung painful obstruction, add Rhizoma Pinelliae Ternatae (*ban xia*), Radix Asteris Tatarici (*zi wan*), Semen Pruni Armeniacae (*xing ren*) and Herba Ephedrae (*ma huang*).

For kidney painful obstruction, add Radix Angelicae Pubescentis (*du huo*), Ramulus Cinnamomi Cassiae (*gui zhi*), Cortex Eucommiae Ulmoidis (*du zhong*), Radix Achyranthis Bidentatae (*niu xi*), Radix Astragali Membranacei (*huang qi*) and Rhizoma Dioscoreae Hypoglaucae (*bei xie*).

Prescriptions

Ledebouriella Decoction (*fáng fēng tāng*)

防風湯

Radix Ledebouriellae Divaricatae (*fang feng*)......1 *liang*[1]
Radix Glycyrrhizae Uralensis (*gan cao*)............1 *liang*
Radix Angelicae Sinensis (*dang gui*)..............1 *liang*
Sclerotium Poriae Cocos Rubrae (*chi fu ling*).......1 *liang*
Ramulus Cinnamomi Cassiae (*gui zhi*)............1 *liang*
Herba Ephedrae (*ma huang*).....................5 *qian*
Radix Scutellariae Baicalensis (*huang qin*).........3 *qian*
Radix Gentianae Qinjiao (*qin jiao*)................3 *qian*
Radix Puerariae (*ge gen*).........................3 *qian*

Grind into a powder, mix 5 *qian* with a bowl of water and wine, 3 Fructus Zizyphi Jujubae (*da zao*), and 5 slices of Rhizoma Zingiberis Officinalis Recens (*sheng jiang*). Boil down to half the volume, drain, and drink warm.

Powder that Sagely Unblocks as Desired
(*rú yì tōng shèng sǎn*)

如意通聖散

Radix Angelicae Sinensis (*dang gui*)
Pericarpium Citri Reticulatae (*chen pi*)
Herba Ephedrae (*ma huang*)
Honey-toasted Radix Glycyrrhizae Uralensis
    (*zhi gan cao*)

Radix Ligustici Chuanxiong (*chuan xiong*)

Pericarpium Papaveris Somniferi (*ying su ke*)

Flos Caryophylli (*ding xiang*)

Take equal amounts of the above ingredients. Toast and brown on a low flame, mix 5 *qian* with 2 bowls of water, boil down to 1 bowl, drain, and drink warm. For lower back pain, or lower limb pain, add Os Tigris (*hu gu*), Myrrha (*mo yao*) and Gummi Olibanum (*ru xiang*).

Cinnamon Core Powder (*guì xīn sǎn*)

桂心散

Cortex Cinnamomi Cassiae Rasus (*gui xin*)

Radix Rhapontici seu Echinops (*lou lu*)

Radix Clematidis (*wei ling xian*)

Radix Ligustici Chuanxiong (*chuan xiong*)

Radix Angelicae Dahuricae (*bai zhi*)

Radix Aucklandiae Lappae (*mu xiang*)

Radix Angelicae Sinensis (*dang gui*)

Bombyx Batryticatus (*jiang can*)

Lumbricus (*di long*)

Take 5 *qian* of each ingredient and grind into a fine powder. Take 2 *qian* each time in a little warm wine.

Myrrh Powder (*mò yào sǎn*)

沒藥散

Myrrha (*mo yao*) . . . . 2 *liang*
Os Tigris (*hu gu*) . . . . 4 *liang*

Grind into a fine powder, and take 5 *qian* twice a day in a little warm wine.

Tiger Bone Pill (*hǔ gǔ wán*)

虎骨丸

Os Tigris (*hu gu*) . . . . 4 *liang*
Excrementum Trogopterori seu
   Pteromi (*wu ling zhi*) . . . . 1 *liang*
Bombyx Batryticatus (*jiang can*) . . . . 1 *liang*
Radix Clematidis (*wei ling xian*) . . . . 1 *liang*
Lumbricus (*di long*) . . . . 1 *liang*
Fructus Liquidambaris Taiwanianae (*lu lu tong*) . . . . 1 *liang*
Radix Aconiti Carmichaeli Praeparata
   (*zhi chuan wu*) . . . . 2 *liang*
Semen Juglandis Regiae (*hu tao ren*) . . . . 2.5 *liang*

Grind into a fine powder, boil with flour in wine to a mush, then make pills the size of Semen Sterculiae Scaphigerae (*pang da hai*). Take 10 to 15 pills twice a day with warm wine on an empty stomach.

Ten-Fresh Special Pill (*shí shēng dān*)

十生丹

Rhizoma Gastrodiae Elatae (*tian ma*)

Radix Ledebouriellae Divaricatae (*fang feng*)

Radix et Rhizoma Notopterygii (*qiang huo*)

Radix Angelicae Pubescentis (*du huo*)

Radix Aconiti Carmichaeli Praeparata (*zhi chuan wu*)

Radix Aconiti Kusnezoffii Praeparata (*zhi cao wu*)

Radix Polygoni Multiflori (*he shou wu*)

Radix Angelicae Sinensis (*dang gui*)

Cortex Erythrinae (*hai tong pi*)

Take equal amounts of the above ingredients [all fresh, i.e., not prepared]. Grind into a fine powder, warm up with honey to make pills that weigh 1 *qian*. Chew 1 pill with tea.

One-Tael Gold Special Pill (*yī lí jīn dān*)

一厘金丹

Radix Aconiti Kusnezoffii Praeparata
   (*zhi cao wu*) . . . . 1 *liang*
Excrementum Trogopterori seu Pteromi
   (*wu ling zhi*) . . . . 1 *liang*
Lumbricus (*di long*) . . . . 5 *qian*
Semen Momordicae Cochinchinensis (*mu bie zi*) . . 5 *qian*
Fructus Liquidambaris Taiwanianae (*lu lu tong*) . . . 1 *liang*
Treated China ink (*duan xi mo*) . . . . 5 *qian*
Gummi Olibanum (*ru xiang*) . . . . 5 *qian*
Myrrha (*mo yao*) . . . . 1 *liang*
Radix Angelicae Sinensis (*dang gui*) . . . . 1 *liang*
Secretio Moschus (*she xiang*) . . . . 1 *qian*

Grind into a fine powder, make pills with glutinous rice the size of Semen Sterculiae Scaphigerae (*pang da hai*). Take 2-3 pills with warm wine.

Frankincense Powder to Respond to Pain
   (*rǔ xiāng yìng tòng sǎn*)

乳香應痛散

Gummi Olibanum (*ru xiang*) . . . . 5 *qian*
Myrrha (*mo yao*) . . . . 5 *qian*
Excrementum Trogopterori seu Pteromi
   (*wu ling zhi*) . . . . 1 *liang*
Halloysitum Rubrum (*chi shi zhi*) . . . . 1 *liang*
Radix Aconiti Kusnezoffii Praeparata
   (*zhi cao wu*) . . . . 1.5 *liang*

Grind into a fine powder, make pills the size of a pea, take 15 pills twice a day with wine on an empty stomach.

Cimicifuga Decoction (*shēng má tāng*)

升麻湯

Rhizoma Cimicifugae (*sheng ma*)	3 *liang*
Sclerotium Poriae Cocos Pararadicis (*fu shen*)	1 *liang*
Radix Ginseng (*ren shen*)	1 *liang*
Radix Ledebouriellae Divaricatae (*fang feng*)	1 *liang*
Cornu Rhinoceri (*xi jiao*)	1 *liang*
Cornu Antelopis (*ling yang jiao*)	1 *liang*
Radix et Rhizoma Notopterygii (*qiang huo*)	1 *liang*
Cortex Cinnamomi Cassiae Tubiformis (*guan gui*)	5 *qian*

Grind into a powder, mix 4 *qian* with 2 bowls of water, 2 crushed slices of ginger and a little bamboo sap, Succus Bambusae (*zhu li*). Boil down to 1 bowl and drink warm.

Magically Effective Astragalus Decoction
(*shén xiào huáng qí tāng*)

神效黃耆湯

Fructus Viticis (*man jing zi*)	2 *qian*
Pericarpium Citri Reticulatae (*chen pi*)	2 *qian*
Radix Ginseng (*ren shen*)	8 *qian*
Honey-toasted Radix Glycyrrhizae Uralensis (*zhi gan cao*)	1 *liang*
Radix Paeoniae Lactiflorae (*bai shao*)	1 *liang*
Radix Astragali Membranacei (*huang qi*)	2 *liang*

Grind into a powder and take 5 *qian* at a time. Mix in 2 bowls of water and boil down to 1 bowl, drain, and drink warm before going to bed.

Five-Accumulation Powder (*wǔ jī sǎn*)

五積散

[See formulas at end of chapter 5.]

Five-Ingredient Powder with Poria (*wǔ líng sǎn*)

五苓散

[See formulas at end of chapter 5.]

Fixed Kidney Decoction (*shèn zhuó tāng*)[2]

腎著湯

Sclerotium Poriae Cocos (*fu ling*)	4 *liang*
Rhizoma Atractylodis Macrocephalae (*bai zhu*)	4 *liang*
Radix Glycyrrhizae Uralensis (*gan cao*)	2 *liang*
Rhizoma Zingiberis Officinalis (*gan jiang*)	2 *liang*

Grind into a powder, mix five *qian* with two bowls of water, boil down to half the volume, and drink warm three times a day.

Kidney Trickle Decoction (*shèn lì tāng*)

腎瀝湯

Ootheca Mantidis (*sang piao xiao*)
Cornu Rhinoceri (*xi jiao*)
Tuber Ophiopogonis Japonici (*mai men dong*)
Cortex Acanthopanacis Gracilistylus Radicis (*wu jia pi*)
Cortex Eucommiae Ulmoidis (*du zhong*)
Caulis Mutong (*mu tong*)
Radix Platycodi Grandiflori (*jie geng*)
Radix Paeoniae Rubrae (*chi shao*)
[Dosage and preparation is not specified.]

Five-Painful Obstruction Decoction from
Essential Readings (*wǔ bì tāng*)

五痹湯

Radix Ginseng (*ren shen*)	1 *qian*
Sclerotium Poriae Cocos (*fu ling*)	1 *qian*
Radix Angelicae Sinensis (*dang gui*)	1 *qian*
Radix Paeoniae Lactiflorae (*bai shao*)	1 *qian*
Radix Ligustici Chuanxiong (*chuan xiong*)	1 *qian*
Rhizoma Atractylodis Macrocephalae (*bai zhu*)	1 *qian*
Fructus Schisandrae Chinensis (*wu wei zi*)	50 seeds
Herba cum Radice Asari (*xi xin*)	7 *fen*
Radix Glycyrrhizae Uralensis (*gan cao*)	5 *fen*
Rhizoma Zingiberis Officinalis Recens (*sheng jiang*)	1 slice

Decoct and take between meals.

Chapter Notes

1. Note on measurements: one *liang* (37.5g) equals 10 *qian*; one *qian* equals 10 *fen*. With respect to the formulas drawn from Zhang Zhong-Jing's *Essentials from the Golden Cabinet* and *Discussion of Cold-induced Disorders,* there is some controversy regarding the meaning of the terms of measurement. The prevailing view is that, at the time they were written, one *liang* was equivalent to three grams. Another view, however, is that one *liang* was equivalent to 37.5 grams, as in later periods. During Zhang's time there were 16 *liang* in one *jin* , and four *fen* in one *liang*.

2. This formula is drawn from *Essentials from the Golden Cabinet.* It is also known as Licorice, Ginger, Poria, and Atractylodis Macrocephalae Decoction (*gan cao gan jiang fu ling bai zhu tang*).

CHAPTER THIRTY-THREE

Precepts for Physicians
(Yi men fa lü)
C. 1658 by YU CHANG

From "On Wind Attack"
(DIVISION 3)

WIND PAINFUL OBSTRUCTION

Of the four wind-attack disorders, one is called wind painful obstruction.[1] Although they are all of a similar type, in reality there are differences among them. Wind affects the yang first, while painful obstruction affects the yin first. However, since painful obstruction results from the combination of wind, cold and dampness, it is impossible to distinguish them. Nonetheless, when wind predominates, it is moving painful obstruction, because wind is mobile by nature; when cold predominates, it is severe painful obstruction, because cold controls contraction and urgency; when dampness predominates, it is fixed painful obstruction, because dampness controls heaviness and stagnation.

When the pernicious influence invades, there are five superficial [cases] and five deep [cases]; it is necessary to analyze them correctly. When it is at the bone level, the limbs are heavy and cannot be raised; when it is in the sinews, there is flexion but no extension; when it is in the flesh, there is numbness; when it is in the vessels, the blood congeals and does not flow; when it is in the skin, it creates cold. In all five cases, the pernicious influences are in the body and there is no pain. Those that are painful follow the blood vessels to ascend and descend, as well as the cold that congeals the humors which permeate the intramuscular spaces and lead to pain. Although it bears a different name, encompassing painful obstruction,[2] it does not belong to an attack on the blood vessels.

If bone painful obstruction does not heal, after renewed attacks of pernicious influences it may settle into the kidneys. If sinew painful obstruction does not heal, after renewed attacks of pernicious influences it may settle into the liver. If vessel painful obstruction does not heal, after renewed attacks of pernicious influences it may settle into the heart. If muscle painful obstruction does not heal, after renewed attacks of pernicious influences it may settle into the spleen. If skin painful obstruction does not heal, after renewed attacks of pernicious influences it may settle into the lungs. In each of these five cases, there is no direct penetration into the five yin organs. The five yin organs have their corresponding diseases; when the illness is long-standing and is not eliminated, it settles internally in the corresponding organ. In addition, pathogenic wind, cold and dampness become entangled and impair each other; they are not as mobile as wind. This is why they only resemble a wind attack.

[Inner] Classic describes in much detail different types of painful obstruction, but does not mention formulas to treat them. Essentials from the Golden Cabinet (Jin gui yao lue) supplements it by talking about 1) blood painful obstruction; 2) chest painful obstruction; 3) fixed kidneys; and 4) triple burner painful obstruction.

Referring to blood painful obstruction, *Essentials from the Golden Cabinet* says that it targets people with weak bones and abundant muscles and skin. When they overexert themselves with sweating, and go to bed tossing and turning, they allow themselves to be attacked by a slight wind, and the disease is contracted. The pulse is only slightly choppy at the distal position, and a little tight at the middle position. The needling principle is to lead the yang qi and harmonize the pulse. When the tightness goes away, health will return.

In blood painful obstruction the yin and yang are weak, the distal and middle pulses are weak, and the proximal pulse is a little tight. Externally the body lacks feeling and there is a certain similarity with wind painful obstruction. Prescribe Astragalus and Cinnamon Twig Five-Substance Decoction (*huang qi gui zhi wu wu tang*).

Essentials from the Golden Cabinet discusses chest painful obstruction, pulse and characteristics; it also clearly lists the therapeutic methods.[3]

In the fixed kidney disease[4] from *Essentials from the Golden Cabinet*, the patient has a very heavy sensation in the body, and feels cold in the lumbar region, as if sitting in water. While this condition is similar to a water [condition], there is an absence of thirst, abundant urination, and a normal appetite. This illness belongs to the lower burner, and it occurs after sweating upon exertion and keeping the wet and cold clothes on when these occur over a very long period. There is a cold and heavy sensation in the lower back and below, with heaviness in the abdomen as if carrying 5,000 gold coins. Prescribe Licorice, Ginger, Poria, and Atractylodes Macrocephala Decoction (*gan cao gan jiang fu ling bai zhu tang*) for it.

Essentials from the Golden Cabinet also mentions treatment of the three painful obstructions, although at present it is mistakenly considered to be under the category of panarthralgia with yellow sweat. It states that the various limbs and different joints are painful, the body has lost weight, the feet are edematous as if they were about to fall off, there is vertigo, nausea and shortness of breath. It recommends Cinnamon Twig, Peony, and Anemarrhena Decoction (*gui zhi shao yao zhi mu tang*).

Precepts

In treating painful obstruction, those who are not clear on its principles and lump all the various types together, indiscriminately treating them as if they were all wind problems, are medical criminals. It is not that wind is not present in painful obstruction, but it enters into the yin level, clumps with cold and dampness, and disturbs the blood vessels. In this way the body's yang cannot communicate with the yin, which results in painful obstruction.

Many old formulas used Herba Ephedrae (*ma huang*) and Radix Angelicae Dahuricae (*bai zhi*) because Herba Ephedrae (*ma huang*) can unblock the yang qi, and Radix Angelicae Dahuricae (*bai zhi*) can promote the movement of the nutritive and protective [qi]. When these herbs are added to those from Four-Substance Decoction (*si wu tang*) and Four-Gentlemen Decoction (*si jun zi tang*), it is not solely because they can release the exterior.

As for the method of purging the interior, it has never been used because the herbs that purge the interior are all bitter and cold. After using them the yang would be more blocked, leading the painful obstruction to enter the various organs, thereby causing many lethal conditions. Can we neglect to carefully analyze these conditions and be especially careful?

Prescriptions

Astragalus and Cinnamon Twig Five-Substance Decoction (*huáng qí guì zhì wǔ wù tāng*)

黃蓍桂枝五物湯

[See formulas at end of chapter 5.]

Licorice, Ginger, Poria, and Atractylodes Macrocephala Decoction (*gān jiāng líng zhú tāng*)

甘薑苓朮湯

[See formulas at end of chapter 7.]

Cinnamon Twig, Peony, and Anemarrhena Decoction (*guì zhī shào yào zhī mǔ tāng*)

桂枝芍藥知母湯

[See formulas at end of chapter 5.]

Four-Substance Decoction (*sì wù tāng*)

四物湯

[See formulas at end of chapter 5.]

Four-Gentlemen Decoction (*sì jūn zǐ tāng*)

四君子湯

Radix Ginseng (*ren shen*) . . . . 2 *qian*[5]
Rhizoma Atractylodis Macrocephalae (*bai zhu*) . . . . 2 *qian*
Sclerotium Poriae Cocos (*fu ling*) . . . . 2 *qian*
Radix Glycyrrhizae Uralensis (*gan cao*) . . . . 6 *fen*

Make a decoction, adding 3 slices of fresh ginger and 2 jujubes.

Chapter Notes

1. *Editors' note:* In this text the four wind-attack problems are hemilateral withering *(piān kū)*, wind paralysis *(fēng fèi)*, wind choking *(fēng yì)* and wind painful obstruction *(fēng bì)*.

2. See chapter 27 of *Divine Pivot*, most of which is translated in chapter 25 of this book.

3. *Editors' note:* This refers to chapter 20 of that book.

4. *Editors' note:* This refers to chapter 6 of that book.

5. Note on measurements: one *liang* (37.5g) equals 10 *qian*; one *qian* equals 10 *fen*; one *sheng* equals approximately 200ml.

CHAPTER THIRTY-FOUR

Acupuncture for Painful Obstruction Disorders

THROUGHOUT THE HISTORY of Chinese medicine, acupuncture has been an important modality for the treatment of painful obstruction disorders. The first group of selections in this chapter is drawn from division 229 of the Qing dynasty work, *Medical Section of the Grand Compilation of Ancient and Contemporary Works (Gu jin tu shu ji cheng yi bu)*. The second group of selections is from the Ming work, *Great Compendium of Acupuncture and Moxibustion (Zhen jiu da cheng)*

Basic Questions *(Su wen)*
C. 200 B.C.–100 A.D.

FROM "SUMMARY OF DEEP PUNCTURES"
(CHAPTER 55)

When the disease is in the sinews, the sinews are contracted, the joints are painful, and movement is impossible. This is called painful obstruction of the sinews. Needle the sinews, between the muscle layers, without hitting the bone. When the condition is resolved, the sinews become warmer and the disease ceases.

When the illness is in the skin and muscles, the skin and muscles are painful. This is called painful obstruction of the muscles, and the injury is from cold and dampness. Needle the big and small interstices, and needle deeply several times to generate heat; take care not to injure the sinews and bones, as these injuries would create an abscess. If the modifications are accompanied by a production of heat in all the interstices, the disease ceases.

When the disease is in the bones, the bones are heavy, the person cannot get up, and the bones and marrow are sore and painful. The cold qi arrives and it is called painful obstruction of the bones. Needle deeply, taking care not to injure the vessels nor the muscles. The needle's path is through the big and small interstices. When the bones have warmed up, the disease ceases.

FROM "ON ECCENTRIC NEEDLING"
(CHAPTER 63)

In all cases of painful obstruction that move around without a fixed place, needle the painful area, in the flesh intervals. Do this a number of times equal to the number of the lunar day, as this number corresponds to the abundance or weakness of qi. If we exceed it, there is a sloughing of qi, and if we do not reach it, the qi is not drained. For problems on the left choose the right, for those on the right choose the left. If the disease is not better, repeat with the same technique: needle once on the first day of the month, twice on the second day, increasing the number of needlings by one each day until fifteen times on the fifteenth, then fourteen times on the sixteenth day, and thereafter decreasing the number by one each day.

Divine Pivot (Ling shu)

C. 200 B.C.–100 A.D.

FROM "LONG LIFE AND PREMATURE DEATH, HARDNESS AND SOFTNESS (MODELED ON THE [SIX] SOUND PIPES)" (CHAPTER 6)

When the disease is in the yang, it is called wind; when it is located in the yin, it is called painful obstruction; when the yin and the yang are both affected, it is wind painful obstruction. When the disease has form but no pain, it belongs to the yang category; when it is painful but has no form, it belongs to the yin category. When it has no form and it is painful, it means that the yang is becoming exhausted and is being injured by the yin; we must then treat the yin rapidly and avoid attacking the yang....

When the patient has been sick for nine days, needle him three times and then stop; when the disease has lasted for a month, needle ten times and then stop. According to distance and proximity, this technique is used to weaken it. When the painful obstruction is chronic and cannot be eliminated from the body, examine the collaterals and bleed them.

FROM "FUNCTIONS OF NEEDLES (MODELED ON THE [SEVEN] STARS)" (CHAPTER 7)

There are five types of punctures, corresponding to the five organs: the first one is called half-puncture (*bàn cì* 半刺): needling is superficial, withdrawal is rapid, it does not injure the muscles, it feels as light as a feather, it gets the skin qi. This corresponds to the lungs.

The second one is called leopard-pattern puncture (*bào wén cì* 豹文刺): it consists of needling on the right and the left, in front and behind, in order to penetrate the vessels and get the blood of the channels and collaterals. This corresponds to the heart.

The third one is called barrier puncture (*guān cì* 關刺): the principle is to perform a direct puncture, on both sides, along the sinews in order to get the painful obstruction from the sinews; take care not to induce bleeding. This corresponds to the liver....

The fourth one is called joined valley puncture (*hé gǔ cì* 合谷刺): it consists of "chicken scratching" to the left and right, needling between the intramuscular spaces, in order to get the painful obstruction from the muscles. This corresponds to the Spleen.

The fifth one is called transport puncture (*shū cì* 輸刺): the principle is to go in and out directly and deeply to the bone. This gets the painful obstruction from the bone. It corresponds to the kidneys.

FROM "CHANNELS AND VESSELS" (CHAPTER 10)

The Yellow Emperor said, "All the collaterals cannot go through the main joints, they have to use other pathways to go in and out. When they gather at the level of the skin, their meeting points appear on the outside. This is the reason why the collateral vessels must be needled on their knots (*jié* 節). In cases of blood overabundance, despite the absence of knots, treat them rapidly in order to expel the pathogenic influence from the blood; allowing it to remain inside may create painful obstruction."

FROM "THE FOUR SEASONS' QI" (CHAPTER 19)

When painful obstruction is not gotten rid of, and the long-term cold does not cease, needle ST-36 (*zu san li*) immediately.

FROM "THE FIVE PATHOGENIC INFLUENCES" (CHAPTER 20)

When the pathogenic influence is in the kidneys, the illness manifests itself as pain in the bones and a yin painful obstruction. A yin painful obstruction is not perceived on palpation, the abdomen is bloated, the lower back is painful, bowel movements are difficult, the shoulders, back and neck are painful, there is intermittent vertigo; needle KI-1 (*yong quan*) and BL-60 (*kun lun*); if there is blood stasis, it must be completely expelled.

FROM "INVERSION DISORDERS" (CHAPTER 24)

When there are headaches for which needling is inefficient, this is the bad consequence of a great painful obstruction. When this occurs as a daily crisis it can be improved, but not cured.

FROM "DISCUSSION ON BLOOD IN THE COLLATERALS" (CHAPTER 39)

When the yin and the yang are affected and gather to generate painful obstruction, it circulates abundantly inside the channels, and flows outside into the collaterals. When this is the case, the yin and the yang both have surplus in excess, even if you let out a large amount of blood; if not, it will not be possible to generate a deficiency [i.e., disperse the excess].

FROM "ON PROHIBITIONS AND PRESCRIPTIONS" (CHAPTER 48)

When the carotid pulse is tight, this is severe painful obstruction; when this pulse is consistently irregular (*dài* 代), it means that the pain is intense or intermittent. When overabundant, drain it; when deficient, tonify it. When it [the pulse] is tight and there is pain, needle the intramuscular spaces; when it is consistently irregular, needle the blood collaterals and add herbs to the treatment. When it is collapsed, use moxa. When it is neither overabundant nor deficient, treat the channel; this technique is called channel puncture.

When the radial pulse is tight, this is severe painful obstruction. When it is consistently irregular, this means that the intermittent pain is interspersed with quiet periods. When overabundant, drain it; when deficient, tonify it. When it [the pulse] is tight, needle first and then apply moxa; when it is intermittent, needle the blood collaterals and later regulate it. When it is sunken, use moxa. When sunken, the vessel blood connects with the middle; when the middle has stuck blood, the blood is cold, so moxa it. When it is neither overabundant nor deficient, treat the channel; this technique is called channel puncture.

FROM "THE TWENTY-FIVE TYPES OF PEOPLE ACCORDING TO YIN AND YANG" (CHAPTER 64)

The Yellow Emperor asked, "How should we needle the yin and the yang?"

Qi Bo answered, "Palpate the radial and carotid pulses in order to determine the yin and yang balance; palpate to find out if there is congealing and roughness in the channels. If there are knots and no fluidity, it means that there is severe painful obstruction throughout the body; when it is intense, there is no circulation so congealing and roughness develop. With congealing and roughness, bring the qi there to warm it, and when the blood is harmonized, we can stop the treatment. When there are knots in the collaterals, the vessels contract and the blood cannot move; if they are dredged, the blood circulates. That is why it is said that [when] there is excess qi above, it must be led and brought down. When the qi is deficient above,

we must push and warm it up. When there is stagnation and it does not arrive, we must meet it [i.e., needle the area of stagnation].

"We must understand the channels and conduits in order to master it [the treatment]. When heat and cold are struggling, we must lead [qi and blood] in order to restore proper circulation. When there is meandering blood without knots, we must normalize [i.e., select the appropriate treatment]. We must first understand clearly the twenty-five types of people, the localization of the qi and blood, left or right, and above or below, in order to needle appropriately and heal the condition."

Thousand Ducat Prescriptions (*Qian jin yao fang*)

C. 650 by SUN SI-MIAO

TB-2 (*ye men*) treats pain in the arm.

SI-9 (*jian zhen*) treats paresthesia and numbness of the upper limb with inability to lift it.

CV-7 (*yin jiao*) treats contractures of the arms and legs.

LU-11 (*shao shang*) treats insensitivity of the upper limb.

"Anterior axilla" (*qian ye*)[1] treats contractures of the medial aspect of the arm with inability to lift the upper limb.

LU-5 (*chi ze*) treats painful contractures of the upper limb with inability to extend it.

LI-11 (*qu chi*) treats inability of the upper limb to lift heavy weights, contractures of the wrist, pain in the elbow with difficulty in extending and flexing. It also treats insensitivity of the upper limb.

LI-5 (*yang xi*) treats heavy feeling in the arm with contractures of the elbow.

TB-13 (*nao hui*), TB-6 (*zhi gou*), LI-11 (*qu chi*), SI-4 (*wan gu*) and LI-12 (*zhou liao*) treat painful obstruction of the elbow joint, heavy and tired feeling in the arm, painful contractures of the armpit, and difficulty flexing or extending the elbow.

TB-10 (*tian jing*) treats pain in the shoulder with painful obstruction, atrophy and insensitivity, inability to flex or extend, and paresthesia and numbness.

LI-13 (*qu yuan*) treats painful obstruction of the scapular region.

SP-9 (*yin ling quan*) treats painful obstruction of the legs.

GV-16 (*feng fu*) and GV-2 (*yao shu*) treat insensitivity of the legs.

GB-38 (*yang fu*), GB-35 (*yang jiao*) and GB-34 (*yang ling quan*) treat insensitivity of the hip and knee bones.

BL-67 (*zhi yin*) treats wind and cold ascending from the fifth toe, causing ascending and descending painful obstruction of the vessels.

ST-44 (*nei ting*) and GB-30 (*huan tiao*) treat pain in the calf with inability to flex or extend.

"Amidst yang"(*yang jian*),[2] GB-30 (*huan tiao*) and BL-56 (*cheng jin*) treat calf painful obstruction with insensitivity.

KI-1 (*yong quan*) and KI-2 (*ran gu*) treat pain in the five toes and inability to place the feet on the ground.

For pain in the hip with inability to move, use and retain the filiform needle to induce cold; taking into account the lunar cycle to determine the number of punctures relieves the pain instantly.

LR-3 (*tai chong*) treats pain in the medial aspect of the knee and the anterior aspect of the ankle.

ST-34 (*liang qiu*), LR-8 (*qu quan*) and GB-33 (*xi yang guan*) treat contractures of the tendons with inability to flex or extend the knee and inability to walk.

ST-35 (*du bi*) treats pain in the knee with insensitivity; this point is also said to treat insensitivity of the knee and difficulty in kneeling down.

ST-31 (*bi guan*) treats cold in the knee with insensitivity, atrophy, painful obstruction, and inability to flex or extend it.

GB-31 (*feng shi*) treats flaccidity, atrophy, and painful obstruction, pain in the calf with coldness and insensitivity.

GB-32 (*zhong du*) treats the cold pathogenic influence located in the intramuscular spaces with painful suffering, painful obstruction and insensitivity.

GB-33 (*xi yang guan*) treats pain in the lateral aspect of the knee with inability to flex or extend, calf painful obstruction, and insensitivity.

GB-39 (*xuan zhong*) treats edema-inducing damp painful obstruction, contractures of the hip tendons, and pain in the leg.

LR-8 (*qu quan*) treats violent painful obstruction which radiates toward the inferior aspect of the patella.

GB-34 (*yang ling quan*) treats painful obstruction of the hip which radiates toward the lateral aspect of the knee with pain, insensitivity, and contractures of the tendons.

GB-39 (*xuan zhong*) treats pain in the hip, painful instability of the knee joint with painful obstruction and insensitivity, contractures of the tendons, and soreness of various joints.

SP-7 (*lou gu*) treats chronic damp painful obstruction with inability to walk.

SP-5 (*shang qiu*) treats painful obstruction of the bones with irritability and a sensation of fullness [in the chest].

GB-41 (*zu lin qi*) treats painful obstruction of the body with cold sensation and chills.

Every time there is insensitivity in the body, start by needling BL-64 (*jing gu*), followed by draining LR-4 (*zhong feng*) and GB-39 (*xuan zhong*).

For panarthralgia, applying moxa twenty-seven times at the painful location yields good results.

Outline of Medicine
(*Yi xue gang mu*)
1515 by YU TUAN

For white tiger panarthralgia, apply moxa on the tips of both the medial and lateral malleoli.

For generalized diffuse pain that goes up and down, comes and goes without order, needle GB-38 (*yang fu*).

For generalized diffuse pain, we can needle the painful spot without paying attention to the channels. Avoid the sinews and bones. These points are called heavenly resonances (*tiān yìng* 天應).

For pain in the shoulder, needle LI-15 (*jian yu*), LI-10 (*shou san li*) and TB-5 (*wai guan*).

For pain in the shoulder with paresthesia and numbness, needle LI-15 (*jian yu*), GB-21 (*jian jing*) and LI-11 (*qu chi*).

For painful paresthesia and numbness of the shoulder, needle LI-15 (*jian yu*), LI-9 (shang lian) and LI-4 (*he gu*); if no result, then needle GB-21 (*jian jing*) and LU-7 (*lie que*).

For pain in the arm radiating toward the wrist, drain by needling TB-2 *(ye men)* through to TB-4 *(yang chi)*, and TB-3 *(zhong zhu)* through to SI-4 *(wan gu)*.

For pain in the medial aspect of the arm, needle LU-8 *(jing qu)* 0.1 unit deep (this point is forbidden for moxa), HT-4 *(ling dao)* 0.1 unit deep, 0.3 unit parallel to the skin, and HT-3 *(shao hai)* 0.5 unit.

For weariness of the arm with contractures, needle LI-12 *(zhou liao)*, GB-11 *(tou qiao yin)*, LU-5 *(chi ze)*, SI-2 *(qian gu)* and SI-3 *(hou xi)*.

For pain in the wrist, needle LI-5 *(yang xi)* and LI-11 *(qu chi)*.

For lack of strength in the wrist with pain, needle SI-4 *(wan gu)* parallel to the skin, 0.3 unit deep; drain in cases of pain, tonify in cases of weakness. Drain or tonify LI-11 *(qu chi)* according to the same principles.

For contractures of the five fingers, needle LI-3 *(san jian)* 0.1 unit deep (drain first, then tonify by applying moxa), SI-2 *(qian gu)* 0.1 unit deep (drain and then apply moxa).

For pain in the five fingers, needle TB-4 *(yang chi)*, TB-5 *(wai guan)* and LI-4 *(he gu)*.

For pain in the pelvic girdle with wind in the lower limbs, needle GB-30 *(huan tiao)* in a lateral recumbent position with the leg flexed, 3.5 units deep, tonifying mildly and draining strongly, retaining the needle for eight breaths; drain GB-29 *(ju liao)* and retain the needle for eight breaths, and then bleed BL-40 *(wei zhong)*.

For pain in the pelvic girdle with inversion *(jué* 厥*)* of the legs, needle GB-30 *(huan tiao)*, GB-39 *(xuan zhong)* 0.5 unit deep, retain the needle for three breaths, then apply three moxa cones.

For pain in the pelvic girdle, wind in the lower limbs, inability to turn over, difficult mobilization, needle GB-30 *(huan tiao)* 3.5 units deep and apply moxa five times, GB-31 *(feng shi)* two times seven moxa cones, GB-29 *(ju liao)* 3.5 units deep and apply five times seven moxa cones, BL-40 *(wei zhong)*, BL-60 *(kun lun)*, ST-36 *(zu san li)* and GB-34 *(yang ling quan)*; if there is no marked improvement, needle GB-27 *(wu shu)* and GB-38 *(yang fu)*.

For pain in the lower back and feet, needle BL-40 *(wei zhong)*, BL-60 *(kun lun)* and GV-26 *(ren zhong)*.

For lateral foot wind, needle GB-39 *(xuan zhong)* and LR-3 *(tai chong)*.

For pain in the hip pivot, cold and heat in the leg, and pain in the bones and skin of the lateral aspect of the leg, needle GB-41 *(zu lin qi)* 0.1 unit deep, SP-6 *(san yin jiao)* 0.5 unit deep, and GB-38 *(yang fu)*.

For contractures of the hip tendons, pain in the leg, flaccidity, atrophy and painful obstruction, pain in the calf, coldness in the knee (primarily in the lateral aspect) with inability to flex or extend, damp painful obstruction with mobile edema, needle GB-31 *(feng shi)*, GB-32 *(zhong du)*, GB-33 *(xi yang guan)* and GB-39 *(xuan zhong)*.

For pain in the leg, needle GB-34 *(yang ling quan)*, ST-36 *(zu san li)*, ST-32 *(fu tu)* and ST-33 *(yin shi)*.

For contractures of the thigh and knee radiating toward the flanks accompanied by a green, brown or black color, or a withered aspect resembling dead wood, apply moxa at GB-31 *(feng shi)*, needle GB-34 *(yang ling quan)*, LR-8 *(qu quan)* and BL-60 *(kun lun)*.

For pain in the lateral aspect of the knee and thigh, edema in the gluteal region, lassitude of the calf, contractures of the tendons, atrophy and painful obstruction, or heat in the knee and calf with inability to walk, needle GB-43 *(xia xi)* 0.5 unit deep, ST-31 *(bi guan)*, and GB-37 *(guang ming)* 1 unit deep.

For painful obstruction of the hip radiating toward the knee, painful contractures of the lateral aspect of the hip, lassitude of the calf with trembling and cracking, and diffuse joint pain with inability to walk, needle GB-34 *(yang ling quan)*, GB-39 *(xuan zhong)* and LR-4 *(zhong feng)*.

For pain in the medial aspect of the thigh and knee radiating toward the patella with inability to flex or extend the knee, radiating to the abdomen and leading to a sore throat, needle LR-3 *(tai chong)* 0.5 unit deep, LR-4 *(zhong feng)* and LR-7 *(xi guan)*.

For lassitude and cold in the leg with heat under the foot, inability to stand up for a long period of time, or damp painful obstruction with insensitivity, needle LR-6 *(zhong du)*, ST-42 *(chong yang)*, BL-57 *(cheng shan)* and BL-56 *(cheng jin)*.

For a cold leg, heaviness in the four limbs, shortness of breath with difficulty in speaking, and inability to lie down, needle GV-9 *(zhi yang)* and SP-6 *(san yin jiao)*.

For straw sandal wind,[3] drain BL-60 *(kun lun)* and retain the needle for six breaths, drain KI-3 *(tai xi)* and retain the needle for six breaths, then needle BL-62 *(shen mai)* 0.5 unit deep, tonifying mildly, draining strongly, and retain the needle for two breaths; it is forbidden to apply moxa at this point.

For straw sandal wind with pain in the instep, needle BL-60 *(kun lun)* through to KI-3 *(tai xi)*, needle SP-5 *(shang qiu)* 0.5 unit deep. Apply moxa and drain. Another method consists of needling BL-60 *(kun lun)*, GB-40 *(qiu xu)*, SP-5 *(shang qiu)* and KI-6 *(zhao hai)*. If there are no results, needle LR-3 *(tai chong)* and ST-41 *(jie xi)*.

For insensitivity of the instep with atrophy and limping, difficulty in getting up from a seated position, pain in the hip and foot, needle GB-37 *(guang ming)* 0.5 unit deep and direct the needle parallel to the skin, and GB-40 *(qiu xu)* 0.5 unit deep perpendicular to the skin.

For redness, swelling and pain in the lateral malleolus, drain BL-62 *(shen mai)* 0.5 unit deep.

For wind that circles the ankles, needle LI-11 *(qu chi)*; for painful swelling of the lateral ankle, puncture the minute collaterals at the leg lesser yang level at the fifth toe, 0.3 unit deep; in case of painful edema of the medial malleolus, add SP-2 *(da du)* puncturing 0.3 unit deep; in case of painful edema of the anterior aspect of the ankle, needle LR-2 *(xing jian)* 0.6 unit deep.

For pain in the anterior bone of the main big toe joint [first phalange], needle LR-3 *(tai chong)* and vibrate the needle by tapping it to induce bleeding.

For pain in the five toes with inability to rest the foot on the ground, needle KI-1 *(yong quan)* 0.2 unit deep, and KI-2 *(ran gu)* 0.1 unit deep.

For pain in the hundred joints with no apparent etiology, use the pyramid needle to puncture and bleed GB-39 *(xuan zhong)*.

Introduction to Medicine
(Yi xue ru men)

1575 by LI ZHAI-JIAN

For wind-damp-cold painful obstruction, needle GB-30 *(huan tiao)*, GB-34 *(yang ling quan)*, TB-8 *(san yang luo)* and GV-1 *(chang qiang)*. For loss of sensation, pain and pruritus, burn corn-sized moxa balls on top of the needle three to five times, and stop as soon as the sensitivity to pain returns.

Great Compendium of Acupuncture and Moxibustion
(Zhen jiu da cheng)

1601 by YANG JI-ZHOU

[The following selections are acupuncture odes and songs collected in the Ming dynasty work, *Great Compendium of Acupuncture and Moxibustion*. Many of these selections were originally published in earlier works. Here we have not attempted to translate their poetic language, but simply to lay out the point prescriptions. When the commentaries for a selection are not redundant, we have included them as well.]

FROM "ODE OF ONE-HUNDRED CONDITIONS"

Stiff neck due to a cold-damage: LI-7 *(wen liu)* and LR-14 *(qi men)*.

Stiff neck with aversion to wind: BL-65 *(shu gu)* and BL-10 *(tian zhu)*.

Spasms: GB-25 *(jing men)* and GB-40 *(qiu xu)*.

Stubborn paresthesia and numbness in the arms: HT-3 *(shao hai)* and LI-10 *(shou san li)*.

Pain in the flanks and ribs: ST-13 *(qi hu)* and CV-20 *(hua gai)*.

Fullness in the chest with stiff neck: KI-25 *(shen cang)* and CV-21 *(xuan ji)*.

Pain in the back radiating toward the lower back: BL-30 *(bai huan shu)* and BL-40 *(wei zhong)*.

Stiff spine: ST-28 *(shui dao)* and GV-8 *(jin suo)*.

Pain in the lower limbs: SI-3 *(hou xi)* and GB-30 *(huan tiao)*.

FROM "ODE OF XI HONG"

Intolerable pain in the arm, shoulder and back: LI-4 *(he gu)*, LR-3 *(tai chong)*.

Functional disruption of the upper limbs: LI-11 *(qu chi)* and LI-4 *(he gu)*, where the puncture must be very accurate.

Five types of elbow pain: LU-5 *(chi ze)*, LU-9 *(tai yuan)*.

Lower back pain: BL-40 *(wei zhong)*.

Swelling of the foot and knee: BL-67 (*zhi yin*).

Lower back pain due to qi stagnation with inability to remain in the upright position: SP-11 (*heng gu*), SP-2 (*da du*).

Breaking-type lower back pain with tinnitus: ST-36 (*zu san li*), and tonify or drain GB-42 (*di wu hui*).

Upper back and shoulder pain due to wind consumption: LI-3 (*san jian*), BL-23 (*shen shu*).

If we needle GB-21 (*jian jing*), we must combine it with ST-36 (*zu san li*); otherwise, the qi will not be regulated.

Knee pain: warm needle GB-34 (*yang ling quan*).

Lower back pain with contractures of the feet: BL-40 (*wei zhong*).

Pain in the foot with swelling of the knee: ST-36 (*zu san li*), GB-39 (*xuan zhong*), GB-34 (*yang ling quan*), SP-9 (*yin ling quan*), SP-6 (*san yin jiao*).

Paresthesia and numbness of the toes: LR-3 (*tai chong*).

Cramps with blurry vision: BL-57 (*cheng shan*), BL-60 (*kun lun*).

Wind-cold and cold painful obstruction that are difficult to cure: warm needle GB-30 (*huan tiao*) and GV-2 (*yao shu*).

Pain in the hip and lower limb: drain ST-36 (*zu san li*) and separate stagnant qi from the lower by needling KI-7 (*fu liu*).

Long-term cold-damage with pain in the shoulders and back: TB-3 (*zhong zhu*).

Unremitting pain in the shoulder radiating toward the navel: LI-10 (*shou san li*); if there is a heavy numb sensation after needling, drain the point and do not retain the needle after the qi sensation has been obtained.

FROM "ODE OF THE JADE DRAGON"

Leg qi: ST-36 (*zu san li*), GB-39 (*xuan zhong*), SP-6 (*san yin jiao*).

Lower limb fatigue: GB-31 (*feng shi*), ST-33 (*yin shi*).

Painful swelling of the knees: SP-9 (*yin ling quan*), GB-34 (*yang ling quan*).

Cough and paravertebral thoracic pain: GV-12 (*shen zhu*).

Severe stoop: GB-20 (*feng chi*), GB-39 (*xuan zhong*).

Flaccidity of the tendons causing the body to lean forward: GV-26 (*ren zhong*), LI-11 (*qu chi*).

Severe foot pain: SP-5 (*shang qiu*), ST-41 (*jie xi*), GB-40 (*qiu xu*).

Sinew contractions making them useless: LU-5 (*chi ze*).

Difficulty in moving the hands and wrist: SI-4 (*wan gu*).

Pain in the upper back and shoulder: GB-27 (*wu shu*) and "Back Seam" (*bei feng*).[4]

Painful contractures of the elbow: LU-5 (*chi ze*), LI-11 (*qu chi*).

Wind-dampness in both shoulders: LI-15 (*jian yu*).

Swelling and redness of the arms: TB-3 (*zhong zhu*), TB-2 (*ye men*).

Grabbing pain in the shoulder: GB-21 (*jian jing*).

Wrenching pain in the lumbar spine that is difficult to control: GV-26 (*ren zhong*), BL-40 (*wei zhong*).

Swollen feet with difficulty in walking: KI-3 (*tai xi*), BL-60 (*kun lun*), BL-62 (*shen mai*).

Heaviness and pain in the calves and feet: M-LE-28 (*kuan gu*),[5] M-LE-16 (*xi yan*), LR-7 (*xi guan*).

Difficulty in walking: ST-36 (*zu san li*), LR-4 (*zhong feng*), LR-3 (*tai chong*).

Pain in the lower limbs due to wind-dampness: GB-29 (*ju liao*), GB-30 (*huan tiao*), BL-40 (*wei zhong*).

FROM "ODE OF THE ESSENTIALS OF PENETRATING MYSTERIES"

Difficulty in walking: LR-3 (*tai chong*).

Pain and stiffness in the spine and upper back: GV-26 (*ren zhong*).

Neck stiffness due to wind damage: GV-16 (*feng fu*).

Spasms of the elbow: LI-11 (*qu chi*).

Lassitude of the four limbs: KI-6 (*zhao hai*).

Stiffness of the head and nape: CV-24 (*cheng jiang*).

Painful cramps of the sinews: BL-57 (*cheng shan*).

Painful ankle and foot: BL-60 (*kun lun*).

Pain in the thigh and knee: ST-33 (*yin shi*).

Knee swelling and eye diseases: LR-2 (*xing jian*).

Pain in the elbow with contracture of the sinews: LU-5 (*chi ze*).

Insensitivity in the arms: GB-21 (*jian jing*).

Pain in the lower limbs: M-LE-28 (*kuan gu*).[6]

Lower back pain: BL-23 (*shen shu*).

FROM "ODE OF DIVINE LIGHT"

Contracture of the lower limbs: ST-33 (*yin shi*).

[All] five types of lower back pain: BL-40 (*wei zhong*).

Difficulty in mobilizing the hips: drain GB-40 (*qiu xu*).

Pain due to pathogenic wind: ST-35 (*du bi*).

Pain in the feet: BL-60 (*kun lun*).

Ankle pain: BL-61 (*pu shen*).

Lower limb cramps and chronic hemorrhoids: BL-57 (*cheng shan*).

Inability to extend the fingers: TB-3 (*zhong zhu*).

Leg qi: needle the four yin Heel and yang Heel vessel points [KI-6 (*zhao hai*) and BL-62 (*shen mai*)]; SP-9 (*yin ling quan*) and GB-34 (*yang ling quan*) can also treat this condition, as well as the yin Heel and yang Heel vessel points and ST-36 (*zu san li*).

FROM "SONG OF THE JADE DRAGON"

Painful stiffness in the back of the neck with difficulty in looking backward; the pain is similar to a toothache: start by tonifying and draining CV-24 (*cheng jiang*), and then needle GV-16 (*feng fu*).

COMMENTARY: CV-24 (*cheng jiang*) should be drained and GV-16 (*feng fu*) should not be needled deeply.

Painful stiffness of the spine and back: drain GV-26 (*ren zhong*). This point is also indicated for wrenching lower back pain. In addition, lower back pain disorders can be treated at BL-40 (*wei zhong*).

COMMENTARY: Moxa is forbidden at BL-40 (*wei zhong*), but bleeding the small vessels is permitted. Caution should be exercised in weak patients.

Lower back pain due to weakness of the kidneys: apply moxa frequently at BL-23 (*shen shu*) bilaterally.

Thigh and buttock wind: GB-30 (*huan tiao*); one can also needle GB-29 (*ju liao*) combined with bleeding BL-40 (*wei zhong*).

COMMENTARY: Applying moxa at GB-29 (*ju liao*) will cause contraction of the sinews.

Lower limb weakness with difficulty in standing in the upright position due to wind-dampness: warm GB-31 (*feng shi*) and ST-33 (*yin shi*) with moxa.

COMMENTARY: Tonify first, and then drain.

Pain in both legs: M-LE-28 (*kuan gu*).

Redness and swelling of both knees with inability to walk: M-LE-16 (*xi yan*), LR-7 (*xi guan*).

Leg qi due to damp-cold, becoming unbearable: first needle ST-36 (*zu san li*) and SP-6 (*san yin jiao*), and then add GB-39 (*xuan zhong*).

Straw-sandal wind with swelling and redness of the feet: BL-60 (*kun lun*), BL-62 (*shen mai*), KI-3 (*tai xi*).

Pain of the dorsum of the foot: needle obliquely and bleed GB-40 (*qiu xu*); then needle ST-41 (*jie xi*) and SP-5 (*shang qiu*) in accordance with the principles of tonification and draining. If symptoms are aggravated and there is difficulty in walking, needle LR-3 (*tai chong*), ST-36 (*zu san li*) and LR-4 (*zhong feng*).

Redness and swelling of the knees, crane's knee wind: needle GB-34 (*yang ling quan*) through to SP-9 (*yin ling quan*).

Lack of strength in the wrist with pain and difficulty in grasping objects: needle SI-4 (*wan gu*); do not overlook the importance of tonification and draining.

Acute pain in both arms radiating toward the chest: needle GB-21 (*jian jing*), where the true qi concentrates, and which should be tonified more than drained.

Shoulder and back wind with pain radiating toward the arm: needle M-BW-39 (*bei feng*).[7] GB-27 (*wu shu*) also treats lower back pain.

Contracture of both elbows with difficult mobilization: drain LI-11 (*qu chi*), LU-5 (*chi ze*).

COMMENTARY: LI-11 (*qu chi*) should be drained; moxa should not be used.

Swelling, pain, and redness of the shoulder due to a struggle between cold and dampness: needle LI-15 (*jian yu*), where moxa can also be applied.

Contracture of the sinews and difficulty in extending the hands: LU-5 *(chi ze)*.

Swelling and redness of the forearm and wrist: drain TB-2 *(ye men)*, TB-3 *(zhong zhu)*.

COMMENTARY: TB-2 *(ye men)* must be needled transversely through to TB-4 *(yang xi)*.

For diffuse pain, this is not an ordinary condition, and the painful points must be analyzed; if sinews and bones are involved, the puncture must be shallow, and the use of moxa restricted.

FROM "SONG OF OVERCOMING JADE"

Shoulder[8] pain: GB-21 *(jian jing)*.

Stiff neck: CV-24 *(cheng jiang)*.

Swollen knees: LR-2 *(xing jian)*.

Contracture of the sinews: LU-5 *(chi ze)*.

Difficulty in walking: LR-4 *(zhong feng)*, LR-3 *(tai chong)*.

Pain in the dorsum of the foot: SP-5 *(shang qiu)*.

Foot wind: BL-40 *(wei zhong)*.

Pain in both hands with difficulty in grasping objects: LI-11 *(qu chi)*, LI-4 *(he gu)*, LI-15 *(jian yu)*.

Pain in the arms and back: LI-10 *(shou san li)*.

Lower back pain: M-BW-26 *(zhong kong)*.[9]

Cramps and pain in the thigh and buttocks with difficulty in walking: drain GB-30 *(huan tiao)*, GB-31 *(feng shi)*, ST-33 *(yin shi)*.

Swelling of the knees from no apparent cause: moxa M-LE-16 *(xi yan)*, ST-36 *(zu san li)*.

Cramps in both buttocks: BL-57 *(cheng shan)*.

Leg qi: KI-7 *(fu liu)*.

Pain in the malleolus: moxa BL-60 *(kun lun)*; GB-39 *(xuan zhong)* and GB-40 *(qiu xu)* may also be selected.

Lower back pain due to injury of the kidneys with frequent urination: BL-23 *(shen shu)*.

FROM "SONG ON SELECTING POINTS FOR MISCELLANEOUS DISEASES"

For wind diseases located in the hand: TB-10 *(tian jing)*, GB-21 *(jian jing)*, LI-1 *(shang yang)*, LU-11 *(shao shang)*, LI-2 *(er jian)*, LI-3 *(san jian)*.

Pain in the fingers radiating to the shoulder: LI-4 *(he gu)*, LR-3 *(tai chong)*.

Pain in the shoulder radiating to the navel: LI-10 *(shou san li)*.

Pain in the upper back behind the heart: TB-3 *(zhong zhu)*.

For lower back pain, GB-30 *(huan tiao)* and BL-40 *(wei zhong)* are miraculous points; if the pain radiates toward the back, add BL-60 *(kun lun)*; if the pain radiates toward the thigh, tonify SI-4 *(wan gu)* and drain ST-36 *(zu san li)*; if the pain radiates toward the feet, drain GB-30 *(huan tiao)* and needle LR-2 *(xing jian)* and GB-31 *(feng shi)*.

Various knee and foot pains: LR-2 *(xing jian)*, ST-36 *(zu san li)*, BL-62 *(shen mai)*, BL-63 *(jin men)*.

Leg cramps with visual disturbances: KI-2 *(ran gu)*, BL-57 *(cheng shan)*.

Difficulty in walking: first needle GB-39 *(xuan zhong)* and then ST-38 *(tiao kou)*.

Lassitude with paresthesia and numbness of the lower limbs: tonify KI-3 *(tai xi)*.

Pain in the sole of the foot and heel: BL-61 *(pu shen)*, ST-44 *(nei ting)*.

COMMENTARY: Drain BL-61 *(pu shen)* for plantar pain, and drain ST-44 *(nei ting)* for heel pain.

Pain in the lower limb radiating toward the flank and axilla: GB-30 *(huan tiao)*, GB-34 *(yang ling quan)*.

Wind-cold-damp painful obstruction: needle GB-30 *(huan tiao)*, and then use warm needles at GB-34 *(yang ling quan)* and ST-36 *(zu san li)*.

FROM "SONG OF ELEVEN SETS OF POINTS FOR MISCELLANEOUS DISEASES"

Scapular and thoracic pain with pain in the upper arm: needle LI-11 *(qu chi)* and LI-4 *(he gu)* 0.7 unit deep; if there are no results, needle LU-5 *(chi ze)* 1 unit deep and then LI-3 *(san jian)* 0.7 unit deep; HT-8 *(shao fu)* and GV-16 *(feng fu)* may also be needled 0.7 unit deep.

Elbow pain: needle LI-11 *(qu chi)*, LU-8 *(jing qu)*, LI-4 *(he gu)* 0.5 unit deep; if this treatment does not work, add LI-3 *(san jian)* to a depth of 0.5 unit; if there is pain due to qi stagnation in the channel with fever and chills, needle PC-5 *(jian shi)* briefly.

Pain in the lower back, hips and thighs due to a focal accumulation of qi:[10] needle M-LE-28 (kuan gu) 0.7 unit deep, GB-31 (feng shi) and ST-36 (zu san li) 1 unit and 0.3 unit deep, drain SP-6 (san yin jiao) 1 unit deep, needle LR-2 (xing jian) 0.5 unit deep. For the illness to be cured, the needling technique must be synchronized with the patient's breathing.

Pain in the elbow and knee: needle LI-11 (qu chi) 1 unit deep on the side opposite the affected side; if this rule is followed, the draining power of the qi is miraculous. For pain in the knees, needle M-LE-16 (xi yan) 2 units deep; for ST-36 (zu san li) and SP-6 (san yin jiao), manipulate the needle seven times. As long as the cause of the illness has been carefully determined, the efficacy of the treatment is very rapid.

FROM "HEAVEN AND STARS SECRET SONG OF LORD CHANG-SANG"

Painful obstruction and contractures of the arm: LI-15 (jian yu).

Cramps in the legs with blurry vision: first BL-57 (cheng shan), then the medial malleolus.

Painful leg qi: first GB-21 (jian jing), then ST-36 (zu san li) and GB-34 (yang ling quan).

Lower back pain with tinnitus: first GB-39 (xuan zhong), then ST-38 (tiao kou) and ST-42 (chong yang).

Wind-damp-cold painful obstruction: first GB-30 (huan tiao), then GB-34 (yang ling quan).

Painful contractures of the fingers: LU-11 (shao shang).

FROM "SONG TO KEEP UP ONE'S SLEEVE"

Disorders affecting the head and face: BL-67 (zhi yin).

Disorders of the leg and foot: GV-16 (feng fu).

Disorders of the chest and heart: drain HT-8 (shao fu).

Disorders of the umbilical area and abdomen: LR-8 (qu quan).

Various disorders of the shoulder and back: TB-3 (zhong zhu).

Pain and stiffness of the lower back and knee: KI-8 (jiao xin).

Pain in the flank and thigh: SI-3 (hou xi).

Swelling in the hip and knee: drain LR-3 (tai chong).

For crane's knee wind with difficulty in walking, LU-5 (chi ze) can alleviate the pain in the bones and sinews; LI-11 (qu chi) may also be selected, depending on the origin of the illness. GV-16 (feng fu) can be added to ensure a complete cure of the disorder.

Contractures of the arm: deeply needling LU-5 (chi ze) eliminates the insensitivity.

Acute wind with contractures of the upper and lower back: needle LI-11 (qu chi) 1.5 units deep.

Chronic pain in the knees and feet: BL-60 (kun lun), KI-3 (tai xi).

Wind painful obstruction, atrophy or inversion: BL-11 (da zhu), LR-8 (qu quan).

Inability to fully extend both lower limbs and flanks: needle TB-6 (zhi gou) 0.7 unit deep.

Radical cure for lumbar weakness: BL-40 (wei zhong).

FROM "THE VARIOUS WINDS"

Inability to flex the elbow: SI-4 (wan gu).

Legs lacking in gloss and luster: LI-9 (shang lian).

Contracture of the elbow from wind-stroke: PC-6 (nei guan).

Wind painful obstruction: TB-10 (tian jing), LU-5 (chi ze), HT-3 (shao hai), BL-40 (wei zhong), GB-38 (yang fu).

Wind consumption: LR-8 (qu quan), BL-28 (pang guang shu).

Wind pouring:[11] GV-20 (bai hui), BL-18 (gan shu), BL-20 (pi shu), BL-23 (shen shu), BL-28 (pang guang shu).

Pain from wind-stroke: GB-41 (zu lin qi), GV-20 (bai hui), GB-21 (jian jing), LI-15 (jian yu), LI-11 (qu chi), TB-10 (tian jing), PC-5 (jian shi), PC-6 (nei guan), LI-4 (he gu), GB-31 (feng shi), ST-36 (zu san li), ST-41 (jie xi), BL-60 (kun lun), KI-6 (zhao hai).

FROM "PAINFUL OBSTRUCTION AND INVERSION"

Wind painful obstruction: LU-5 (chi ze), GB-38 (yang fu).

Accumulation painful obstruction and phlegm painful obstruction: BL-17 (ge shu).

Cold inversion: LU-9 (*tai yuan*), TB-2 (*ye men*).

Inversion with atrophy: GB-40 (*qiu xu*).

Cold painful obstruction: LI-11 (*qu chi*), LU-7 (*lie que*), GB-30 (*huan tiao*), GB-31 (*feng shi*), BL-40 (*wei zhong*), SP-5 (*shang qiu*), LR-4 (*zhong feng*), GB-41 (*zu lin qi*).

Inversion of the four extremities: LU-5 (*chi ze*), SI-8 (*xiao hai*), TB-6 (*zhi gou*), SI-2 (*qian gu*), ST-36 (*zu san li*), SP-6 (*san yin jiao*), LR-8 (*qu quan*), KI-6 (*zhao hai*), KI-3 (*tai xi*), ST-44 (*nei ting*), LR-2 (*xing jian*), SP-2 (*da du*).

From "Head and Face Problems"

Headache with stiffness: ST-6 (*jia che*), GB-20 (*feng chi*), GB-21 (*jian jing*), HT-3 (*shao hai*), SI-3 (*hou xi*), SI-2 (*qian gu*).

Head and nape pain: GV-20 (*bai hui*), GV-19 (*hou ding*), LI-4 (*he gu*).

Headache with stiff neck, heaviness with inability to raise the head, hyperextension of the spine, and inability to look backward: CV-24 (*cheng jiang*) (drain first and then tonify) and GV-16 (*feng fu*).

From "Chest, Upper Back, and Flank Problems"

Painful obstruction of the chest: LU-9 (*tai yuan*).

Stifling sensation and pain in the chest and upper arms: GB-21 (*jian jing*).

Chest and flank pain: TB-10 (*tian jing*), TB-6 (*zhi gou*), PC-5 (*jian shi*), PC-7 (*da ling*), ST-36 (*zu san li*), SP-3 (*tai bai*), GB-40 (*qiu xu*), GB-38 (*yang fu*).

Upper back and shoulder soreness and pain: BL-12 (*feng men*), GB-21 (*jian jing*), TB-3 (*zhong zhu*), TB-6 (*zhi gou*), SI-3 (*hou xi*), SI-4 (*wan gu*), BL-40 (*wei zhong*).

Supraclavicular pain: LU-9 (*tai yuan*), LI-1 (*shang yang*), GB-41 (*zu lin qi*).

Pain in the flanks radiating toward the spine: BL-18 (*gan shu*).

Painful contracture of the back, neck, and arm: GV-14 (*da zhui*).

Upper and lower back stiffness with inability to rotate the trunk: GV-2 (*yao shu*), BL-13 (*fei shu*).

Pain in the lumbar spine: BL-40 (*wei zhong*), KI-7 (*fu liu*).

Lower and upper back stoop: GB-20 (*feng chi*), BL-12 (*feng men*).

Thoracic contracture: LU-8 (*jing qu*).

Pain in the back and both shoulders: LI-2 (*er jian*), LI-1 (*shang yang*), BL-40 (*wei zhong*), BL-60 (*kun lun*).

Unilateral severe painful obstruction of the flank and back: LU-10 (*yu ji*), BL-40 (*wei zhong*).

Upper back pain: GB-40 (*qiu xu*), LU-10 (*yu ji*), BL-60 (*kun lun*), BL-64 (*jing gu*).

Spinal and paravertebral stiffness and pain: BL-40 (*wei zhong*).

Upper and lower back pain with difficulty in rotation: TB-16 (*tian you*), GB-20 (*feng chi*), LI-4 (*he gu*), BL-60 (*kun lun*).

Pain in the spine with inability to flex or extend: LI-4 (*he gu*), KI-7 (*fu liu*), BL-60 (*kun lun*).

Stiffness of the vertebral column with generalized pain and inability to rotate: GV-15 (*ya men*).

Chest pain that radiates to the flanks: needle LR-14 (*qi men*) first, and then LR-13 (*zhang men*), GB-40 (*qiu xu*), LR-2 (*xing jian*), KI-1 (*yong quan*).

Painful obstruction and pain in the shoulders: LI-15 (*jian yu*), TB-10 (*tian jing*), LI-11 (*qu chi*), SI-5 (*yang gu*), TB-1 (*guan chong*).

From "Arms, Legs, Lower Back, and Axillary Problems"

Pain in the arm with inability to raise it: LI-11 (*qu chi*), LU-5 (*chi ze*), LI-15 (*jian yu*), HT-3 (*shao hai*), LU-9 (*tai yuan*), TB-4 (*yang chi*), LI-5 (*yang xi*), SI-5 (*yang gu*), SI-2 (*qian gu*), LI-4 (*he gu*), TB-2 (*ye men*), TB-5 (*wai guan*), SI-4 (*wan gu*).

Cold sensation in the arm: LU-5 (*chi ze*), HT-7 (*shen men*).

Pain in the medial aspect of the arm: LU-9 (*tai yuan*).

Pain in the lateral aspect of the arm: SI-5 (*yang gu*).

Tremors of the wrist: PC-3 (*qu ze*).

Axillary pain: HT-3 (*shao hai*), PC-5 (*jian shi*), HT-8 (*shao fu*), GB-38 (*yang fu*), GB-40 (*qiu xu*), GB-41 (*zu lin qi*), BL-62 (*shen mai*).

Weariness of the elbow: TB-10 (*tian jing*), LI-11 (*qu chi*), PC-5 (*jian shi*), LI-5 (*yang xi*), TB-3 (*zhong zhu*), SI-5 (*yang gu*), LU-9 (*tai yuan*), SI-4 (*wan gu*), LU-7 (*lie que*), TB-2 (*ye men*).

Lack of strength in the wrist: LU-7 (*lie que*).

Pain in the arm and elbow: LI-15 (*jian yu*), LI-11 (*qu chi*), HT-5 (*tong li*), LI-10 (*shou san li*).

Contracture of the elbow: LU-5 (*chi ze*), LI-15 (*jian yu*), HT-3 (*shao hai*), PC-5 (*jian shi*), PC-7 (*da ling*), SI-3 (*hou xi*), LU-10 (*yu ji*).

Lassitude and heaviness of the shoulders and arms: TB-6 (*zhi gou*).

Pain in the arm and elbow with inability to flex the fingers: LI-11 (*qu chi*), LI-10 (*shou san li*), TB-5 (*wai guan*), TB-3 (*zhong zhu*).

Paresthesia, numbness, and insensitivity of the arm and hand: TB-10 (*tian jing*), LI-11 (*qu chi*), TB-5 (*wai guan*), LU-8 (*jing qu*), LU-9 (*tai yuan*), TB-6 (*zhi gou*), LI-5 (*yang xi*), SI-4 (*wan gu*), LI-9 (*shang lian*), LI-4 (*he gu*).

Pain and cold sensation in the arm: GB-21 (*jian jing*), LI-11 (*qu chi*), LI-9 (*shang lian*).

Contracture of the fingers: LI-11 (*qu chi*), SI-5 (*yang gu*), LI-4 (*he gu*).

Hot hands: PC-8 (*lao gong*), LI-11 (*qu chi*), PC-3 (*qu ze*), PC-6 (*nei guan*), LU-7 (*lie que*), LU-8 (*jing qu*), LU-9 (*tai yuan*), PC-9 (*zhong chong*), HT-9 (*shao chong*).

Swelling and redness of the arms: LI-11 (*qu chi*), HT-5 (*tong li*), TB-3 (*zhong zhu*), LI-4 (*he gu*), LI-10 (*shou san li*), TB-2 (*ye men*).

Wind painful obstruction with contracture of the elbow and inability to raise it: LU-5 (*chi ze*), LI-11 (*qu chi*), LI-4 (*he gu*).

Spasms of the arms, wind concealed rash,[12] throat painful obstruction, fullness in the chest and flanks, laxity of the tendons at the level of the arms with lack of strength, and very dry skin: LI-11 (*qu chi*) (first drain and then tonify), LI-15 (*jian yu*), LI-10 (*shou san li*).

Irritability and pain in the shoulder and upper arm: LI-15 (*jian yu*), GB-21 (*jian jing*), LI-11 (*qu chi*).

Pain in all five fingers: TB-5 (*wai guan*).

Contracture of the hand and pain in the fingers: LU-11 (*shao shang*).

Heat in the palms of the hands: LU-7 (*lie que*), LU-8 (*jing qu*), LU-9 (*tai yuan*).

Swelling of the axilla and elbow: LU-5 (*chi ze*), SI-8 (*xiao hai*), PC-5 (*jian shi*), PC-7 (*da ling*).

Swelling below the axillary region: GB-38 (*yang fu*), GB-40 (*qiu xu*), GB-41 (*zu lin qi*).

Lower back pain: GB-21 (*jian jing*), GB-31 (*feng shi*), ST-33 (*yin shi*), ST-36 (*zu san li*), BL-40 (*wei zhong*), BL-57 (*cheng shan*), GB-38 (*yang fu*), BL-60 (*kun lun*), GV-2 (*yao shu*), BL-23 (*shen shu*).

Icy-cold sensation in the legs: ST-33 (*yin shi*).

Wrenching lower back pain and pain in both flanks: LU-5 (*chi ze*), LI-11 (*qu chi*), LI-4 (*he gu*), LI-10 (*shou san li*), SP-9 (*yin ling quan*), CV-7 (*yin jiao*), LR-2 (*xing jian*), ST-36 (*zu san li*).

Lower back pain with difficulty in moving: GB-31 (*feng shi*), BL-40 (*wei zhong*), LR-2 (*xing jian*).

Painful stiffness of the lumbar spine: GV-2 (*yao shu*), BL-40 (*wei zhong*), KI-1 (*yong quan*), BL-27 (*xiao chang shu*), BL-28 (*pang guang shu*).

Pain in the lumbar region and feet: GB-30 (*huan tiao*), GB-31 (*feng shi*), ST-33 (*yin shi*), BL-40 (*wei zhong*), BL-57 (*cheng shan*), BL-60 (*kun lun*), BL-62 (*shen mai*).

Pain in the medial aspect of the thigh and knee: BL-40 (*wei zhong*), ST-36 (*zu san li*), SP-6 (*san yin jiao*).

Weariness and pain in the knees and legs: GB-30 (*huan tiao*), GB-34 (*yang ling quan*), GB-40 (*qiu xu*).

Pain in the knees and feet: BL-40 (*wei zhong*), ST-36 (*zu san li*), LR-8 (*qu quan*), GB-34 (*yang ling quan*), GB-31 (*feng shi*), BL-60 (*kun lun*), ST-41 (*jie xi*).

Swelling of the knee, thigh and leg: BL-40 (*wei zhong*), ST-36 (*zu san li*), GB-38 (*yang fu*), ST-41 (*jie xi*), BL-57 (*cheng shan*).

Sensation of sitting in water: GB-38 (*yang fu*).

Lower limb atrophy: KI-7 (*fu liu*).

Wind painful obstruction with paresthesia and numbness of the foot and calf: GB-30 (*huan tiao*), GB-31 (*feng shi*).

Numbness and painful obstruction of the lower limbs: GB-30 (*huan tiao*), GB-34 (*yang ling quan*), GB-38 (*yang fu*), KI-3 (*tai xi*), BL-67 (*zhi yin*).

Leg qi: GB-21 *(jian jing)*, M-LE-16 *(xi yan)*, GB-31 *(feng shi)*, ST-36 *(zu san li)*, BL-57 *(cheng shan)*, LR-3 *(tai chong)*, GB-40 *(qiu xu)*, LR-2 *(xing jian)*.

Hip pain: GB-30 *(huan tiao)*, GB-34 *(yang ling quan)*, GB-40 *(qiu xu)*.

Sensations of cold and heat in the legs: ST-36 *(zu san li)*, BL-40 *(wei zhong)*, GB-34 *(yang ling quan)*, KI-7 *(fu liu)*, KI-2 *(ran gu)*, LR-4 *(zhong feng)*, SP-2 *(da du)*, SP-1 *(yin bai)*.

Swelling of the foot: BL-57 *(cheng shan)*, BL-60 *(kun lun)*, KI-2 *(ran gu)*, ST-39 *(xia ju xu)*, GB-31 *(feng shi)*, M-LE-28 *(kuan gu)*.

Icy-cold feet: BL-23 *(shen shu)*.

Chills in the whole body with lassitude of the legs: BL-57 *(cheng shan)*, BL-63 *(jin men)*.

Cold legs and feet: KI-7 *(fu liu)*, BL-62 *(shen mai)*, ST-45 *(li dui)*.

Contracture of the foot: BL-23 *(shen shu)*, GB-34 *(yang ling quan)*, GB-38 *(yang fu)*, GB-39 *(xuan zhong)*.

Diffuse joint pain: GB-38 *(yang fu)*.

Swelling of the calf: BL-57 *(cheng shan)*, BL-60 *(kun lun)*.

Flaccidity of the foot: GB-34 *(yang ling quan)*, ST-42 *(chong yang)*, LR-3 *(tai chong)*, ST-39 *(xia ju xu)*.

Weakness of the foot: BL-40 *(wei zhong)*, ST-36 *(zu san li)*, BL-57 *(cheng shan)*.

Painful swelling of both knees: LR-7 *(xi guan)*, BL-40 *(wei zhong)*, ST-36 *(zu san li)*, ST-33 *(yin shi)*.

Straw-sandal wind of the heel: BL-60 *(kun lun)*, GB-40 *(qiu xu)*, SP-5 *(shang qiu)*, KI-6 *(zhao hai)*.

Inability to walk: ST-36 *(zu san li)*, LR-8 *(qu quan)*, BL-40 *(wei zhong)*, GB-38 *(yang fu)*, SP-6 *(san yin jiao)*, KI-7 *(fu liu)*, ST-42 *(chong yang)*, KI-2 *(ran gu)*, BL-62 *(shen mai)*, LR-2 *(xing jian)*, BL-20 *(pi shu)*.

Pain and lassitude of the ankle: BL-40 *(wei zhong)*, BL-60 *(kun lun)*.

Pain in the sole of the foot: BL-60 *(kun lun)*.

Contracture of the foot tendon with heaviness of the foot, panarthralgia of the knee which presents like crane's knee wind, aversion to wind, and inability to get out of bed during crises: GB-31 *(feng shi)*.

Lower back pain with difficulty in standing for long periods, heaviness and soreness of the legs and knees to the point where the limbs cannot be raised: BL-59 *(fu yang)*.

Heaviness and intolerable pain in the lower back to the point where it is difficult to rotate or get out of bed, cold painful obstruction, contracture of the foot tendons with inability to flex or extend: apply simultaneously three moxa cones to the four points located on either side of the knee crease on both legs, with two people blowing continuously on them until they go out. For example, when the moxa is applied at midday, if there is borborygmus at night, or if the patient is able to take a few steps, the condition will be cured.

Lower back pain and inability to get up: BL-61 *(pu shen)*.

Diseases from the knee up: moxa GB-30 *(huan tiao)*, GB-31 *(feng shi)*.

Diseases from the knee down: moxa ST-35 *(du bi)*, LR-7 *(xi guan)*, ST-36 *(zu san li)*, GB-34 *(yang ling quan)*.

Diseases from the ankle up: moxa SP-6 *(san yin jiao)*, GB-39 *(xuan zhong)*, BL-60 *(kun lun)*.

Diseases from the ankle down: moxa KI-6 *(zhao hai)*, BL-62 *(shen mai)*.

Pain in the leg: M-LE-28 *(kuan gu)*.

Leg qi: apply 50 to 100 cones of moxa at GB-31 *(feng shi)*, needle ST-32 *(fu tu)* to a depth of 0.3 unit (moxa is forbidden at this point), and apply moxa at M-LE-16 *(xi yan)* (50 cones), ST-36 *(zu san li)* (100 cones), LI-9 *(shang lian)*, LI-8 *(xia lian)* (100 cones), GB-39 *(xuan zhong)*.

Knee sinew cramps that are intolerable: apply moxa above the ankle during attacks; apply moxa on the medial side for medial problems and vice versa.

Chronic leg cramps for many years for which medicine has been ineffective: BL-57 *(cheng shan)* (14 moxa cones).

FROM "ASSEMBLED ESSENTIALS OF TREATING CONDITIONS"

No. 39. Paresthesia and numbness of the arm and hand with insensitivity: LI-15 *(jian yu)*, LI-11 *(qu chi)*, LI-4 *(he gu)*.

CAUSE OF THE DISEASE: this affliction is due to cold and dampness contending with each other and leading to qi stagnation and blood stasis. For relapse, needle GB-21 *(jian jing)* and LU-7 *(lie que)*.

No. 40. Cold, wind, soreness, and pain in the hand and arm: GB-21 (*jian jing*), LI-11 (*qu chi*), LI-10 (*shou san li*), LI-8 (*xia lian*).

CAUSE OF THE DISEASE: sleeping in a cold environment, causing the cold pathogenic influence to invade the channels and collaterals. For relapse, needle LI-13 (*shou wu li*), LU-8 (*jing qu*), LI-9 (*shang lian*).

No. 41. Pain, swelling, and redness of the arm: LI-13 (*shou wu li*), LI-11 (*qu chi*), HT-5 (*tong li*), TB-3 (*zhong zhu*).

CAUSE OF THE DISEASE: clogging and stagnation of blood and qi obstructing the channels and vessels. For relapse, needle LI-4 (*he gu*) and LU-5 (*chi ze*).

No. 43. Contracture and spasm of the hand and arm, and the sinews in both hands are so tight that they cannot open up: TB-4 (*yang chi*), LI-4 (*he gu*), LU-5 (*chi ze*), LI-11 (*qu chi*), TB-3 (*zhong zhu*).

CAUSE OF THE DISEASE: invasion of dampness while sleeping outside, or invasion of wind-dampness while walking in the heat, or sleeping outside after sexual activity or consumption of alcohol. For relapse, needle LI-15 (*jian yu*), TB-3 (*zhong zhu*), LI-10 (*shou san li*), LU-11 (*shao shang*).

No. 44. Swelling, redness, pain in the shoulder and back: LI-15 (*jian yu*), BL-12 (*feng men*), TB-3 (*zhong zhu*), BL-11 (*da zhu*).

CAUSE OF THE DISEASE: loosening of the interstices and pores promotes the invasion through the skin of pathogenic wind, which combines with pathogenic cold, leading to coagulation and stagnation of blood and qi. For relapse, needle BL-43 (*gao huang shu*), BL-13 (*fei shu*), LI-15 (*jian yu*).

No. 49. Paresthesia and numbness of both feet: GB-38 (*yang fu*), GB-35 (*yang jiao*), GB-39 (*xuan zhong*), LR-2 (*xing jian*).

CAUSE OF THE DISEASE: dampness invading the channels which is not eliminated, or excessive sexual activity, or excessive consumption of alcohol, leading to disruption of the harmony between cold and heat. For relapse, needle BL-60 (*kun lun*), GB-39 (*xuan zhong*), GB-40 (*qiu xu*).

No. 50. Swelling, redness and pain in both knees: LR-7 (*xi guan*), BL-40 (*wei zhong*).

CAUSE OF THE DISEASE: either from a spleen person contracting dampness with the spreading of phlegm and congested fluids, or pathogenic cold entering the channels and collaterals after a dysenteric disorder; or from the spreading of a cold-induced disorder. For relapse, needle GB-34 (*yang ling quan*), CV-12 (*zhong wan*), ST-40 (*feng long*).

No. 51. Inability to walk: GB-40 (*qiu xu*), LR-2 (*xing jian*), BL-60 (*kun lun*), LR-3 (*tai chong*).

CAUSE OF THE DISEASE: sexual intercourse while drunk, such that the kidney channel is exhausted, leading first to weakness in the legs, and then to an inability to walk. If the above is ineffective, needle ST-36 (*zu san li*), GB-38 (*yang fu*), SP-6 (*san yin jiao*), KI-7 (*fu liu*).

No. 52. Weak and powerless legs: SP-4 (*gong sun*), ST-36 (*zu san li*), GB-39 (*xuan zhong*), BL-62 (*shen mai*).

CAUSE OF THE DISEASE: pathogenic dampness flowing into the channels and contending with the blood and qi; or excessive sexual activity injuring the essence and the qi; or excessive walking injuring the sinews and bones. For relapse, needle BL-60 (*kun lun*) and GB-38 (*yang fu*).

No. 54. Swelling, redness, and pain in the dorsum of the foot: LR-3 (*tai chong*), GB-41 (*zu lin qi*), LR-2 (*xing jian*), ST-44 (*nei ting*).

CAUSE OF THE DISEASE: consumption and overwork, or washing with [excessively] hot water, which prevents the blood and qi from circulating. For relapse, needle GB-40 (*qiu xu*), BL-60 (*kun lun*).

No. 55. Straw-sandal wind:[13] KI-6 (*zhao hai*), GB-40 (*qiu xu*), SP-5 (*shang qiu*), BL-60 (*kun lun*).

CAUSE OF THE DISEASE: consumption and overwork leads to stagnation of pathogenic dampness, thus generating a sensation of cold, or if the patient takes a cold foot bath after a long walk in the heat. For relapse, needle LR-3 (*tai chong*), ST-41 (*jie xi*).

No. 56. Wind pain with inability to rotate and difficulty in walking: GB-30 (*huan tiao*), GB-31 (*feng shi*), BL-60 (*kun lun*), GB-29 (*ju liao*), ST-36 (*zu san li*), GB-34 (*yang ling quan*).

CAUSE OF THE DISEASE: excessive sexual activity, lying down on the cold and damp ground inducing damp-cold to invade the channels, or trauma or wrenching causing lower back pain with limited range of motion. If ineffective, needle GB-27 (*wu shu*), GB-38 (*yang fu*), TB-6 (*zhi gou*).

No. 57. Lower back pain and leg pain: BL-40 *(wei zhong)*, GV-26 *(ren zhong)*.

No. 58. Lower back pain due to kidney deficiency: BL-23 *(shen shu)*, BL-40 *(wei zhong)*, KI-3 *(tai xi)*, BL-30 *(bai huan shu)*.

No. 59. Lower back pain and stiffness: GV-26 *(ren zhong)*, BL-40 *(wei zhong)*.

No. 60. Wrenching lower back and flank pain: LU-5 *(chi ze)*, BL-40 *(wei zhong)*, GV-26 *(ren zhong)*.

CAUSE OF THE DISEASE: excessive sexual activity injuring the kidney channel and leading to a drying up of the essence and blood; kidney deficiency lower back pain; or disruption of the blood and qi subsequent to walking while carrying a heavy load; or invasion of pathogenic heat preventing the blood from returning to its source; or a number of different causes leading the qi to attack both flanks and causing pain. If the treatment fails, needle BL-60 *(kun lun)*, BL-65 *(shu gu)*, TB-6 *(zhi gou)*, GB-34 *(yang ling quan)*.

No. 111. Flank pain due to a cold-induced disorder: TB-6 *(zhi gou)*, LR-13 *(zhang men)*, GB-34 *(yang ling quan)*.

No. 112. Chest and flank pain due to a cold-induced disorder: PC-7 *(da ling)*, LR-14 *(qi men)*, CV-17 *(tan zhong)*, PC-8 *(lao gong)*.

No. 151. Paresthesia and numbness of the four limbs: LI-15 *(jian yu)*, LI-11 *(qu chi)*, LI-4 *(he gu)*, SI-4 *(wan gu)*, GB-31 *(feng shi)*, BL-60 *(kun lun)*, LR-2 *(xing jian)*, ST-36 *(zu san li)*, GB-39 *(xuan zhong)*, BL-40 *(wei zhong)*, HT-4 *(ling dao)*, GB-34 *(yang ling quan)*. For this condition one should tonify more and drain less. For swelling and redness of the limbs, drain more and tonify less.

Chapter Notes

1. *Editors' note:* We have been unable to determine which point is meant by *qián yè*.

2. *Editors' note:* We have been unable to determine which point is meant by *yáng jiān*.

3. *Editors' note:* Straw-sandal wind *(cǎo xié fēng)* is a disorder marked by vesicles or sores in the area around the heel. There may also be swelling, pain or itching, and it may extend down to the sole.

4. *Editors' note:* The point *bèi fēng* is also known as *jiǎ fēng* ("scapular seam"). This is a miscellaneous point located lateral to the inferior angle of the scapula, at the tip the posterior axillary fold. We are unaware of any numbering scheme which includes this point.

5. *Editors' note:* The point *kuān gǔ* ("thigh bone") has two locations in the literature. One is of a single point on each side, located on the lateral aspect of the thigh, 1 unit lateral to ST-34 *(liang qiu)*. The other is of two points on each side, located 1.5 units lateral and medial to the same point.

6. *Editors' note:* Ibid.

7. *Editors' note:* See n. 4 above.

8. *Editors' note:* The original has hip *(bì)*. However, the commentary explains that the context makes it much more likely that shoulder is intended.

9. *Editors' note:* This point is *zhōng kōng* ("central space"). The commentary says that it is located 3 units inferior and lateral to BL-23 *(shen shu)*. In other sources it is located 3.5 units lateral to the spinous process of the fifth lumbar vertebra.

10. *Editors' note:* Modern Chinese commentators believe that the word *bì*, usually translated as "focal distention," refers here to one of the five accumulations *(jí)*, in this case that of the Spleen.

11. *Editors' note:* Modern Chinese commentators interpret the phrase "wind pouring" *(fēng zhǔ)* to mean a condition marked by moving pain and spasms of the skin and flesh.

12. *Editors' note:* "Wind concealed rash" *(fēng yǐn zhěn)* refers to urticarious eruptions.

13. *Editors' note:* See n. 3 above.

CHAPTER THIRTY-FIVE

Acupuncture for Lower Back Pain

Throughout the history of medicine in China, acupuncture has been an important modality for the treatment of lower back pain. The following are selections from various works that are included in division 188 of the Qing dynasty work, *Medical Section of the Grand Compilation of Ancient and Contemporary Works (Gu jin tu shu ji cheng yi bu)*.

Basic Questions *(Su wen)*

FROM "NEEDLING HEAT"
(CHAPTER 32)

In spleen heat disease, the struggle with heat causes lower back pain with an inability to flex or extend, abdominal fullness, diarrhea, and pain in both cheeks. These symptoms are exacerbated during *jia* and *yi* days [1 and 2]. There is profuse sweating during *wu* and *ji* days [5 and 6]. When the qi rebels, death will occur during *jia* and *yi* days. Needle the leg greater yin and leg yang brightness.

In kidney heat disease, there is lower back pain with lassitude of the calves, polydypsia with body heat. The symptoms are exacerbated during *wu* and *ji* days. There is profuse sweating during *ren* and *gui* days [9 and 10]. When the qi rebels, death will occur during *wu* and *ji* days. Needle the leg lesser yin and leg greater yang.

FROM "NEEDLING MALARIAL DISORDERS" (CHAPTER 36)

Leg greater yang malarial disorder causes lower back pain with heaviness of the head. Cold rises up from the back. Needle and bleed BL-40 *(wei zhong)*.

Leg terminal yin malarial disorder causes lower back pain with lower abdominal fullness and difficulty in urination. Needle the leg terminal yin.

Kidney malarial disorder causes a shivering cold and the lumbar spine is painful and bent. Needle the leg greater yang and lesser yin.

If the disease starts with lumbar spine pain, begin by needling and bleeding BL-40 *(wei zhong)*.

Divine Pivot *(Ling shu)*

FROM "PATHOLOGICAL MANIFESTATIONS OF THE ORGANS DUE TO PATHOGENIC QI" (CHAPTER 4)

In small intestine disease, the lower abdomen is painful, the lower back pain radiates toward the testes, there is a pressing need to defecate and urinate, there is heat in front of the ear, or intense cold, or intense heat on top of the shoulders, or heat in the space between the second and fifth finger, or the pulse is hidden. According to these symptoms, this is an arm greater yang disorder. Needle ST-39 *(xia ju xu)*.

From "Endings and Beginnings" (Chapter 9)

When the disease is on top, treat it at the bottom; when it is at the bottom, treat it above. When it is located in the head, treat it at the feet. When it centers in the lower back, treat it at the popliteal fossa.

From "Channels and Vessels" (Chapter 10)

The divergence of the leg lesser yin is called KI-4 *(da zhong)*. It diverges and goes to the greater yang and its divergence follows that channel and ascends to below the pericardium, externally linking up with the lumbar spine. When this channel is affected, its qi rebels causing irritability and a stifling sensation. In cases of excess, there is obstruction [of bowel movements and urination]; in cases of deficiency, there is lower back pain. Choose from where it diverges [KI-4 *(da zhong)*].

From "Five Pernicious Influences" (Chapter 20)

When a pernicious influence is in the kidneys, it causes pain in the bones and yin painful obstruction. Yin painful obstruction is not felt upon palpation; there is abdominal distention, lower back pain, difficult bowel movements, pain in the shoulders, upper back and neck, and occasional vertigo. Treatment consists of needling KI-1 *(yong quan)* and BL-60 *(kun lun)*; if you observe blood, get all of it.

From "Inversion Disorder" (Chapter 24)

In headaches caused by a inversion disorder *(jué 厥)* the nape hurts first and the lumbar spine responds; first needle BL-10 *(tian zhu)* and then choose the leg greater yang.

From "Miscellaneous Disorders" (Chapter 26)

In case of an inversion disorder encircling the vertebral column with pain extending to the vertex, a heavy, sinking sensation in the head, blurry vision, and stiffness in the lumbar spine, treat the leg greater yang at the level of the blood vessels in the popliteal fossa.

In case of heart pain radiating toward the lumbar spine with a desire to vomit, treat the leg lesser yin.

From "Licentious Pathogens Leading to Dreams" (Chapter 43)

When the kidney qi is abundant, there are dreams in which the lumbar and thoracic spine become disassociated and lose their interconnection [a sensation of being estranged from one's own lower back]; in this type of abundance, needle the corresponding point by draining it and [the problem] will immediately cease.

Systematic Classic of Acupuncture and Moxibustion *(Zhen jiu jia yi jing)*

From "Contraction of Disease by Kidneys and Small Intestine Developing Abdominal Distention and Lower Back Pain Radiating to the Upper Back and Lower Abdomen while Pulling on the Testicles" (Division 9, Chapter 8)

For lower back pain and ascending cold with a spine that is tense and rigid with excess, use GV-1 *(chang qiang)* as the main point.

For lower abdominal pain that pulls toward the genital area and radiates to the lumbar spine, and hernial pain that surges up to the heart, a rigid lumbar spine, dark urine, and dry mouth, use BL-27 *(xiao chang shu)* as the main point.

For pain of the lumbar spine with contracture radiating toward the back and lower abdomen, difficulty flexing and extending, inability to rest on one's back, atrophy and heaviness of the lower limbs, inability to raise the buttocks, dark red urine, insensitivity with a sensation of cold in lower back and below, and inability to get up from a sitting position, use BL-28 *(pang guang shu)* as the main point.

For lower back pain with inability to flex or extend, use BL-29 *(zhong lu shu)* as the main point.

For lower back and leg pain with a sensation of cold, a tendency to lean forward, and retraction of the testicles, use BL-31 *(shang liao)* as the main point.

For lower back pain with inability to flex or extend, insensitivity in the lower back and below, cold in the lumbar and thoracic spine, BL-32 *(ci liao)* is the main point; begin by needling ST-12 *(que pen)*, then GV-1 *(chang qiang)*, and finally BL-31~34 *(ba liao)*.

For lower back pain with difficult defecation, urgent morning diarrhea, with cold in the lumbar-coccygeal region, use BL-33 (*zhong liao*) as the main point.

For lower back pain with vertebral tension, fullness in both flanks, and a hard and tense lower abdomen, use BL-52 (*zhi shi*) as the main point.

For lower back pain with aversion to wind, a full and hard lower abdomen, urinary blockage with a heavy sensation in the perineum followed by an inability to urinate, use BL-53 (*bao huang*) as the main point.

For lower back pain with cold in the sacrum, difficult flexing and extending with tension, pain in the external genital organs with heaviness in the perineum, and an inability to urinate, use BL-54 (*zhi bian*) as the main point.

For lower back pain pulling toward the testicles, lower abdomen and buttocks, and sudden inability to straighten oneself up after bending forward, needle ST-30 (*qi chong*).

For lower back pain with inability to turn to the side, use LR-13 (*zhang men*) as the main point.

For lower back pain with inability to remain in the standing position for long, or to flex or extend the trunk, use GB-25 (*jing men*) and LR-2 (*xing jian*) as the main points.

For pain in the lower back, abdomen and lower abdomen, use BL-34 (*xia liao*) as the main point.

For lower back pain with an inability to flex or extend, use SP-9 (*yin ling quan*) as the main point.

For lower back pain, fullness in the lower abdomen, difficult urination as in urinary blockage, wasting and emaciation, focusing on fears and anxieties, qi deficiency, and an uncomfortable sensation in the abdomen, use LR-3 (*tai chong*) as the main point.

For pain in the lower back and lower abdomen, use LR-9 (*yin bao*) as the main point.

For lower back pain with difficult defecation, use KI-1 (*yong quan*) as the main point.

For lower back pain radiating along the lumbar spine comparable to pain occurring during defecation; in cases of excess, there is obstruction [of defecation and urination], shivering, lumbar spine pain with twisting, rolling of the eyes, a strong desire to lie down, and heat in the mouth; in cases of deficiency, there is lower back pain with cold extremities, and irritability of the heart region with a stifling sensation: use KI-4 (*da zhong*) as the main point.

For lower back pain radiating along the medial border of the spine, needle KI-7 (*fu liu*), and do not bleed during spring; if excessive bleeding is induced, it may cause a deficiency that cannot be restored [to normal]. This is the same as for the leg lesser yin pain noted above.

For lower back pain with inability to lift the foot and to sit down for a moment, as if stumbling down after getting out of a cart, and a burning sensation in the calf, use BL-62 (*shen mai*) as the main point.

For lower back pain with a sensation like little awls inside, painful swelling (one should not cough, as coughing might induce a contraction of the tendons), diffuse joint pain at the top or at the bottom with no particular location, cold and heat attacks, use GB-38 (*yang fu*) as the main point.

For lower back pain with inability to lift the heel and pain in the posterior aspect of the calf with atrophy of the foot, use BL-61 (*pu shen*) as the main point.

For lower back pain ascending along both sides of the spine to the head with visual disturbances and vertigo, use BL-40 (*wei zhong*) as the main point; this corresponds to needling and bleeding the leg greater yang cleft point [BL-63 (*jin men*)].

For lower back pain with an ability to flex but an inability to extend. With extension there is a fear of falling over. This results from attempting to lift a heavy weight and is related to bad blood (*è xuè* 惡血); use BL-37 (*yin men*) as the main point. This is lower back pain from the vessel of the collateral of the penetrating vessel.

Lower back pain, yin cold with intense pain in the coccyx, buttocks, and hips: in cases of deficiency, there is agitation of the blood, and in cases of excess, there is a combination with heat [fever], hemorrhoidal pain, swelling of the coccyx and buttocks area, and fecal incontinence; use BL-36 (*cheng fu*) as the main point.

Thousand Ducat Prescriptions (*Qian jin yao fang*)

For thoracolumbar pain, needle the blue and red collaterals located in the popliteal and inguinal folds; the cure is obtained after bleeding them.

In cases of lumbar pain with inability to flex or extend, ask the patient to stand up, measure the distance between the ground and the umbilicus with a bamboo stick and cut it at that length, then use this stick to measure the spine and apply moxa at its upper extremity. Use one moxa cone for each year of the patient's life. Once completed, hide the bamboo stick.

For lower back pain, burn ten moxa cones at the border of the white skin in the transverse fold at the level of the heel.

We can also burn seven moxa cones at the level of the foot greater yang which is located below the lateral malleolus.

We can also apply seven moxa cones at the level of the "lower back eye holes" which are located to the left and right of the coccyx.

We can also apply moxa at the level of BL-31~34 *(ba liao)* points and on the tip of the lateral malleolus.

For abrupt lower back pain, apply seven moxa cones at the level of the coccyx, as well as 1 unit to its left and right.

For a sensation of fullness of the five yin organs and six yang organs of the chest and abdomen, with back pain, vomiting, regurgitation of food, difficult urination, wasting, and shortness of breath, apply moxa at BL-22 *(san jiao shu)*; the number of cones is equal to the age of the patient.

For abdominal diseases with lumbar pain, cold in the bladder, diarrhea, intense thirst, apply moxa at M-BW-21 *(xia ji shu)*;[1] the number of moxa cones is determined by the age of the patient.

For overexertion, coldness, rebellious qi, cold painful obstruction in the lumbar and hip region, and difficulty in flexing and extending the lower limbs, apply a hundred moxa cones at the level of the yang heel [vessel] below the lateral malleolus, in the space where you can fit a finger.

For difficult thoracolumbar rotation, tight sinews, painful obstruction, and contractures of the sinews, apply moxa at the level of the twenty-first vertebra; the number of moxa cones is determined by the age of the patient.

GV-11 *(shen dao)*, "Middle of the Valley" *(gu zhong)*,[2] GV-2 *(yao shu)*, GV-1 *(chang qiang)*, BL-11 *(da zhu)*, BL-46 *(ge guan)*, CV-9 *(shui fen)*, BL-20 *(pi shu)*, BL-27 *(xiao chang shu)* and BL-28 *(pang guang shu)* are points used to treat urgent tightness of the lumbar spine.

GV-2 *(yao shu)*, BL-28 *(pang guang shu)*, GV-1 *(chang qiang)*, ST-30 *(qi chong)*, BL-31 *(shang liao)*, BL-34 *(xia liao)* and GB-29 *(ju liao)* treat lower back pain.

"Will Gate" *(zhi men)*[3] and GB-25 *(jing men)* treat painful contracture of the lumbar spine.

BL-27 *(xiao chang shu)*, BL-29 *(zhong lu shu)* and BL-30 *(bai huan shu)* treat lumbar spine hernial pain.[4]

BL-32 *(ci liao)*, BL-53 *(bao huang)* and BL-56 *(cheng jin)* treat lower back pain with aversion to cold.

ST-36 *(zu san li)*, ST-33 *(yin shi)*, GB-38 *(yang fu)* and LR-5 *(li gou)* treat lower back pain with inability to turn around to look back.

BL-65 *(shu gu)*, BL-58 *(fei yang)* and BL-56 *(cheng jin)* treat breaking-type lower back pain.

BL-62 *(shen mai)*, LR-3 *(tai chong)* and the yang heel[5] treat lower back pain with inability to straighten oneself up.

BL-60 *(kun lun)* treats vertebral stiffness and a heavy sensation in the back and coccyx.

BL-55 *(he yang)* treats lumbar pain radiating to the abdomen.

BL-40 *(wei zhong)* treats lower back pain encircling the spine all the way to the head with dizziness. Every time there is pain in the lumbar region and a corresponding pain in the lower limb, bleed this point; even in the case of a chronic or lingering condition, the patient will be able to get up.

KI-4 *(da zhong)*, SP-3 *(tai bai)*, SP-9 *(yin ling quan)* and LR-2 *(xing jian)* treat lower back pain with inability to flex or extend.

BL-36 *(cheng fu)* treats cold pain in the lumbar region, coccyx and buttocks.

KI-1 *(yong quan)* treats lower back pain radiating toward the abdomen with urgent bowel movement.

KI-10 *(yin gu)* treats pain in the internal aspect of the spine.

BL-46 *(ge guan)*, BL-54 *(zhi bian)* and BL-64 *(jing gu)* treat pain with aversion to cold, stiffness of the spine, and difficulty flexing or extending.

Confucians' Duties to Their Parents
(Ru men shi qin)

Both BL-23 *(shen shu)* points are located 1.5 units on either side of the fourteenth vertebra; apply five moxa cones to treat lower back pain with inability to flex or extend, difficulty in rotation, chills and fever, an appetite that is at least doubled, wasting, dark yellow complexion, or blurred vision. They are also useful in treating cold disorders or qi consumption in men and women.

Both BL-29 *(zhong lu shu)* points are located 1.5 units on either side of the eleventh vertebra; apply five moxa cones to treat lower back pain with inability to flex or extend, pain encircling the spine, sensitivity to pressure both at the top and at the bottom. If the pain spreads between the neck and this point, moxibustion is efficacious.

GV-2 *(yao shu)* is located below the [spinous process of the] twenty-first vertebra in a hollow; apply five moxa cones to treat lower back pain with inability to stand up for a long period of time, coldness and insensitivity in the area located between the lower back and the feet, difficulty in sitting down and getting up, lower back pain with inability to get up, contractures, inability to lean forward with a heavy sensation in the lumbar area like a piece of rock, and difficulty in moving.

Teachings of [Zhu] Dan-Xi
(Dan xi xin fa)

For a crooked lower back with an inability to straighten up, needle GV-26 *(ren zhong)*.

Outline of Medicine
(Yi xue gang mu)

In chapter 41, "Needling Lower Back Pain," of *Basic Questions*, three needling methods for leg greater yang lower back pain radiating toward the neck and the coccyx are presented: bleed BL-40 *(xi zhong)*; the other two methods consist of bleeding points on the leg greater yang channel.

This classic also states that when the pathogenic influence is located in the kidneys, there is abdominal bloating with lower back pain, difficult defecation, pain in the shoulders, back and neck, and intermittent vertigo. The treatment consists of needling KI-1 *(yong quan)* and BL-

60 *(kun lun)*; if there is blood, we must use the bleeding technique—this is the method for bleeding the leg greater yang and lesser yin.

This classic also specifies that when the leg greater yang is disturbed, the disease rises to the head and triggers pain. We must then determine the state of the greater yang—excess, deficiency, cold, heat, inversion—to be able to apply the appropriate treatment—tonification, draining, rapid needling, retained needle, moxibustion—in order to harmonize the condition.

The needling technique used for leg lesser yin lower back pain radiating on either side of the spine is to extract blood from the leg lesser yin. The classic states that the divergence of the leg lesser yin is KI-4 *(da zhong)*, which travels behind the malleolus, goes around it, from which a divergence travels to the leg greater yang. When affected and in the case of deficiency, there will be lower back pain, and we must select its divergence [KI-4 *(da zhong)*] which corresponds to tonifying the leg lesser yin collateral.

There are four needling methods for lower back pain with inability to flex or extend; three of them correspond to the lesser yang, yang brightness, and the transverse collaterals; bleeding is indicated in all three cases. The classic says that when the leg terminal yin Liver channel is disturbed, there is disease with lower back pain, with inability to flex or extend, and we must determine if this is a state of deficiency, excess, cold, heat or inversion—to decide among tonification, draining, rapid needling, retained needle, moxibustion—in order to harmonize the condition.

To treat lower back pain radiating toward the lower abdomen, weighing down on the flanks, with inability to straighten oneself up, select points located in the interosseous spaces in the sacrum.

Three chapters speak about lower back pain in *Basic Questions*, this being one of them. Chapter 63, "On Eccentric Needling," states that for lower back pain radiating to the abdomen, pulling on the flanks, and making it impossible to breathe with the trunk erect, needle M-BW-23 *(yao yi)* at the juncture of the lower back and sacrum, above the buttocks, a number of times corresponding to the lunar phase. Results are instantaneous; the disease ceases immediately. For problems on the left choose the right, for those on the right choose the left. Chapter 60, "On Bony Hollows," recommends that in treating lower back pain that prevents movement and rotation, with an acute sensation radiating down to the testicles, needle the eight sacral foramina and the areas of pain. The eight holes are distributed between the lower back and the coccyx. These three chapters generally share a similar appearance and differ in small details, but they represent the same method.

When the leg terminal yin is disturbed, then the person comes down with lower back pain with inability to flex or extend; we must then determine if this is a state of deficiency, excess, cold, heat or inversion in order to harmonize the condition. This corresponds to the same symptomatology, but with a different treatment method.

There are three needling methods for lower back pain with visual disturbances; treating the flourishing yang vessel is one of them. If the pain radiates toward the shoulders with urinary leakage, needle the dispersed vessel at the level of the lateral aspect of BL-40 *(wei zhong)* in the space separating the sinews and the bones: this is BL-39 *(wei yang)*. If the pain radiates to the neck with spinal stiffness and a tendency to fall down, bleed BL-40 *(wei zhong)* on the leg greater yang.[7]

Introduction to Medicine
(Yi xue ru men)

For slight lower back pain, bleeding BL-40 *(wei zhong)* brings a rapid cure; if the pain is intense, tonify GB-30 *(huan tiao)* and drain BL-40 *(wei zhong)*. For long-term cases, all are tonified.

If the lower back pain causes thoracic pain, needle BL-60 *(kun lun)* and BL-40 *(wei zhong)*.

For lower back pain radiating toward the legs, tonify SI-4 *(wan gu)* and drain ST-36 *(zu san li)*.

When the lower back pain radiates to the feet, tonify GB-30 *(huan tiao)* and drain GB-31 *(feng shi)*, LR-2 *(xing jian)* and ST-36 *(zu san li)*.

GV-4 *(ming men)* is used to treat lower back pain due to kidney deficiency in the elderly.

Chapter Notes

1. *Editors' note:* This point is located below the spinous process of the third lumbar vertebra.
2. *Editors' note:* We have been unable to determine which point is meant by *gǔ zhōng*.
3. *Editors' note:* We have been unable to determine which point is meant by *zhì mén*.
4. *Shàn* covers several concepts, the most common of which is hernial disorder, but it also refers to ulcerations of the external genital organs, as well as abdominal pain with difficult urination and defecation.
5. *Editors' note:* Usually, when yang heel *(yáng qiáo)* refers to a point, it means the vessel's confluent point, BL-62 *(shen mai)*. Because that cannot be the case here, we are unable to determine which point is intended, or if the reference is instead to the vessel.
6. *Editors' note:* This paragraph is adapted from chapter 41 of *Basic Questions*. See the translation in chapter 24 for more details.

Appendix
Supplemental Materia Medica

THIS APPENDIX CONTAINS descriptions of materia medica found in the text but which are not among those included in such widely used texts as *Chinese Herbal Medicine: Materia Medica (Revised Edition)* edited by Dan Bensky and Andrew Gamble. Since readers may be unfamiliar with these medicinal substances, we present basic information about them here in an abbreviated version of the format used in that book. The materia medica are arranged in alphabetical order based on their *pinyin* names. Please note that for a few of the substances mentioned in this book, little significant information was available to us, and they were thus not included in this appendix.

bái jiāo xiāng
白膠香
PHARMACEUTICAL NAME: Resina Liquidambaris
BOTANICAL NAME: *Liquidambar taiwaniana* Hance.
FAMILY: hamamelidaceae
ALTERNATE NAME: *fēng guǒ zhī*
ENGLISH: sweetgum resin
LITERAL ENGLISH TRANSLATION: "white gummy fragrance"
PROPERTIES: acrid, bitter, neutral
CHANNELS ENTERED: Spleen, Lung
ACTIONS & INDICATIONS:

• Invigorates the Blood, cools the Blood, relieves Toxicity, and stops pain: for painful sores, hidden rashes, toothache, vomiting blood, and nosebleeds.
CAUTIONS & CONTRAINDICATIONS: None noted.
DOSAGE: 3-6g internally. Often used in topically-applied plasters and powders.
NOTE: This is the resin from the tree that produces Fructus Liquidambaris Taiwanianae (*lu lu tong*).

chēng liǔ
檉柳
PHARMACEUTICAL NAME: Ramulus et Folium Tamaricis
BOTANICAL NAME: *Tamarix chinensis* Lour., *T. juniperina* Bge., or *T. ramosissima* Ledeb.
FAMILY: tamaricaceae
ALTERNATE NAME: *shān chuān liǔ*
ENGLISH: tamarix stems and leaves
LITERAL ENGLISH TRANSLATION: "west river willow"
PROPERTIES: acrid, neutral
CHANNELS ENTERED: Lung, Stomach, Heart
ACTIONS & INDICATIONS:
• Induces sweating and vents rashes: for the early stages of measles when there is incomplete expression of the rash, or when Wind-Cold externally hampers the expression of the rash, leading to the rash Toxin collapsing internally.
• Scatters and dispels Wind: for itching from Wind rash

and externally-contracted cough. When combined with herbs that dispel Wind-Dampness, it can be used for Wind-Damp painful obstruction.

CAUTIONS & CONTRAINDICATIONS: Do not use after the rash of measles has already been expressed. If too large a dosage is given, the person may become irritable.

DOSAGE: 3-9g. Can be used externally as a wash or steam.

chuān shān lóng
穿山龍

PHARMACEUTICAL NAME: Rhizoma Dioscoreae Nipponicae

BOTANICAL NAME: *Dioscorea nipponica* Mak.

FAMILY: dioscoreaceae

ENGLISH: Japanese yam

LITERAL ENGLISH TRANSLATION: "mountain-piercing dragon"

PROPERTIES: bitter, slightly cold

CHANNELS ENTERED: Liver, Kidney

ACTIONS & INDICATIONS:

• Dispels Wind, eliminates Dampness, invigorates the Blood and stops pain: for pain from Wind-Dampness in the sinews and bones, or trauma injuring the Blood leading to stasis.

• Dispels Phlegm and stops coughing: for relatively mild cases of coughing from Hot Phlegm.

CAUTIONS & CONTRAINDICATIONS: None noted.

DOSAGE: 9-30 g

dīng gōng téng
丁公藤

PHARMACEUTICAL NAME: Radix et Caulis Erycibes Obstusifoliae

BOTANICAL NAME: *Erycibe obtusifolia* Benth.

FAMILY: convolvulaceae

ENGLISH: erycibe root and stem

LITERAL ENGLISH TRANSLATION: "spike duke vine"

PROPERTIES: acrid, warm, toxic

CHANNELS ENTERED: None noted.

ACTIONS & INDICATIONS:

• Releases the exterior, expels Wind-Dampness, eliminates painful obstruction, reduces swellings, and alleviates pain: for Wind-Damp painful obstruction, hemiplegia, and pain from trauma.

CAUTIONS & CONTRAINDICATIONS: Contraindicated during pregnancy. Side effects may include severe sweating that does not stop, and numbness of the extremities. The antidote is Radix Glycyrrhizae Uralensis (*gan cao*) with honey.

DOSAGE: 3-6g in decoctions. Also used externally and in medicinal wines.

guǐ jiàn yǔ
鬼箭羽

PHARMACEUTICAL NAME: Appendix Euonymi Alati

BOTANICAL NAME: *Euonymus alatus* (Thunb.) Sieb.

FAMILY: celastraceae

ENGLISH: winged spindle tree, euonymus

LITERAL ENGLISH TRANSLATION: "ghost arrow feather"

PROPERTIES: bitter, cold

CHANNELS ENTERED: Liver

ACTIONS & INDICATIONS:

• Breaks up blood stasis, unblocks the menses: for amenorrhea, postpartum abdominal pain, and lower back pain.

• Kills parasites: for abdominal pain from parasitic accumulation.

CAUTIONS & CONTRAINDICATIONS: Contraindicated during pregnancy.

DOSAGE: 4.5-9g

hēi dà dòu
黑大豆

PHARMACEUTICAL NAME: Semen Glycine Max

BOTANICAL NAME: *Glycine max* (L.) Merr.

FAMILY: fabaceae

ENGLISH: soybean

LITERAL ENGLISH TRANSLATION: "black big bean"

PROPERTIES: sweet, neutral

CHANNELS ENTERED: Spleen, Kidney

ACTIONS & INDICATIONS:

• Invigorates the Blood and promotes urination: for floating edema.

• Dispels Wind: for leg qi due to Wind Toxin, muscular tetany due to Wind obstruction.

• Relieves Toxicity: for abscesses and carbuncles.

• Also relieves materia medica poisoning.

DOSAGE: 9-30g

lǎo guàn cǎo
老鹳草

PHARMACEUTICAL NAME: Herba Erodii seu Geranii

BOTANICAL NAME: *Erodium stephanianum* Willd. or *Geranium wilfordii*. Maxim. In various parts of China other species of *Geranium* are used.

FAMILY: geraniaceae

ENGLISH: cranesbill, erodium, geranium
LITERAL ENGLISH TRANSLATION: "old stork herb"
PROPERTIES: acrid, bitter, neutral
CHANNELS ENTERED: Liver, Large Intestine
ACTIONS & INDICATIONS:
• Dispels Wind, eliminates Dampness, relaxes the sinews, and invigorates the collaterals: for Wind-Damp painful obstruction, numbness and paresthesia, as well as sore and painful sinews and bones.
• Stops diarrhea: for Damp-Heat dysenteric disorders.
CAUTIONS & CONTRAINDICATIONS: None noted.
DOSAGE: 9-60g. Larger doses are for when used alone.

lù xián cǎo
鹿衔草
PHARMACEUTICAL NAME: Herba Pyrolae Rotundifoliae
BOTANICAL NAME: *Pyrola rotundifolia* L.
FAMILY: pyrolaceae
ALTERNATE NAME: *lù hán cǎo*
ENGLISH: pyrola
LITERAL ENGLISH TRANSLATION: "deer bit herb"
PROPERTIES: sweet, bitter, warm
CHANNELS ENTERED: Liver, Kidney
ACTIONS & INDICATIONS:
• Dispels Wind-Dampness and strengthens the sinews and bones: for Wind-Damp painful obstruction and weakness of the sinews and bones. Often used in the elderly. Also used for bone spurs.
• Tonifies the Kidneys and moistens the Lungs: for lower back pain accompanied by cold, painful feet from Kidney deficiency. Also for chronic cough from Lung deficiency, chronic dryness, or Kidneys failing to grasp the Qi.
• Stops bleeding: for various types of bleeding, including nosebleeds, vomiting blood, and excessive menstruation.
• Nourishes the Heart and restrains sweating: for palpitations with night sweats.
CAUTIONS & CONTRAINDICATIONS: None noted.
DOSAGE: 15-30g

mián huā zǐ
棉花子
PHARMACEUTICAL NAME: Semen Gossypii
BOTANICAL NAME: *Gossypium hirsutum* L. or *G. herbaceum* L.
FAMILY: malvaceae
ENGLISH: cotton seeds

PROPERTIES: sweet, warm
CHANNELS ENTERED: None noted.
ACTIONS & INDICATIONS:
• Tonifies the Qi and raises the sunken: for prolapse or enuresis usually due to sunken middle Qi. As such, it is used as a substitute for Radix Astragali Membranacei *(huang qi)* in some areas of China.
• Warms the Kidneys: for impotence.
CAUTIONS & CONTRAINDICATIONS: Contraindicated in patients with Fire due to yin deficiency.
DOSAGE: 6-12g. Sometimes used externally in fumigation.

qiāng láng
蜣螂
PHARMACEUTICAL NAME: Catharsius
ZOOLOGICAL NAME: *Catharsius molossus* L. In some parts of China, *Xylotropes dichotomus* L. is used.
ENGLISH: dung beetle, cartharsius
PROPERTIES: salty, cold, toxic
CHANNELS ENTERED: Liver, Stomach, Large Intestine
ACTIONS & INDICATIONS:
• Arrests tremors and convulsions: for seizures and tremors.
• Breaks up Blood stasis and unblocks the bowels: for abdominal masses and other problems due to severe Blood stasis, especially when there is constipation.
• Attacks Toxin: for a wide variety of problems when the strategy is to "attack Toxin with Toxin."
CAUTIONS & CONTRAINDICATIONS: Contraindicated during pregnancy.
DOSAGE: 1-2g

qié gēn
茄根
PHARMACEUTICAL NAME: Radix Solani Melongenae
BOTANICAL NAME: *Solanum melongena* L.
FAMILY: solanaceae
ALTERNATE NAMES: *bái qié gēn, qié mǔ*
ENGLISH: eggplant root
PROPERTIES: sweet, acrid, cold
CHANNELS ENTERED: None noted.
ACTIONS & INDICATIONS:
• Dispels Wind and Dampness: used for painful obstruction, especially for Wind-predominant painful obstruction.

- Treats Blood and reduces swellings: for such problems as bloody painful urinary dysfunction, bleeding from the rectum, and bloody dysenteric disorders.
- Also used for chilblain and toothache.

CAUTIONS & CONTRAINDICATIONS: None noted.

DOSAGE: 9-18g in decoctions. Can be used externally as a poultice or wash.

qīng fēng téng
青風藤

PHARMACEUTICAL NAME: Caulis et Rhizoma Sinomenii Acuti

BOTANICAL NAME: *Sinomenium acutum* (Thunb.) Rehd. In some parts of China, *Sabia japonica* Maxim. is used.

FAMILY: aristolochiaceae

ALTERNATE NAME: *qīng fēng téng*

ENGLISH: sinomenium

LITERAL ENGLISH TRANSLATION: "green wind vine"

PROPERTIES: acrid, bitter, warm

CHANNELS ENTERED: Liver, Spleen

ACTIONS & INDICATIONS:

- Dispels Wind-Dampness and unblocks the channels and collaterals: for acute Wind-Damp joint pain, especially when the joint is swollen, red, and painful. Also for stasis and swelling due to trauma

CAUTIONS & CONTRAINDICATIONS: Note that in Japan this plant is often used in place of Radix Stephaniae Tetrandrae *(han fang ji)*.

DOSAGE: 9-15g

rù dì jīn niú
入地金牛

PHARMACEUTICAL NAME: Radix seu Ramulus et Folium Zanthoxyli Nitidi

BOTANICAL NAME: *Zanthoxylum nitidum* (Roxb.) DC.

FAMILY: rutacae

ALTERNATE NAME: *liǎng miàn zhēn*

ENGLISH: shiny bramble, zonthoxylum nitidum roots, stems, and leaves

LITERAL ENGLISH TRANSLATION: "enter earth golden ox"

PROPERTIES: acrid, slighlty warm, slightly toxic

CHANNELS ENTERED: Liver, Stomach

ACTIONS & INDICATIONS:

- Dispels Wind, unblocks the collaterals, reduces swelling, and stops pain: for Wind-Damp pain, throat painful obstruction, pain from trauma, burns, and stomach pain.

CAUTIONS & CONTRAINDICATIONS: This herb should not be prescribed in excess. Too large a dosage can lead to dizziness, lightheadedness, vomiting, and stomachache. By tradition, sour foods should be avoided when taking this herb.

DOSAGE: 9-15g

shēn jīn cǎo
伸筋草

PHARMACEUTICAL NAME: Herba cum Radice Lycopodii Clavati

BOTANICAL NAME: *Lycopodium clavatum* L. In some parts of China, *Smilax nipponica* Miq. is used.

FAMILY: lycopodiaceae

ENGLISH: running pine, staghorn clubmoss

LITERAL ENGLISH TRANSLATION: "extend sinew herb"

PROPERTIES: bitter, acrid, warm

CHANNELS ENTERED: Liver, Spleen, Kidney

ACTIONS & INDICATIONS:

- Dispels Wind and scatters Cold, eliminates Dampness and swelling, relaxes the sinews, and invigorates the collaterals: for painful obstruction due to Wind, Cold, and Dampness, especially of the joints; numbness of the skin; weakness of the extremities; trauma and contusions.

CAUTIONS & CONTRAINDICATIONS: Contraindicated during pregnancy and in case of hemorrhage.

DOSAGE: 9-15 g

shǔ qū cǎo
鼠曲草

PHARMACEUTICAL NAME: Herba Gnaphalii Affinis

BOTANICAL NAME: *Gnaphalium affine* D. Don

FAMILY: compositae

ALTERNATE NAME: *shǔ ěr*

ENGLISH: cudweed, gnaphalium

LITERAL ENGLISH TRANSLATION: "rat crooked herb"

PROPERTIES: sweet, neutral

CHANNELS ENTERED: Lung

ACTIONS & INDICATIONS:

- Transforms Phlegm and stops coughing: for coughing with profuse sputum, wheezing, and Wind-Cold colds.
- Dispels Wind-Dampness: for pain in the sinews and bones.

CAUTIONS & CONTRAINDICATIONS: None noted.

DOSAGE: 6-15g

xú cháng qīng
徐長卿

PHARMACEUTICAL NAME: Herba cum Radix Cynanchi
  Paniculati

BOTANICAL NAME: *Cynanchum paniculatum* (Bge.) Kitag.

FAMILY: asclepiadaceae

ALTERNATE NAME: *liáo diāo zhú*

ENGLISH: cynanchum paniculatum

LITERAL ENGLISH TRANSLATION: "slow long-lasting
  minister"

PROPERTIES: acrid, warm

CHANNELS ENTERED: Liver, Stomach

ACTIONS & INDICATIONS:

• Dispels Wind and stops pain: for pain including Wind-
  Damp painful obstruction, pain from trauma, abdominal pain, or toothache. Because this herb is relatively
  effective in dispelling Wind and stopping pain, it can be
  used for pain from Wind-Dampness, Cold congealing,
  Qi stagnation, or Blood stasis. Recently used for post-
  operative pain and the pain associated with tumors.

• Dispels Wind and stops itching: for skin problems such
  as eczema, urticaria, or stubborn cases of tinea.

• Also used topically for poisonous snake bite.

CAUTIONS & CONTRAINDICATIONS: Use with caution in
the debilitated.

DOSAGE: 3-10g in decoctions, 1.5-3g in powders. Do not
decoct for long, as it is aromatic.

xún gǔ fēng
尋骨風

PHARMACEUTICAL NAME: Rhizoma seu Herba
  Aristolochiae Mollissimae

BOTANICAL NAME: *Aristolochia mollissima* Hance.

FAMILY: aristolochiae

ENGLISH: root or entire plant of hairy birthwort or artis-
  tolochia mollissima

LITERAL ENGLISH TRANSLATION: "seek bone wind"

PROPERTIES: acrid, bitter, neutral

CHANNELS ENTERED: Liver

ACTIONS & INDICATIONS:

• Dispels Wind, unblocks the collaterals, and stops pain:

for Wind-Damp painful obstruction with numbness
and paresthesia and spasms of the sinews. Also for pain
secondary to trauma.

• Also used for stomachache or toothache.

CAUTIONS & CONTRAINDICATIONS: Some sources suggest
that this herb should not be used when there is internal
Heat from yin deficiency.

DOSAGE: 9-15g. Can be used in tinctures or linaments.

zhú jié xiāng fù
竹節香附

PHARMACEUTICAL NAME: Radix Anemones Raddeanae

BOTANICAL NAME: *Anemone raddeana* Reg.

FAMILY: ranunclulaceae

ALTERNATE NAME: *liǎng tóu jiān*

ENGLISH: anemone

LITERAL ENGLISH TRANSLATION: "bamboo node aromatic appendage"

PROPERTIES: acrid, hot, toxic

CHANNELS ENTERED: None noted.

ACTIONS & INDICATIONS:

• Dispels Wind-Dampness, reduces abscesses: for Wind-
  Damp painful obstruction, abscesses, and sores.

CAUTIONS & CONTRAINDICATIONS: Signs of toxicity are
said to be similar to those caused by aconite.

DOSAGE: 1.5-3 g

zǐ bái pí
梓白皮

PHARMACEUTICAL NAME: Cortex Catalpae Ovatae
  Radicis

BOTANICAL NAME: *Catalpa ovata* G. Don

FAMILY: bignoniacee

ENGLISH: catalpa bark or root bark

PROPERTIES: bitter, cold

CHANNELS ENTERED: Stomach, Gallbladder

ACTIONS & INDICATIONS:

• Clears Heat, resolves Toxicity, and kills parasites: for
  seasonal febrile diseases, jaundice, sores, and pruritis.

CAUTIONS & CONTRAINDICATIONS: None noted.

DOSAGE: 1.5-3g. Also used topically as a powder or wash.

Bibliography

Academy of Traditional Chinese Medicine, Guangzhou College of Traditional Chinese Medicine. *Jian ming zhong yi ci dian (Concise Dictionary of Traditional Chinese Medicine)*. Beijing: People's Health Publishing Company, 1980.

Amor, B., et al. *Révision accélérée*. Paris: Maloine, 1986.

Anonymous. *Huang di nei jing ling shu yi shi (Translated and Annotated Yellow Emperor's Inner Classic: Divine Pivot)*. Edited by Nanjing College of Traditional Chinese Medicine. Shanghai: Shanghai Science and Technology Press, 1986.

Anonymous. *Huang di nei jing su wen yi shi (Translated and Annotated Yellow Emperor's Inner Classic: Basic Questions)*. Edited by Nanjing College of Traditional Chinese Medicine. Shanghai: Shanghai Science and Technology Press, 1981.

Auteroche, B., and P. Navailh. *Le Diagnostic en médecine chinoise*. Paris: Maloine, 1983.

Baldry, P. E. *Acupuncture, Trigger Points, and Musculoskeletal Pain*. Edinburgh: Churchill Livingstone, 1989.

Beijing Institute of Traditional Chinese Medicine. *Zhong yi ji chu (Fundamentals of Traditional Chinese Medicine)*. Shanghai: Shanghai Science and Technology Press, 1980.

Bézange-Beauquesne, L., et al. *Plantes médicinales des régions tempérées*. Paris: Maloine, 1980.

Bruhat M.-A. "La ménopause." *Impact Médecin — Les Dossiers du Practicien* (1990): 54-5.

Cahiers du G.R.I.O. *Ostéoporoses actualités* 10, nos.1-11 (1987), no. 12 (1990).

Cazin, F.-J. *Traité pratique et raisonné des plantes médicinales indigènes*. Paris: Labé, 1958.

Chamfrault, A. *Traité de médecine chinoise*. Vol. 1. Angoulême: Coquemard, 1964.

Chamfrault, A., and Nguyen Van Nghi. *Traité de médecine chinoise*. Vol. 6. Angoulême: Coquemard, 1969.

Chao Yuan-Fang. *Zhu bing yuan hou lun jiao shi (Collected and Annotated Discussion of the Origins of Symptoms of Disease)*. Edited by Nanjing College of Traditional Chinese Medicine. Beijing: People's Health Publishing Company, 1982.

Chen Dazhong and Xia Xiang. *Les maladies bi et algies articulaires.* Rennes: Congrès de Vannes, Cercle sinologique de l'Ouest, 1985.

Chen Meng-Lei, et al., ed. *Gu jin tu shu ji cheng yi bu quan lu (Complete Medical Section of the Compendium of Ancient and Modern Charts and Books).* Vol. 6. Beijing: People's Health Publishing Company, 1983.

Chevalier, J., and A. Gheerbrant. *Dictionnaire des symboles.* Paris: Seghers, 1974.

Christiansen, C., and B. Riis. "L'Ostéoporose postménopausique, une menace silencieuse." Trans. G.R.I.O. Vedbaek, Denmark: Fondation Européenne contre l'ostéoporose et les maladies osseuses, 1990.

Chung, C. *Ah Shih Point: An Illustrated Diagnostic Guide to Clinical Acupuncture.* Taipei: Chen Kwan Book Company, 1983.

Cummings, Stevens R., et al. "Epidemiology of Osteoporosis and Osteoporotic Fractures." *Epidemiology Reviews* 7 (1985).

Cygler, B. *La Tête et le cou.* Paris: La Tisserande, 1987.

Denis, A. *Le Pied douloureux [Folio rheumatologica].* Geneva: Documenta Geigy, 23, 1974.

Desouter, B. "Le bi." *La reveu des séminaires d'acupuncture de l'A.F.E.R.A.* 1 (1987): 29-42.

Despeux, C., trans. *Shang Han Lun: Traité des "coups de froid."* Paris: La Tisserande, 1987.

Despeux, C., trans. *Sun Si Miao, Traité d'acupuncture.* Paris: Guy Trédaniel, 1987.

Dubois, J.-C. "Traitement des lombalgies en médecine chinoise." *Meridiens* (1985): 69-70, 131-45.

Duron, Laville, Méry, Borsarello. *Bioénergétique et médecine chinoise.* Vol. 1. Paris: Maisonneuve, 1978.

Eyssalet, J.-M., G. Guillaume, and Mach Chieu. *Diététique énergétique et médecine chinoise.* Sisteron: Présence, 1984.

Faubert, A. *Traité didactique d'acupuncture traditionnelle.* Paris: Guy Trédaniel, 1977.

Fournier, P. *Le Liver des plantes médicinales et vénéneuses de France.* Paris: Lechevalier, 1947.

Grison, J., trans. *Nan Jing, Les 81 difficultés de l'acupuncture.* Paris: Masson, 1979.

Guillaume, G. "Examen de la main." *Reveu française d'acupuncture* 34 (1983): 33-7.

Guillaume, G. "*Jin ye,* Liquides organiques." *Reveu française d'acupuncture* 38 (1984): 33-41.

Guillaume, G. "Liquides organiques et Glaires, une approche énergétique de la goutte." *Actes du 5eséminaire de la S.A.A.* (1985): 3-8.

Guillaume, G. "Why Western Protocols are Unsuitable for Assessing the Effects of Acupuncture." *American Journal of Acupuncture* 10, no. 2 (1991): 153-56.

Guillaume, G. "Phytothérapie et rhumatologie." In *Encyclopédie des Médecines Naturelles.* Paris: Editions Techniques, 1991.

Guillaume, G., and Mach Chieu. *Pharmacopée et médecine traditionelle chinoise.* Sisteron: Présence, 1987.

Hackett, G.-S. *Ligament and Tendon Relaxation Treated by Prolotherapy.* Springfield: C. C. Thomas, 1958.

Hernandez, M. "Apport des travaux de Travell et de Hackett en acupuncture." In *Mémoire d'acupuncture.* Paris: A.F.E.R.A., 1986.

Hunan College of Traditional Chinese Medicine. *Zhong yi zhen duan xue (Traditional Chinese Medical Diagnosis).* Zhengzhou: Henan Science and Technology Press, 1985.

Huang Wen-Dong, et al. *Shi yong zhong yi nei ke xue (Practical Traditional Chinese Internal Medicine).* Shanghai: Shanghai Science and Technology Press, 1985.

Huang-Fu Mi. *Zhen jiu jia yi jing jiao shi (Collected and Annotated Systematic Classic of Acupuncture and Moxibustion).* Edited by Shangdong College of Traditional Chinese Medicine, et al. Beijing: People's Health Publishing Company, 1980.

Husson, A., trans. *Huang Di Nei Jing Su Wen*. Paris: A.S.M.A.F., 1973.

Institut Ricci. *Dictionnaire français de la langue chinoise*. Paris: Kuangchi Press, 1976.

Kespi, J.-M. *Acupuncture*. Paris: Maisonneuve, 1982.

Kespi, J.-M. *Cliniques*. Paris: La Tisserande, 1988.

Lafont, J.-L. "La Notion de bi." *Méridiens* (1981): 55-6, 185-95.

Laurent, P. *La Théorie des jing luo*. Rennes: Cercle sinologique de l'Ouest, 1986.

Leclerc, H. *Précis de phytothérapie*. Paris: Masson, 1976.

Li Zhong-Cai, *Yi zong bi du (Essential Readings for Those in the Medical Lineage)*. Shanghai: Shanghai Health Publishing, 1983.

Maspero, H. *Le Taoïsme et les religions chinoises*. Paris: Gallimard, 1969.

Ming Wong. *Les Massages en médecine traditionnelle chinoise*. Paris: Masson, 1984.

Nguyen Van Nghi. *Pathogénie et pathologie énergétiques en médecine chinoise*. Marseille: Don Bosco, 1971.

Nguyen Van Nghi. *Art et pratique de l'acupuncture et de la moxibustion selon Zhen Jiu Da Cheng*. 2 vol. Marseille: N.V.D., 1982.

Nguyen Van Nghi. "Affections rheumatismales - les Pei." *Mensuel du médecin acupuncteur* 91 (1982): 819-24.

Nguyen Van Nghi. "Les Huit Règles de diagnostic en médecine chinoise." *Mensuel du médecin acupuncteur* 94 (1982): 937-47.

Perrot, E., and R. Paris. *Les Plantes médicinales*. Paris: P.U.F., 1974.

Porkert, M. *The Theoretical Foundations of Chinese Medicine*. Cambridge: MIT Press, 1980.

Renier J.-C. "L'Ostéoporose." Impact Médecin—Les dossiers du practicien (1990): 79.

Requena, Y. *Le Diagnostic morpho-typologique de la main en acupuncture*. Marseille: Solal, 1986.

Rochat de la Vallée, E. *Symphonie corporelle*. Paris: Institut Ricci, (no date cited).

Roudler, J., et al. "The Epstein-Barr Virus Glycoprotein GP 110, A Molecular Link between HLA DR4, HLA DR1 and Rheumatoid Arthritis." *Scandinavian Journal of Immunology* 27 (1988): 367-71.

Roustan, C. *Traité d'acupuncture de l'université de Shanghai*. 3 vol. Paris: Masson, 1979.

Roux, H., A. Luxembourg, and J. Roudier. *Immunorhumatologie*. Marseille: Solal, 1989.

Savigny, N., and G. Andres. "La Ménopause." *Revue Franéaise d'Acupuncture* 31 (1982): 49-55.

Schatz, J., C. Larre, and Rochat de la Vallée. *Aperçus de médecine chinoise traditionnelle*. Paris: Maisonneuve, 1979.

Schnorenberger, J. "Les effets syndromiques des points d'acupuncture." *Revue Française d'Acupuncture*, nos. 63-6 (1990-91).

Simon, L., et al. *Rhumatologie*. Paris: Abrégés Masson, 1989.

Soulié de Morant, G. *L'acuponcture chinoise*. Paris: Maloine, 1979.

Soulié de Morant, G. *Traité de chiromancie chinoise*. Paris: Trédaniel, 1978.

Taillandier, J. "Les Muscles et les Méridiens." *La revue des séminaires d'acupuncture de l'A.F.E.R.A.* 1 (1987): 43-61.

Taillandier, J. "Le Membre supérieur." *La revue des séminaires d' acupuncture de l' A.F.E.R.A.* 1 (1987): 63-100.

Travell, J., and D. Simons. *Myofascial Pain and Dysfunction: The Trigger Point Manual*. Baltimore: Williams & Wilkins, 1984.

Wang Su-Yen and Hsu Hong-Yen, trans. *Chin Kuei Yao Lueh, Prescriptions from the Golden Chamber*. Long Beach: Oriental Healing Arts Institute, 1983.

Wong, P.C.N. "Fracture Epidemiology in a Mixed Southeast Asian Community (Singapore)." *Clinical Orthopedics* 45 (1966): 55-61.

Yang Ji-Zhou. *Zhen jiu da cheng (Great Compendium of Acupuncture and Moxibustion).* Edited by Heilongjiang Province Traditional Chinese Medicine Research Institute. Beijing: People's Health Publishing Company, 1984.

Zhang Cong-Zhen. *Ru men shi qin jiao zhu (Collated and Annotated Confucians' Duties to Their Parents).* Edited by Zhang Hai-Qin. Zhengzhou: Henan Science and Technology Press, 1984.

Zhang Zhong-Jing. *Jin gui yao lue fang lun (Essentials from the Golden Cabinet).* Beijing: People's Health Publishing Company, 1978.

Zhang Zhong-Jing. *Shang Han Lun: Traité des "coups de froid".* Translated by D. Despeux. Paris: La Tisserande, 1987.

Zhang Zhong-Jing. *Synopsis of Prescriptions from the Golden Chamber.* Translated by Luo Xiwen. Beijing: New World Press, 1987.

Zhejiang College of Traditional Chinese Medicine. *A Handbook of Traditional Chinese Gynecology.* Translated by Zhang Ting-Liang. Boulder, Colorado: Blue Poppy Press, 1987.

Acupuncture Point Index

C

G

. . . .

Herb Index

The Chinese materia medica in this book are listed here by their pharmaceutical names.
European plant extracts are listed by their Latin and English names.

Formula Index

Note: In the entries below, bold numbers indicate pages
on which the ingredients of the formulas are listed.

General Index

C

N

Pathogenic influences. *See also specific pathogenic influences*
  diagnosis, 356
  factors promoting invasion, 98–99
Pathogenic invasion, classic description, 313–14
Pattern, Cause, Pulse and Treatment (Zheng yin mai zhi), 121
Pattern of disease *(zheng)*, 51
A Peek at the Eight Methods and Efficacious Formulas (Ba fa xiao fang ju yu), 72
Pelvic pain, 276
Pelvic stagnation, 161, 164–65
Pelvis
  bony lesions in hip pain, 275
  energetic balance in women, 147
  prenatal Qi, 176
Penetrating vessel
  in foot, 292
  governing spine, 185
  illustration, 28, 187
  in knee, 282, 286
  in lower back pain, 117, 200
  in menopause, 178
  pathways, 185
  in sciatica, 213
Pensiveness, 40
Pernicious influences. *See* Etiology of disease, traditional, pernicious influences; *see also* Pathogenic influences
Pes cavus, 294
Pes planus. *See* Flat foot
Peyronie's disease, 261, 295
Phenobarbital, 83
Phlegm
  with Blood stasis, 60–62, 69, 84, 99
  in disease pathogenesis, 42
  expulsion, 69, 71
  in lower back pain, 111, 115
  in painful obstruction, 59, 61–62
  from pathogenic Dampness, 100
  patterns, 60
  production by Spleen, 118
  stagnation pain, 47–48
  turbid, in collaterals, 173
Phlegm-Cold, 183
Phthisis, 157
Phytotherapy. *See* Herbal therapy
Plantar calluses, 293
Plantar heel, 295
Plantar neuralgia. *See* Morton's neuroma
Plum-pit Qi syndrome, 37
Polyarteritis nodosa, 58, 89
Polyarticular painful syndromes
  acupuncture, 159, 160—67
  atrophic disorders, 165
  channel disorders

acute, 163
chronic, 163
curious vessels, 164–65
diagnosis, 162–63
greater yang axis, 162–63
primary channels, 163–64
disruption in Five Revolutions, 166–67
edema, 162
emotional disorders in, 162
knee pain, 160
limited range of motion, 160
mechanisms, 160–62
moving joint pain, 162
Organ pathology, 165–66
with paresthesia, 165
sudden painful obstruction, 166
symptomatic treatment, 159
therapeutic approaches, 159
triggering mechanisms, 159
vertebral complications, 160
Polyfibromatosis, hereditary, 261
Polymyositis, 58, 88–89
Popliteal cyst, 283
Postural imbalance, 284, 293–94
Practical Traditional Chinese Internal Medicine (Shi yong zhong yi nei ke xue), 51
Precepts for Physicians (Yi men fa lü), 57, 72, 115, **305**, **351–53**
Pregnancy, 126, 147
Pregnancy complications, 161
Prescriptions of Universal Benefit from My Practice (Pu ji ben shi fang), 102
Primary channels
  function, 7
  illustrations, 9–17
  in lower back pain, 204
Progesterone-stimulating plants, 180
Prostate disorders, 213
Protective Qi, 324
Psoriatic arthritis, 296
Pubic symphysis disorders, 275
Pulmonary catarrh, 157
Pulse. *See also specific conditions, pulse, e.g.,* Lower back stiffness, pulse changes
  choppy, 120, 214
  floating and choppy, 119
  floating and lax, 62
  floating and rapid, 119
  floating and tight, 118
  rapid, 81, 89, 172
  rapid and forceful, 102
  rapid and thin, 102
  slippery, 118
  slippery and rapid, 206